YOGA, TAI CHI
MASSAGE, THERAPIES & HEALING REMEDIES

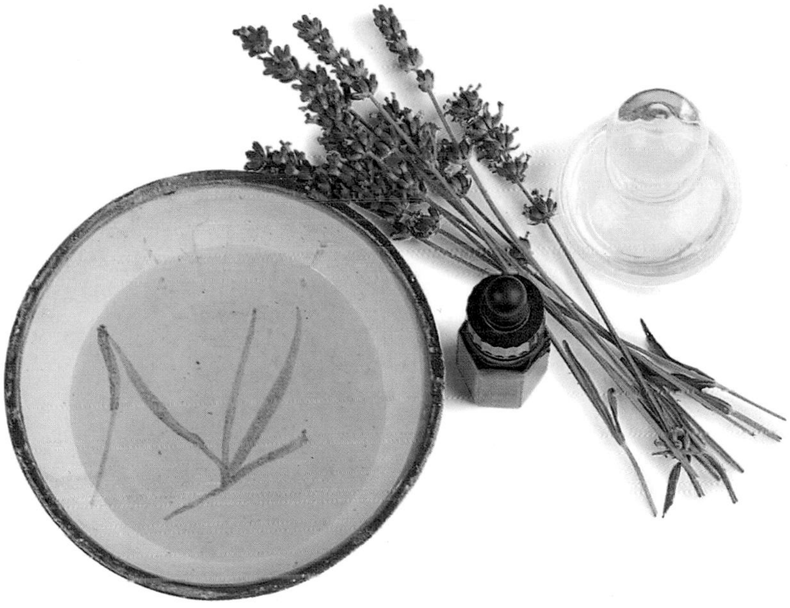

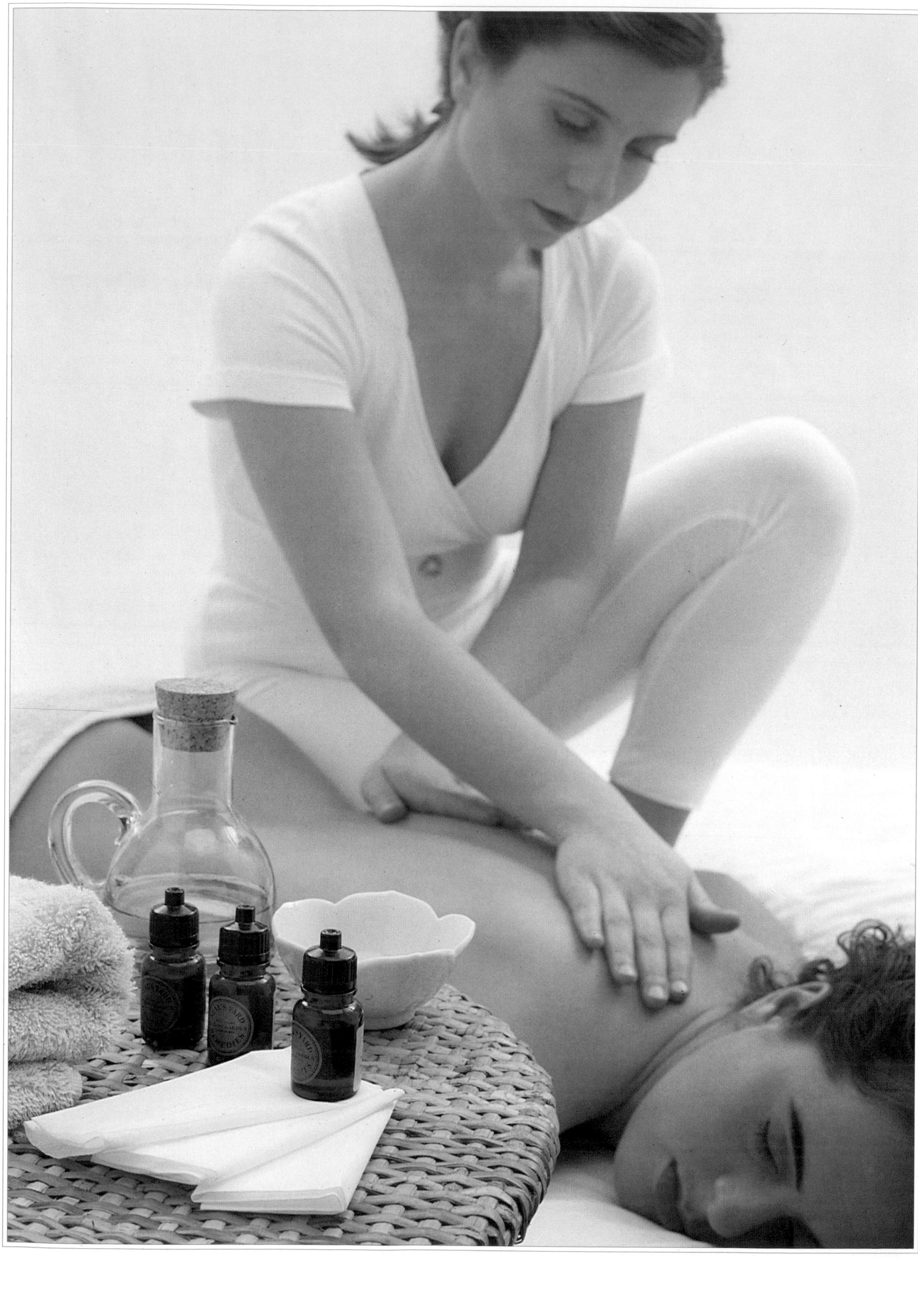

YOGA, TAI CHI
MASSAGE, THERAPIES & NATURAL REMEDIES

natural ways to health, relaxation and vitality: a complete practical guide

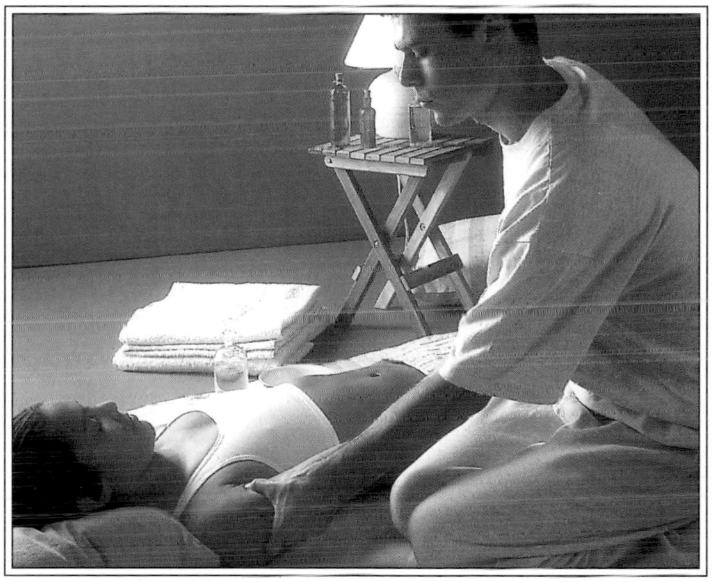

MARK EVANS B Phil., FNIMH

HERMES HOUSE

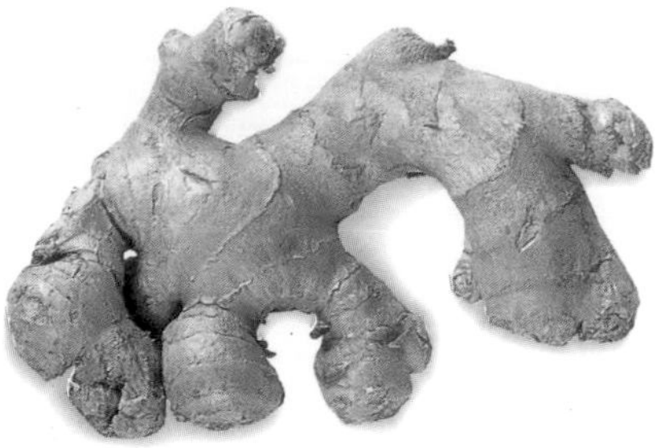

This edition is published by Hermes House

Hermes House is an imprint of Anness Publishing Ltd
Hermes House, 88–89 Blackfriars Road, London SE1 8HA
tel. 020 7401 2077; fax 020 7633 9499; info@anness.com

A CIP catalogue record for this book is available from the British Library.

Publisher: Joanna Lorenz
Editorial Managers: Helen Sudell, Joanne Rippin
Designer: Nigel Partridge
Photographers: Sue Atkinson, Simon Bottomley, Dave Jordan, Don Last and Lucy Mason,
Other chapters supplied by: John Hudson (Meditation), Michèle MacDonnell (Alexander Technique), Carole McGilvery (Aromatherapy), Jimi Reed (Massage), Kate Shapland (Fitness and Exercise) and Paul Tucker (T'ai Chi)
Additional text supplied by: Andrew Ackroyd, Felicity Roma Bowers, Karine Butchart, Suzanne Franzen, Anne Gains, Clare Harris and Paul Harvey
Exercise advisor: Dean Hodgkin

3 5 7 9 10 8 6 4 2

The majority of this volume was previously published as: *The Guide to Natural Living*

Important Notice

The advice given in this book is appropriate in most cases. However, it cannot take into account specific individuals' reactions. Neither the author nor the publishers can accept any responsibility for claims arising from the inappropriate use of any remedy or healing treatment. For further advice, and before beginning any treatment suggested herein, read page 121 for information pertaining to certain conditions and herb restrictions.

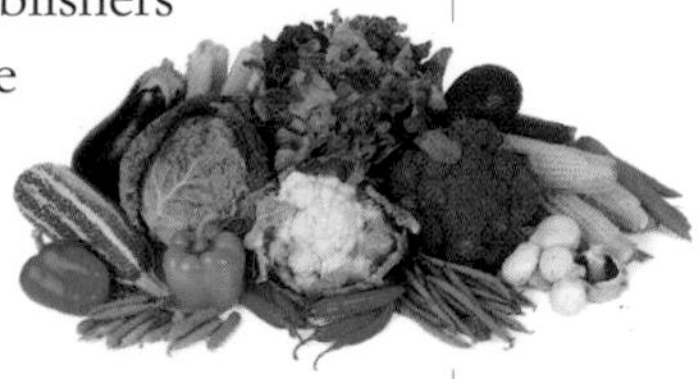

CONTENTS

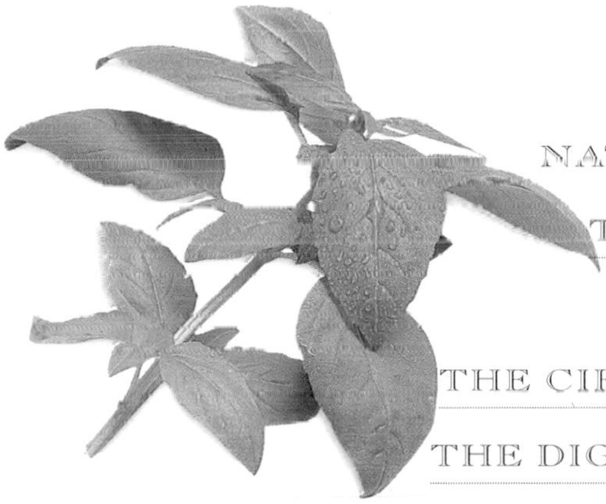

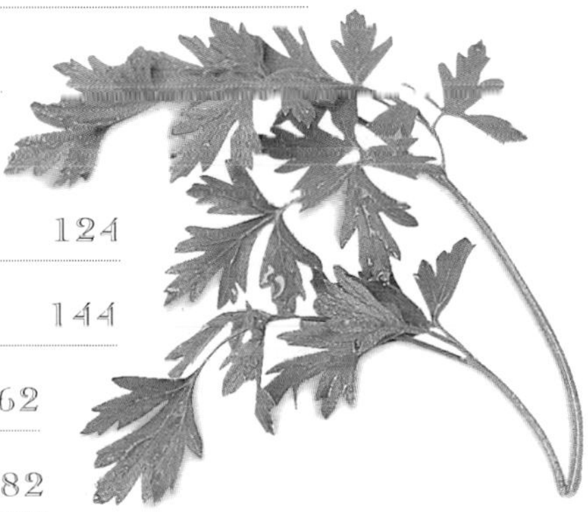

NATURAL REMEDIES

Health is, or should be, the most natural state of being. The origins of the word are linked with those of wholeness and healing, and it is that complete sense of harmony, of being whole, that brings true health. This is also the ultimate aim of the natural healing systems, those that adopt a holistic view rather than the reductionist perspective that is evident in much of conventional modern medicine.

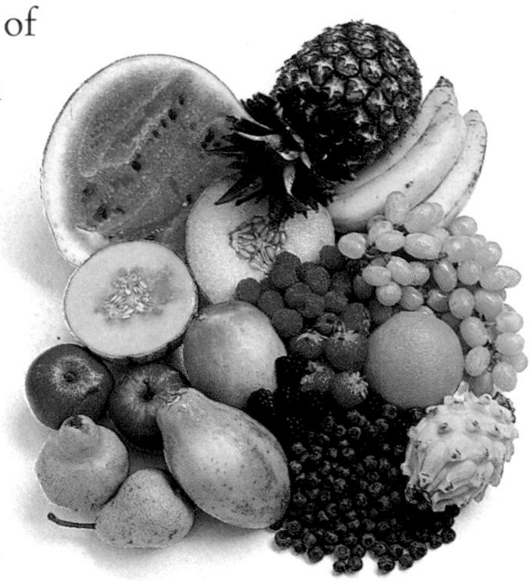

In the last 10 years or so, there has been a great revival of interest in natural therapies, both as a recognition of their tremendous value and also as a move away from some of the side-effects and impersonal approaches of allopathic medicine. In this section of the book, we are looking at how natural therapies can be used at home, as self-help remedies, for a variety of common complaints; it should not be forgotten, however, that in professional practice more complex or chronic conditions can also be treated by alternative or complementary medicine, and if in doubt over any problem do seek qualified advice.

Many traditions of natural medicine extend back over several centuries, with an impressive accumulation of practical knowledge. For this section we have focused on four main therapies, which not only have such an established tradition but also have good standards of training, clinical research data and widespread acceptance. They are aromatherapy, herbalism, homeopathy and naturopathy.

ABOVE: Fresh fruit is an excellent natural source of vitamins.

OPPOSITE: Herbs can be grown successfully in ordinary garden flower beds, giving off wonderful scents as well as providing a useful source of herbal medicines.

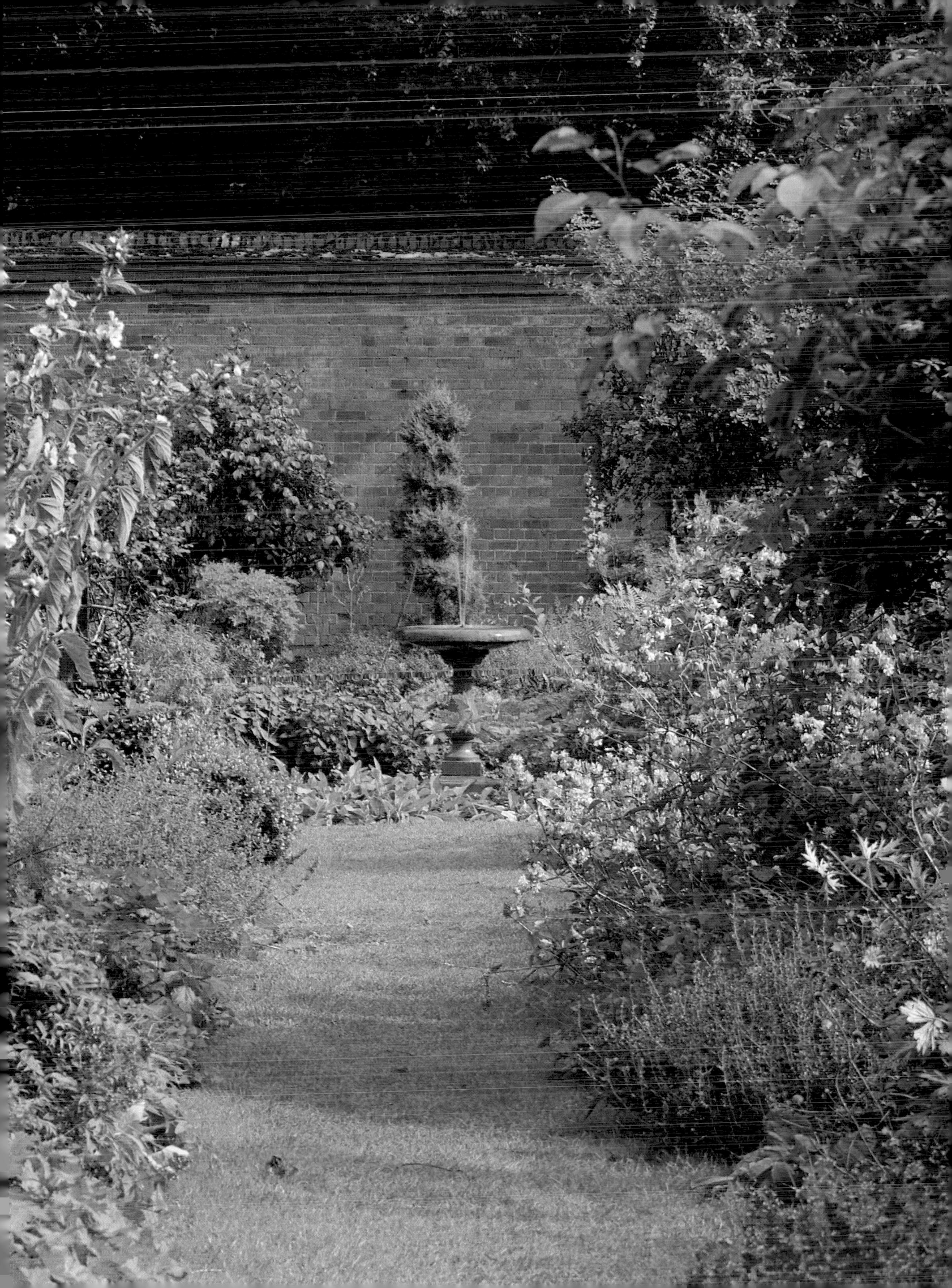

AROMATHERAPY

The use of pure essential oils from plants dates back many centuries, and the history of aromatherapy is in many ways part of the history of herbal medicine as a whole. The Arabic countries are credited with first discovering the process of distillation of oils, around a thousand years ago, and since then their use has spread both eastwards through the Indian sub-continent and westwards into Europe. Much modern research has taken place, for example, in France, ranging from perfumery applications to medicinal uses as powerful anti-infective agents.

Essential oils are highly concentrated substances – pure oil of Rose, for instance, may require 5,000 roses to make just 5 ml (1 tsp) of oil! For this reason they should be treated with respect and used sparingly – small is definitely better (and cheaper). In large doses many essential oils can become somewhat irritating to the skin, and a few are quite toxic if not used correctly. See general warning on page 121.

Since a large part of their effect on our moods and emotional states occurs through our sense of smell, it is important not to use any individual oil for too long, as they become tolerated and less useful. As a general rule, do not use an oil on a daily basis for more than 10 days. Similarly, do not inhale or mix too many oils together at one time; the olfactory centre in the brain becomes confused and an excess of essences can cause headaches or even nausea. Three or at the most four oils should be the maximum; two may be better.

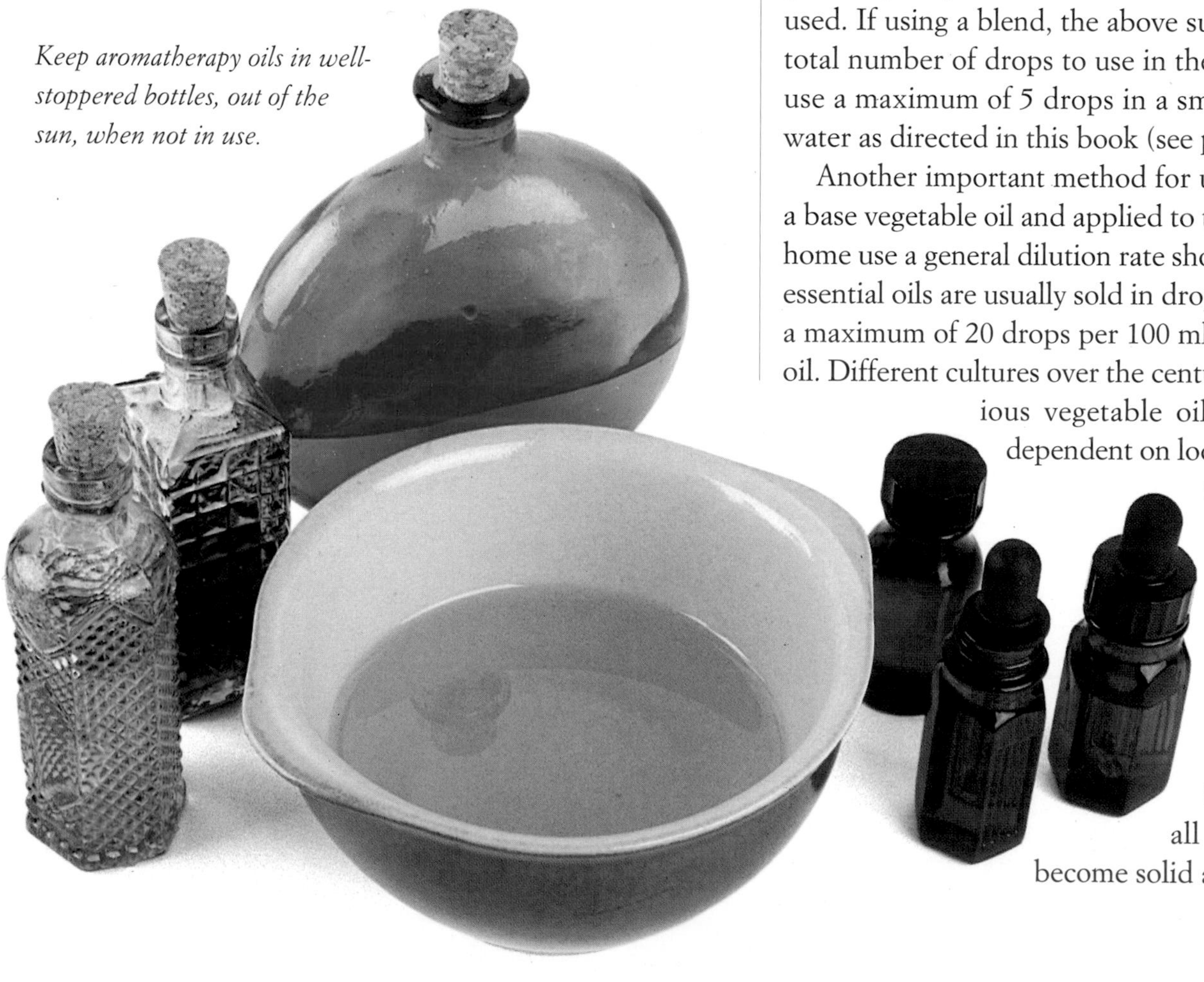

Keep aromatherapy oils in well-stoppered bottles, out of the sun, when not in use.

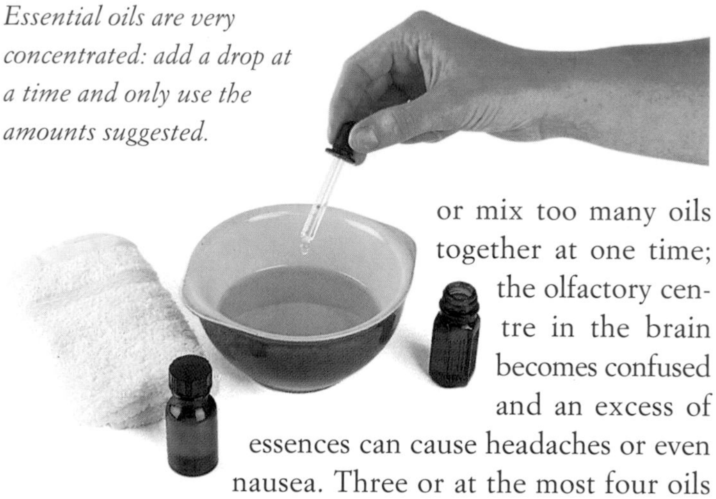

Essential oils are very concentrated: add a drop at a time and only use the amounts suggested.

A common way to use essential oils for self-treatment is in the bath. Place 6 drops on the surface of the bath water just before entering. The drops quickly form a thin film over the surface which adheres to the skin and is partially absorbed, helped by the warmth of the water. For oils such as Peppermint, which can make the skin tingle if used in large amounts, just add 3-4 drops, whereas with a mild and generally very safe oil such as Lavender, 10 drops can be used. If using a blend, the above suggestions represent the total number of drops to use in the bath. For compresses, use a maximum of 5 drops in a small bowl of hot or cold water as directed in this book (see page 15).

Another important method for using oils is diluted into a base vegetable oil and applied to the skin in massage. For home use a general dilution rate should be 1 per cent; since essential oils are usually sold in dropper bottles, this means a maximum of 20 drops per 100 ml (4 fl oz/½ cup) of base oil. Different cultures over the centuries have favoured various vegetable oils for massage, mostly dependent on local availability. Probably the most versatile oil is that of Sweet Almond; it is absorbed well into the skin and helps to nourish the skin, too. Other good base oils are Grapeseed, Sunflower and Safflower; the lightest oil of all is Coconut, but it may become solid at cool temperatures.

HERBALISM

Herbal medicine is the most widespread of all forms of medicine across the world, both historically and even today. At some time all cultures have used herbalism as the main system of treatment; its origins are essentially the origins of mankind itself. Probably the earliest herbal tradition comes from India. Medical knowledge from there spread into China on the one hand and into the Middle East on the other. The philosophy underlying Ancient Egyptian, and later Graeco-Roman, medicine has many similarities with both the old Ayur-Vedic system from northern India and traditional Chinese medicine.

Modern Western herbal medicine stems from the knowledge of the Greeks, with a strong input from the Native American tradition too. Increasingly, research being carried out today often confirms centuries-old empirical knowledge. Around 80 per cent of the world's population still relies on herbal medicine for their health needs, and even within conventional Western medicine up to 20 per cent of drugs are derived from plants in one way or another.

Herbs are almost certainly the most popular method of self-help in minor complaints, and introduce people to natural medicine. Throughout this book you will find references to how to take herbs internally; the easiest method is to make a tea, using a rough rule of 5 ml (1 tsp) per person plus the same for the teapot (many of the most popular herbs are available in tea bags, simply use one of these). If using fresh herbs, for example Lemon Balm *(Melissa officinalis)* you can use double the above amounts.

For stronger, more medicinal brews, you need to make either an infusion or a decoction (see page 12). For either an infusion or a decoction, the standard dose is 100-150 ml (4-5 fl oz/½-⅔ cup) – approximately a medium-sized teacupful – three times a day.

These infusions and decoctions can also be used to make a compress or poultice (see page 15). Once again, if using fresh herbs you can use more, perhaps 50 per cent more of each herb.

Many of the herbs found in gardens today have been used by herbalists for over two thousand years.

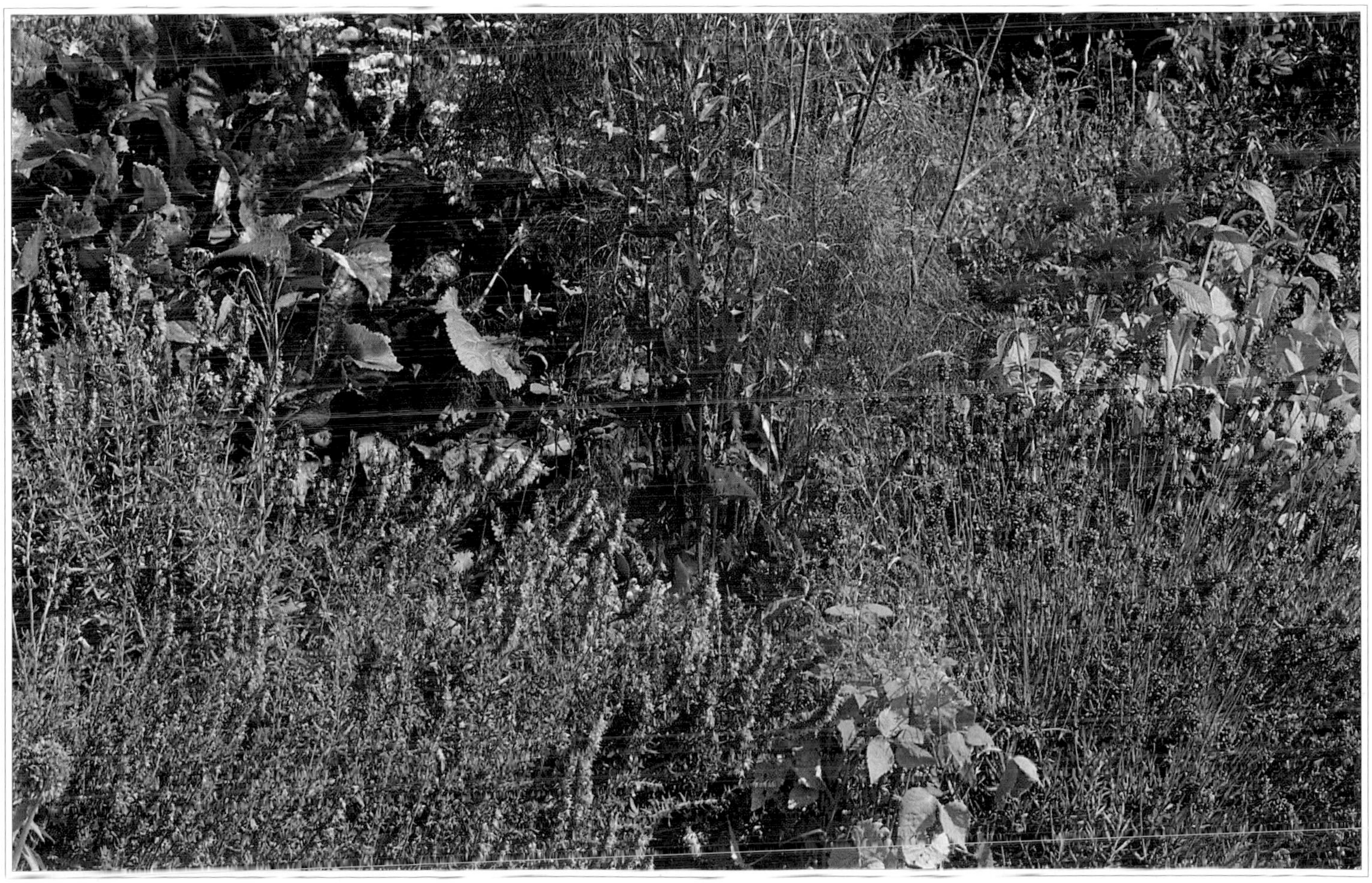

MAKING AN INFUSION

An infusion is made by pouring boiling water over an amount of the herb, to extract the properties. It is suitable for leaves and flowers, whose parts are easily extracted.

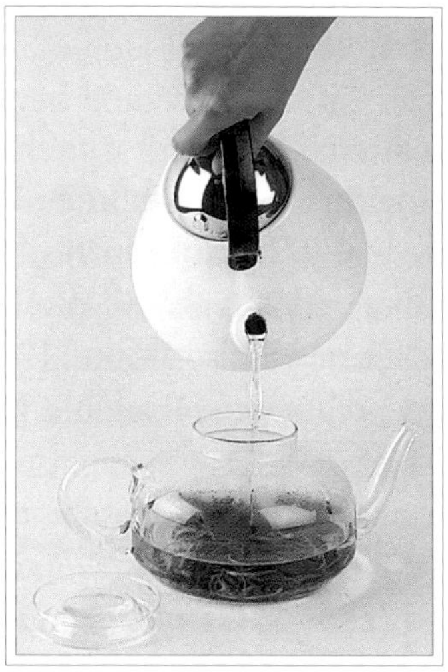

1 Place the herb in a teapot with a close-fitting lid. Pour in boiling water. Leave to infuse for up to 10 minutes.

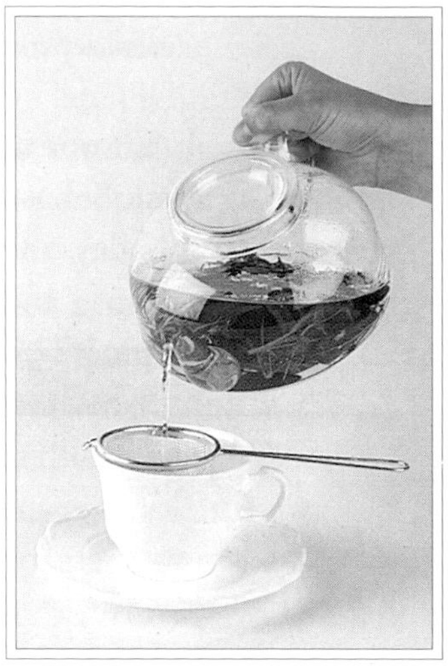

2 Strain through a sieve or strainer into a cup. Store the remainder in a jug, preferably in the fridge.

Standard Quantities

25 g (1 oz) dried herb or 50 g (2 oz) fresh herb to 500 ml (16 fl oz/2 cups) boiling water.

Standard Doses

One teacup (approximately 150 ml (5 fl oz/⅔ cup)) 3 times a day.

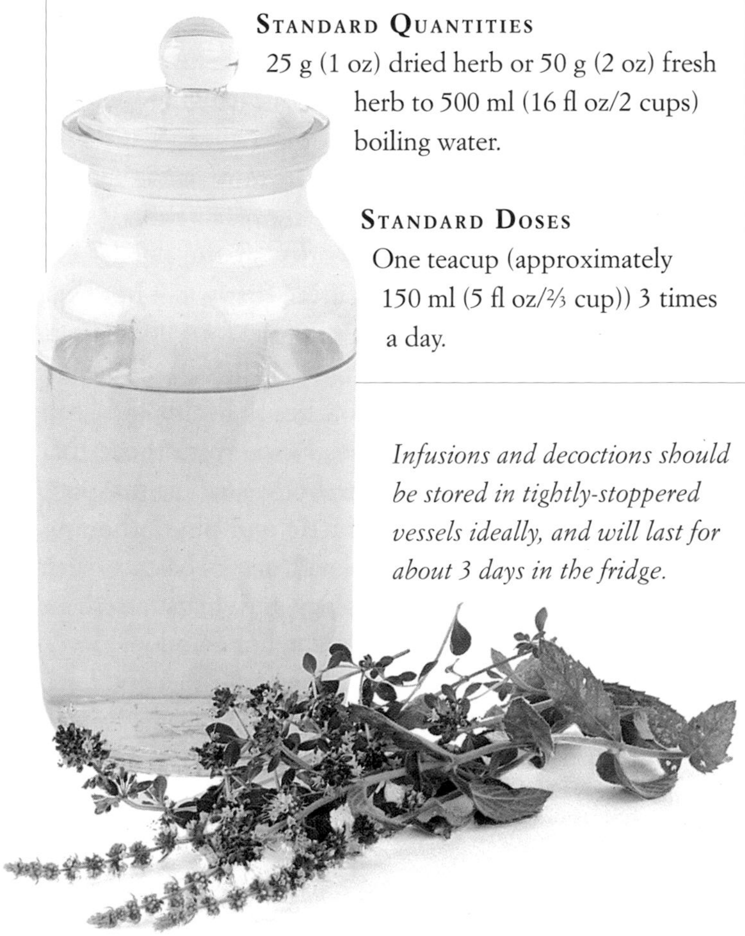

Infusions and decoctions should be stored in tightly-stoppered vessels ideally, and will last for about 3 days in the fridge.

MAKING A DECOCTION

A decoction involves simmering the herb in water to extract its properties, and is suitable for roots or woody parts that do not easily yield their ingredients in a simple infusion. If combining two plants, where one is a root, say Dandelion (*Taraxacum officinale*), and the other a flower, say Chamomile (*Chamomilla recutita*), use the strained decoction of the former for pouring on to the latter to make the infusion.

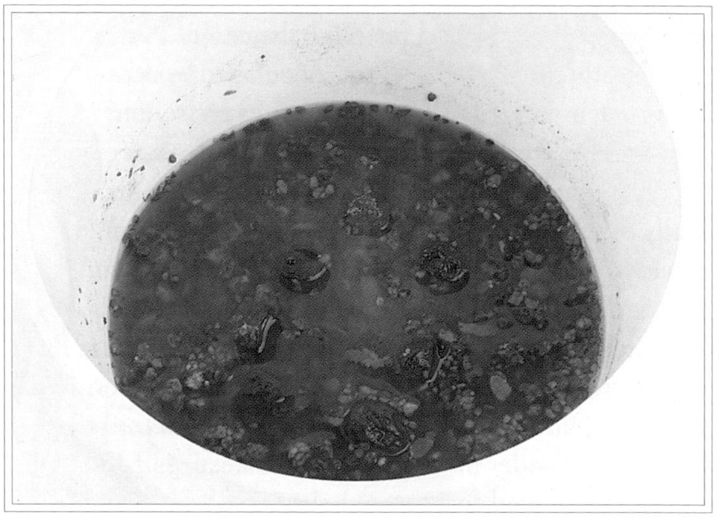

1 Place the herb in a saucepan and pour on cold water. Bring to the boil and simmer, until the liquid is reduced by a third.

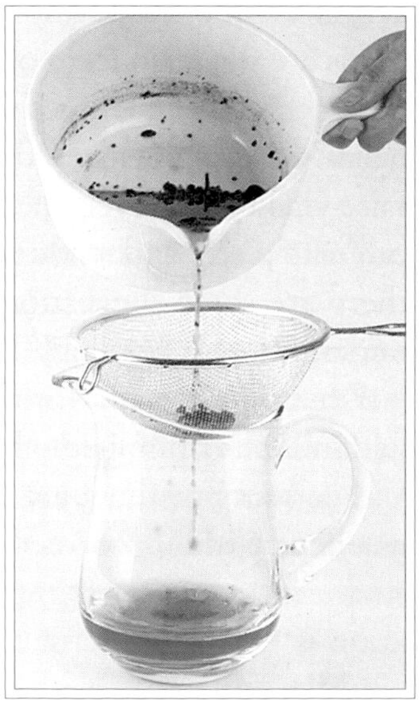

2 Strain through a sieve into a jug, and store in a fridge. It will keep for up to three days.

Standard Quantities

25 g (1 oz) dried herb or 50 g (2 oz) fresh herb to 750 ml (1¼ pt/3⅔ cups) water, reduced to 500 ml (16 fl oz/2 cups) after simmering.

Standard Doses

One teacup (150 ml (5 fl oz/⅔ cup)) 3 times a day.

MAKING A HOT OIL INFUSION

Herbs can be infused in oil, to make an extract for use in massage, or in making creams and ointments. Infused oils may keep for a few months, but will be stronger made in small batches for more immediate use. Hot infused oils may be made from herbs such as Comfrey (*Symphytum officinale*), while flowers such as Marigold (*Calendula officinalis*) or St John's Wort (*Hypericum perforatum*) are better as cold infused oils. Any light oil, such as Sunflower, Safflower or Sweet Almond oil, is a suitable medium to use.

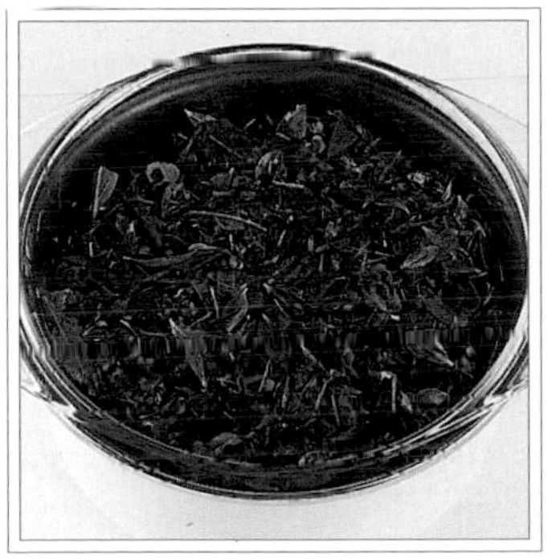

1 Place the herb and oil in a glass bowl, over a saucepan of simmering water, and heat gently for a couple of hours.

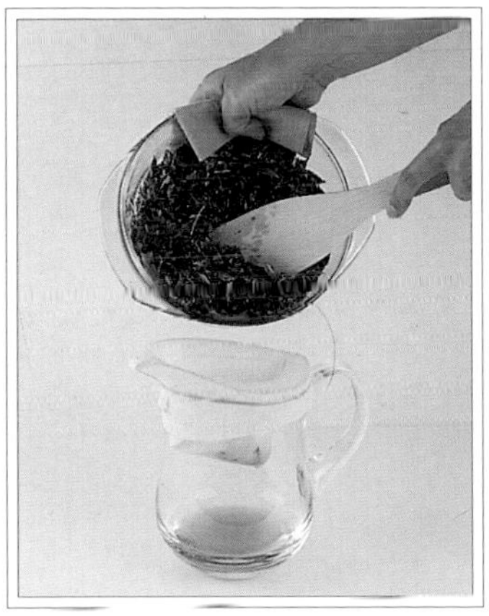

2 Pour through a jelly bag into a clean jug.

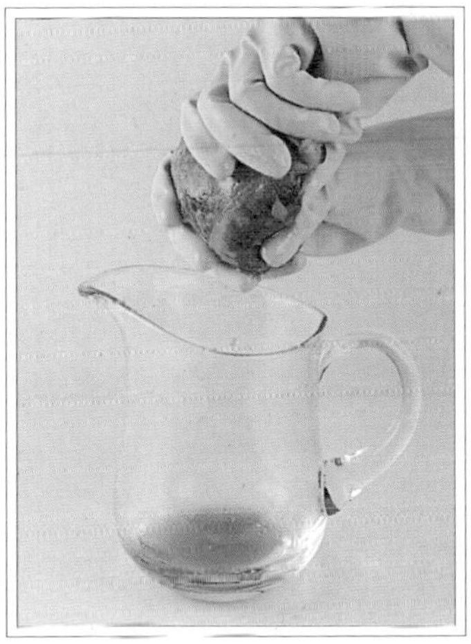

3 Squeeze out as much oil as possible through the bag (wear gloves as the oil is hot), to get a really strong extract.

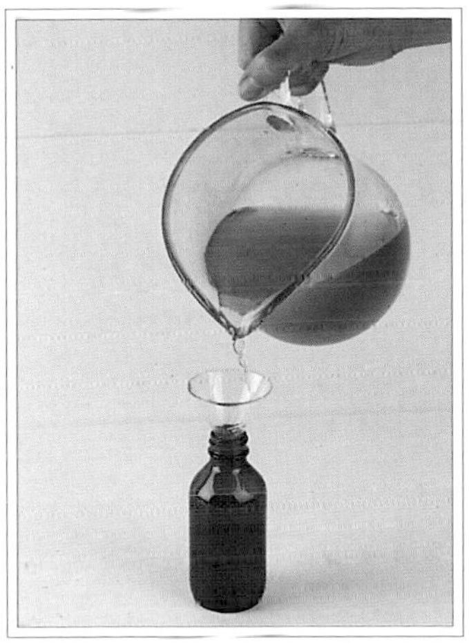

4 Pour into clean, dark bottles. Seal and store. Keep in a cool place and use within 3 months of making.

STANDARD QUANTITIES

250 g (9 oz) dried herb or 500 g (1¼ lb) fresh herb to 500 ml (16 fl oz/2 cups) pure vegetable oil.

MAKING A COLD OIL INFUSION

Some plants contain important medicinal oils which are highly volatile, i.e. they escape with heat, and a cold oil infusion retains their properties much more successfully.

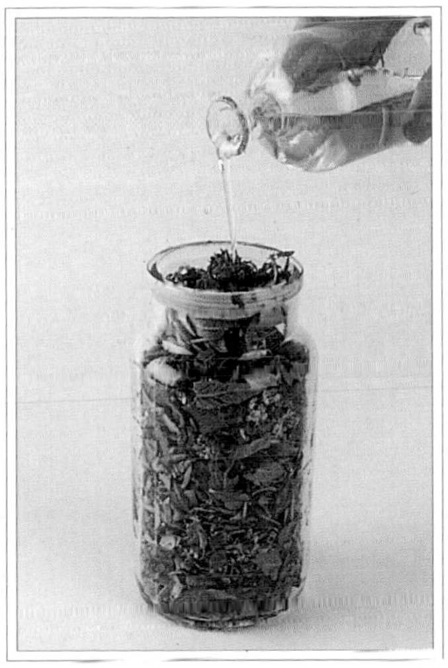

1 Pack a large jar with the herb and cover with oil. Seal and leave in a sunny spot for 2 weeks.

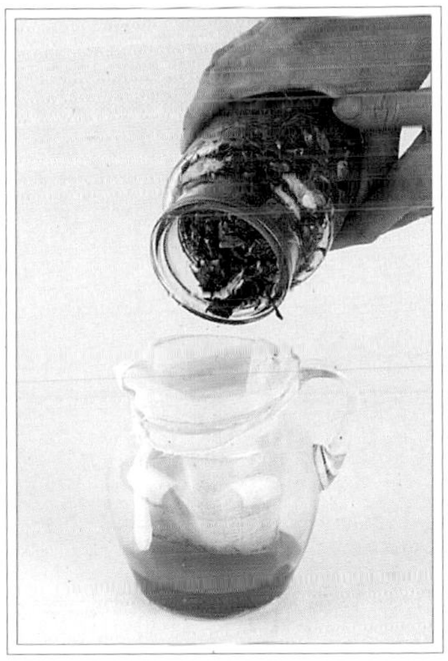

2 Pour slowly through a jelly bag into a clean jug, allowing time for the oil to filter through the fabric.

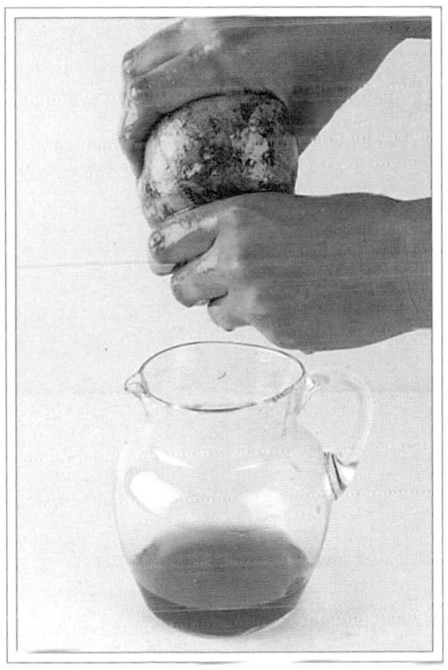

3 Squeeze out as much oil as possible through the bag. To make the infused oil even stronger, repeat steps 1, 2 and 3 with the same oil and new amounts of the herb.

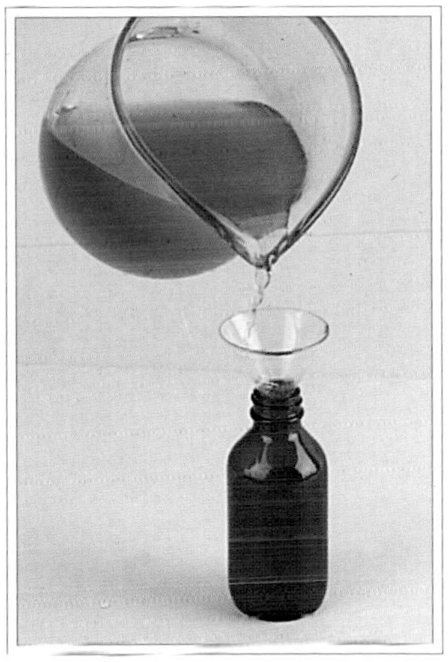

4 Pour into clean, dark bottles. Seal and store. Preferably, use small bottles as when opened the oil starts to deteriorate.

STANDARD QUANTITIES

250 g (9 oz) dried herb or 500 g (1¼ lb) fresh herb to 500 ml (16 fl oz/2 cups) pure vegetable oil.

MAKING A TINCTURE

Many herbs contain active ingredients which are not easily extracted by water, or are destroyed by heat, and a tincture solves these problems as well as preserving the extract. A tincture is an extract of a herb in a mixture of alcohol and water, normally 25 per cent alcohol strength. This is one of the most concentrated extracts from a herb, and the alcohol preserves the medicine for 2 years or more. The alcohol used commercially is ethyl alcohol, but a spirit such as brandy or vodka can be used for home tinctures. Do not use industrial alcohol, isopropyl alcohol or methylated spirits, as they are all poisonous.

Because a tincture is such a concentrated extract, only use where recommended, and for short periods of time. Do not be tempted to increase the dosage.

Caution

If in any doubt about using a tincture, seek professional advice, or stick to the other methods described in this book. Do not give tinctures to children, unless advised, and remember to keep all medicines out of the reach of small children.

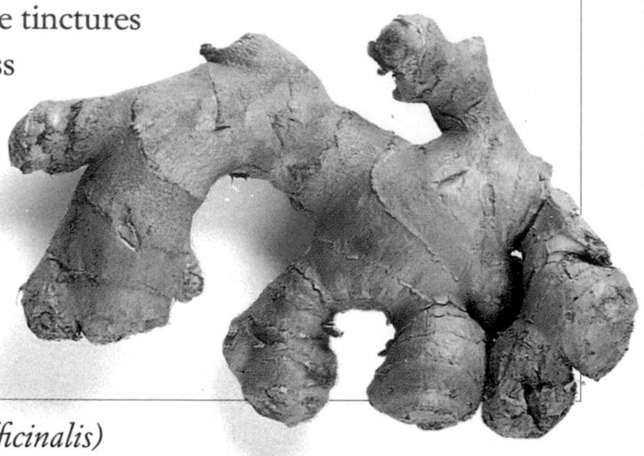

Ginger *(Zingiber officinalis)*

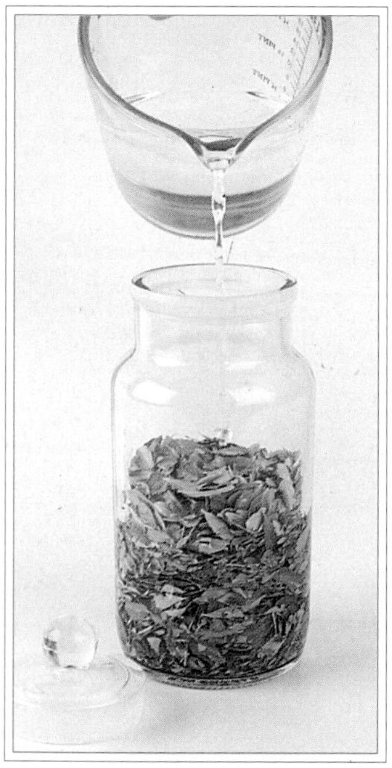

1 Put the herb into a large jar and pour on the alcohol/water mixture. Seal the jar and store in a cool place for two weeks. Shake the jar occasionally.

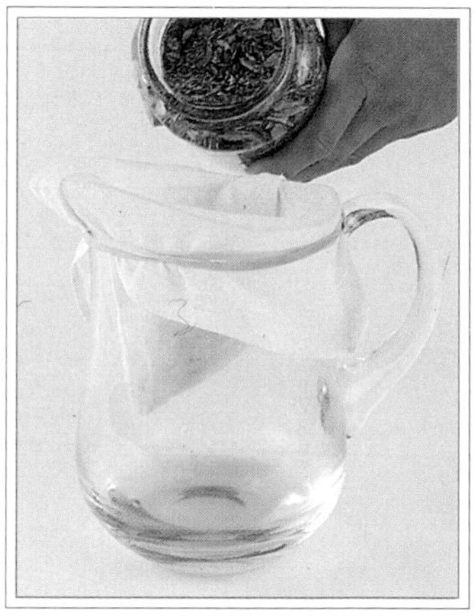

2 Pour mixture through a jelly bag into a clean jug.

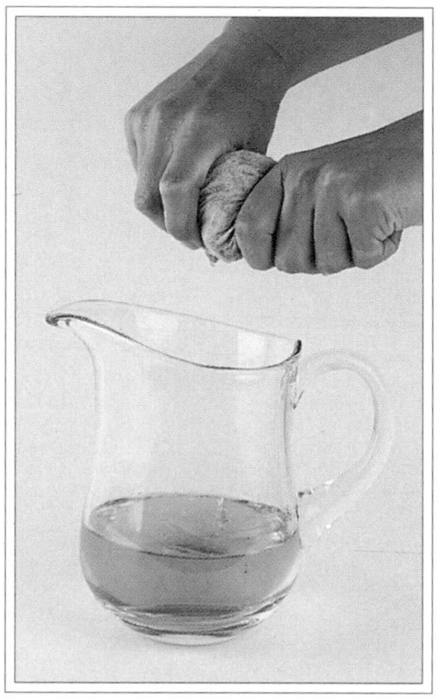

3 Squeeze out the tincture from the bag. Ideally, use a wine press and press the mixture into a clean jug.

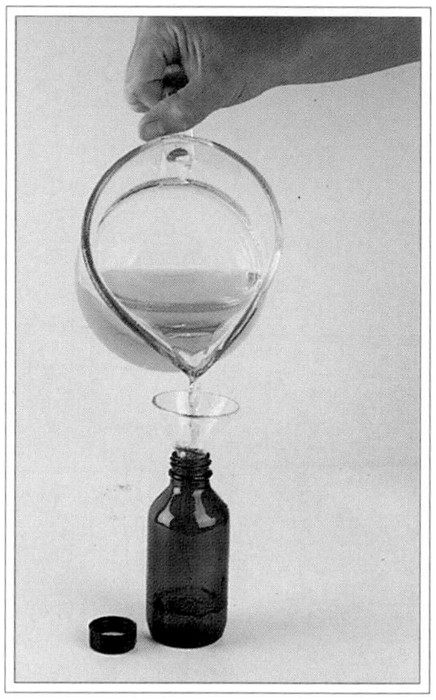

4 Pour the strained liquid into clean, dark bottles. Seal and store. Keep in a cool dry place and label.

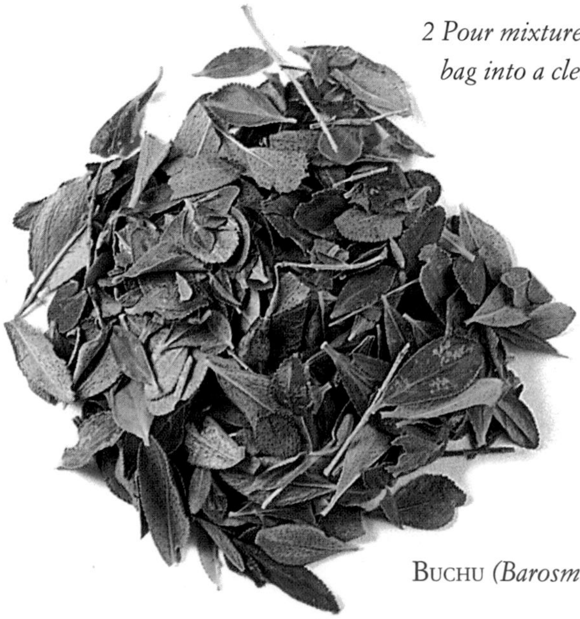

Buchu *(Barosma betulina)*

Standard Quantities

200 g (7 oz) dried herb or 40 g (1½ oz) fresh herb to 1 litre (1¾ pt/4 cups) 25 per cent alcohol/water mix (e.g. if using 40 per cent vodka or brandy, add 375 ml (13 fl oz/1½ cups) water to 600 ml (1 pt/2½ cups) spirit to make a 25 per cent strength).

Standard Doses

Up to 5 ml (1 tsp), three times a day. These may be taken diluted in a little water. For concentrated herbs such as Ginger *(Zingiber officinalis)*, take up to 10 drops, 3 times a day. Preferably take these with water.

WARM AND COLD COMPRESSES

A compress is a way of applying herbal extracts directly to the skin, to reduce the inflammation or promote healing. Usually, an infusion or decoction of the herb is prepared for use in the compress, or simply hot or cold water can be used.

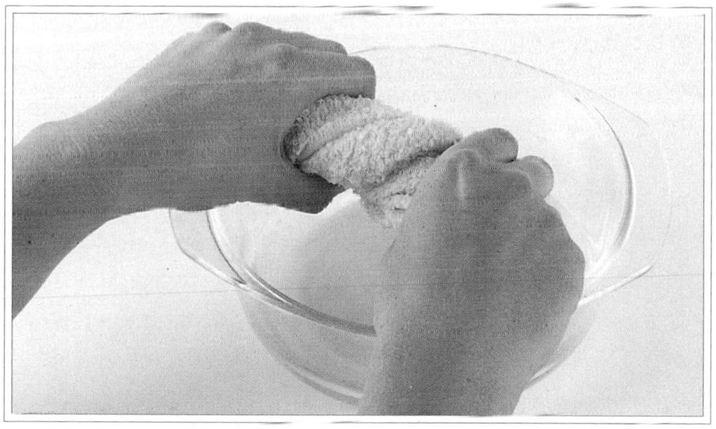

1 Soak a clean cloth or flannel in a hot infusion or hot water.

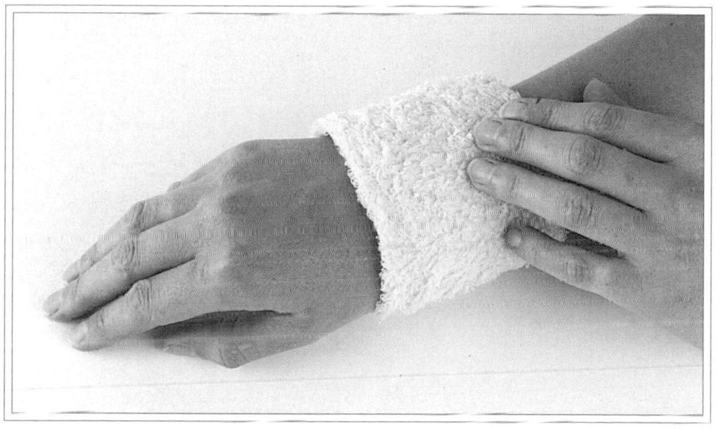

2 Place on the affected area and hold firmly in place – use a towel or bandage to tie in place if kept on for long. The same procedure applies for cold compresses.

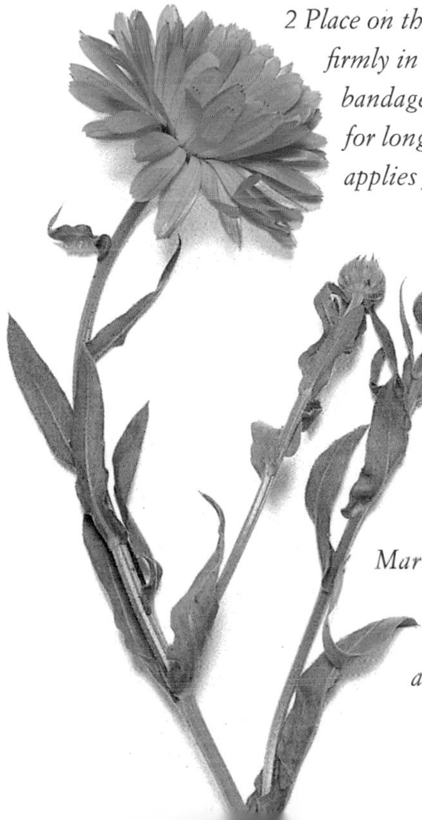

Marigold (Calendula officinalis) *is very soothing for bites and stings.*

POULTICE

A poultice acts in a similar way to a compress, but the herb itself is used, rather than just a liquid extract. Normally poultices are applied hot, and it may be useful to apply a little oil to the skin first, to stop the herb from sticking.

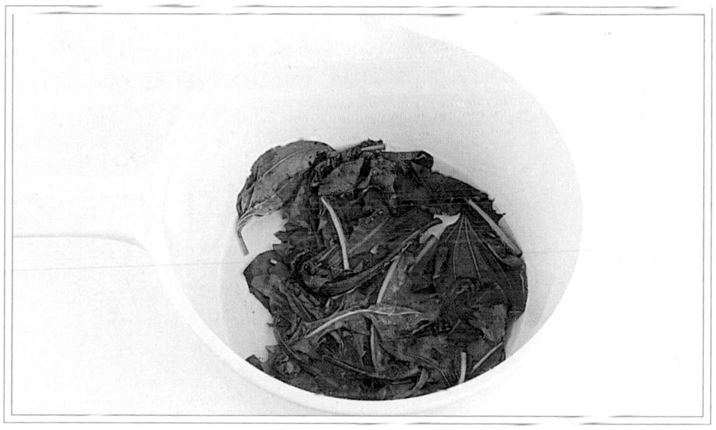

1 Chop up the fresh herb if it is too large, and place sufficient herbs to cover the affected area into a saucepan. Add a little water and simmer for a couple of minutes.

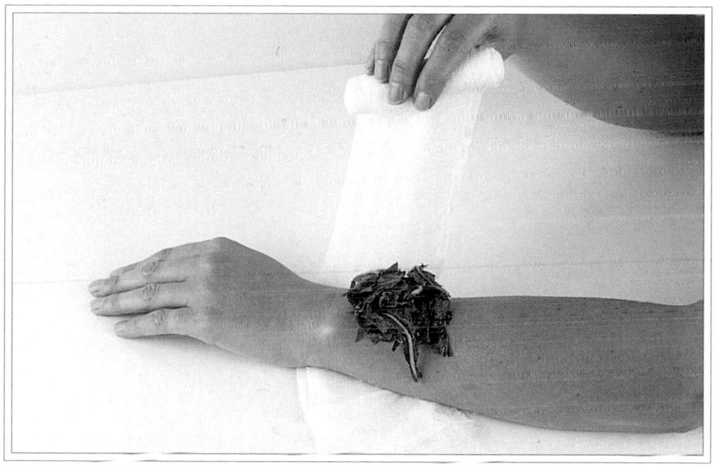

2 Squeeze out any excess moisture and place on the affected area. Cover with a bandage or cotton strips to hold in place.

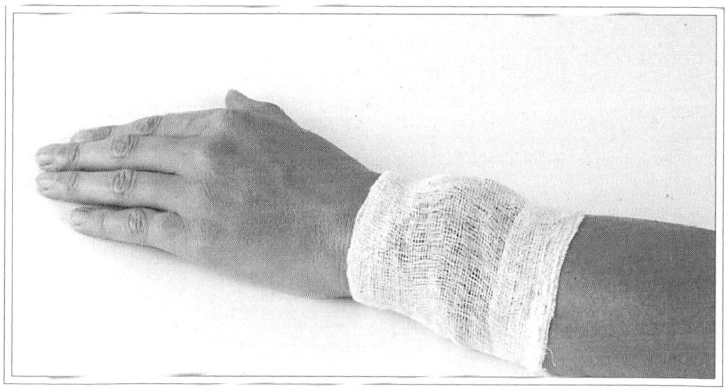

3 Keep in place for 3-4 hours, replacing every hour with a fresh, hot poultice if necessary.

MAKING AN OINTMENT

An ointment contains oils or fats, but not water, and is useful to form a protective layer over the skin. Petroleum jelly or paraffin wax may be used, but a wonderful natural method is to use vegetable oil, such as Sweet Almond or Sunflower, with beeswax. This is also very easy to make at home.

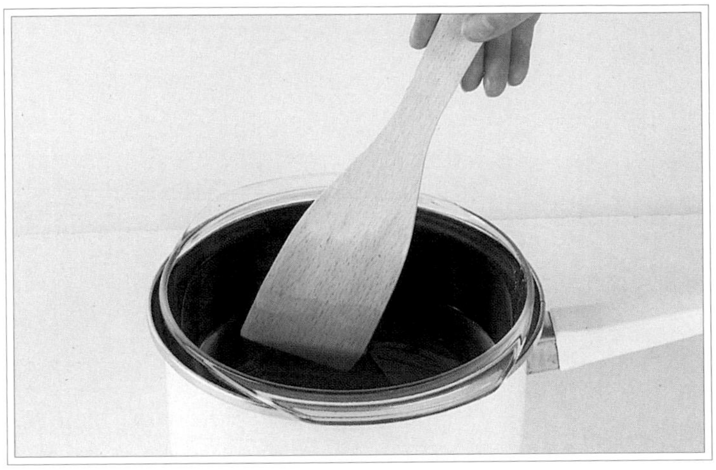

1 Place the beeswax and oil in a glass bowl over a saucepan of water. Bring the water to the boil and simmer until the wax has melted into the oil. Remove from the heat.

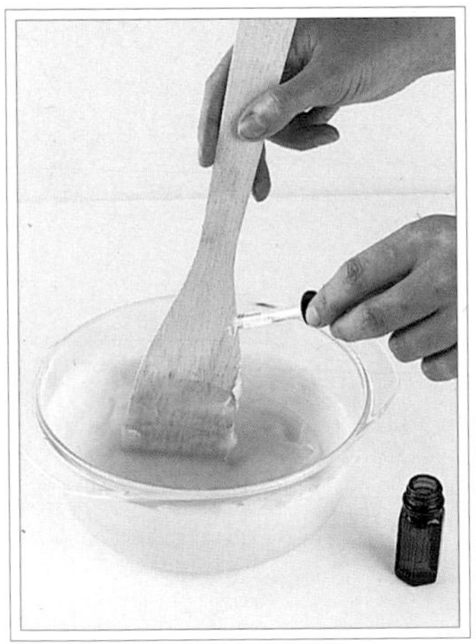

2 Stir continually as the oil/wax mixture cools and stiffens; essential oils may be added at this stage, as recommended, and stirred into the mixture.

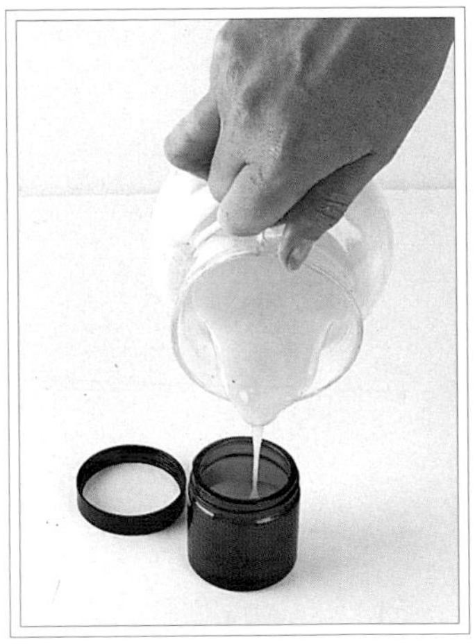

3 Pour or spoon into small, clean ointment jars, seal and store. This may keep for a few months under good conditions, but should be made in small amounts as needed.

STANDARD QUANTITIES

25 g (1 oz) beeswax to 100 ml (4 fl oz/½ cup) vegetable oil. If adding essential oils, use 20-30 drops for this amount, but only 10 drops if skin is very sensitive.

MAKING A CREAM

Making an organic cream is very similar to making an ointment, again using beeswax.

1 Place beeswax and oil in a glass bowl in a saucepan of water (see left). Bring water to the boil and simmer until the wax has melted. Place water in another glass bowl, over a saucepan of simmering water. Remove both glass bowls from the heat.

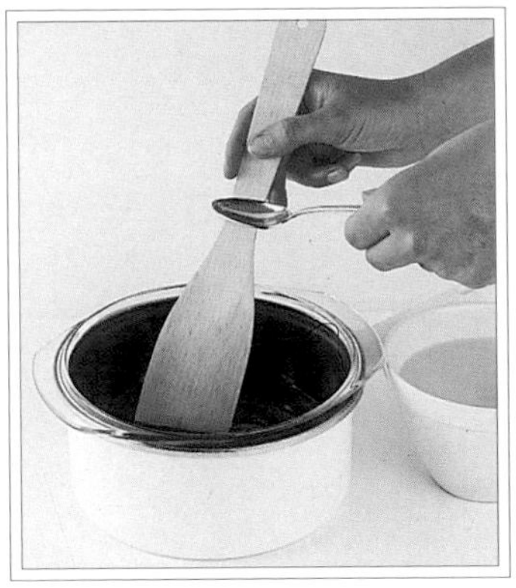

2 Add water to the melted wax/oil mixture, drop by drop, stirring all the time until the cream thickens and cools.

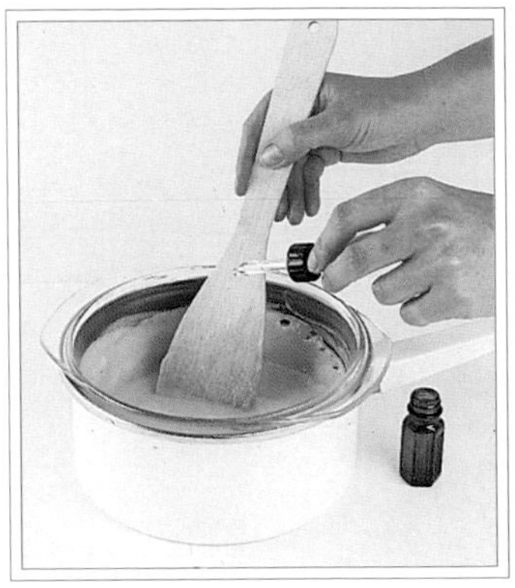

3 At this stage essential oils may be added, as recommended, and gently stirred into the cream.

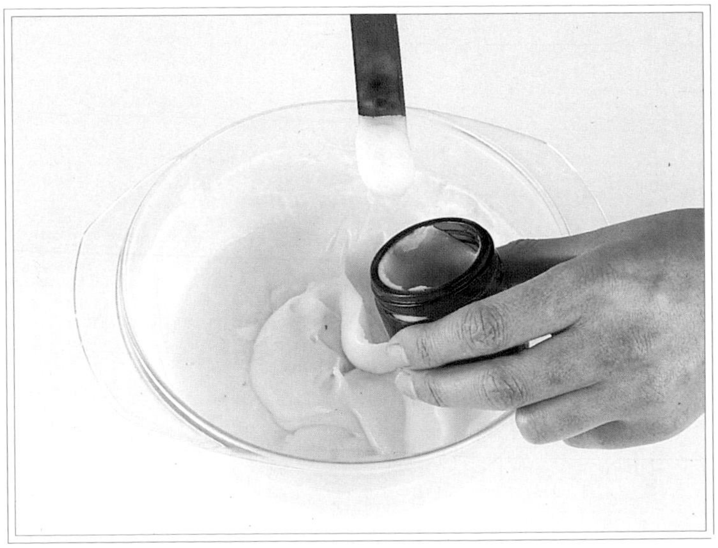

4 Pour or spoon into small, clean ointment jars, seal and store. Make small amounts as required. This cream may keep for a few months under good conditions.

STANDARD QUANTITIES

25 g (1 oz) beeswax, 25 ml (1½ tbsp) water and 100 ml (4 fl oz/½ cup) vegetable oil. If adding essential oils, use 20-30 drops at the most for this amount of cream.

MIXING ESSENTIAL OILS FOR MASSAGE

When essential oils are used for aromatherapy massage, different oils are combined to increase their therapeutic effect. Light vegetable oils such as Sweet Almond, Grapeseed or Sunflower are the best oils to begin with. For home use the general dilution rate should be 1 per cent (i.e. a maximum of 20 drops per 100 ml (4 fl oz/½ cup) of base oil). Once you have mixed your oils, store in a cool, dark place and use them immediately, as they are perishable.

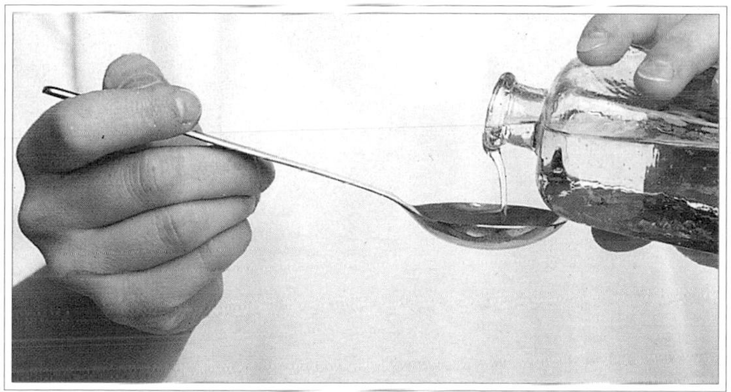

1 Before you begin, wash and dry your hands and make sure that all your utensils are clean and dry. Have your essential oils at the ready, but leave the lids on the bottles until they are required. Carefully measure out approximately 10 ml (2 tsp) of your chosen vegetable oil.

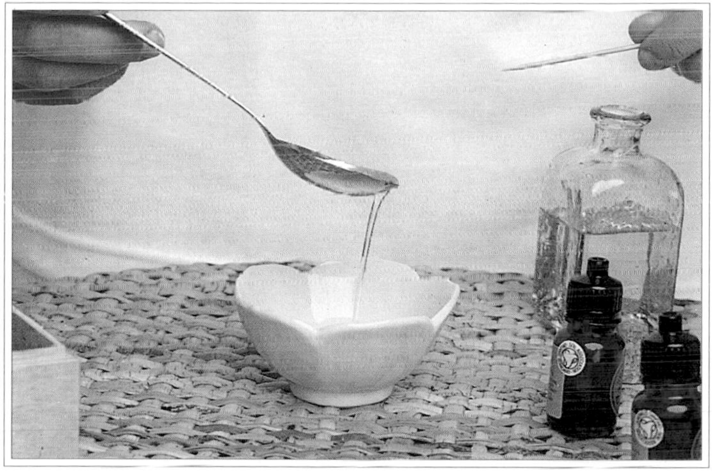

2 Gently pour the vegetable oil into your blending bowl.

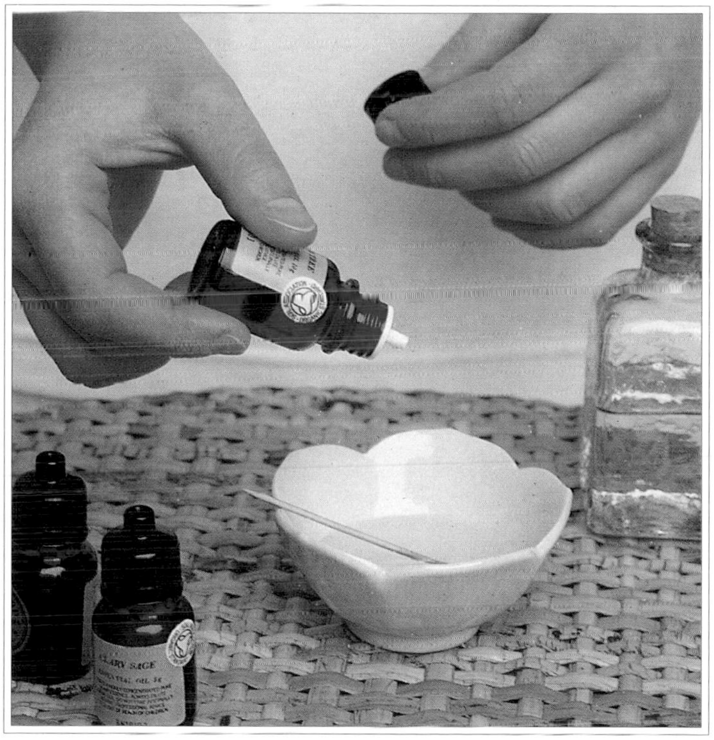

3 Add the essential oil, one drop at a time. Mix gently with a clean, dry cocktail stick or toothpick, to blend.

CAUTION

The essential oil recommendations in this book are extremely safe in the amounts given. If someone has very sensitive skin or lots of allergies then try massaging with just one drop of essential oil per 20 ml (4 tsp) of base oil at first to test for any signs of reaction (rare). If the person is pregnant or may be pregnant, stick to the oils and doses suggested in the chapter on reproduction. If in any doubt, seek medical advice.

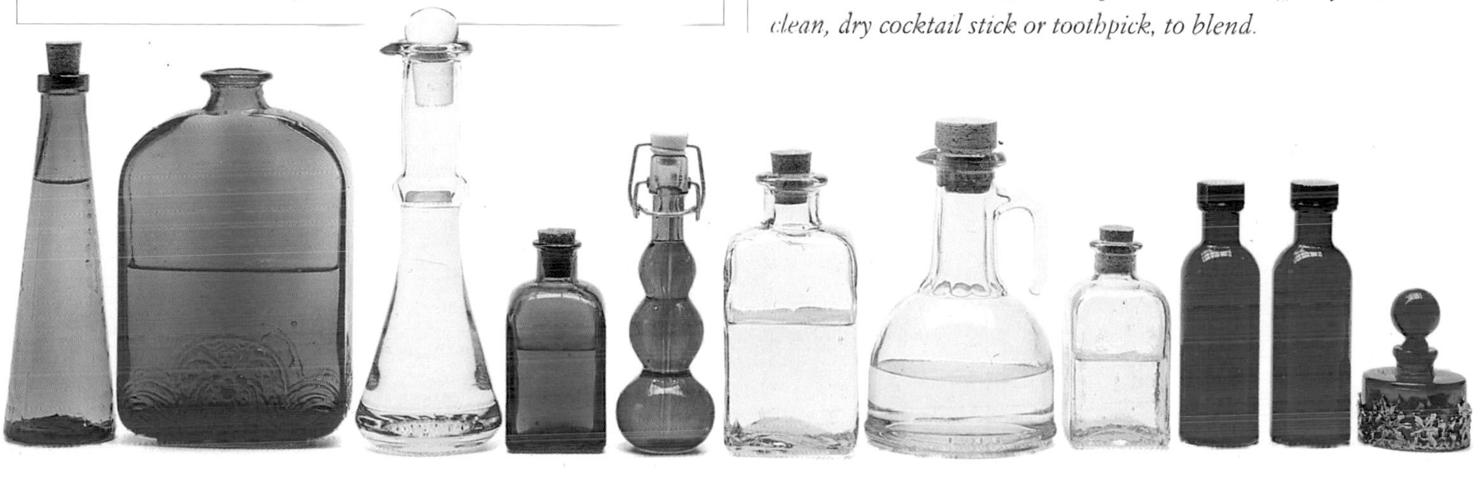

THE NERVOUS SYSTEM

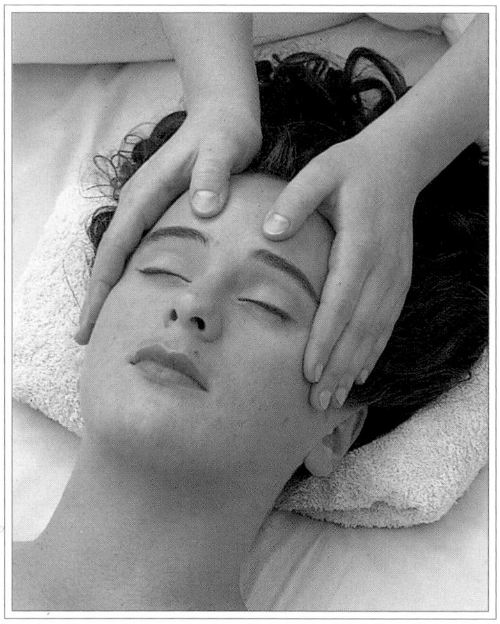

One of the main principles of natural medicine is the holistic approach, taking into account the physical, mental, emotional and indeed spiritual well-being of the person when assessing health; this is most obviously apparent when looking at nervous disorders. Physical symptoms, such as headaches or insomnia, and emotional ones, such as depression, mental strains and stresses, can all weave together to create disease, or simply *dis-ease* – a lack of harmony.

When trying to treat these problems, therefore, it is essential to look at all the reasons for the disorder. One of the first things to do is apply some common sense: is your headache due to an excess of alcohol last night, does your anxiety stem from tomorrow's interview, or your insomnia follow three cups of coffee in the evening? Finding the cause may not solve your immediate problem, but may help you to take preventive steps. In many cases of course, the causes are not so obvious and for persistent or recurring problems professional help should be sought.

Apart from the therapies described in this book, there are many sources of help for nerve-related conditions – since stress is a major factor in much ill-health nowadays, most forms of alternative medicine look at this aspect in their approaches. These might range from counselling and hypnotherapy through to acupuncture and cranial osteopathy. Equally importantly, these should all help to empower *you* to help yourself more effectively, which is the key aim of this book.

ABOVE: Taking time to relax and unwind is important for the overall well-being of our nervous system.

ANXIETY

There are many situations where some level of anxiety is perfectly normal, and a natural response to a stressful situation. It only becomes a problem when the degree of anxiety is out of proportion to the problem, or indeed when there is no objective, external reason for it. Symptoms might include constant feelings of tension, sweating, palpitations, hyper-ventilating and lack of sleep.

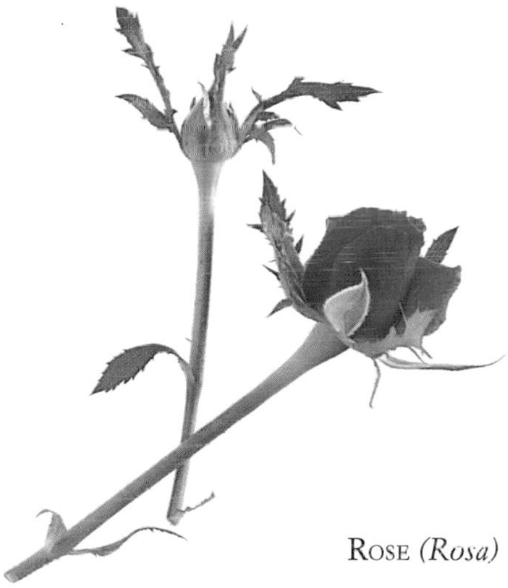

ROSE (*Rosa*)

AROMATHERAPY

There are several oils which have a relaxing, calming effect on the nervous system; probably the nicest way to use them is in the bath (see page 17), where the warm water aids relaxation and helps the oils to be absorbed.

CLARY SAGE: a relaxing, warming and almost euphoric effect, especially helpful where anxiety leads to exhaustion.

LAVENDER: calming, helping to balance the mind and emotions, it is one of the gentlest oils to use.

MELISSA: very soothing and, like Lavender, gentle to the skin.

It is useful where anxiety affects the digestion, and also where hormone imbalance creates tension (see Pre-menstrual Problems, page 71).

ROSE: it is wonderfully relaxing and is also considered one of the finest hormone regulators.

YLANG-YLANG: almost sedating, it slows the heart-rate and excessively rapid breathing. Do not overdo it, as large amounts or prolonged usage can result in a headache.

HERBALISM

Herbal remedies are well suited to relieving anxiety, try using one or more of the following herb teas:

CHAMOMILE (*Chamomilla recutita*): relaxing and good for the digestion; tea bags of it are sold everywhere.

LEMON BALM (*Melissa officinalis*): this can be safely taken over quite a time for mild anxiety; the fresh herb is much nicer tasting, just gather a few sprigs and take a tea morning and night.

LIME BLOSSOM (*Tilia europaea*): a very good evening drink, to soothe the mind and calm the digestion and heart-rate.

SKULLCAP (*Scutellaria lateriflora*): more strongly relaxing, this herb may be easier to find in tablet form.

VALERIAN (*Valeriana officinalis*): a powerful relaxant, relieving mental and physical tension. Better to take in tablet form, or up to 5 ml (1 tsp) of the tincture, as the tea tastes disgusting!

HOMEOPATHY

As always, long-term problems need professional treatment. In the meantime, a choice of these remedies may help.

ACONITE: for a sudden onset of anxiety or fear, perhaps after a fright, with much restlessness.

ARGENTICUM NITRICUM: for tension giving rise to butterflies in the stomach and indigestion, or a constant craving for sweet things.

ARSENICUM ALBUM: if very restless, fearful, no appetite and very finicky about food.

GELSEMIUM: for nervous apprehension, such as pre-exam nerves or stage fright, with weak trembling knees.

NATUROPATHY

Apart from recommending activities like yoga or meditation to help reduce levels of anxiety in the long term, gentle exercise and warm baths may be helpful to ease tensions and calm down. The addition of a Vitamin B complex supplement in the mornings, and calcium in the evenings will help both to feed the nervous system and restore a more natural rhythm to the energy use through the day – one of the reasons for the popularity of milky drinks as a nightcap is that they are rich in calcium, a natural relaxant.

Lime Blossom tea

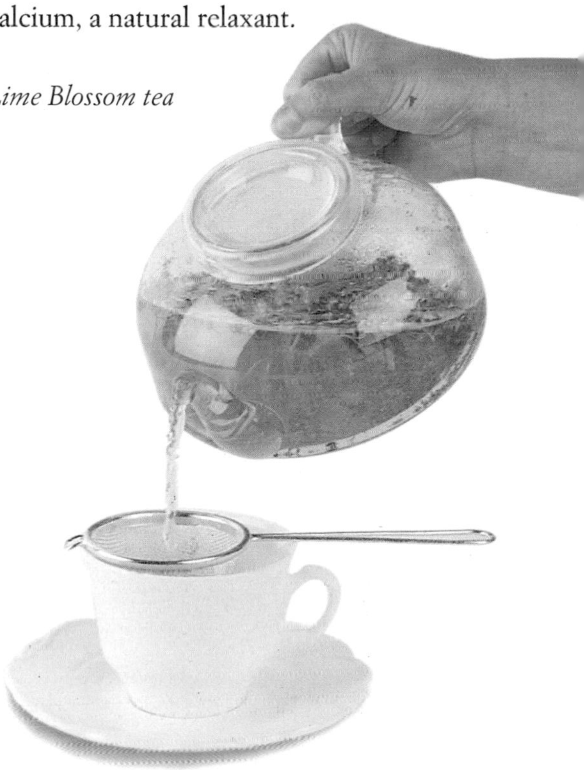

DEPRESSION

Just as with anxiety, depression can be due to several reasons, and its symptoms may be quite varied. Conditions like constipation, headaches, insomnia and loss of appetite can all relate to depression and in deep or continuing instances of depression professional help is essential. This is especially so when there is no obvious reason for the feelings, a condition generally labelled endogenous depression.

AROMATHERAPY

Many oils have quite profound effects on mood, and it may be necessary to change the oil used as symptoms vary. The benefits of aromatherapy massage using diluted essential oils (see page 17), with the caring effect of the direct contact, are the most useful way of treating someone with depression, but oils can also be very helpful in the bath (see page 8).

BERGAMOT: this is one of the most uplifting of oils, with a refreshing citrus fragrance which is appealing to both men and women – and gives Earl Grey tea its distinctive aroma.

CLARY SAGE: this is quite relaxing, but with an uplifting, almost euphoric effect as well; good when chronic tension has led to depression or exhaustion.

GERANIUM: this oil actually comes from varieties of scented pelargonium, and has a tonic effect on the adrenal cortex, which helps to regulate stress hormone production.

NEROLI: this oil, from the blossom of the bitter orange, is very concentrated (and also expensive!) so a little can go a long way. It relaxes and soothes, relieving muscle spasm and the irritability which often goes with a depressed state.

HERBALISM

The traditional approach to depression included looking at all the body systems, in particular liver function, and often bitter herbs were prescribed to stimulate digestion and act as a tonic; a few drops of a tincture (see page 14) of a herb such as Gentian *(Gentiana lutea)* may do the trick in mild cases of depressed spirits. The herbs below can be taken as a tea, or for a stronger effect take as an infusion (see page 12).

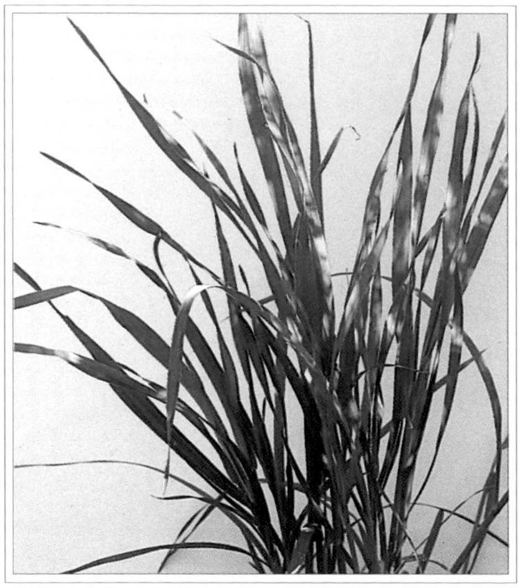

OATSTRAW *(Avena sativa)*

BORAGE *(Borago officinalis)*: an adrenal stimulant and general tonic, best taken as a tea and for short periods only.

OATSTRAW *(Avena sativa)*: an all-round nervous restorative; either use 20 drops of the tincture twice daily, or simply add plenty of oats to the diet, for example, in cereals.

ROSEMARY *(Rosmarinus officinalis)*: excellent where nervous exhaustion leads to depression, also good for headaches and sluggish digestion.

VERVAIN *(Verbena officinalis)*: a relaxing tonic, very useful for the depression of convalescence from an illness, when everything seems a struggle.

HOMEOPATHY

In the short term, look at these remedies.

AURUM METALLICUM: for deep depression and almost suicidal feelings, perhaps following failure in exams or at work.

IGNATIA: this is especially appropriate for depression following a shock or grief, with pent-up, almost hysterical feelings and a lump in the throat .

KALI PHOS: for nervous exhaustion, leaving a lack of mental or physical energy.

PULSATILLA: generally most useful for mild, gentle people who are prone to weepiness, with a rapid change of mood to feeling miserable – this is often a good remedy for children, but seek medical advice first!

NATUROPATHY

One of the first things to do is overhaul the diet, to make sure there is enough nourishment for the nervous system. Reduce coffee, tea, sugar and alcohol intake. Take plenty of wholefoods, possibly increasing protein intake, if the diet has been poor.

Taking more exercise is a positive move, helping to improve circulation, muscle tone and increase oxygen intake. The main difficulty of course is motivation, so support from an exercise class may be more successful than doing it alone.

Supplement the diet with a good general multi-mineral and vitamin supplement to give a wide spectrum of nutrients.

HEADACHES

Headaches can develop for a number of reasons; usually they can be related to some obvious cause such as nasal congestion or sinusitis, eyestrain, fatigue or tension. The majority of headaches are due to stress or worries, with muscle spasms in the neck leading to head pains. These can be made worse by poor posture, and many jobs create special problems – for instance, computer operators often get eyestrain and stiff, aching shoulders or neck muscles, and consequently headaches.

AROMATHERAPY

Many essential oils have some analgesic properties. A useful way of employing the following for headaches is as a cold compress (see page 15), applied to the temples and forehead – use 5 drops in a small bowl of cold water, wring out a flannel or something similar and place on the area. Alternatively, gently massage a couple of drops directly into the temples.

LAVENDER: relaxing, warming and analgesic, one of the gentlest of oils. Where there is neck tension, apply a hot compress to the neck and upper back at the same time (proportions as above for cold compress).

PEPPERMINT: this is very cooling in its effect, and is also very useful for relieving catarrh and nasal congestion. As it has something of a stimulant action, it could be used in equal amounts with Lavender, as described above, on the temples and forehead.

ROSEMARY: this is even more stimulating to the central nervous system, and is excellent for headaches following mental strain and exhaustion, as well as helping to clear the sinuses.

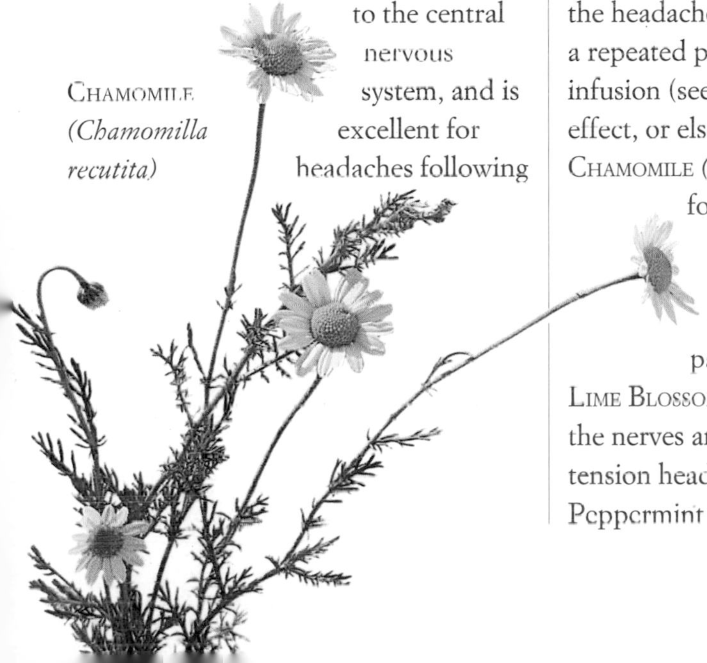

CHAMOMILE (*Chamomilla recutita*)

SEVERE HEADACHES

Causes such as very high blood pressure, meningitis or even brain tumours are much rarer; these of course need professional treatment, and severe, unexplained or persistent headaches should be checked out carefully, but most headaches can be identified and cured at home. Where there has been any kind of accident, for instance a whiplash injury, it makes good sense to consult a manipulative therapist such as a chiropractor or an osteopath.

HERBALISM

At the earliest signs of a headache taking a herbal tea from the choice below can stop it in its tracks; if the headache is more pronounced, or is a repeated problem, try making an infusion (see page 12) for a stronger effect, or else get medical advice.

CHAMOMILE (*Chamomilla recutita*): good for bilious headaches, stemming from over-eating or indigestion, where there is a dull, throbbing pain on top of the head.

LIME BLOSSOM (*Tilia europaea*): soothes the nerves and is very helpful for tension headaches; can be mixed with Peppermint for a more uplifting effect.

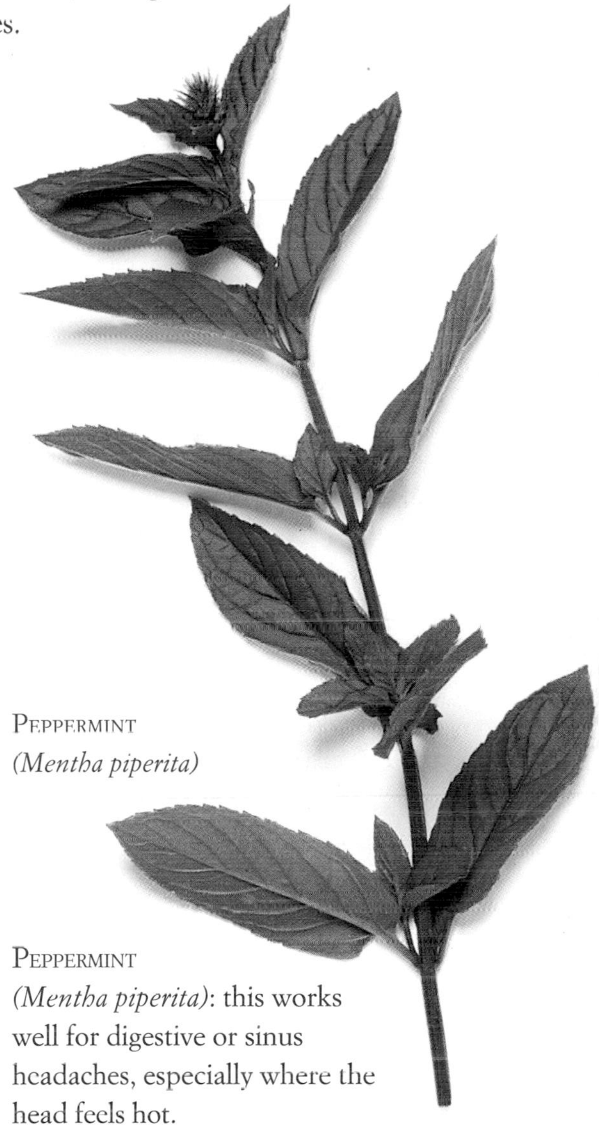

PEPPERMINT (*Mentha piperita*)

PEPPERMINT (*Mentha piperita*): this works well for digestive or sinus headaches, especially where the head feels hot.

ROSEMARY (*Rosmarinus officinalis*): for headaches related to exhaustion or depression, and also for bilious heavy heads. When the headache is due to a hangover, Rosemary and Peppermint tea can do wonders – but prevention is still better than a cure!

HOMEOPATHY

The choice is large, in part due to the many factors which go to produce the individual symptoms.

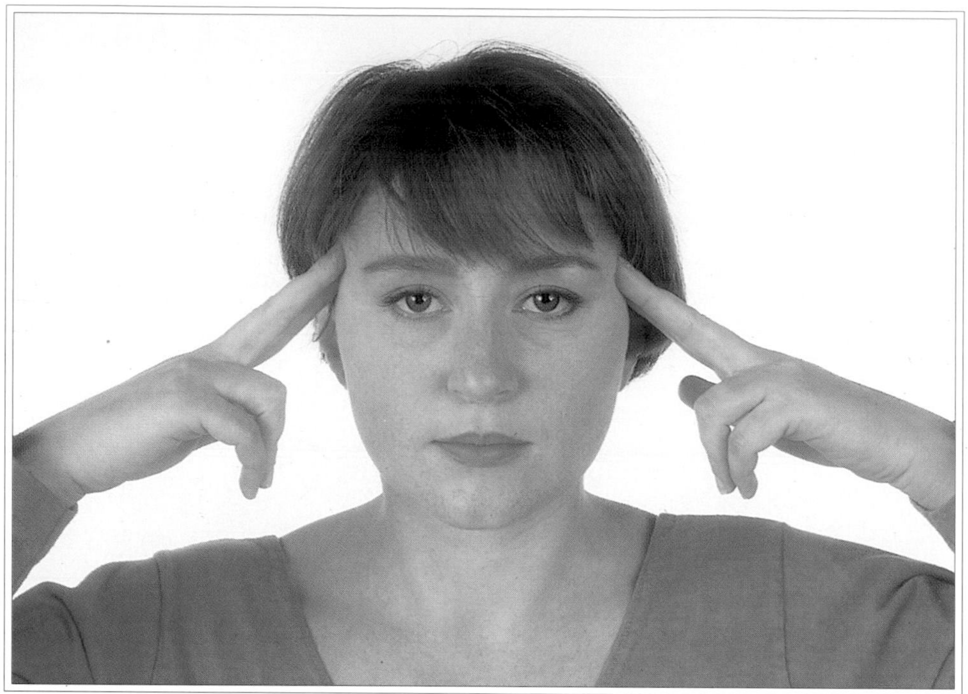

For tension headaches, gently massage the temples with small circling movements.

BELLADONNA: for a burning, violent headache with a hot head; the symptoms are worse with any jarring movement of the head, or loud noises.
BRYONIA: for a severe, splitting headache, only relieved by lying very still or with firm, cool pressure across the forehead.
NUX VOMICA: for a sharp headache, either on waking or after food, with nausea or bilious feelings from over-eating; better if taken when lying down, and keeping warm.
PULSATILLA: good for headaches associated with menstruation, also where brought on by too much rich food; relief seems to come from cool applications to the head and being out in the fresh air.

NATUROPATHY

In general, the naturopathic approach is to look at prevention, by changing lifestyle to reduce the reasons for headaches. Eating a varied wholefood diet, reducing alcohol, coffee and tea, and getting more exercise and fresh air are all likely to help lower the frequency of headaches for regular sufferers. Drink plenty of fluids, as dehydration can be a factor, especially for people working in hot, stuffy atmospheres and, of course, in hangovers. Avoid dramatic changes in diet, such as crash dieting, which upsets blood sugar levels and can contribute to headaches. Sometimes a Vitamin B complex supplement can be useful in relieving mental exhaustion. For hot, congested headaches use cold compresses to the forehead, perhaps combined with a hot footbath to improve circulation.

BENEFITS OF SELF-HELP
Prevention is better than cure so try to adopt some of the measures outlined in this book to maintain good health rather than just waiting to be ill. If you suffer from several complaints, read all the relevant sections for an overall picture of what you can do to improve your general health and be aware of early signs of trouble.

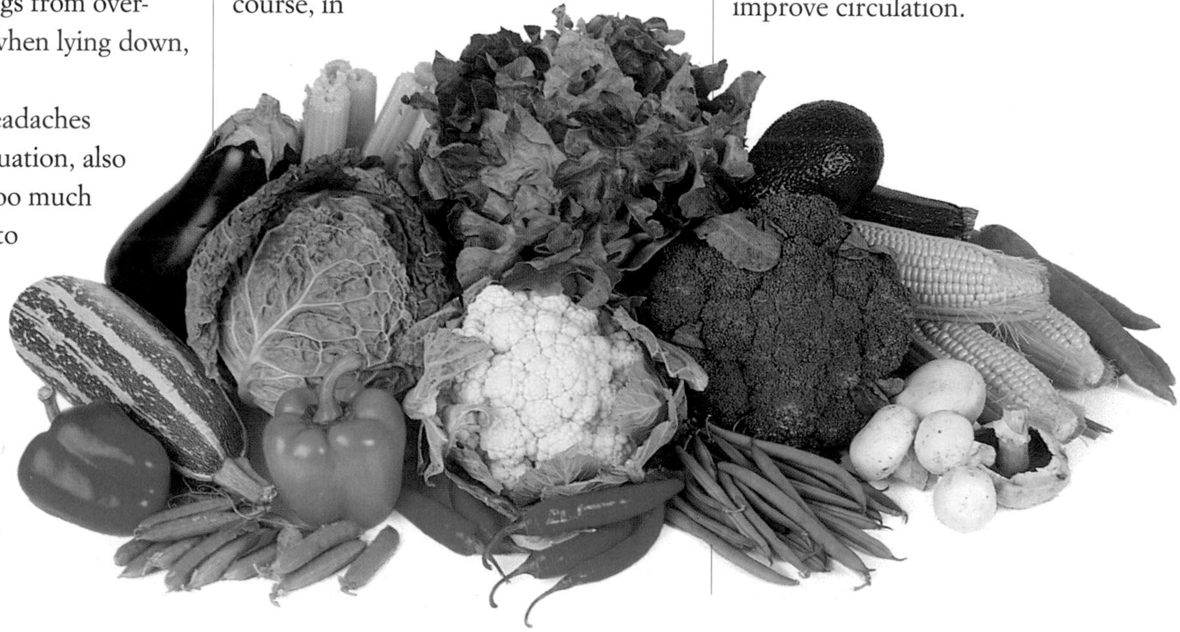

Eating a varied diet of fresh vegetables and wholefoods can ward off many ailments.

INSOMNIA

It is important to distinguish between habitual sleeplessness, repeated night after night, and a temporary problem due perhaps to some worry or anxiety. It is also important not to become obsessed with trying to get a certain amount of sleep; not everyone needs an 8-hour quota – quality is more vital than quantity. People generally need less sleep as they get older, or at least less continuously, so if granny has a day-time snooze and sleeps for less time at night, that is perfectly normal.

AROMATHERAPY

Essential oils are a very pleasant and effective means of unwinding and aiding restful sleep – try using them in the bath (see page 8) – or else putting 2-3 drops on to a paper tissue under the pillow at night. Choose from the following, either using a single oil or a blend; do not use the same oil for more than 2 weeks or you will find it becomes less effective.

CHAMOMILE: calming and relaxing in its effects, it is good where indigestion contributes to broken sleep.

CLARY SAGE: this has a sedating and almost euphoric action, *but* do not use if you have had alcohol as you can quickly get drunk, and have nightmares or a hangover feeling later on.

LAVENDER: not only very soothing, but also analgesic, so if any aches or pains contribute to insomnia, this oil is probably the best remedy.

MARJORAM: relaxing and warming, in large amounts it is quite sedating but can leave you feeling a bit thick-headed the next morning, so do not overdo it.

HERBALISM

An infusion (see page 12) of one or more of these relaxing herbs can help a return to a natural sleep pattern if stress has disturbed it. Other ways of using herbs include herb-filled pillows; traditionally hops were used as they are sedating (but not very pleasant smelling!). Fill a small muslin bag loosely with the appropriate herb and place under your normal pillow. Another old favourite remedy was cowslip wine; this not only tastes better than the infusion but is certainly very relaxing.

CHAMOMILE: *(Chamomilla recutita)*: calms the stomach and the brain, settling the digestion and helping sleep.

HYSSOP *(Hyssopus officinalis)*: a gentle relaxant; also helps to ease nasal congestion and colds, which can cause insomnia.

LEMON BALM *(Melissa officinalis)*: this helps to restore balance to the nervous system, and can be used safely on children. The fresh herb tastes much nicer, and can be drunk as a tea anytime.

LIME BLOSSOM *(Tilia europaea)*: mildly analgesic as well as calming; can soothe headache or other pains.

PASSIONFLOWER *(Passiflora incarnata)*: a strong relaxant or sedative, but without any ill-effects. Many commercial herbal tablets for insomnia contain this herb.

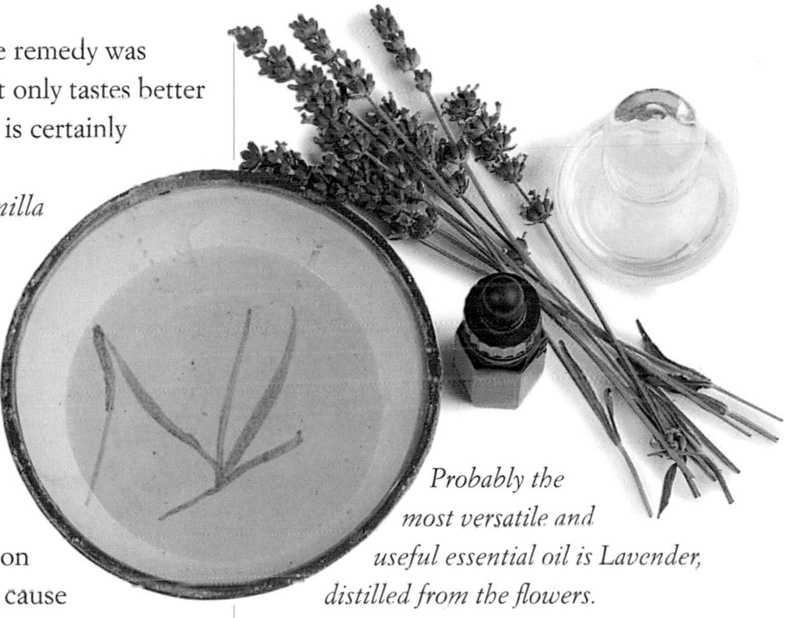

Probably the most versatile and useful essential oil is Lavender, distilled from the flowers.

HOMEOPATHY

In the short term, look at these remedies:

ACONITE: for restlessness associated with sudden upset or fear, and resulting in tossing and turning in bed.

COFFEA: if the mind is completely awake and the brain will not turn off – just as if you had drunk strong coffee.

NUX VOMICA: for insomnia due to overwork or excess food or alcohol, waking around 3 or 4 a.m. for several hours, with disturbed dreams.

SULPHUR: for over-excitement, with the mind full of ideas, and easily awakened by the slightest noise.

NATUROPATHY

In order to get the proper rhythm of energy through the day, it is useful to get plenty of exercise and get fresh air in the daytime. It may help to get up fairly early in the morning as well, to restore this balance. Do not sleep in a stuffy room, or drink coffee, tea or cola at night.

At bedtime, a calcium/magnesium supplement such as dolomite tablets can help to relax, especially if taken with a warm herb tea, or perhaps a hot milky drink if you do not suffer from a lot of catarrh.

MIGRAINE

Anyone who has experienced a migraine will know that it is more than a severe headache. Migraines generally involve acute pains, often over one eye, and perhaps disturbed vision or flashing lights. There may also be nausea or vomiting, and sensitivity to bright light.

AROMATHERAPY

Since the sense of smell is altered and often heightened during a migraine, aromatherapy is definitely best used between attacks; use at the earliest stage of a migraine only if the smell is well tolerated.

A central feature of the natural approach to migraines is to distinguish between a "hot" migraine, where the blood vessels are dilated, and a "cold" migraine, where there is excessive constriction of the blood vessels. In the first type, a cold or perhaps just cool compress (see page 15) across the forehead will give relief and oils of Peppermint or Lavender can be used. For "cold" types of migraine, a hot compress on the forehead or back of the neck may help, using Marjoram.

HERBALISM

Catching the migraine early gives the best chance of success (otherwise try to use these infusions regularly, as a preventive). Choose from the following:

CHAMOMILE *(Chamomilla recutita)*: for dull, throbbing headache with a feeling of queasiness – add a little Ginger *(Zingiber officinalis)* to relieve more severe nausea.

FEVERFEW *(Chrysanthemum parthenium)*: an excellent remedy taken daily to prevent the "cold" type of migraine, where there is a sense of a tight band around the head. This is widely available in tablet form as well.

ROSEMARY *(Rosmarinus officinalis)*: good where stress is a trigger for migraines, and where local warmth gives relief.

NECK MASSAGE FOR MIGRAINE

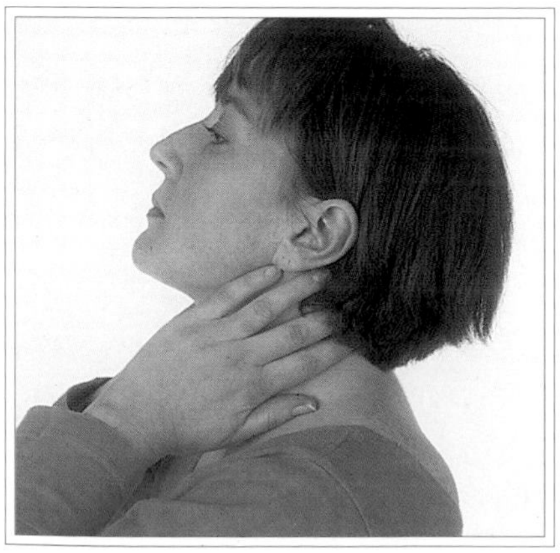

1 For stiff, aching neck muscles massage the neck with firm circular movements. Try to keep the arms relaxed.

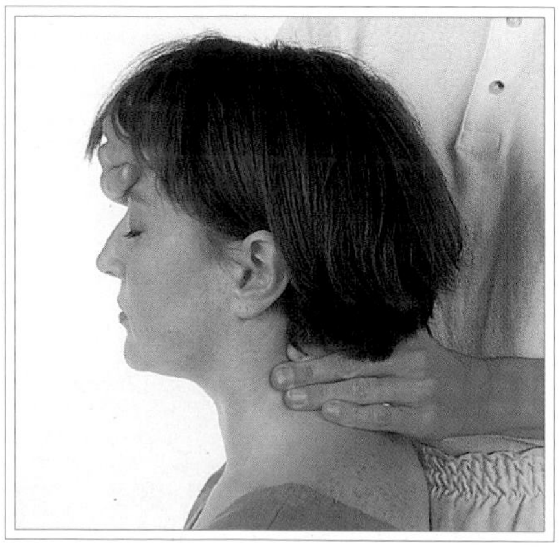

2 Ideally get someone else to massage the neck for you. They can also support your head while they massage.

CAUSES OF MIGRAINE

A migraine can be triggered by all sorts of factors: hormone changes, stress, stuffy atmospheres, noises, smells and certain foods are well-known triggers. Repeated attacks call for professional help; self-help treatments should be largely used as preventive measures.

HOMEOPATHY

During an attack try one of these:

KALI BICH: for an intense headache, preceded by a loss of vision and nausea, made worse in hot weather.

NATRUM MURIATICUM: for a severe, pounding headache with zigzags in front of the eyes, nausea and a pale face. The migraine may also be triggered by menstruation.

SILICA: for pains spreading from the back of the neck over to the eyes, usually right-sided, and often vomiting.

NATUROPATHY

Diet needs to be looked at carefully; try to avoid tea, coffee, alcohol especially red wine, red meat, cheese, chocolate, tomatoes and eggs. Eat plenty of fresh, raw salads and drink lots of fluid, as dehydration can be a factor. Try taking a Vitamin B supplement daily and see if this helps to reduce attacks. In between attacks, exercises to relieve tension in the neck and shoulders can be useful, and also massage of these areas (see left).

NEURALGIA

Neuralgia is a sharp pain originating along the course of one or more nerves, and may come about from a variety of causes; both sciatica and shingles (see pages 26 and 27) give rise to forms of neuralgic pain. Facial neuralgia, affecting one of the trigeminal nerves in the face, can give intense pain, and may relate to stress, migraines or dental problems.

AROMATHERAPY

Using warm compresses (see page 15), including analgesic oils, over the affected areas can give much relief. Choose from Chamomile, Lavender, Marjoram or Rosemary oils – alternate the oil used for recurrent pains, or blend them together for greater effect.

HERBALISM

An infusion (see page 12) of Lavender *(Lavandula vera)* flowers, Lime Blossom *(Tilia europaea)* and Rosemary *(Rosmarinus officinalis)* leaves can be very helpful, not only to ease the pains but to ease tension and tone the nervous system. This mixture can also be used as a warm compress directly over the area.

Two other helpful herbs as infusions are:

ST JOHN'S WORT *(Hypericum perforatum)*: anti-inflammatory and a nervous restorative. The blood-red oil made by infusing the flowers in pure vegetable oil (see page 13) is an excellent local analgesic and healer.

VERVAIN *(Verbena officinalis)*: a relaxant and nervous tonic, very helpful when neuralgia is related to being generally run-down and exhausted.

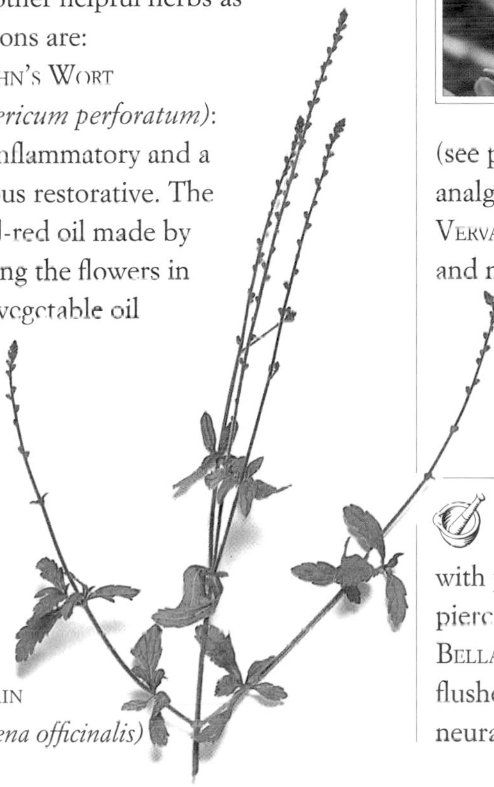

VERVAIN *(Verbena officinalis)*

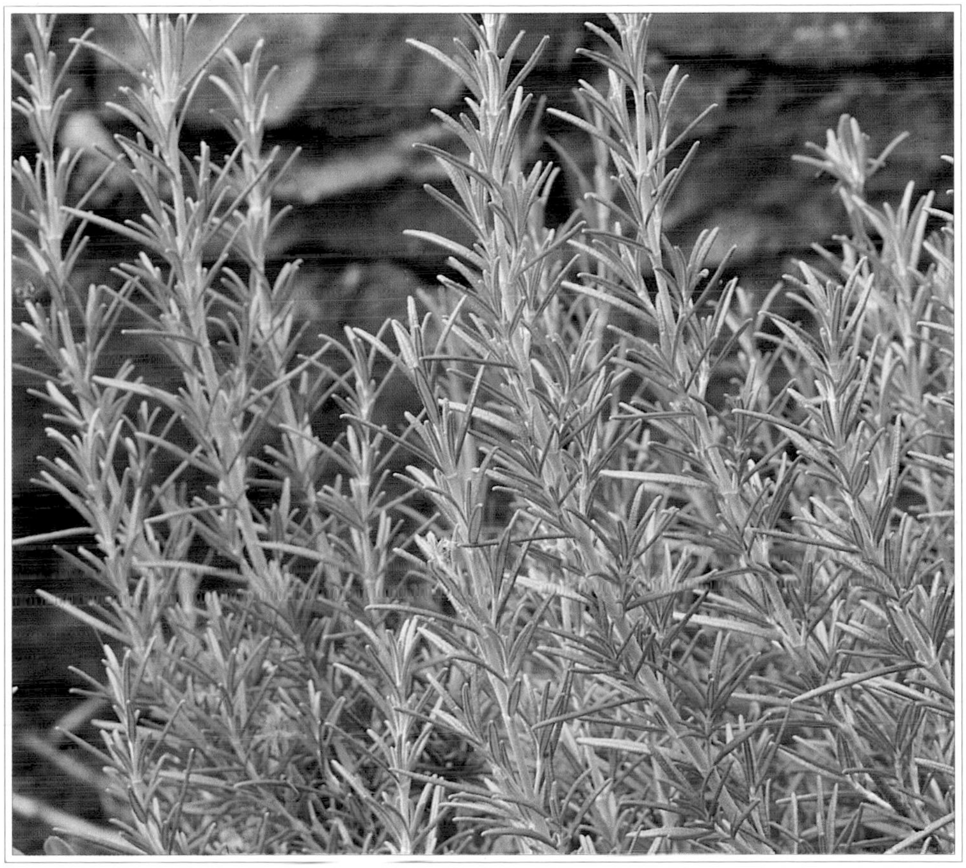

ROSEMARY *(Rosmarinus officinalis)*

HOMEOPATHY

In the short term, try the following:

ACTAEA RAC: for facial neuralgia with pains into the cheekbone and as if piercing the eyeball. Pains ease at night.

BELLADONNA: for a hot, burning and flushed face, with mostly right-sided neuralgic pains and twitching muscles.

GELSEMIUM: for pains radiating from the neck into the face, possibly with some nausea; migraine-related neuralgia.

NATUROPATHY

Simply using alternating hot and cold compresses, 3-4 minutes hot and a maximum 1 minute cold, repeated a few times, can ease the pains. For chronic sufferers a Vitamin B complex supplement can help to nourish the nervous system. In addition, look at ways of reducing stress such as relaxation or yoga classes.

SCIATICA

Pains along some point of the sciatic nerves, running from the low back down either leg to the foot, are a common form of neuralgia (see page 25). The pains may come about from an injury, and treatment from an osteopath or chiropractor should always be considered as one of the best ways to correct the cause. Poor posture, badly designed chairs or even a full back pocket can all cause pressure and pain in the sciatic nerve.

AROMATHERAPY

Initially, use cold compresses (see page 15) with either Chamomile or Lavender oils included. When the pains are less acute, or in longer-lasting sciatic discomfort, try warm compresses as suggested for Neuralgia (see page 25).

These oils are very helpful, diluted 2 per cent in a base oil and slowly massaged into the affected area.

HERBALISM

Chamomile *(Chamomilla recutita)* or Lavender *(Lavandula vera)* are also two useful herbs to take in infusion (see page 12) to ease muscle spasm and inflammation which add to the pains. For acute muscle spasms in the thigh or legs, try making a strong decoction (see page 12) of Cramp Bark (European Cranberry Bush) *(Viburnum opulus)* and using as a warm compress. A small cupful of this may be taken internally as a powerful relaxant.

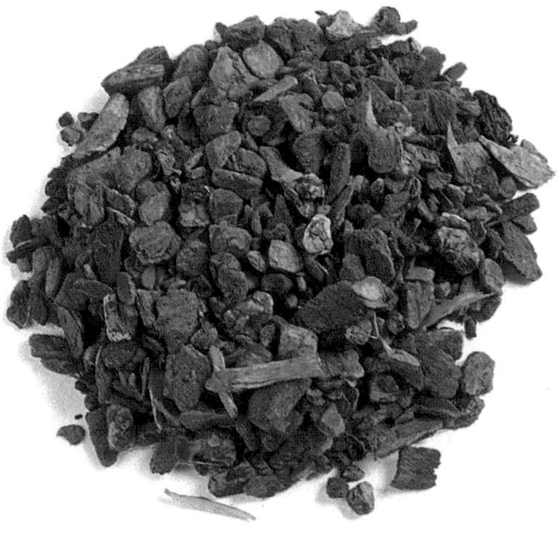

CRAMP BARK (EUROPEAN CRANBERRY BUSH)
(Viburnum opulus)

IMPROVING YOUR POSTURE

Apart from the suggestions listed on this page, you may want to consider help with improving your posture, learning how to move and hold yourself comfortably. The Alexander Technique and the Feldenkrais Technique are two systems that can help here; there are many qualified teachers of both available. Massage is not generally suitable in an acute phase, but in the longer term it is very helpful (see below for self-massage, or find a good massage therapist for best results).

HOMEOPATHY

ARSEN ALB: for intermittent pains shooting from the thigh down to the knee or even ankle.
IGNATIA: for sharp pains in the lower back and upper thighs, eased by walking around.
RHUS TOX: for severe pains in the hip, radiating down to the knee and causing limping. Generally these pains are worse in damp weather.

NATUROPATHY

Hot and cold compresses, as described for Neuralgia (see page 25), may give relief. Gentle exercise is generally useful, but stop if it becomes too painful. Take a serious look at your posture, how you bend, pick things up and so on. It is important to try to keep your back fairly upright, using your legs to bend or to take the weight.

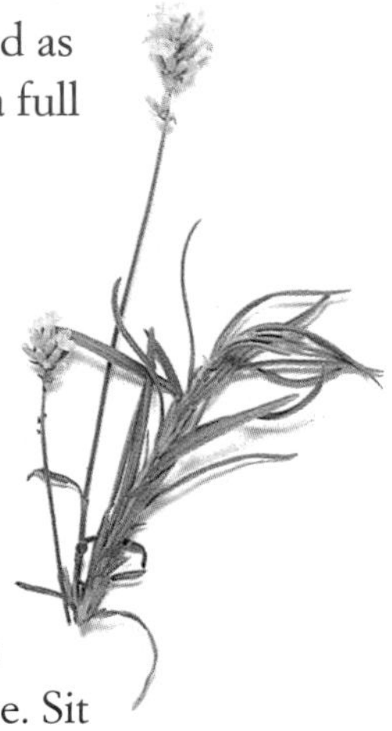

LAVENDER
(Lavandula 'Nana')

Look carefully at all the chairs you use. Sit well back on a chair, and use cushions if necessary to get you into a more comfortable position. In general, avoid staying in one position for too long, as the muscles begin to tighten and stiffen. For example, try to have regular breaks on a long car journey, or walk about for a while on the train.

To help ease sciatic pain, massage diluted essential oils, as recommended, into the buttock and upper thigh with slow circular movements.

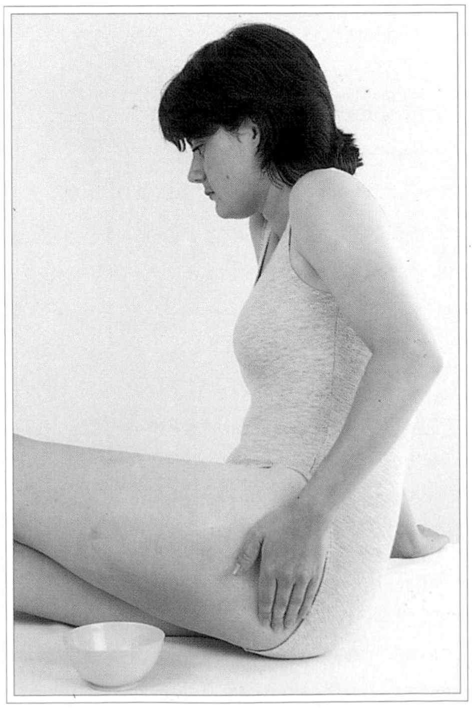

SHINGLES

This condition is brought about by the same virus, *Herpes zoster*, that causes chickenpox; it can lie dormant in the body for years before triggering an attack, often when you are stressed and exhausted. There is usually some pain in the affected area for a day or so before the very painful blisters appear along the pathway of the affected nerves. Sometimes there is considerable pain around the site for weeks, months or even years after the blisters have gone, and this can be treated in the same way as Neuralgia (see page 25).

AROMATHERAPY

A number of essential oils can act locally very powerfully to reduce the pains, dry up the blisters and as direct anti-viral agents. It may be best to use a combination of two or three of these oils; for small areas of blisters paint the oils on neat, once or twice daily, otherwise use them in the bath or diluted in water as a warm compress (see page 15).

Initially, choose from Bergamot, Eucalyptus or Tea Tree oils; if pains persist, use Lavender for its healing and analgesic properties – good combinations are Bergamot and Tea Tree, Bergamot and Lavender, but all the above are useful.

HERBALISM

Lavender oil *(Lavandula vera)*, as described above, is excellent for local use; this can be backed up by taking Lavender flowers as an infusion (see page 12) for their relaxing effect. If there are long-standing pains, after the acute attack has gone (known as post-herpetic syndrome), then a general nerve tonic like Oatstraw *(Avena sativa)* is very helpful – either take 20 drops of the tincture (see page 14) twice daily, or simply include plenty of oats in the diet, for instance as porridge. If depression has set in, an infusion of Rosemary *(Rosmarinus officinalis)* works wonders; drink a cupful in the morning. At the other end of the day, a cup of Lime Blossom *(Tilia europaea)* tea in the evening can help restful sleep.

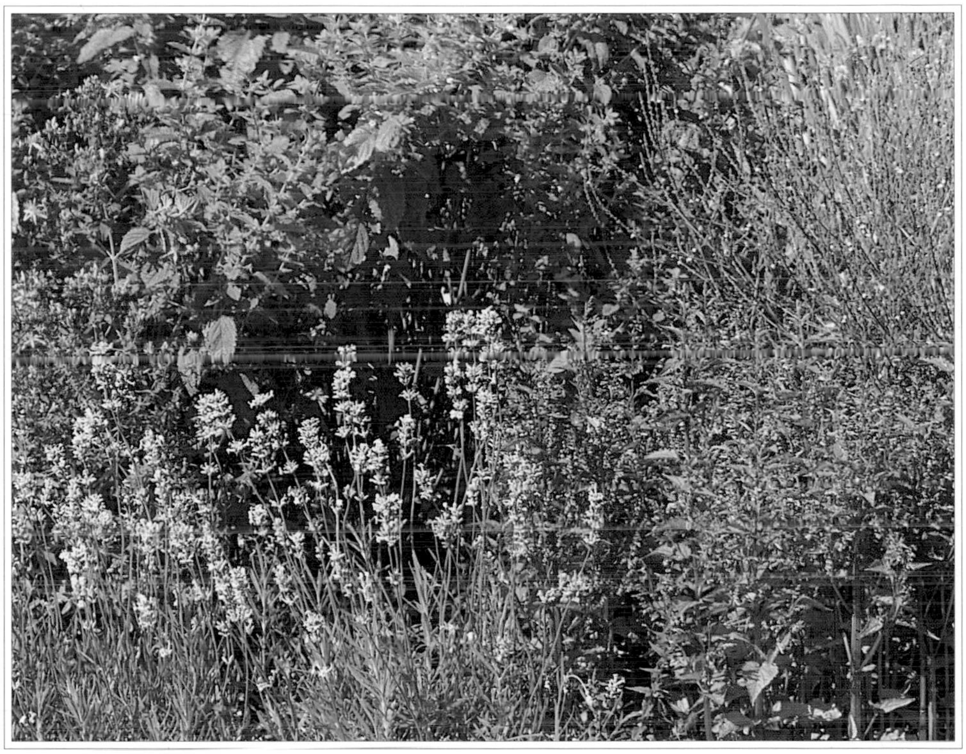

LAVENDER *(Lavandula vera)*

HOMEOPATHY

Some possibilities are:

APIS MEL: where there is a large amount of blistering, with swelling and a burning sensation. Symptoms are eased by cold applications.

ARSEN ALB: for reddened skin, with the blisters merging together and possibly discharging. Symptoms eased by warm applications.

RHUS TOX: for highly inflamed skin, with small white blisters that are intensely painful and itchy; difficult to keep still due to the irritation and discomfort.

NATUROPATHY

In preventive terms, it is advisable to try to steer clear of someone with chickenpox, especially if you are feeling very run-down yourself. Since in real life you may be the one looking after your child with chickenpox, this is not so easy! Spraying the sick room with essential oils (see Aromatherapy above for choice), using 10-15 drops in a 600 ml (1 pt/2½ cups) plant spray filled with water, can help too.

If you feel the first signs of irritation, try rubbing the area with a freshly cut lemon. During an attack of shingles a salt bath may give relief and promote healing and drying of the blisters. Take a Vitamin B complex supplement to nourish the nervous system, and look generally at reducing stress and maintaining a healthy lifestyle.

STRESS

Stress is one of those rather vague terms that is very difficult to define. It is also important to say that stress is not in itself harmful, and a certain amount can be necessary to get us motivated and enjoying life; only when the amount of stress is too much for our systems to cope with does it become a problem. People have a marvellous capacity to adapt to and cope with various sources of stress, but when they get overloaded and nervous or adrenal exhaustion sets in, they can become seriously ill.

AROMATHERAPY

Many oils are of value in helping to reduce the impact of stress. The best way of using them is probably diluted in a vegetable oil and used in massage (see page 17), but if you do not have a willing, and trained, partner then use them in the bath (see page 8).

For more uplifting effects choose from Bergamot, Clary Sage, Geranium or Rosemary, while Lavender or Marjoram are more relaxing. Three luxurious, although expensive, oils which have excellent de-stressing properties (and smell wonderful!) are Jasmine, Neroli (or Orange Blossom) and Rose – use sparingly as they are very concentrated. Jasmine is relaxing and almost euphoric, Neroli is an anti-depressant and is refreshing, and Rose is calming and relaxing.

HERBALISM

For the more agitated aspects of being stressed, choose relaxing infusions such as Lavender *(Lavandula vera)*, Lime Blossom *(Tilia europaea)* or Lemon Balm *(Melissa officinalis)*, or for acute tensions try Valerian *(Valeriana officinalis)* – since this tastes disgusting, it may be better to buy it in tablet form. When exhaustion has set in, infusions of Rosemary *(Rosmarinus officinalis)*, Vervain *(Verbena officinalis)* or Betony *(Stachys betonica)*, or a mixture of all three, will act as a tonic. Oats are helpful to add to the diet, as a nourishment for the nervous system.

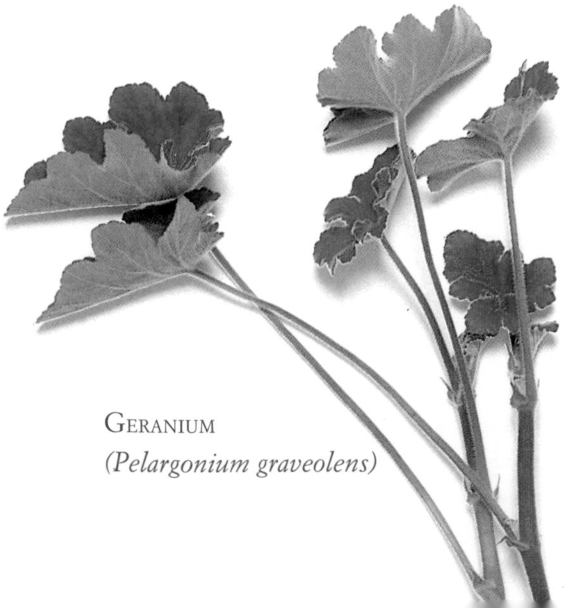

GERANIUM
(Pelargonium graveolens)

HOMEOPATHY

ACONITE: for acute anxiety and mental confusion, with thoughts whizzing round in the head and much restlessness.

CHAMOMILLA: if everything and everybody seems to irritate, and it is

SYMPTOMS OF STRESS

Symptoms of stress vary, see also Anxiety and Depression (pages 19 and 20), but if you experience some or all of the following, you may be over-stressed:

- Constantly on edge, with a very short fuse and ready to explode for no real reason.
- Feeling on the verge of tears much of the time.
- Difficulty in concentrating, decision-making or with memory.
- Always tired even after a full night's sleep.
- Sleep itself is disturbed and unrefreshing.
- A feeling of not being able to cope, it's all too much.
- Poor appetite, or else nibbling without hunger.
- No sense of fun or enjoyment in life.
- Mistrustful of everybody, unable to enjoy company.
- Inability to relax or unwind even if not working.
- Problems in relationships, no interest in sex.
- Always fidgeting or having a nervous habit such as biting your nails or chewing your hair.

The first step to improving the situation is to recognize that you are stressed, and to know what your limits are. Taking active steps to reduce the amount of external stress will of course be helpful, as well as looking at the methods below for easing the effects of the stress on your system. Other steps might include trying a class in relaxation techniques, or yoga, T'ai Ch'i and so on, or having professional massage treatments. Getting regular breaks from a stressful lifestyle will help you to cope better and avoid the situation reaching a crisis point.

Massage for Stiff Necks

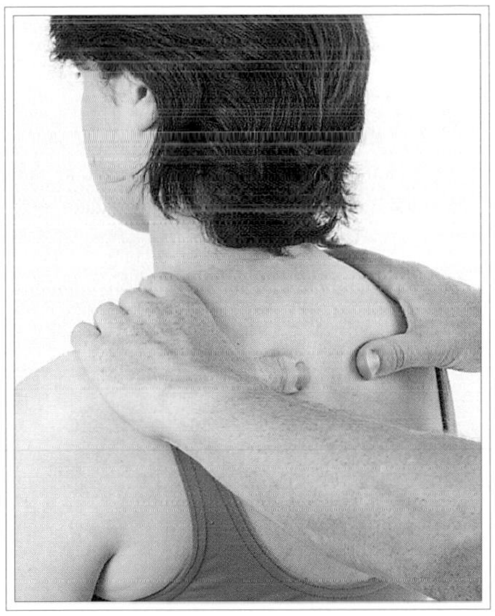

1 Place hands on each shoulder, thumbs on either side of the spine.

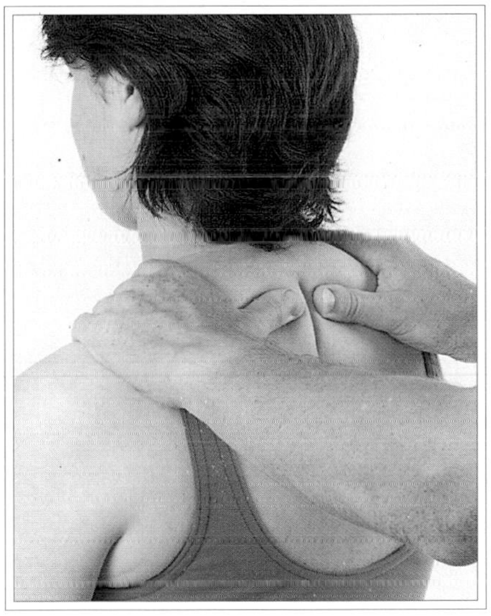

2 Rotate thumbs firmly, lifting and squeezing the shoulder muscles. Relax hands and repeat.

Back Massage to Ease Stress

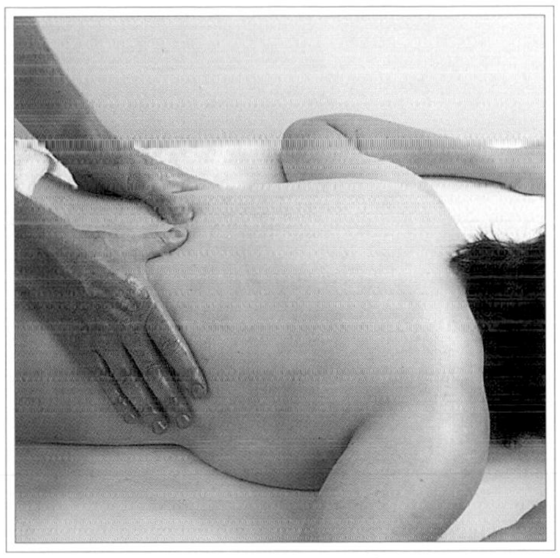

1 To relieve stress and tension, use effleurage, or stroking, on the back. Oil the back and then place hands on lower back with thumbs on either side of the spine.

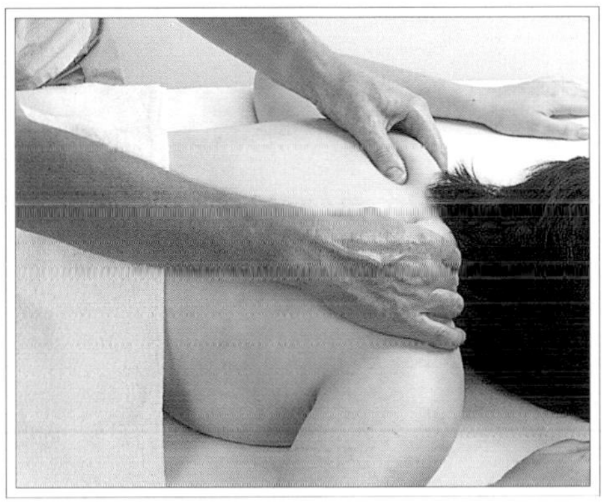

2 Steadily stroke up the back, allow thumbs to move out at the shoulders to join the fingers, and stroke down the side of the back. Bring thumbs to either side of the spine and repeat several times in a slow, relaxing rhythm. Keep the pressure firm, but not too hard.

Neck and Shoulder Exercises

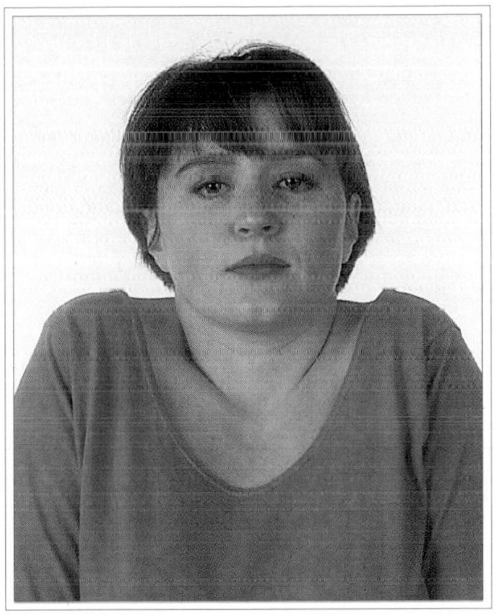

1 Lift shoulders, pressing into the neck Relax and then repeat a few times.

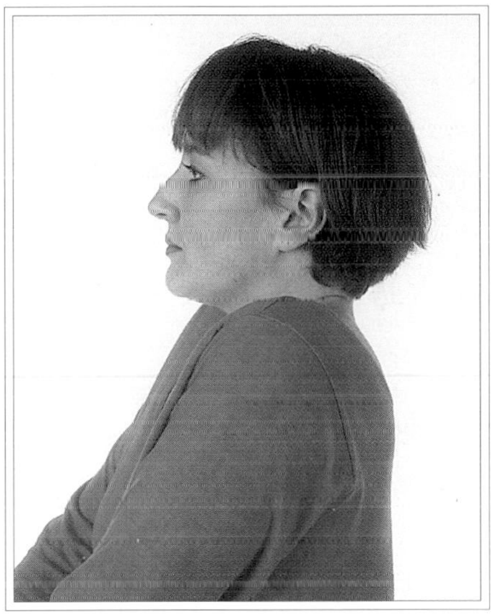

2 Roll the shoulders in a circle. Repeat a few times in a backwards circle, then a few times forwards.

very easy to get into a temper.
IGNATIA: for mood swings, liable to tears and lots of sighing; may bottle things up and get upset suddenly.
KALI PHOS: for prolonged strain, getting fatigued and rather depressed, very jumpy at the least thing. Tends to withdraw from company, doesn't want to go out very much, generally lacks interest in life.

NATUROPATHY

A good plan is to look at basics; overhaul the diet, cutting out all the stimulants such as coffee, tea or cola drinks which only serve to leave you more exhausted when their effects wear off. Also reduce alcohol; it may help you to relax in small amounts but it easily becomes a dangerous habit and has a depressant action in any quantity.

Try to get some exercise; this not only helps to use up excess adrenalin but builds up physical *and* mental stamina. Deeper breathing will also supply more oxygen to the brain, which is the first essential nourishment it needs. It may be useful to add a multi vitamin and mineral supplement to the diet for a while, as the body uses up nutrients faster when under stress.

THE RESPIRATORY SYSTEM

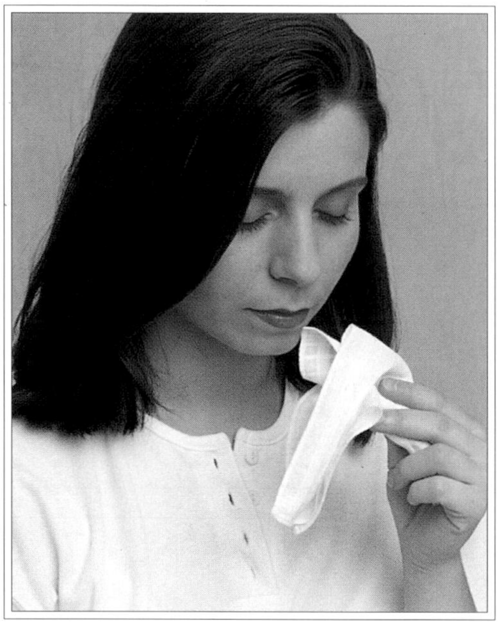

In order to prevent respiratory problems, or to help clear them up more quickly, it is essential to take a wider, holistic view of health. If you live in a relatively mild, damp climate, this will make you more prone to respiratory infections and catarrh; coupled with this, the increase in air pollution this century has added significantly to the burden. However, some internal factors, such as diet, exercise and general health, are also important in affecting our resistance to infections, and the more we pay attention to these internal factors, the healthier we will be.

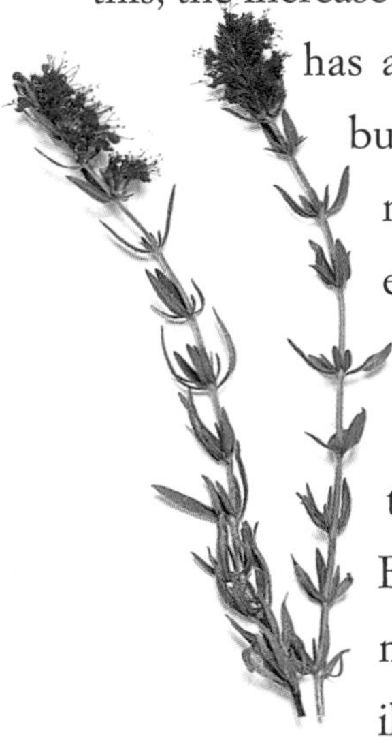

Breathing is one of those bodily functions that normally carry on automatically, but can also be controlled consciously. This is a good illustration of the effect of stress and anxiety on our body, as shallow or over-rapid breathing, nervous coughs and even bronchial spasms can be produced when in an agitated state. Poor posture, lack of exercise or just lack of fresh air, smoking or smoky atmospheres all contribute to an inadequate intake of oxygen and respiratory problems.

Above: The influence of essential oils on our respiratory system can have dramatic effects. Very many essential oils are also extremely pleasing to smell and can help to keep the sinuses clear, for example Lavender (above left)*, Peppermint and Eucalyptus.*

ASTHMA

Asthma is not generally a problem that should simply be tackled at home; it requires professional treatment and attention. Childhood asthma tends to be associated with an allergic response; there may also be hay fever and/or eczema present in the family. In trying to identify the allergens responsible it is often valuable to look further at external factors and also internal ones such as diet, as well as conventional skin testing.

AROMATHERAPY

During an actual attack of asthma, simply sniffing the aroma of a couple of drops of essential oil on a paper tissue may give relief from the spasm of the airways – choose from Lavender, Bergamot, Frankincense or Chamomile. In between attacks, massaging a choice of the above oils, diluted (see page 17), into the chest may help to prevent the spasms and build up of thick mucus which gives the wheezing symptoms.

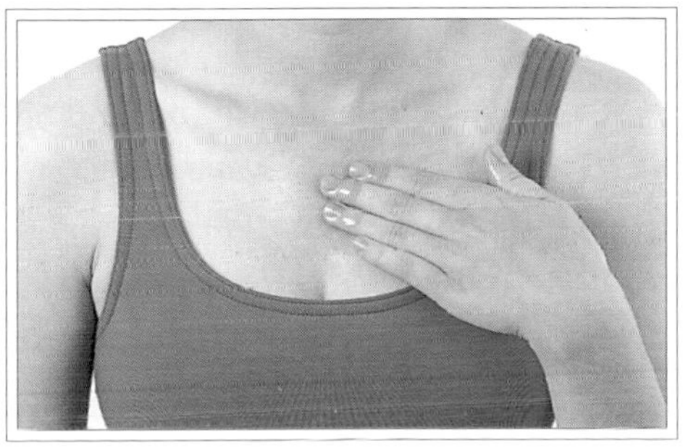

Essential oils, diluted in a base oil as recommended, can be massaged into the chest to relax the airways and ease breathing.

HERBALISM

Professional practitioners may use remedies which directly reduce the allergic response, or dilate the bronchial passageways, depending

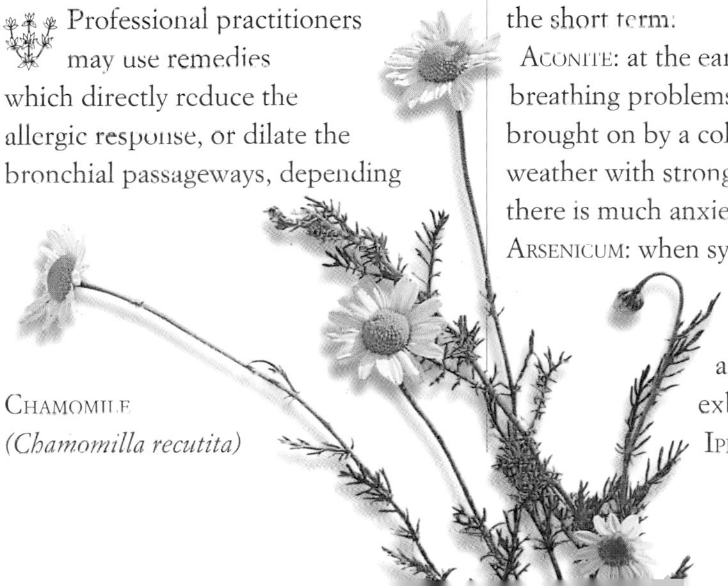

CHAMOMILE *(Chamomilla recutita)*

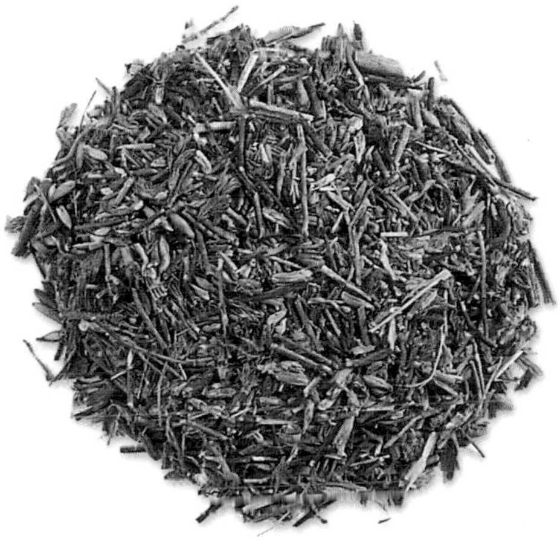

EYEBRIGHT *(Euphrasia officinalis)*

on specific individual needs. In between asthma attacks, taking an infusion (see page 12) of a mixture of Chamomile *(Chamomilla recutita)*, Eyebright *(Euphrasia officinalis)* and Lavender *(Lavandula vera)* may help to relax the airways, tone up the mucous membranes and reduce inflammation and irritability of the bronchi.

HOMEOPATHY

The professional will similarly look to treat each person individually, so only consider the remedies below in the short term.

ACONITE: at the earliest sign of breathing problems, especially if brought on by a cold, or simply cold weather with strong winds, and where there is much anxiety or fear.

ARSENICUM: when symptoms are worse after midnight, with restlessness and a feeling of exhaustion.

IPECACUANHA: where there is wheezing, with a persistent, rattly cough accompanied by a strong feeling of nausea.

NATUROPATHY

For childhood asthma, or where there is a lot of thick mucus, it is well worth trying a change of diet, to exclude cows' milk products for a while, to decrease sugary baking products and sweets (candy), and to increase fresh vegetables and fruit.

Breathing exercises may be of help, especially for later-onset asthma or when exercise seems to aggravate the condition; a simple method of deepening the breathing pattern is to

A useful breathing exercise for asthma is simply to blow up a couple of balloons a day, to deepen the breath and exercise the diaphragm.

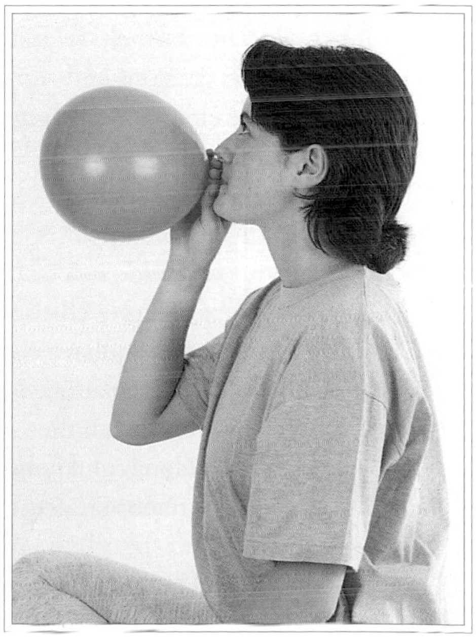

CATARRH

Irritation of the membranes of the nose and throat will encourage production of mucus; where this becomes excessive or prolonged, for example after a cold, then catarrh is the result. When this occurs lower down the airways, bronchial catarrh follows (see Bronchitis, page 33). Nasal catarrh is even more common in damp climates and the same advice is applicable.

AROMATHERAPY

Where there is a lot of nasal congestion, a steam inhalation with essential oils (see page 33) can be instantly effective in giving relief. In the short term Peppermint is excellent, especially combined with Eucalyptus and/or Tea Tree, to loosen thick, sticky mucus and fight any infection present. For longer term catarrhal problems, try using oil of Pine instead of Peppermint, perhaps with Chamomile, Lavender or Tea Tree.

HERBALISM

Apart from using steam inhalations for temporary relief, either with oils as described above or using a handful each of Peppermint *(Mentha piperita)* leaves, Eucalyptus *(Eucalyptus globulus)* leaves and Chamomile *(Chamomilla recutita)* flowers to 1 litre (1¾ pt/4 cups) of boiling water, catarrh can often be very successfully treated with infusions (see page 12) of the following:

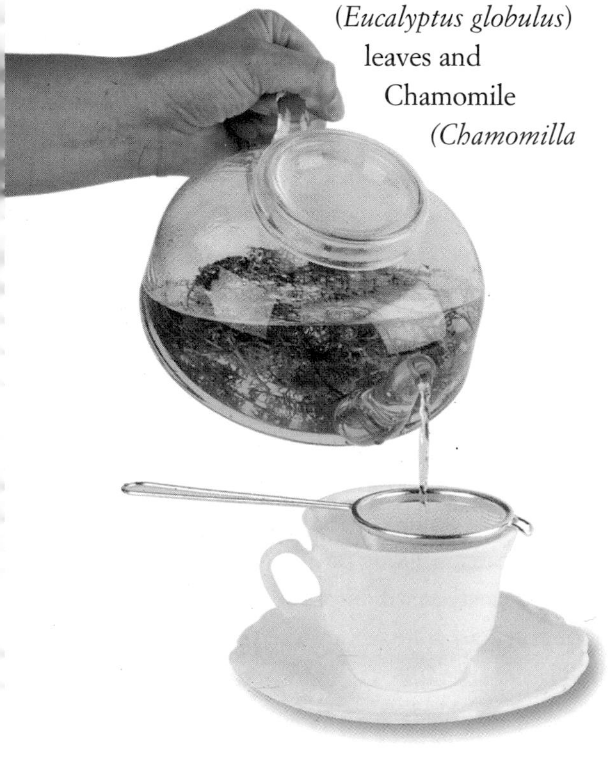

CATMINT *(Nepeta cataria)*: helps to ease nasal congestion and improve the circulation through the nasal passages.
ELDERFLOWER *(Sambucus nigra)*: has an anti-inflammatory effect, reducing swelling of the membranes and easing mucus production.
GOLDEN ROD *(Solidago virgaurea)*: astringent, toning up the membranes and also reducing excess mucus.
HYSSOP *(Hyssopus officinalis)*: loosens up thick phlegm, while calming the breathing; good if there is restlessness and problems with sleeping due to difficulty in breathing.

HOMEOPATHY

Initially think of one of these remedies:
ARSEN ALB: for running, watery catarrh, with a dripping nose.
HYDRASTIS: for a constant post-nasal drip, perhaps associated with blocked Eustachian tubes (connecting to the middle ear), creating a little deafness.
KALI BICH: where there is thick, stringy mucus, which is difficult to shift.
PULSATILLA: in chronic cases, where the catarrh varies at times from clear to a greenish-yellow colour.

Place 25 g (1 oz) dried Chamomile (Chamomilla recutita) *leaves in a teapot and pour on boiling water. Allow to infuse for 5 minutes. Strain and drink a cupful.*

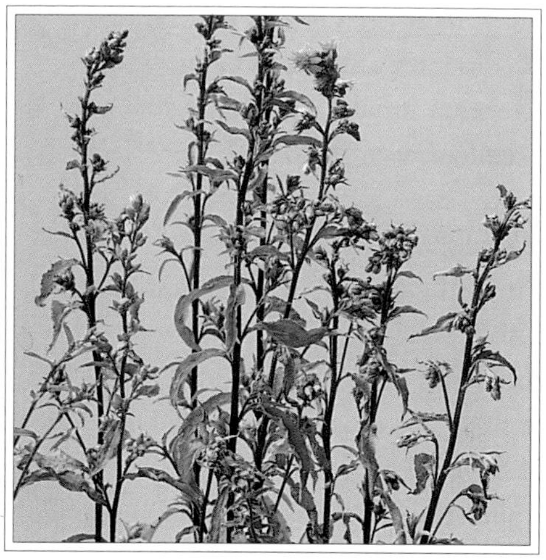

GOLDEN ROD *(Solidago virgaurea)*

NATUROPATHY

Avoid all mucus-forming foods, especially milk and other dairy products, and refined carbohydrates – most breakfasts of cereal and milk fall into this category, as do pastries, cakes and so on. Drinking warm fruit juices can often be helpful. If the catarrh tends to follow on from regular colds, a daily supplement of Vitamin C, up to 500 mg in strength, may need to be taken for a while.

Regular intake of garlic is invaluable in building up resistance to respiratory infections – ideally raw – and since the smell may stop other people coming near you, so colds are harder to catch! Actually, the smelly oil is the most anti-infective part of garlic, and 99 per cent of it is excreted out via the lungs so it works very strongly on the respiratory system. Odourless garlic perles, or capsules, will also work, although not as powerfully as the raw ingredient.

COLDS

Since there are over 200 strains of cold virus, it is not surprising that a cure has not been found. Prevention is better than treatment by far; once a cold has developed, it generally has to run its course. However, treatments can help to relieve symptoms and also stop the cold turning into persistent catarrh or a deeper infection.

AROMATHERAPY

Two methods are most appropriate for using oils to combat cold symptoms and stop complications: steam inhalations (see page 33) and baths. If, in the early stages, the cold is accompanied by a chill, adding 10 drops of Lavender and 5 drops of Cinnamon oil to a warm bath at night will help a lot. More stimulating oils such as Eucalyptus or Tea Tree (10 drops of each) can be used in baths earlier in the day. All the above are valuable in inhalations; a mixture often works better than just one oil.

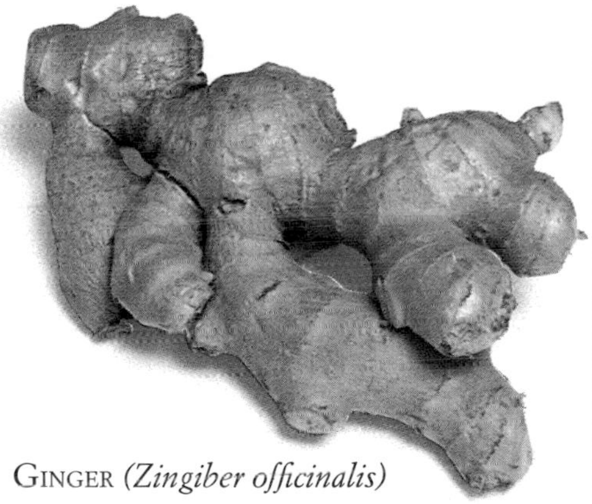

GINGER *(Zingiber officinalis)*

HERBALISM

One of the herbalists' most traditional standbys for colds is still one of the best: use an infusion (see page 12) of equal amounts of Peppermint *(Mentha piperita)*, Elderflower *(Sambucus nigra)* and Yarrow *(Achillea millefolium)*. Taken hot just before going to bed, this will induce a sweat, and if the cold is caught early enough, may stop it altogether. Even if too late for this, it will still be very useful. Other herbs that may be added to the infusion include:

CAYENNE *(Capsicum minimum)*: a favourite North American Indian remedy: use 1.25 ml (¼ tsp) of the powder to really stimulate the circulation.

CINNAMON *(Cinnamomum zeylanicum)*: use a cinnamon stick, and break it into the mixture of herbs, for a gentle, warming and sweat-inducing effect.

GINGER *(Zingiber officinalis)*: grate a small piece of fresh root ginger into the mixture for extra heat.

HOMEOPATHY

ACONITE: for early stages of colds, when starting suddenly, perhaps after exposure to cold winds.

GELSEMIUM: for influenza-like symptoms, feeling chilly and trembling but with a flushed face.

NAT MUR: when there is a lot of sneezing, the nose is sore and inflamed and producing lots of mucus, either watery or like raw egg-white.

Fresh fruit is a natural source of Vitamin C.

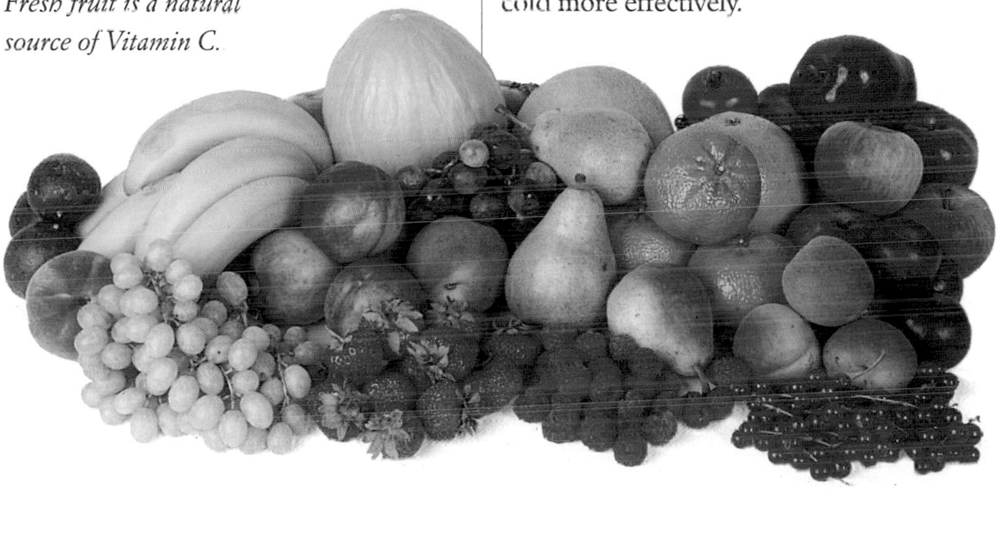

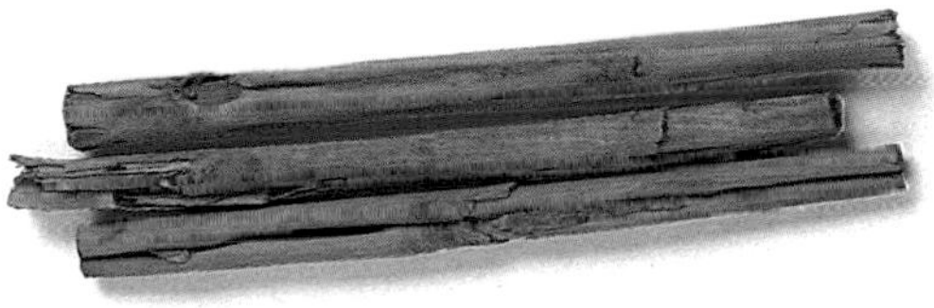

CINNAMON *(Cinnamomum zeylanicum)*

NATUROPATHY

Immediately increase Vitamin C intake; at the earliest stages very high doses of a Vitamin C supplement, up to 2,000 mg, may stop the infection alone, but if left too late, this is not needed and may make the bowels too loose. 500 mg is an ample dose to take regularly until the remaining symptoms clear up. Another useful supplement is sucking zinc lozenges, with up to 20 mg zinc gluconate in them, every 3–4 hours initially (taking *tablets* does not have the same effect).

Eat lots of fresh fruit for natural Vitamin A, B and C, and add plenty of raw garlic to food. Cut out sugary, starchy or milky foods. A short cleansing diet of just fresh fruit and salads, and plenty of liquids such as warm fruit juices or herb teas, will encourage the body to throw off the cold more effectively.

COUGHS

A cough is a natural reflex reaction to any irritation, inflammation or blockage in the airways. It often accompanies an infection such as a cold or bronchitis, but may come about through nervousness, with no direct irritation at all. By keeping the bronchial tubes open and clear, coughing can be of vital importance, and treatment should generally be aimed first at making the cough more effective rather than just suppressing it.

AROMATHERAPY

A useful way to help a cough do its job more effectively is by using oils in a steam inhalation (see page 33); oils can be chosen to soothe the lining of the air passages, fight infection if needed, and loosen mucus to make it easier to be removed.

Soothing oils include Benzoin and Lavender. Many essential oils are antiseptic, especially Thyme and Eucalyptus; to increase expectoration choose Frankincense or Marjoram. In fact all the above oils are helpful for tackling coughs. Choose a blend that you like the smell of – and remember that if the cough does not improve within a few days, seek professional help, especially for children.

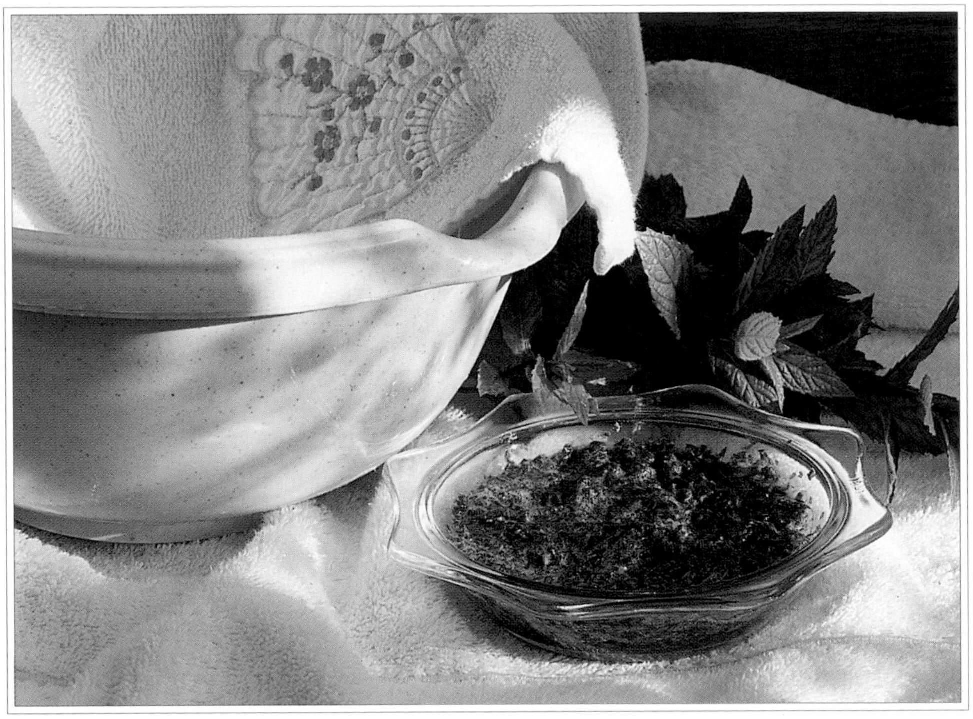

Fresh or dried herbs can be used to make a steam inhalation, to loosen congested mucus and open the airways.

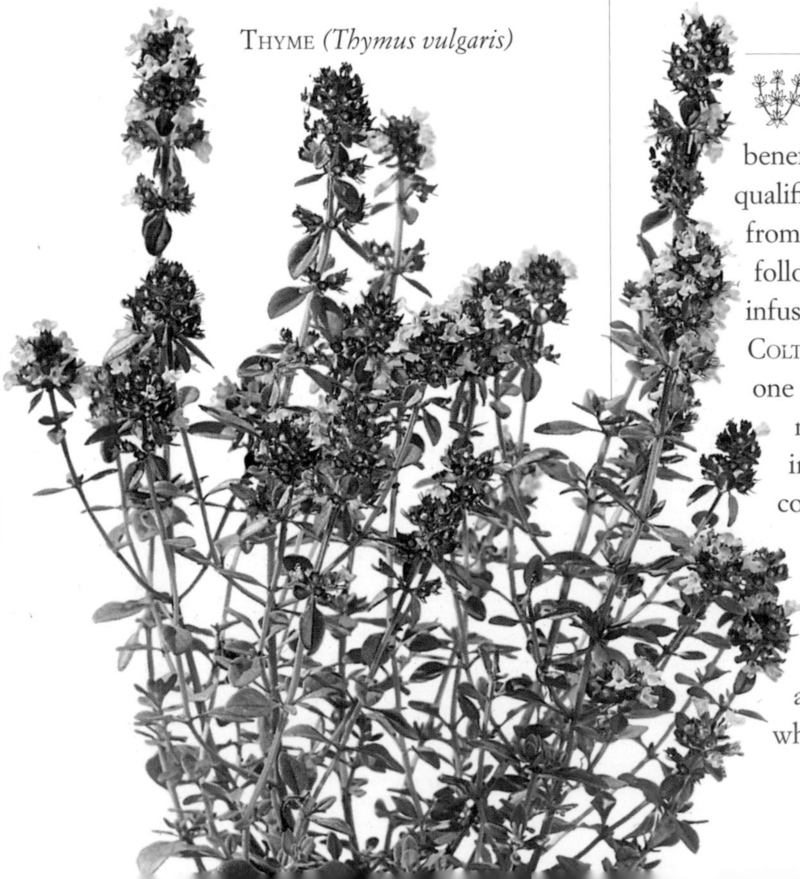

THYME *(Thymus vulgaris)*

HERBALISM

This is an area where herbs are of special benefit; if in doubt get qualified treatment. Choose from one or a mixture of the following, taken as warm infusions (see page 12).

COLTSFOOT *(Tussilago farfara)*: one of the best cough remedies, particularly for irritating, spasmodic coughs. It will soothe, loosen mucus and reduce the spasm.

HYSSOP *(Hyssopus officinalis)*: a calming and relaxing expectorant, when the cough is associated with restlessness and irritation.

MARSHMALLOW *(Althea officinalis)*: a demulcent remedy, which means it is highly soothing to the inflamed tubes. For a harsh, dry and painful cough always include Marshmallow in a mixture, to ease the soreness.

THYME *(Thymus vulgaris)*: powerfully antiseptic, this relieves a dry cough linked with a respiratory infection.

WHITE HOREHOUND *(Marrubium vulgare)*: an expectorant, freeing up thick, sticky mucus and helping it to be removed more effectively.

Types of Cough

It can be useful to divide coughs into two types; when the membranes are hot and dry the cough is painful and non-productive. As mucus is produced, the cough becomes moist, looser and can feel almost choking. The first kind needs soothing, while the latter requires help in removing the excess mucus. Choose the appropriate treatments in each case.

HOMEOPATHY

For short-term treatment of a cough, try a few doses (see page 10) of one of these remedies:

ACONITE: for a dry, short cough which may occur first thing in the morning, or come on after exposure to cold, dry winds.

BRYONIA: for a really spasmodic, dry cough which shakes the whole body and is worse with movement or after eating.

IPECACUANHA: for a moist cough, with some wheezing and a feeling of choking, and often much nausea.

PHOSPHORUS: for a dry, irritating and tickly cough, made worse by changes in temperature.

NATUROPATHY

Initially coughs are often quite dry and painful; taking a little honey from a spoon will help to soothe this. To make the honey much more powerful, try mashing a little chopped raw onion or garlic into it first; it is anti-social but very effective! Cut out all dairy products from the diet, to reduce the catarrh.

Either steam inhalations or a hot compress (see page 15) will encourage expectoration and stimulate the lungs to work better.

Once a cough has been eased, try not to slip back into eating patterns which include a lot of sugar, dairy products, cakes or pastries, as this can lower resistance to infection and help the cough to linger on or even to return in full force.

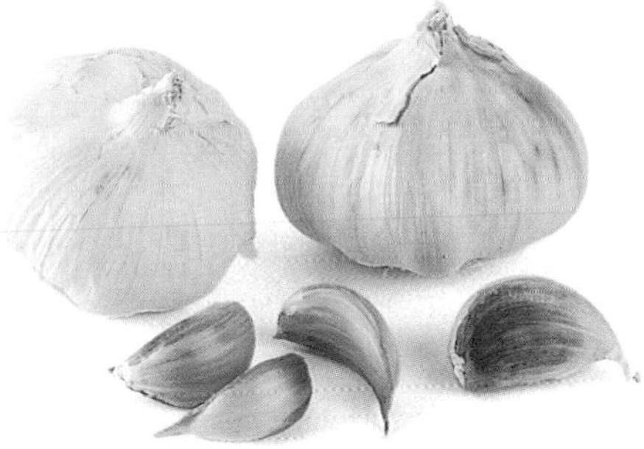

GARLIC *(Allium sativum)*

For children, and for anybody where the cause is unknown, when the cough persists it is important to seek medical advice, as professional help may be needed. Similarly, if the mucus is bright green or yellow this indicates the presence of an infection, and advice should be sought.

Fields of commercially-grown lavender.

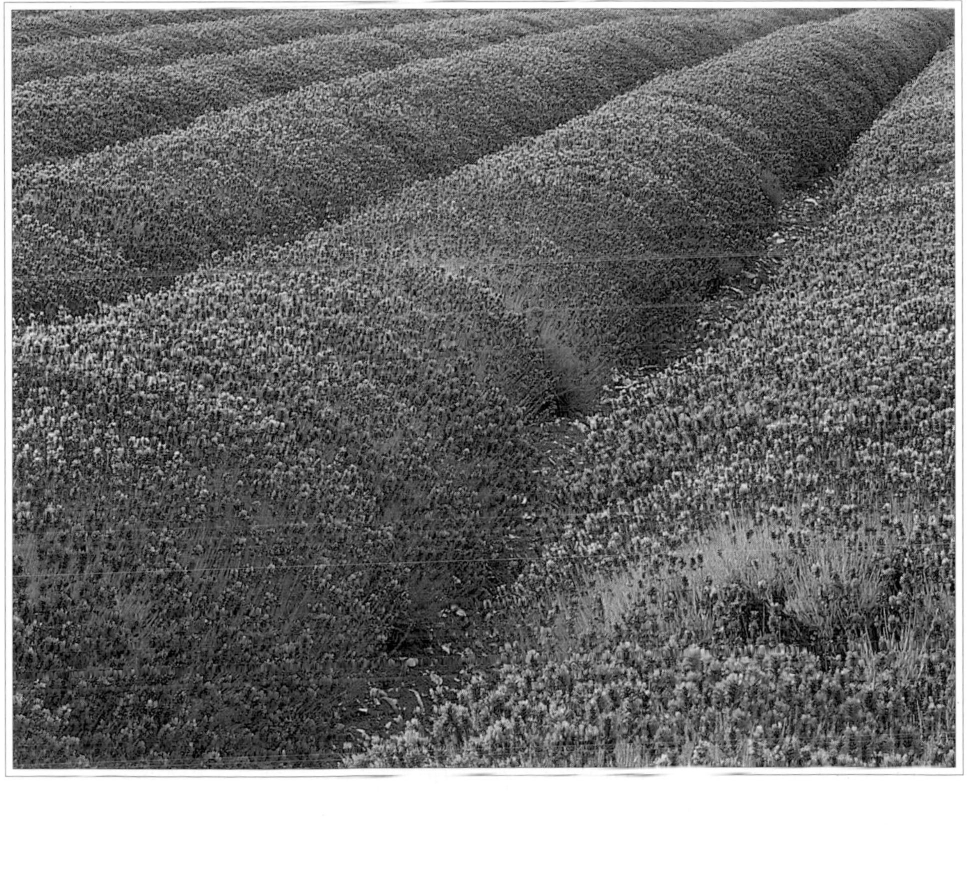

EARACHE

Earaches most often develop through an infection, perhaps following a cold or sinusitis, for instance. Because infections can spread through into the middle or even inner ear, with potentially serious complications, earaches should not be neglected. If an earache is associated with catarrh, this should be treated too. Do *not* put anything into the ear unless it has been examined to ensure that the eardrum is not perforated.

AROMATHERAPY

Use hot compresses (see page 15) over the ear to draw the inflammation outwards, and hopefully help any pus that may be present to come out also. Two very good oils to use are Chamomile and Lavender; a combination of both may be most effective.

HERBALISM

Hot compresses are the most effective home treatment; Chamomile *(Chamomilla recutita)* may be used as an infusion (see page 12) for this purpose too. Taking garlic internally will help to reduce any catarrh and fight infection – if on proper examination the eardrum is not perforated, then a clove of garlic can be crushed into 5 ml (1 tsp) of olive oil; this is warmed to blood temperature and a few drops gently inserted into the ear for an excellent local antibiotic.

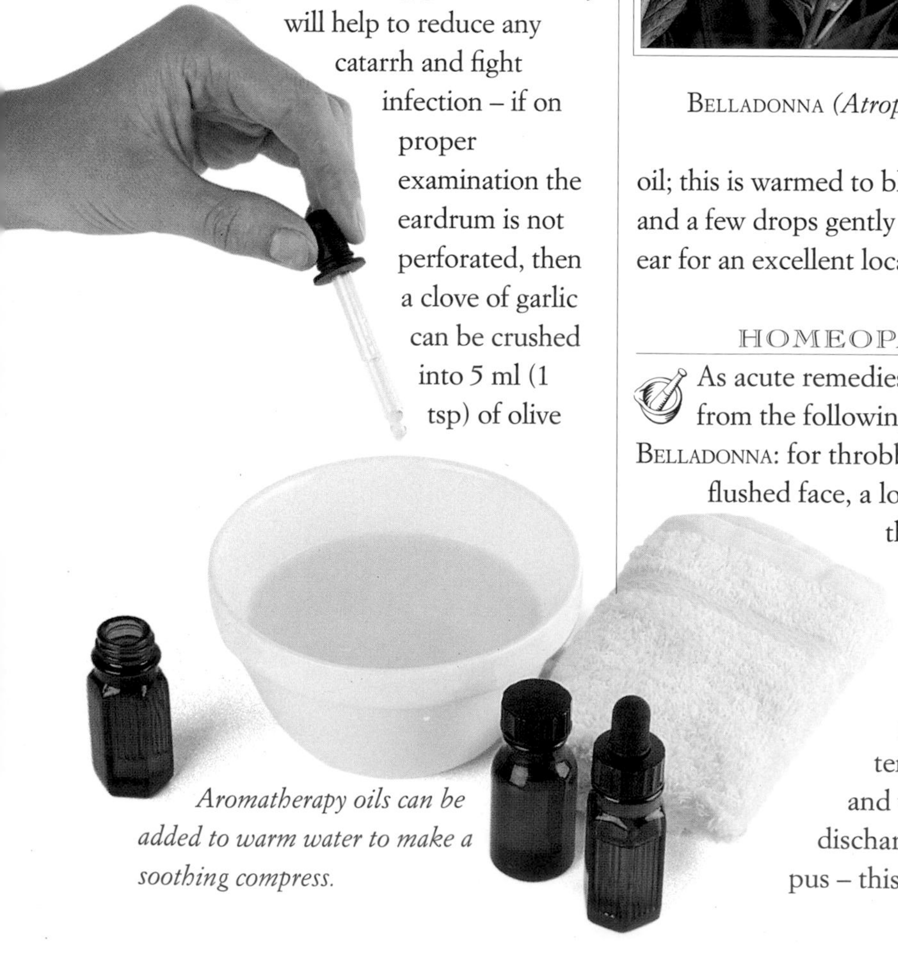

Aromatherapy oils can be added to warm water to make a soothing compress.

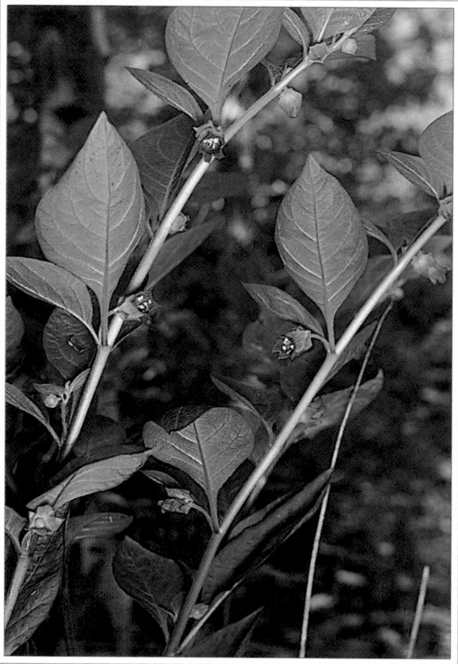

BELLADONNA *(Atropa belladonna)*

HOMEOPATHY

As acute remedies only, choose from the following:
BELLADONNA: for throbbing pains, with a flushed face, a lot of heat around the ear and perhaps a high temperature.
HEPAR SULPH: for a very painful ear, very tender to touch, and which may be discharging offensive pus – this situation requires medical attention quite quickly so do not let it go on unchecked.
PULSATILLA: if there is a lot of thick, green catarrh present, and the earache and congestion is worse in hot rooms or stuffy atmospheres.

EARACHE IN CHILDREN

Earaches, especially in children, need to be treated quickly as an infection within the middle ear can be both painful and damaging. Speedy home help can be very useful to avoid these problems, but get medical help if earache worsens or persists.

NATUROPATHY

Apart from all the local treatments by compress suggested above, follow the advice given for Catarrh (see page 34), especially if there is a pattern of recurring earaches, as prevention should be the primary aim.

CHAMOMILE *(Chamomilla recutita)*

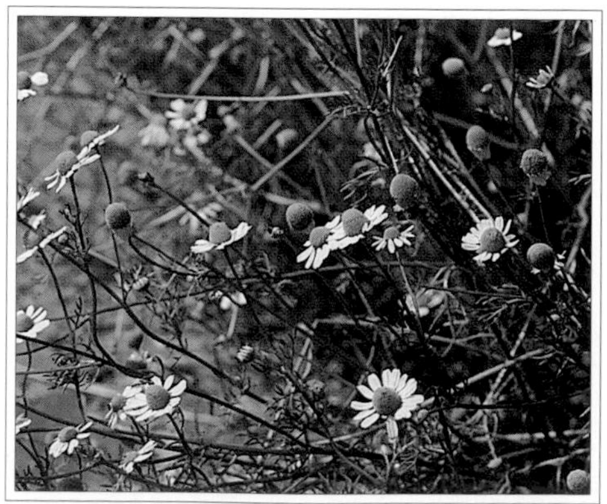

HAY FEVER

Hay fever is an allergic reaction, which can be triggered not just by grass pollens but in some people by various flower or tree pollens too. It is often seen together with other allergic reactions such as asthma and/or eczema, and if it is not relieved by the suggested self-help approaches, then seek qualified treatment. Practitioners may well start to act preventively before the hay fever season.

AROMATHERAPY

Simply sniffing a drop or two of an essential oil may be the best method; steam inhalations (see page 33) can be used but might be too hot for some people. You may well need to vary the oils used through the hay fever season, as they can become less effective if used for too long. Choose from Chamomile, Tea Tree, Pine, Melissa or Eucalyptus.

HERBALISM

Two herbs are very helpful in reducing the symptoms of hay fever: Chamomile *(Chamomilla recutita)* and Eyebright *(Euphrasia officinalis).*

Make an infusion of Chamomile (Chamomilla recutita), *when cool soak a couple of cotton pads and place on the eyes. Rest for 10 minutes with the pads in place.*

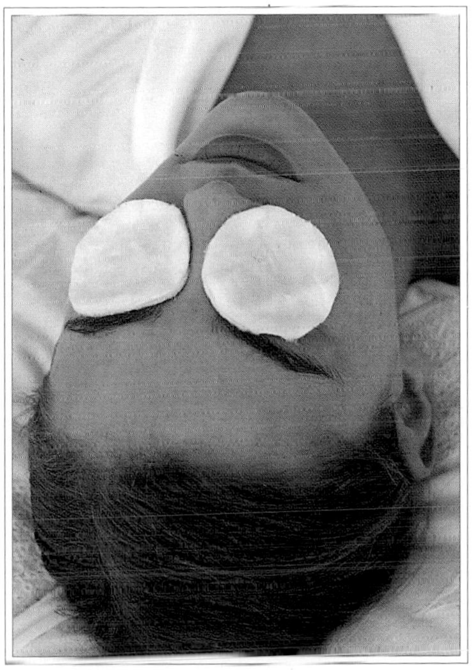

Hayfever Symptoms

The membranes lining the nose are most often affected, with either congestion or else a streaming nose and sneezing; frequently the eyes or throat become inflamed too. An all-year-round allergic reaction, or allergic rhinitis, can be set up, with symptoms triggered by mould spores, house dust, fur and car exhaust fumes, for instance.

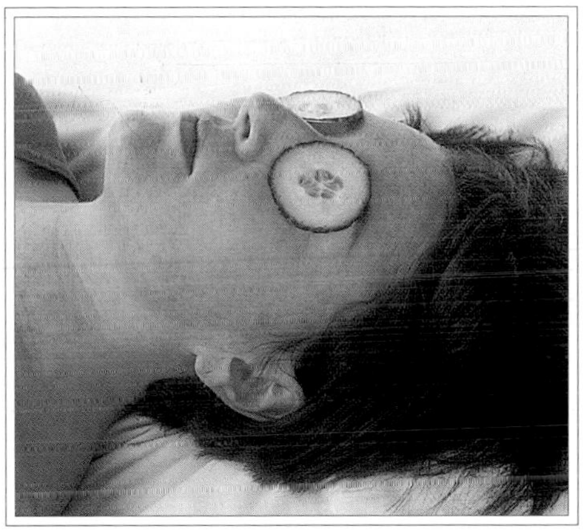

Slices of cucumber may be used on tired, sore eyes in the same way as herb pads.

They can both be used in two ways: firstly, as a tea taken 2 or 3 times a day (in severe cases try an infusion for stronger effect, see page 12) to reduce the inflammation and excess mucus, and, secondly, by soaking pads of cotton wool in a cooled infusion and placing on the eyelids to soothe sore, irritated eyes.

Where the mucus is very watery, alternative internal infusions to the above, or additions to them are:

Ground Ivy *(Glechoma hederacea)*: very astringent, reducing excess mucus and drying out the secretions.

Ribwort *(Plantago lanceolata)*: also anti-catarrhal and astringent, toning up and healing the membranes.

HOMEOPATHY

Sometimes it can be worth using Mixed Pollens themselves in homeopathic dilution, before symptoms have started. Otherwise choose from:

Allium cepa: for a burning nasal discharge; the eyes will run too (think of your reaction to cutting up onions!).

Arsen alb: if the eyes are burning, with tears that feel hot. If the nose runs, that too will feel burning, sneezing gives no relief to the irritation.

Euphrasia: if the nose runs profusely, with lots of watery mucus, although it may block at night; the eyes feel sore and gritty, with burning tears.

NATUROPATHY

Reduce mucus production by cutting out dairy products (also see Catarrh, page 34), and when the symptoms are severe, take high levels of Vitamin C (up to 2,000 mg per day, unless diarrhoea occurs) to act as a natural anti-histamine.

Rinse out the eyes with an eyebath, using cool distilled water or a proprietary eyewash, to give temporary relief – you can also ease the nose by sniffing up distilled water to wash out the pollens.

INFLUENZA

Anyone who has had influenza will know that it is a more serious complaint than simply having a bad cold. Different viral strains produce differing symptoms, but generally there is a fever, aching muscles, headache and general weakness. Sometimes there may also be a harsh cough. In older, frail people it can seriously debilitate.

AROMATHERAPY

Several oils have considerable anti-viral activity, and help to boost the immune system. It is important though to use them at the earliest sign of influenza for maximum benefit. Either use them in the bath or as steam inhalations (see pages 8 and 33); it may also be a good idea to fumigate the house with oils at the same time, to help prevent everyone else getting the infection. This is best done by either putting 2-3 drops on a radiator to evaporate or else adding around 10 drops to a small plant spray filled with water, frequently spraying the room.

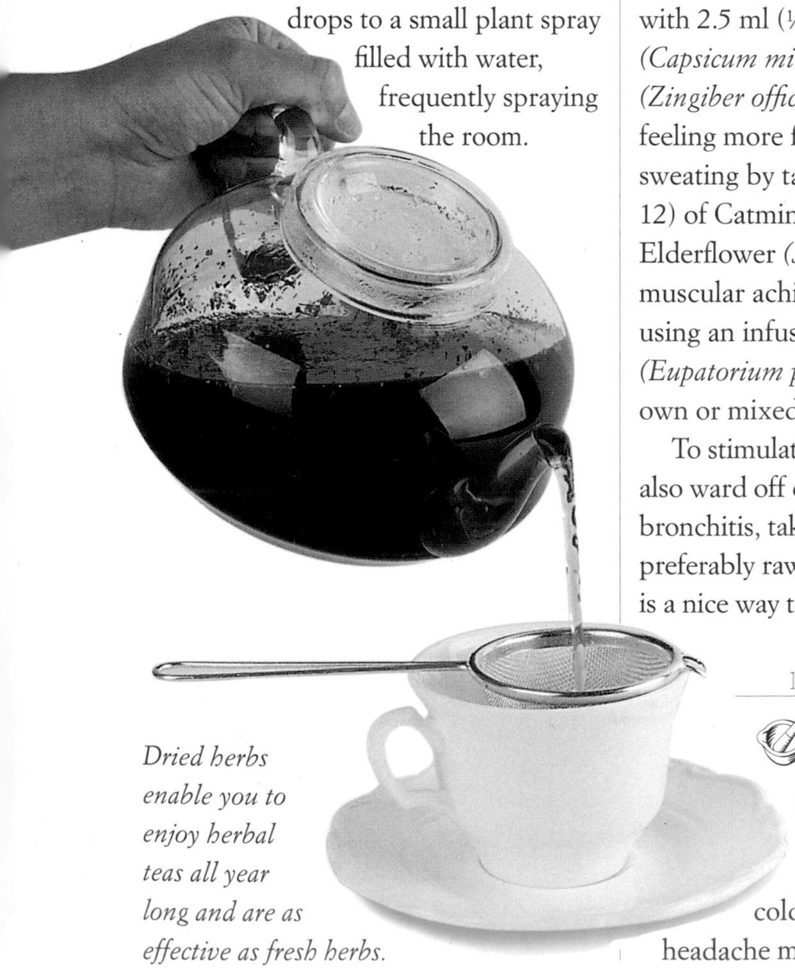

Dried herbs enable you to enjoy herbal teas all year long and are as effective as fresh herbs.

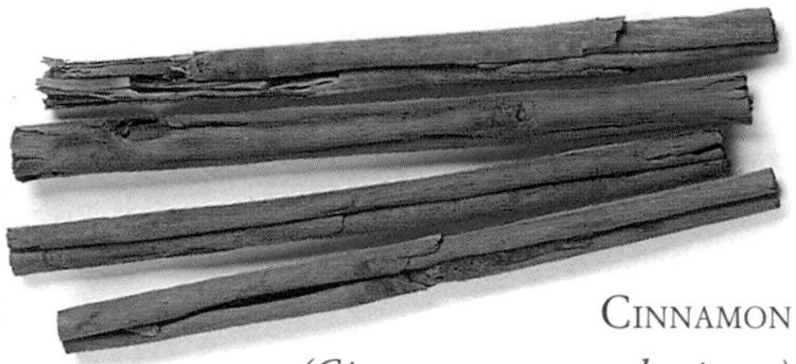

CINNAMON
(Cinnamomum zeylanicum)

Choose from Tea Tree, Eucalyptus, Lemon or Lavender oils.

HERBALISM

In the early stages of a chilled feeling, use a warming tea such as Cinnamon *(Cinnamomum zeylanicum)* – break a stick into a teapot – perhaps with 2.5 ml (½ tsp) of Cayenne *(Capsicum minimum)* or ground Ginger *(Zingiber officinalis)* added. When feeling more feverish, you can provoke sweating by taking infusions (see page 12) of Catmint *(Nepeta cataria)* and/or Elderflower *(Sambucus nigra)*. The deep muscular aching can be relieved by using an infusion of Boneset *(Eupatorium perfoliatum)*, either on its own or mixed with either of the above.

To stimulate the immune system, and also ward off complications such as bronchitis, take plenty of garlic, preferably raw – hot garlic bread or toast is a nice way to take it for all the family.

HOMEOPATHY

Choose from these remedies if not able to get professional treatment:

BRYONIA: if feeling very hot and dry, thirsty for cold drinks, aching all over, headache made worse by movement.

GELSEMIUM: for a hot head and face, but with chills that go up and down the back; burning headache but without any real sense of thirst.

NUX VOMICA: for thoroughly chilled feelings, cannot get warm at all, limbs and back are aching, stomach upset.

NATUROPATHY

At an early stage try having a hot bath to which you add 30–60 ml (2–4 tbsp) of Epsom Salts, then go straight to bed.

Generally restrict the diet, drinking fruit juices until the feverish period has passed, and then starting on fruit, vegetables and whole grains at first. If very hot and sweaty, try applying a cool compress to the chest and trunk.

Immediately the symptoms start, it is advisable to take high levels of Vitamin C to boost the immune system, around 3,000-4,000 mg to start with, reducing over 3-4 days to 500 mg until completely better.

INFLUENZA STRAINS

Influenza occurs in bouts of epidemic proportions, with periodic changes in the viral strains responsible. This makes vaccination programmes more difficult and less effective. Influenza can be a real killer, and attention to good health to prevent the onset of serious symptoms is essential, especially for older people in winter.

LARYNGITIS

Laryngitis is an acute inflammation of the larynx and vocal chords, leading to a very sore throat, hoarseness and even loss of voice. It may follow on from a cold or other infection, or be due to overstraining the voice by shouting, severe coughing or irritations such as smoke or dust.

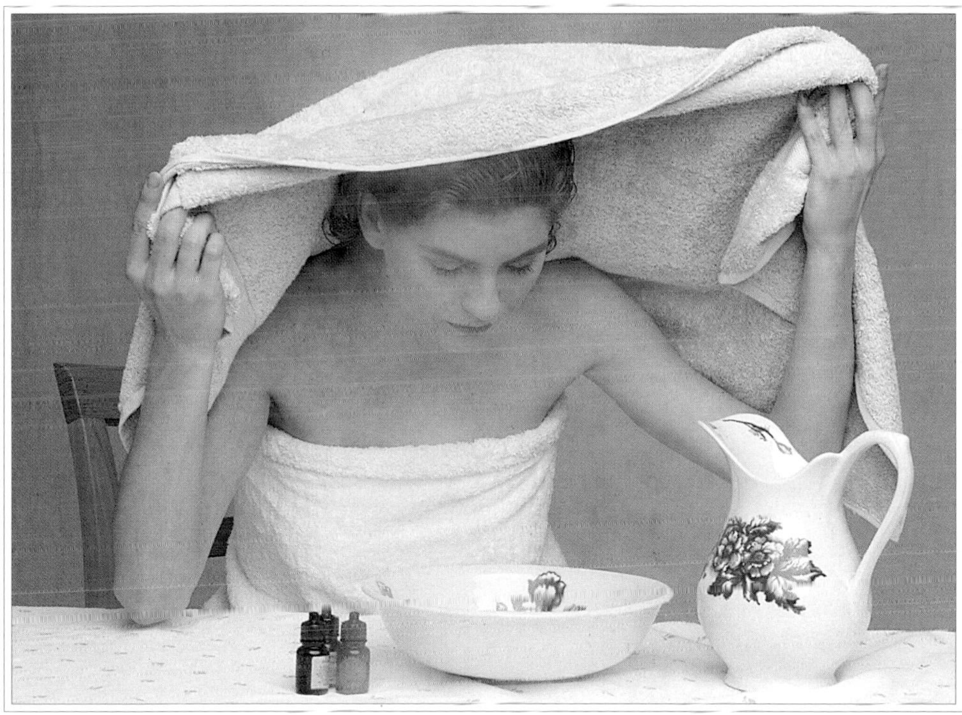

Holding a towel over your head will concentrate the herbal vapours and delay the effects of evaporation.

AROMATHERAPY

The best method for treatment is undoubtedly steam inhalation (see page 33); the natural choice of oil is probably Benzoin, but you could also use Sandalwood or Thyme. As the oils vaporize with the steam, they soothe the dry, inflamed membranes and ease the breathing as well as being highly antiseptic.

HERBALISM

Local treatment is by gargle; there are a number of useful herbs for this, they are most effective as tinctures (see page 14), otherwise use cooled infusions (see page 12). Choose from these astringent herbs: Sage *(Salvia officinalis)*, Thyme *(Thymus vulgaris)*, Agrimony *(Agrimonia eupatoria)* or Raspberry Leaf *(Rubus idaeus)*, which will help to tone up the puffy membranes. For a very soothing effect, add Marshmallow *(Althea officinalis)* to the gargle, or take 10 ml (2 tsp) of a decoction (see page 12) of the root 3 or 4 times a day.

HOMEOPATHY

One of these remedies should be suitable in the short term:

ACONITE: for sudden laryngitis following exposure to cold, dry winds, with a high temperature and a dry cough.

CAUSTICUM: for a hoarse voice, which may go completely, with a burning, raw throat and irritating cough.

PHOSPHORUS: if you cannot talk louder than a whisper, symptoms may have been brought on by overuse of the voice; with a dry cough and a desire for cold drinks and ice-cream.

NATUROPATHY

Cut out dairy produce to reduce excess catarrh, and take plenty of fruit juices. Try placing a cold compress (see page 15) around the throat, if the problem has been around for a while, it may be an idea to use a hot compress followed by a cold one. Sucking zinc gluconate lozenges not only soothes the throat but directly tackles any infection; in addition to fruit and juices it may be useful to take 500 mg of Vitamin C for a few days, or fresh lemon juice and honey drinks.

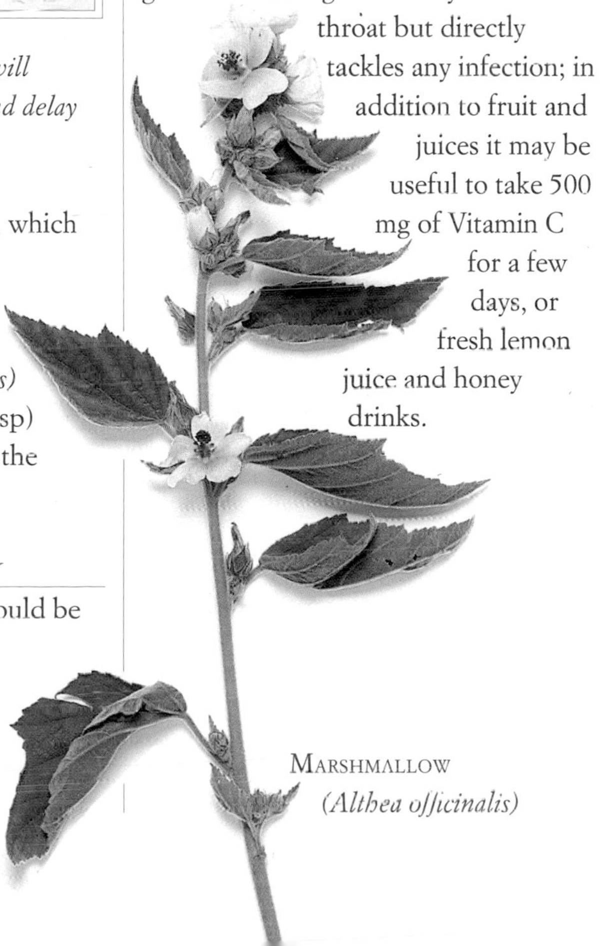

MARSHMALLOW *(Althea officinalis)*

SINUSITIS

The sinus cavities are air spaces in the bones of the skull, behind, above and below the eyes. They act as a kind of sound-box, helping the voice to resonate. Like the nasal passages they are lined with mucous membranes, and an infection in the nose or throat can spread to the sinuses; acute sinusitis can be very painful and needs prompt treatment. Chronic sinusitis may be linked to allergic reactions such as hay fever.

AROMATHERAPY

Steam inhalations (see page 33) are the best way to work directly on the membranes, loosening thick mucus and fighting infection. Choose from oils of Chamomile, Eucalyptus, Lavender, Peppermint, Pine, Thyme or Tea Tree; a combination may be best, or else change around the oils. In acute sinusitis, the inhalations can be taken 4 times a day to ease the pain and relieve the congestion, reducing to once daily as the symptoms ease, until the sinuses have cleared up.

HERBALISM

Apart from steam inhalations as outlined above, using infusions internally (see page 12) can help to reduce the catarrh and inflammation. Look at the following herbs (see also Catarrh, page 34):

CATMINT *(Nepeta cataria)*: reduces nasal congestion and helps to liquefy the thick, sticky mucus.
ELDERFLOWER *(Sambucus nigra)*: reduces inflammation by improving circulation through the area, clears long-term catarrh, and eases congestion.
GOLDEN SEAL *(Hydrastis canadensis)*: has an astringent effect, cooling and toning up swollen, inflamed membranes. As this herb is quite expensive and difficult to find loose, it may be easier to take in tablet form, up to 500 mg a day.

It is also often very valuable to take plenty of garlic, either raw or as garlic perles, to fight any infection.

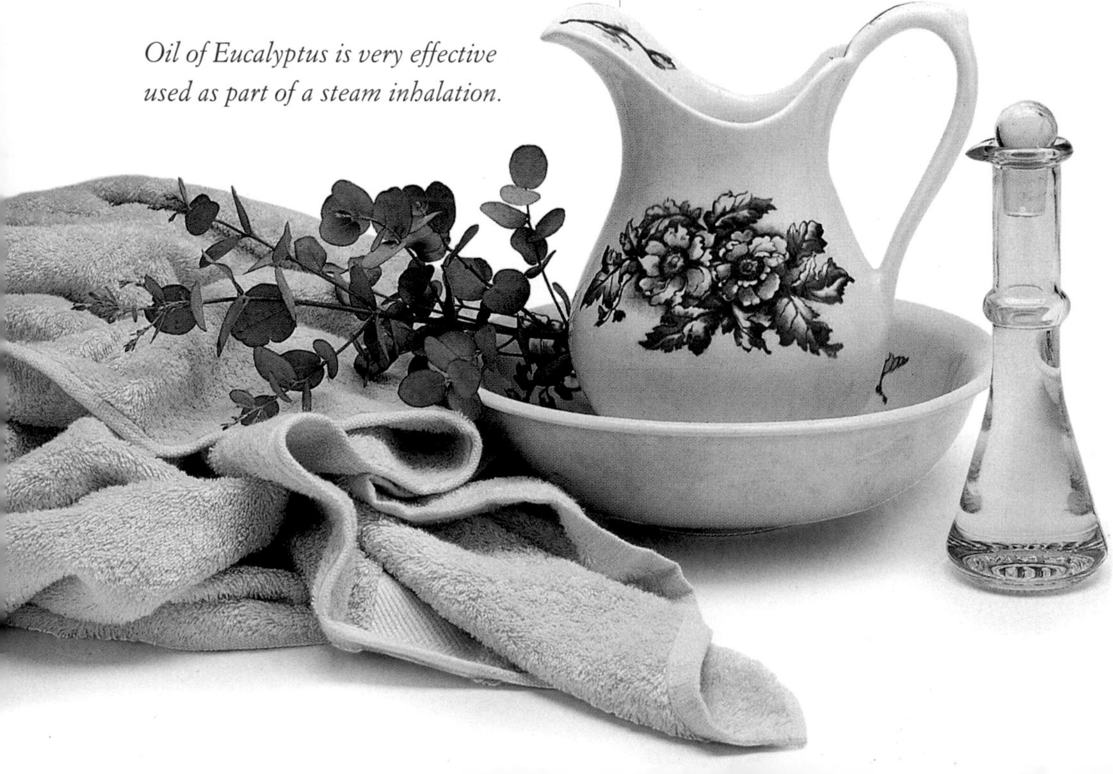

Oil of Eucalyptus is very effective used as part of a steam inhalation.

HOMEOPATHY

Try to match the remedy to the symptom pattern – look also at suggestions for Catarrh, Colds or Hay Fever (pages 34, 35 and 39).

HEPAR SULPH: for painful swelling of the nasal cavities, tender to the touch, with infected, yellow mucus discharge.
NAT MUR: a profuse, watery discharge, sneezing and a frontal headache are typical symptoms calling for this remedy.
SILICA: for a dry, blocked nose and a severe headache, perhaps with bouts of sneezing; worse with cold and better with warmth.

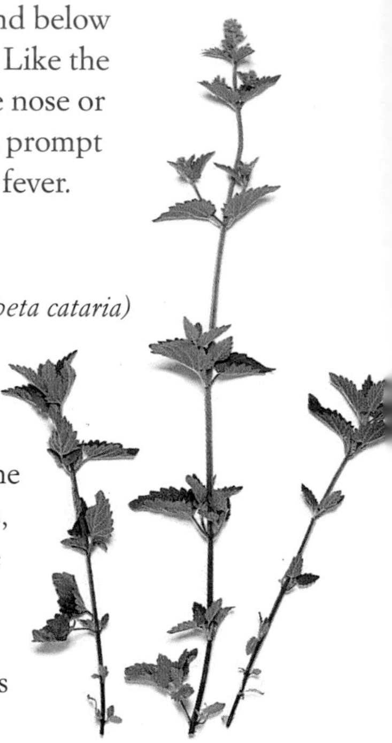

CATMINT *(Nepeta cataria)*

NATUROPATHY

Immediately cut out all dairy products, and restrict white flour, pastries, cakes and so on. Eat plenty of fresh fruit and vegetables. Avoid smoky atmospheres, and do not fly when nasal passages are acutely inflamed or blocked, as the changes in air pressure can given severe pain and could damage the eardrum.

Use alternating hot and cold light compresses (see page 15) or just splashes of water around the nose; start with hot water for about 3 minutes and then cold for no more than 1 minute, repeating 2 or 3 times. This will reduce congestion and inflammation, and thus ease the pains. Using an inhalation can be a helpful back-up to this.

SORE THROATS

Sore throats are more and more common nowadays, with increased airborne pollution, smoky, dry atmospheres in air-conditioned buildings and so on. The irritation can range from an annoying tickle to a rasping soreness, and may be linked to other infections. Where the throat inflammation, or pharyngitis, also extends down to the larynx, the voice may be affected – see also Laryngitis and Tonsillitis (pages 41 and 44).

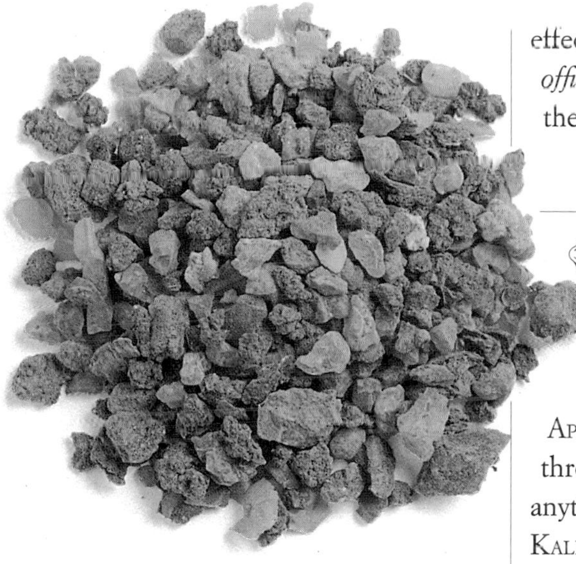

MYRRH *(Commiphora molmol)*

AROMATHERAPY

Use steam inhalations (see page 33) with oils such as Benzoin, Lavender or Thyme. One drop *only* of essential oil of Lemon on 2.5 ml (½ tsp) of honey acts as a powerful local antiseptic, as well as being soothing.

HERBALISM

If possible, use the following herbs as tinctures for gargling; if unavailable then use cooled infusions (see page 12): Agrimony *(Agrimonia eupatoria)*, Sage *(Salvia officinalis)*, and Thyme *(Thymus vulgaris)* are all astringent, toning up the membranes, the latter two also being quite antiseptic. For a more powerful effect try using a tincture (see page 14) of Myrrh *(Commiphora molmol)*, together with one or more of the others. If making infusions, add two broken liquorice sticks to give a more soothing effect, or else use Marshmallow *(Althea officinalis)* leaf in equal amounts with the other herb(s).

HOMEOPATHY

The choice is wide, depending on the causes and the nature of the symptoms. It is advisable to look at other headings in this section too.

APIS MEL: for a red, swollen, burning throat and difficulty in swallowing anything.

KALI BICH: for sharp pains, relieved by swallowing, although there may also be a feeling of a "frog-in-the-throat" which is not relieved. The throat is especially dry and sore first thing in the mornings, with some sticky mucus.

MERC SOL: for a painful and raw throat, with a lot of watery, possibly unpleasant-smelling saliva.

NATUROPATHY

For adults and older children the diet can be restricted to fruit juices only for a day or two at most; younger children and infants will be unlikely to cope with this, so simply reduce the dairy foods and give plenty of fruit juices. If the throat is swollen and feels very hot, try a cold compress (see page 15) around it. If available, suck zinc lozenges. Rest the voice and keep in a warm atmosphere.

In modern offices the dry air leads to frequent sore throats. Sip liquids often, and try to make the air more moist if possible, for example with plants.

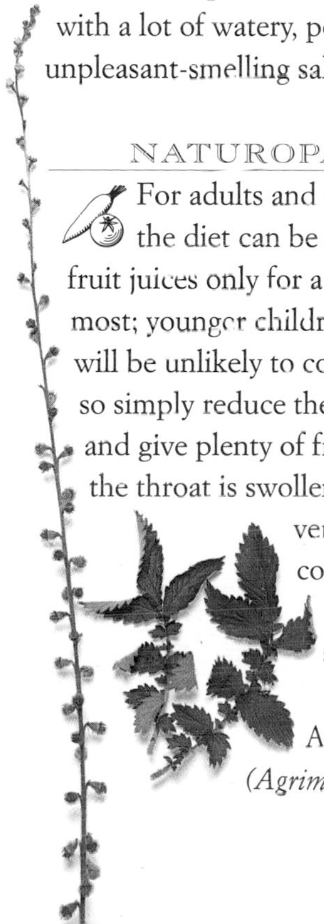

AGRIMONY *(Agrimonia eupatoria)*

OCCUPATIONAL HAZARDS

Many occupations involve excessive use of the voice e.g. teaching, and sore throats are commonplace. The regular use of herbal gargles can ease this discomfort, and help to prevent loss of voice or an actual infection. Keeping the throat moist by drinking liquids often, helps too.

SAGE *(Salvia officinalis)*

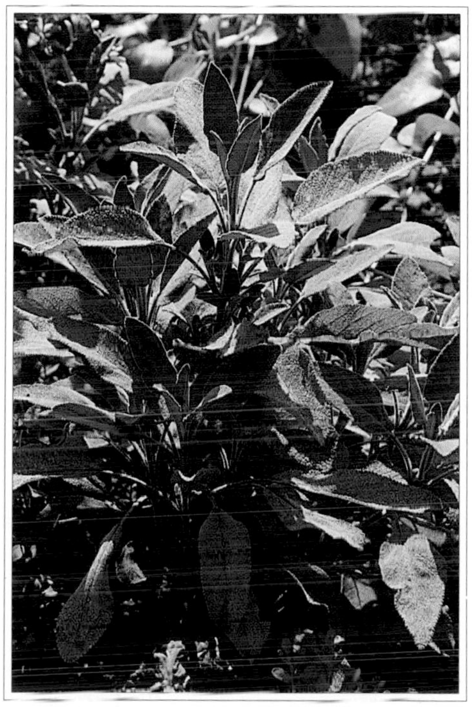

TONSILLITIS

Inflammation and infection of the tonsils most often occurs in children or younger adults; it used to be the fashion to remove the tonsils but unless they become chronically badly infected and act as a focus for other infections, it is now considered better to keep them. They act as an early warning sign of lowered vitality, and if this first line of defence is lost, then more deep-seated conditions can occur in later life.

AROMATHERAPY

Essential oils are not for internal use, unless under qualified treatment, and are rather unpleasant for local treatment. In tonsillitis they are best used as supportive treatment, using steam inhalations (see page 33) of Benzoin, Eucalyptus or Thyme to ease inflammation and fight general infection.

HERBALISM

All the herbs mentioned under Sore Throats (see page 43) for gargling are excellent here too, especially Myrrh *(Commiphora molmol)*, Thyme *(Thymus vulgaris)* and Sage *(Salvia officinalis)*. For repeated bouts of tonsillitis take garlic daily, either perles/capsules or fresh. Another essential herb to use for chronic

GARLIC *(Allium sativum)*

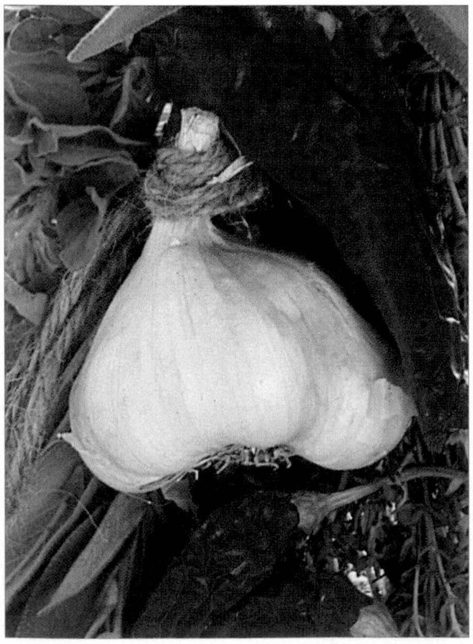

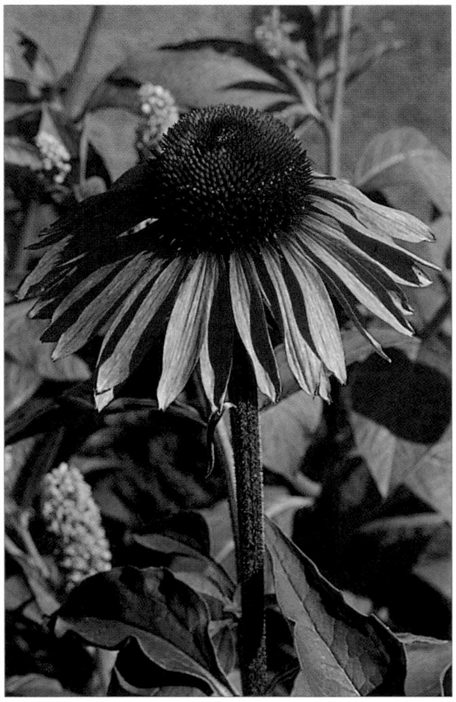

CONE FLOWER *(Echinacea angustifolia)*

tonsillitis is Cone Flower *(Echinacea angustifolia* or *E. purpurea)*; this boosts the immune system and may be taken in tablets or else as a tincture (see page 14), 20 drops twice daily.

HOMEOPATHY

Remedies applicable to tonsillitis include:

ACONITE: for sudden onset of inflammation, with hot, red and burning tonsils and thirst for cold drinks.

HEPAR SULPH: for pain on swallowing, as if something is stuck in the throat, tonsils swollen and discharging a yellow pus.

LYCOPODIUM: for chronic swelling of the tonsils, which look as if they are pitted with small white discharging ulcers; cold drinks make the sensation worse.

NATUROPATHY

The tonsils' actions, in trapping and removing infective bacteria that would otherwise cause deeper problems, means that they are more easily infected themselves. This can produce an infection of the adenoids too, with nasal congestion.

Where these symptoms occur, it is helpful to cut out dairy projects for a while. In any case, take plenty of fluids, especially fruit juices. Freshly-squeezed lemon juice, with a little honey, is a local antiseptic. Repeated attacks of tonsillitis are often a sign of lowered health in general, and may need professional treatment.

THYME *(Thymus vulgaris)*

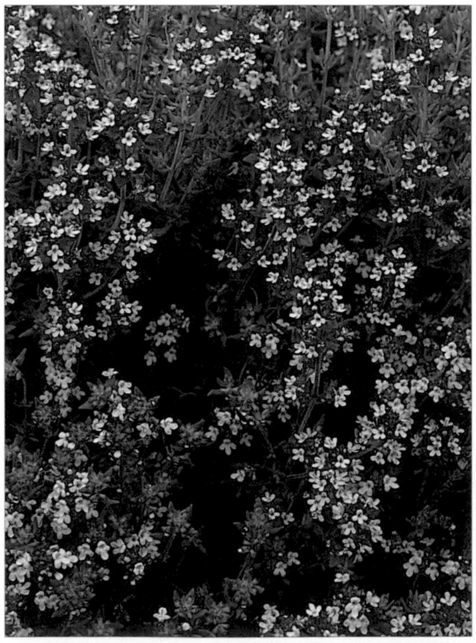

WHOOPING COUGH

This highly infectious bacterial infection tends to occur in epidemics every few years. Thick, sticky mucus gives rise to a spasmodic cough and the difficulty in inhaling with this gives the characteristic whooping sound. It is mostly seen in children, and in babies it can be serious, so get professional help as soon as possible. Symptoms can linger on for several weeks, so continue to help breathing by the measures listed below.

AROMATHERAPY

Relief for the condition is most dramatic with steam; either use inhalations (see page 33) or with infants simply hold them near steam, such as a basin filled with piping hot water or near a hot bath (make sure they do not touch very hot water). Very good oils to add to the steam are Cypress, Lavender and Tea Tree.

HERBALISM

Start to give herbal teas/infusions at the first sign of coughing – do not wait for the respiratory distress that can set in with the whoop. Use steam to free the mucus, as mentioned above. In young infants and babies, diluted teas should be strong enough; older children may need infusions (see page 12), again diluted (for dosages see page 9). Look at these herbs, and use a blend of the most appropriate:

Keep all medicines and aromatherapy oils out of the reach of small children.

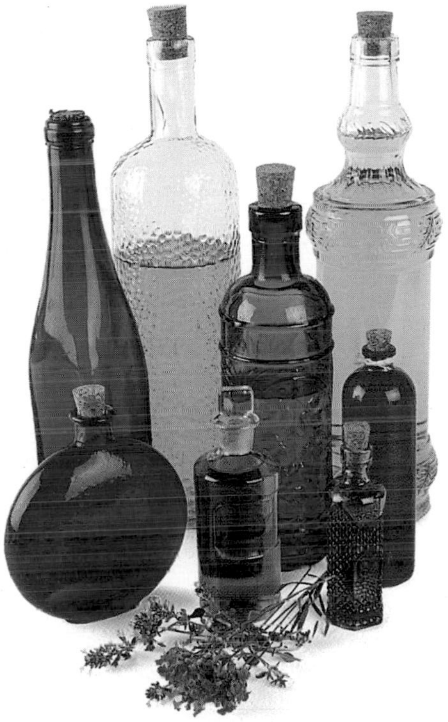

CHAMOMILE *(Chamomilla recutita)*: helps to calm the person down, reduces catarrh and accompanying nausea.
COLTSFOOT *(Tussilago farfara)*: one of the best cough remedies, helping to ease the spasmodic nature of the cough.
LAVENDER *(Lavandula vera)*: a relaxing expectorant, soothing the cough and breathing and also generally calming.
THYME *(Thymus vulgaris)*: highly antiseptic, soothing the dry cough that may herald the start of the problem.
WHITE HOREHOUND *(Marrubium vulgare)*: good expectorant, loosening the sticky mucus and reducing spasm.

An alternative treatment that can work wonders is to chop or crush two cloves of garlic into 15 ml (1 tbsp) of honey and leave for a couple of hours, or even overnight. Give up to 5 ml (1 tsp) either neat or diluted in a little warm water, 4 times a day.

HOMEOPATHY

Ideally seek qualified advice for this ailment, but a remedy often used for the characteristic rapid paroxysmal cough is Drosera. Often the bout of coughing can result in vomiting. If children have been in contact with whooping cough, it can be worth trying this remedy as a prophylactic: give 3 doses of 30c dilution (see page 10) in a 24-hour period.

SELF-HELP MEASURES

Anyone who has heard the distinctive whooping sound will always remember whooping cough. Early treatment is most helpful; self-help measures such as steam treatments can speedily relieve symptoms, but babies and tiny infants should ideally be professionally checked as well.

NATUROPATHY

Keep the fluid intake high, especially if there is vomiting with the coughing bouts; also give only small amounts of light food rather than big meals. Avoid dairy products in order to lessen mucus production, and give easily digested foods.

For older children, supplementing diet with 500 mg Vitamin C daily for a couple of weeks will help to boost the immune system – reduce or stop if diarrhoea develops.

Try to keep the diet light, wholesome and low in dairy foods for quite a while after the initial symptoms have eased, as any build-up in mucus can cause more problems for several weeks.

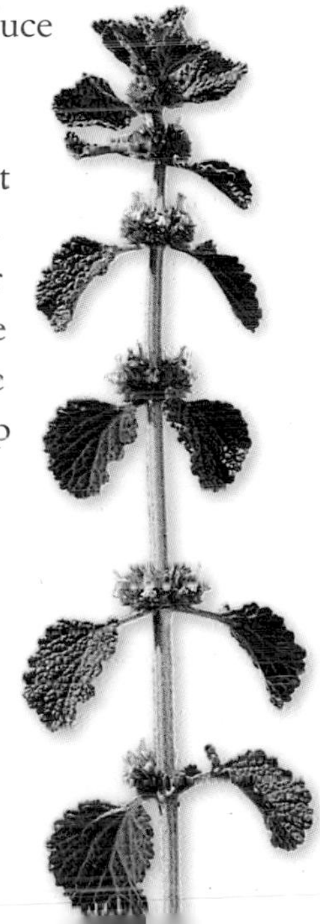

WHITE HOREHOUND *(Marrubium vulgare)*

THE CIRCULATORY SYSTEM

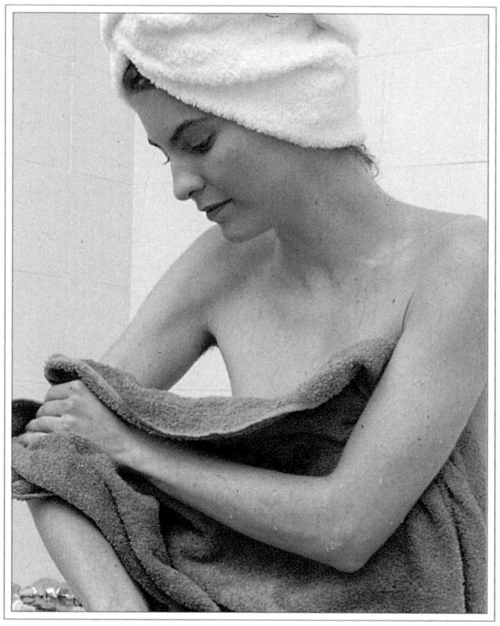

Circulation is absolutely vital for health; the blood transports oxygen and all our other nutrients around the body to all the cells, and carries away the waste materials from cellular activity. Without good circulation we simply do not have the fuel to provide enough energy for health. In cooler climates many people suffer from poor circulation, and lowered immune systems can often follow.

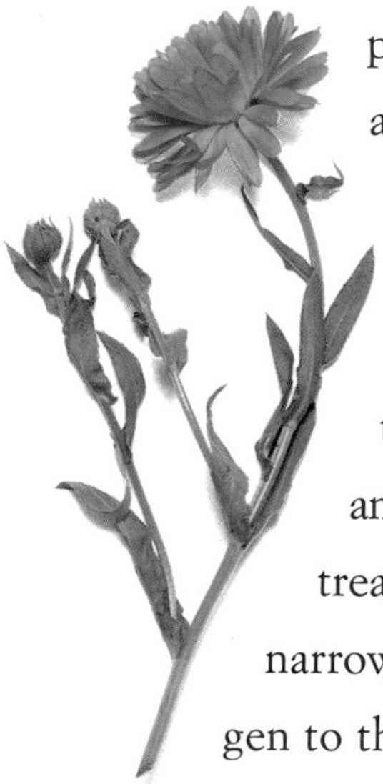

Disorders of circulation can occur in the heart or in the blood vessels; the former are not suitable for self-treatment, and for any prolonged or serious circulatory problems it is best to get professional treatment. For example, angina is a cramping of the heart muscles due to narrowing or obstruction of the coronary arteries. When the supply of oxygen to the cardiac muscles does not meet any extra demand, perhaps when walking uphill, the characteristic cramp and pains of angina occur for a short while. Resting eases the pain after a few minutes. Angina can be relieved by taking infusions of Lime Blossom *(Tilia europaea)*, but full professional treatment needs to look at individual causes as well as the health of the heart.

Above: Alternating hot and cold baths is a useful self-help measure for improving circulation. Herbs such as Marigold (Calendula officinalis) *(*above left*) and Witch Hazel* (Hamamelis virginiana) *can also help astringe and tone swollen veins.*

CHILBLAINS

For people with poor peripheral circulation, living in cool, damp climates often creates chilblains. When circulation is reduced in cold weather, the oxygen supply to the fingers and toes is restricted to the point that the skin cells are damaged and swelling, redness and itching occurs. Warmer weather improves the condition, but using radiant heat, such as warming by the fire, can tend to aggravate the swelling and burning itchy sensation.

AROMATHERAPY

Only use oils locally if the skin is unbroken; otherwise an inflamed reaction may be set off. Massage the affected areas with warming oils such as Black Pepper, Ginger or Marjoram, using a vegetable oil containing a maximum of 3 per cent essential oil. For longer term treatment during the winter months, add oils of Cypress, Juniper, Pine or Rosemary to baths (see page 8 for dilutions), or use them diluted in a base oil as above for regular brisk massage of the hands and feet.

HERBALISM

Locally, use a footbath to which is added a decoction (see page 12) of fresh Ginger root *(Zingiber officinalis)*, using up to 15 g (½ oz) per 750 ml (1¼ pt/ 2⅔ cups) of water, or add a tea made from ground Ginger, or for maximum circulatory-stimulating effect Cayenne *(Capsicum minimum)*. Do not use the latter if the skin is broken.

Handbaths, or footbaths, are good ways to improve circulation to the extremities. Place hands in a bowl of hot water, with essential oils added as recommended.

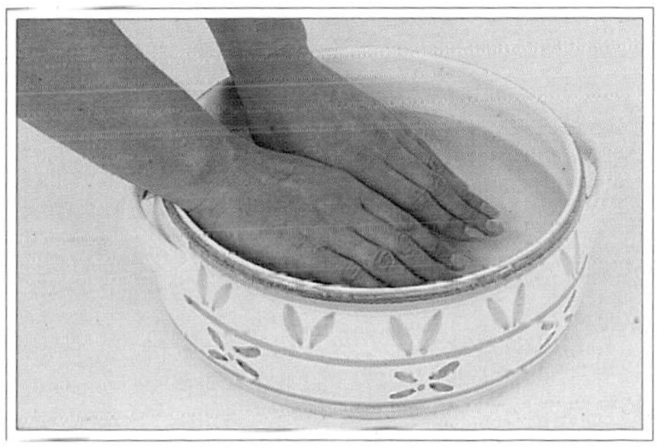

Ginger Decoction

Ginger can be made into a tea, but a stronger medicine is made from a decoction.

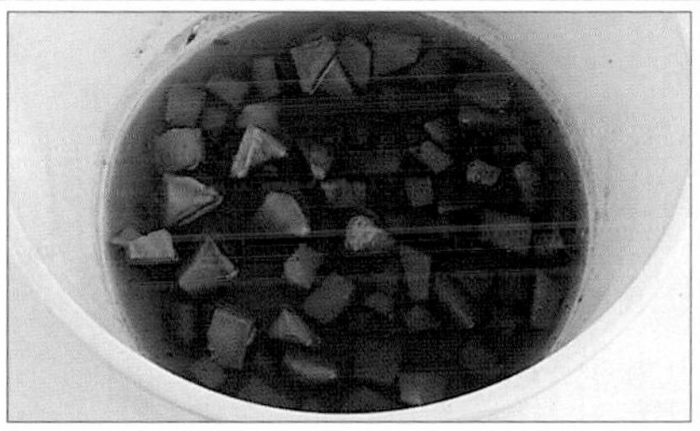

1 Simmer 15 g (½ oz) chopped rhizome in 750ml (1¼ pt/2⅔ cups) water until the liquid is reduced to about 600 ml (1 pt/2½ cups).

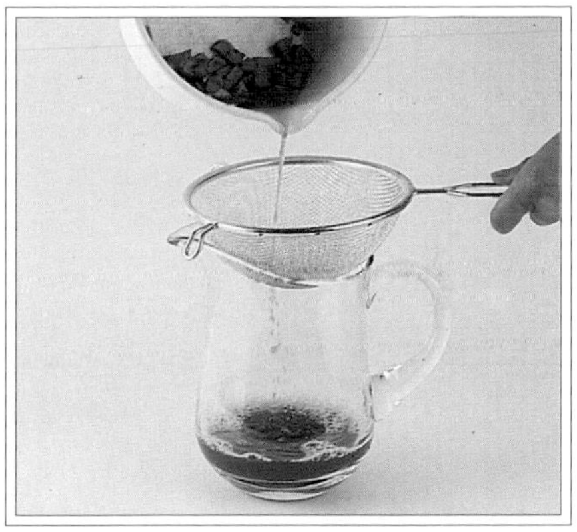

2 Strain through a sieve and store in a jug. Give in doses of 5-20 ml (1 tsp -1½ tbsp), three times a day. It will keep in the fridge for 3 days.

Internally, teas from the above herbs will generally improve circulation. For a gentler effect on the extremities use an infusion (see page 12) of Yarrow *(Achillea millefolium)*, this dilates the tiny blood vessels in the hands and feet, helping them to warm.

HOMEOPATHY

Since treatment may be needed for a couple of weeks or so, use low potencies such as 6c (see page 10).

AGARICUS: if the symptoms are worse when cold, and there is itching and burning with redness of the skin.

CALCAREA CARBONICA: if there is relief from cold, the feet in particular feeling damp and cold to the touch.

PETROLEUM: if, as well as burning and itching, there is chapping and cracking of the skin; typically the fingers get splits at the tips.

NATUROPATHY

Use alternating hot and cold foot or handbaths, using warm rather than too hot water, for about 4 minutes, and then cold for up to 1 minute. Make sure the feet or hands are well dried. Repeat for 10-15 minutes, nightly for a week if needed. Giving the hands or feet a brisk friction-rub daily will also help the circulation

Increase Vitamin C in the diet by eating more fresh fruit and potatoes; if you suffer badly from chilblains, take a supplement of Vitamin C, up to 1 mg until better, possibly together with 300–400 iu of Vitamin E to improve the elasticity of the blood vessels.

FEVER

The raising of the body temperature, usually in response to an infection, is something that natural medicine sees as generally a positive healing attempt by the body. Most of our vital processes are stimulated by the higher temperature, and conversely many infective organisms cannot survive as well, so the fever response is one that can be aided rather than instantly suppressed.

AROMATHERAPY

In order to encourage sweating at the stage of resolving the fever, a warm bath with a maximum of 10 drops of one of these oils may help – if bathing is not appropriate, use them at 1 per cent dilution in a little vegetable oil and massage the back or chest. Chamomile, Cypress, Lavender or Tea Tree are good choices. For a more cooling effect use 5 drops of oils of Eucalyptus, Lavender or Peppermint in a small bowl of tepid water and sponge the upper back, neck and chest.

HERBALISM

If at the early, shivery stage of an infection, use a tea with Ginger *(Zingiber officinalis)* – 2.5 ml (½ tsp) ground ginger, or peel and grate a small piece of fresh root – and Cinnamon *(Cinnamomum zeylanicum)* – 2.5 ml (½ tsp) ground cinnamon, or half a cinnamon stick.

When the fever makes you hot and restless, sweating can be provoked by taking a hot infusion (see page 12) of Elderflower *(Sambucus nigra)*. (At normal temperatures this will not make you sweat.) Other suitable infusions to relieve the symptoms are: Boneset *(Eupatorium perfoliatum)*, Catmint *(Nepeta cataria)*, Peppermint *(Mentha piperita)* and Yarrow *(Achillea millefolium)*, while Lime Blossom *(Tilia europaea)* can be added to aid the dilation of the blood vessels and assist general relaxation. Hyssop *(Hyssopus officinalis)* is another excellent herb to calm the system; a tea may be taken frequently while symptoms prevail.

Catmint *(Nepeta cataria)*

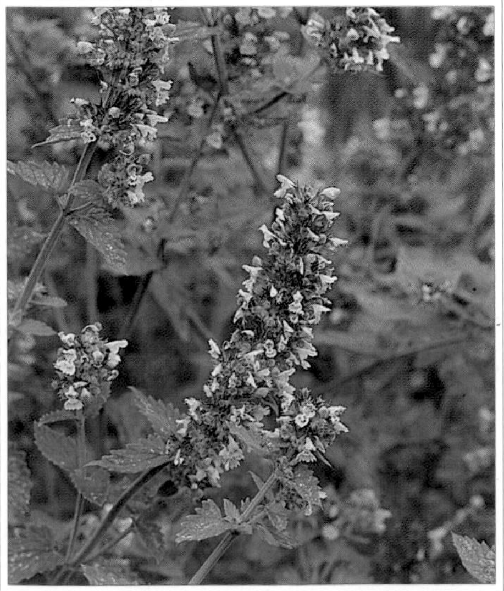

Checking the Temperature

By taking the temperature, and checking on feelings of heat or cold, the stages of the fever can be noted and treatment given. Initially, our internal thermostat is turned up, making us feel cold and shivery; as circulation is boosted and we reach the higher levels, we can feel more comfortable, although with a raised temperature. If the process goes too high, or the infection is not controlled, the thermostat is reset back to normal and we feel feverish and hot. Sweating reduces the temperature. Body temperatures around 38°C (100-101°F) often give the best results in fighting infection. Children's temperatures often go higher, and so may an adult's; if left for too long this can make us feel very unwell and cooling may then be needed, either by inducing sweating or through sponging with tepid water. If in doubt get professional help.

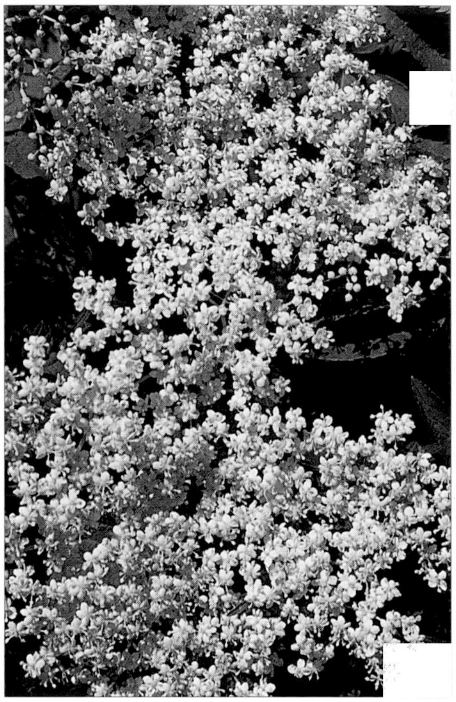

Elderflower *(Sambucus nigra)*

HOMEOPATHY

As with herbalism, there are many homeopathic remedies available and the cause/exact reaction needs to be sorted out first. A few to choose from, in mild feverish states are:

ACONITE: for dry, burning skin and great restlessness and agitation; symptoms may come on quickly.
BELLADONNA: for a high temperature, with a hot, very red face and a racing pulse. In extreme fever cases the person may also be delirious and highly excitable.
EUPATORIUM PERFOLIATUM: for an influenza-type of fever, with chills followed on by heat, aching muscles and maybe sweating.
FERRUM PHOS: for milder fevers, with less obvious causes; a hot, throbbing head and frequent sweating.

NATUROPATHY

Avoid active exercise; take plenty of rest but do not swaddle in heavy bedclothes; keep the room aired.

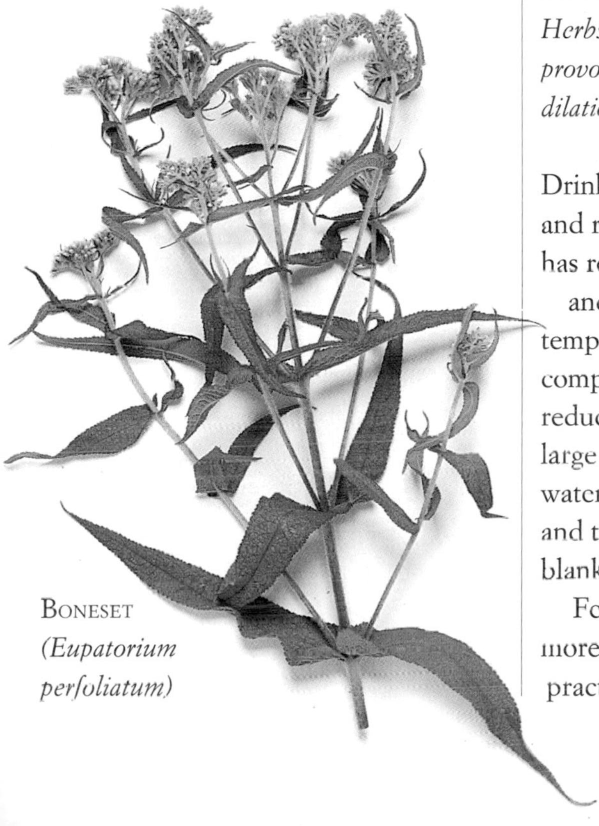

BONESET
(Eupatorium perfoliatum)

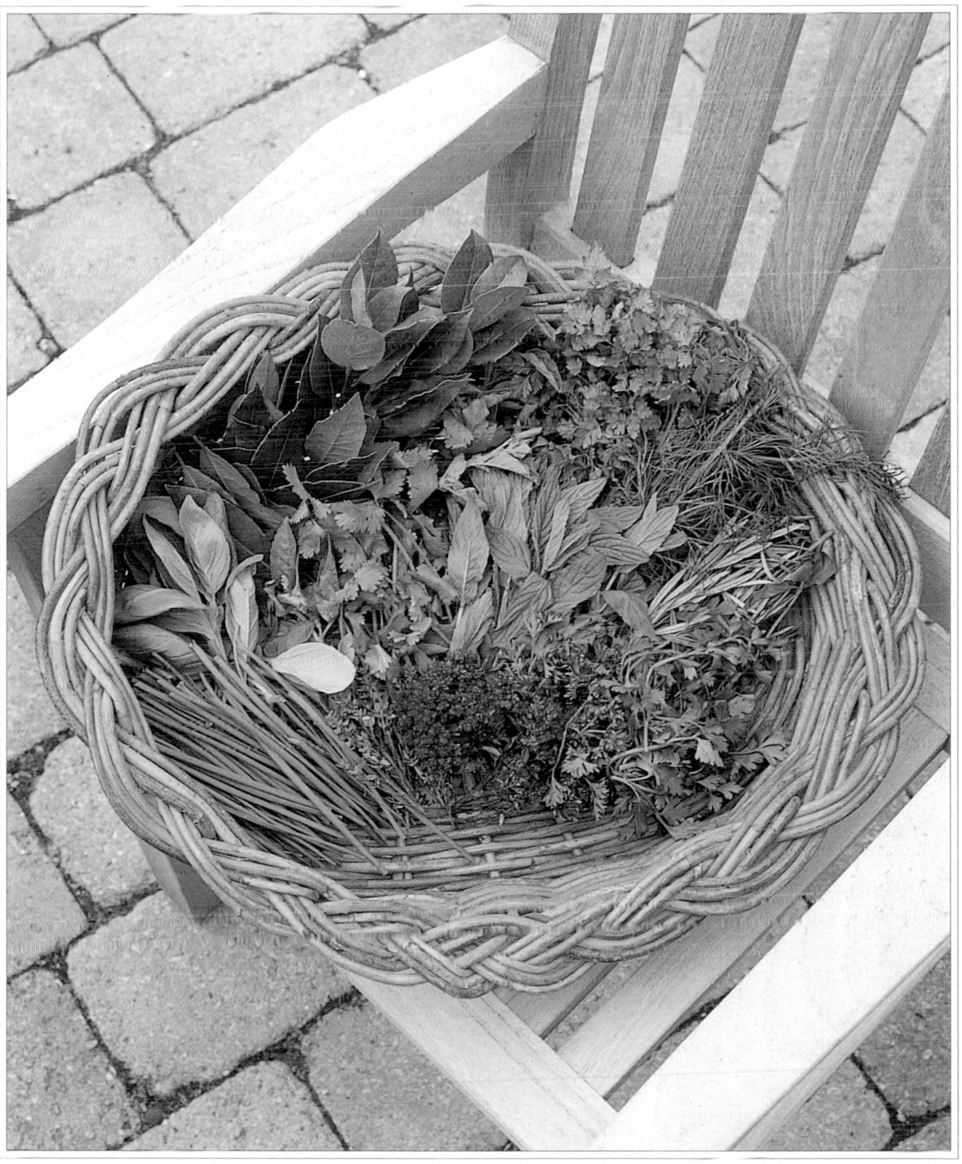

Herbs can help combat a fever by either provoking sweating, or by aiding the dilation of the blood vessels.

Drink fruit juices, herb teas or water, and restrict food until the temperature has returned to normal. Sponge the face and chest with tepid water if the temperature is too hot. A cold pack or compress around the trunk will also reduce excessive heat; use something large like a towel wrung out in cold water and wrapped around the body and then wrap in a larger, dry towel or blanket.

Feverish conditions used to be much more common, and traditional practitioners such as herbalists developed quite sophisticated techniques to deal with them. They have become rarer nowadays, but natural measures remain very important in helping to cope with a fever. If the temperature rises to the point where someone becomes delirious or even has a convulsion, get urgent medical aid. Young children can be quite prone to convulsions, but this is rarer as we get older.

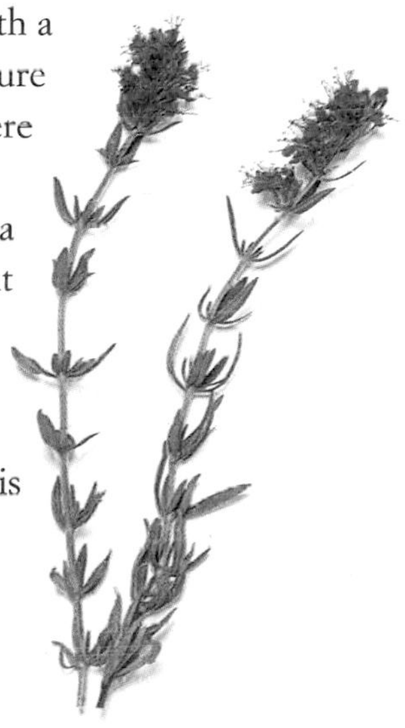

HYSSOP
(Hyssopus officinalis)

HAEMORRHOIDS

Haemorrhoids, or piles, are swollen veins in the rectum due to a restricted local blood supply and congestion in the pelvic cavity. Occasionally they may protrude externally, and can give rise to bleeding especially with a bowel movement. Piles can occur during pregnancy due to the increased pressure, but are often associated with chronic constipation, when frequent straining to empty the bowels causes extra pressure on the veins.

AROMATHERAPY

Using oils such as Cypress or Juniper in the bath can help to stimulate pelvic circulation; also adding a couple of drops of either to a bowl of cool water and then using this for a compress (see page 15) may help too. Massage of the abdomen (see right) with a 2 per cent dilution of oils of Marjoram or Rosemary can help ease constipation and relieve haemorrhoids.

Pilewort *(Ranunculus ficaria)*

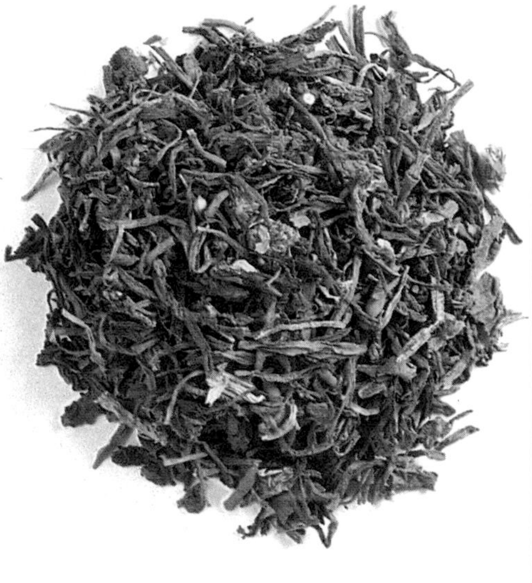

HERBALISM

Local treatment can help to astringe and tone the swollen veins. Use commercial creams made with extract of Pilewort *(Ranunculus ficaria)*, Horse Chestnut *(Aesculus hippocastanum)* or Marigold *(Calendula officinalis)*, or use a compress of distilled Witch Hazel *(Hamamelis virginiana)*; the tincture (see page 14) is much more astringent, if available use this diluted at the rate of 15 ml (1 tbsp) to a small bowl of warm water.

Prolong bleeding from piles can eventually lead to anaemia. Drinking Nettle *(Urtica dioica)* tea may relieve this, but take steps to avoid constipation too.

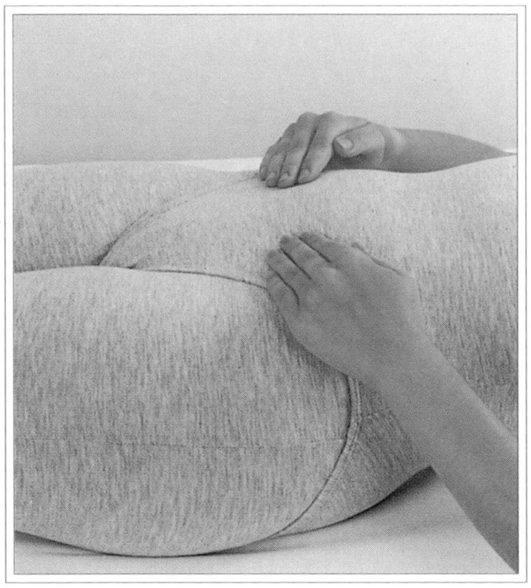

Press fingers steadily into the low abdomen, and massage with small circular movements, to release tension and improve local circulation.

HOMEOPATHY

Some possible remedies are:

Aesculus: for a dry itching and stinging sensation, and a tendency for the veins to prolapse and protrude externally.

Hamamelis: for a burning soreness, often with bleeding.

Sulphur: for hot, burning and itching in the anus; the pains are made worse by standing and better when lying.

NATUROPATHY

Practitioners in all of the therapies are likely to give dietary advice, and it is sensible to ensure you eat plenty of fresh vegetables and fruit to give adequate fibre and ease constipation, see also Constipation (page 57). Hot and cold compresses or even hot/cold baths will improve local circulation and reduce congestion; ice packs may be useful to reduce swelling at times. Exercise is also helpful to get the circulation going; ideally get individual advice. Avoid long periods of standing.

Witch Hazel *(Hamamelis virginiana)*

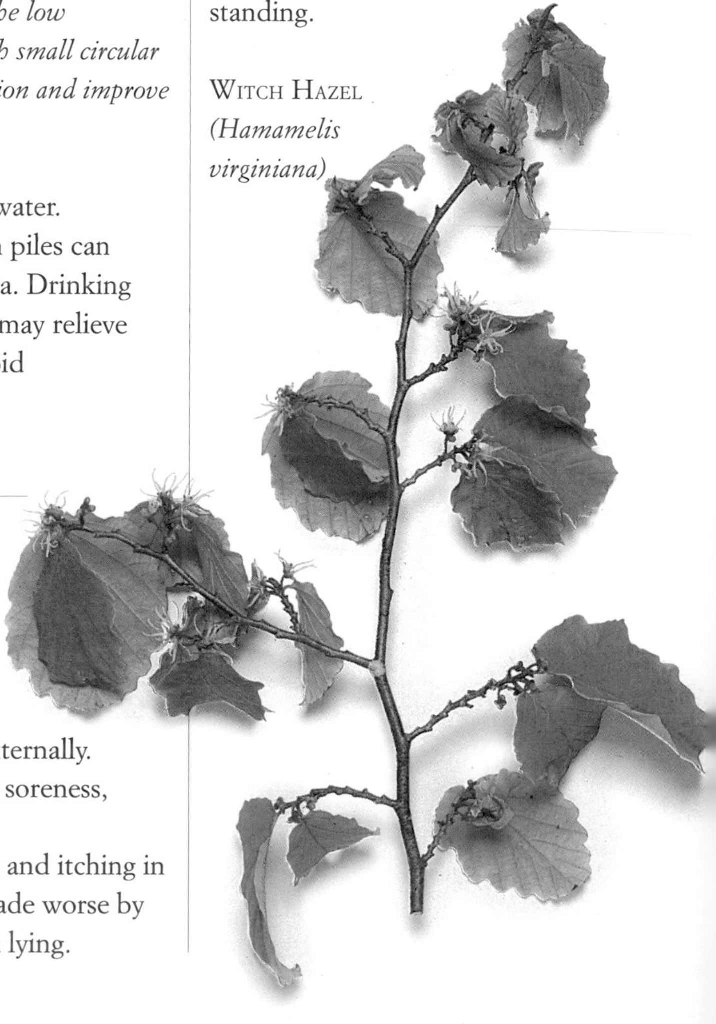

POOR CIRCULATION

Poor circulation to the extremities is quite common in cooler climates, and particularly in elderly people or those who do very little exercise. (See also Chilblains, page 47). Poor circulation can lead on to more serious conditions such as phlebitis or thrombosis, so it should not be neglected, and professional medical help should be sought if in any doubt.

Hand Massage

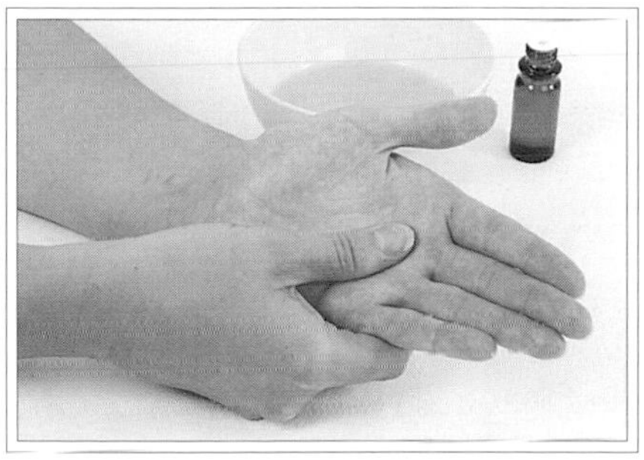

1 Place some base oil in a bowl, with essential oils added as recommended. Massage into palms of hands with a steady circular movement.

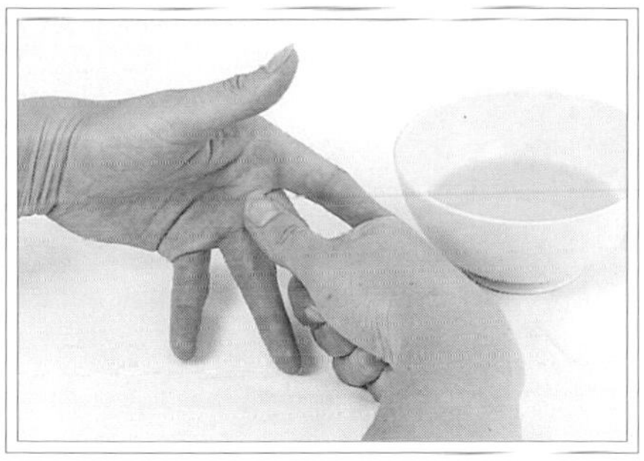

2 Squeeze down the fingers to stretch and loosen them, pushing towards the palm. Repeat steps 1 and 2 several times.

Foot Massage

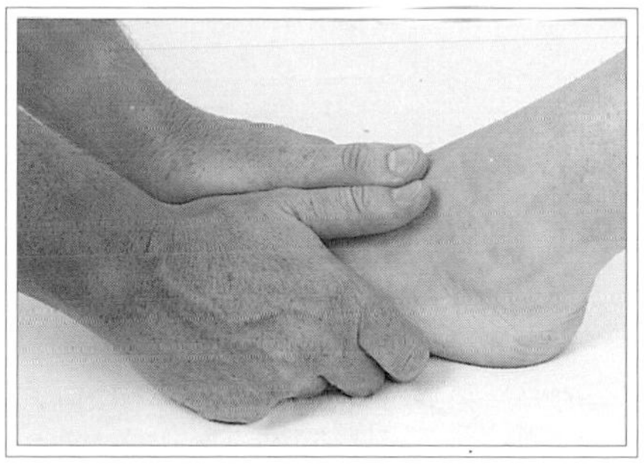

1 To stretch the feet, place hands with thumbs on top of the foot, keeping a firm grip with both of the hands.

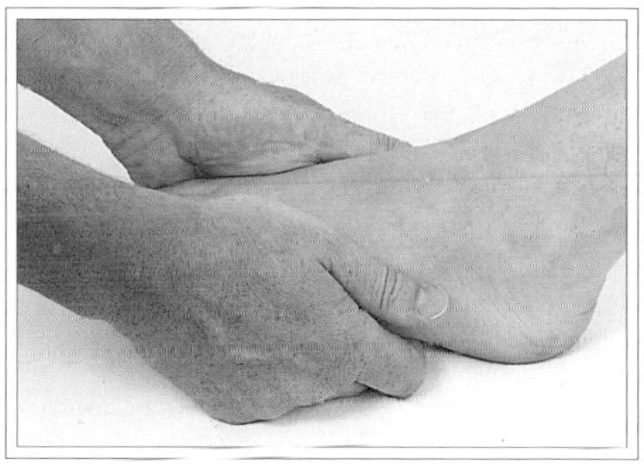

2 Move thumbs outward, as if breaking a piece of bread (be gentle with your partner!); repeat movement several times.

AROMATHERAPY

Massage the hands or feet with diluted oils such as Black Pepper, Lavender, Marjoram or Rosemary. These can be added to a warm footbath for a stronger short-term treatment. Use a maximum of 10 drops in total, and try a blend of 2 or 3 of these oils. Avoid if skin is broken, get advice first.

HERBALISM

Take hot herbal teas regularly to aid peripheral circulation; choose from Elderflower *(Sambucus nigra)*, Ginger *(Zingiber officinalis)*, Lime Blossom *(Tilia europaea)*, Nettle *(Urtica dioica)* or Yarrow *(Achillea millefolium)*. Daily intake of garlic stimulates blood flow too, and cayenne pepper is the strongest circulatory stimulant, perhaps simply use in cooking for this effect as well as its flavour.

HOMEOPATHY

To improve circulation, the following remedies may be of help in the short term, but if symptoms persist and the fingers and toes become numb, then seek professional medical advice:

SECALE: For cold hands and feet with a burning sensation. The rest of the body also feels cold, and the fingers and

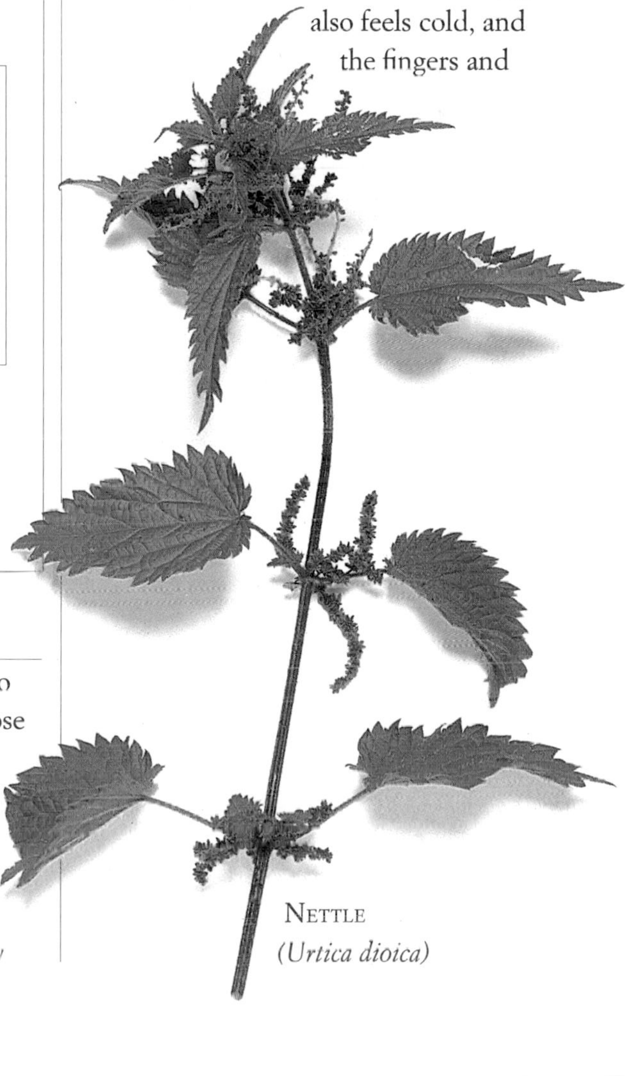

NETTLE
(Urtica dioica)

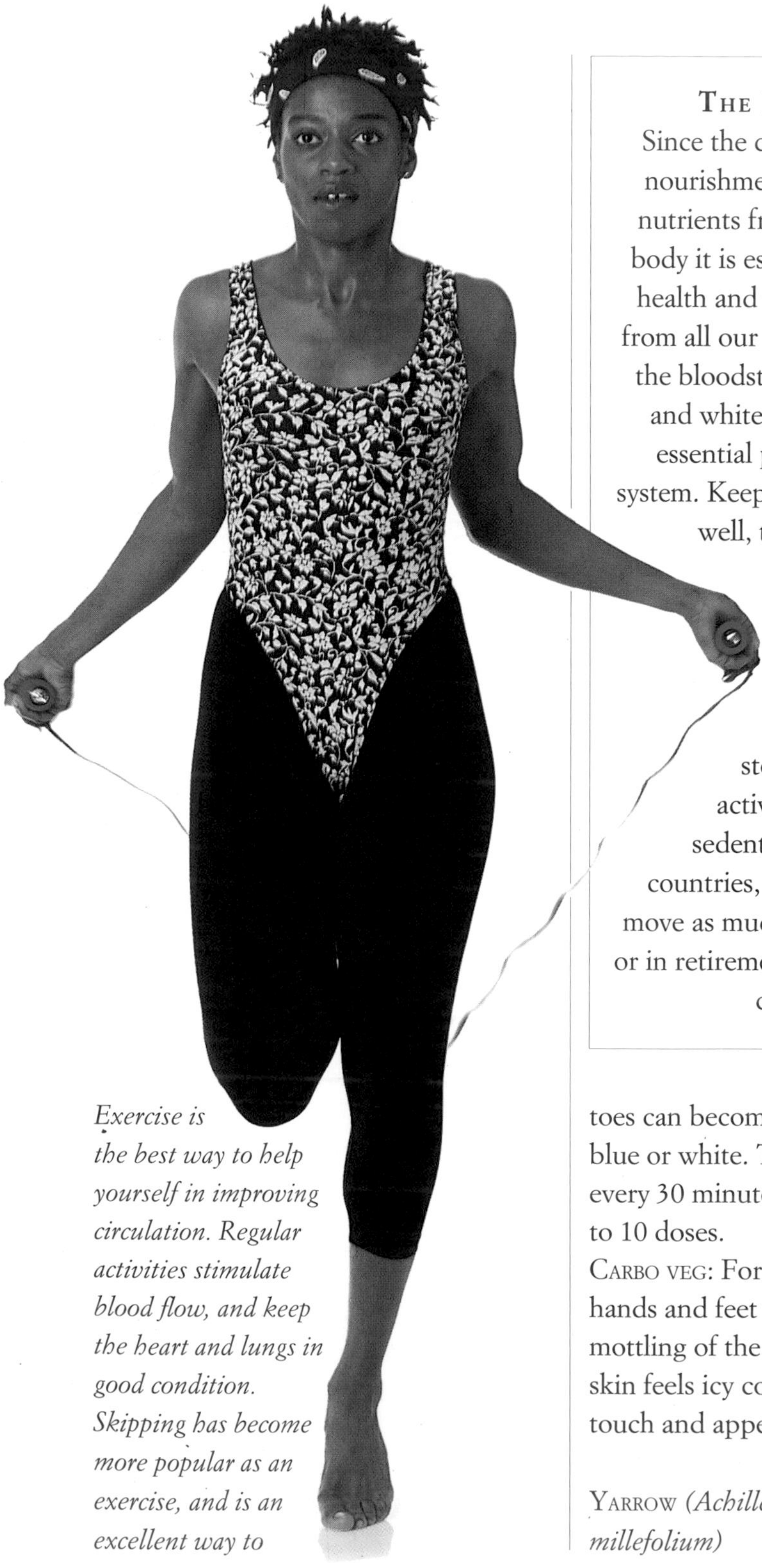

Exercise is the best way to help yourself in improving circulation. Regular activities stimulate blood flow, and keep the heart and lungs in good condition. Skipping has become more popular as an exercise, and is an excellent way to keep warm.

The Bloodstream

Since the circulation transports nourishment, both oxygen and nutrients from food, around the body it is essential for our overall health and vitality. Waste matter from all our cells is carried away in the bloodstream for elimination, and white blood cells form an essential part of our immune system. Keeping circulation flowing well, therefore, should be a priority for everyone.

As we get older, circulation tends to slow down and this is exaggerated if we stop exercising or being active. With increasingly sedentary lifestyles in many countries, it is very important to move as much as possible at work, or in retirement, to combat reduced circulation.

toes can become quite blue or white. Take 6c every 30 minutes for up to 10 doses.
CARBO VEG: For cold hands and feet with a mottling of the skin. The skin feels icy cold to the touch and appears blue,

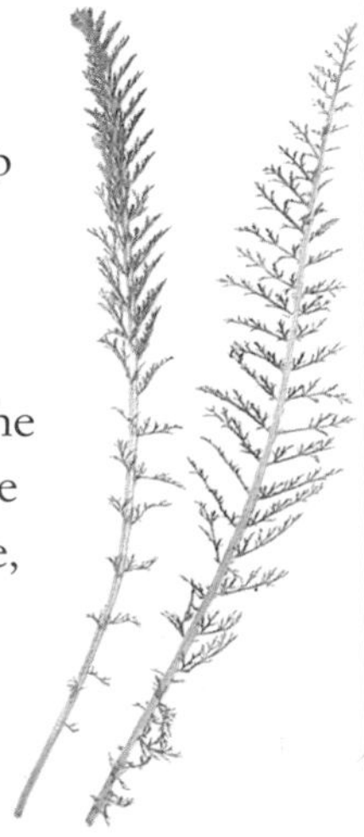

YARROW *(Achillea millefolium)*

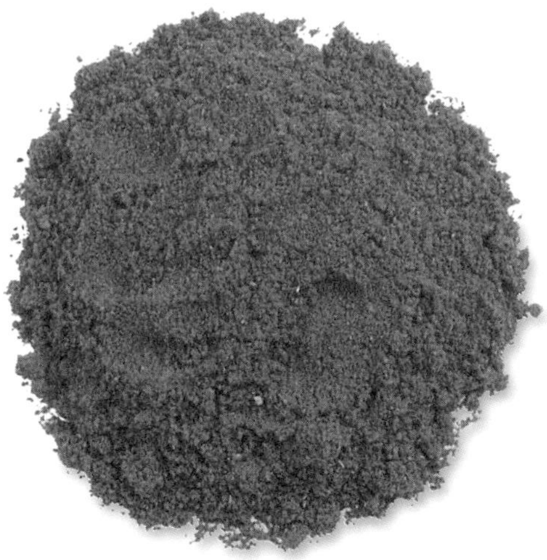

CAYENNE *(Capsicum minimum)*

with prominent veins. Skin can also appear blotchy.

NATUROPATHY

Various substances constrict the peripheral blood vessels, most notably caffeine and nicotine, so reducing or cutting out coffee and tobacco will help greatly. Exercise is another essential, wherever possible, and in colder weather keep the wrists and ankles warm as well as the hands and feet themselves. Additional amounts of Vitamin C (up to 500 mg per day) and Vitamin E (up to 400 iu per day) can boost circulation and aid the elasticity of the blood-vessel walls.

Caution

Do not increase the doses from those suggested here: it is likely to do more harm than good.

VARICOSE VEINS

Swollen veins most often occur in the lower legs, but can happen elsewhere, see also Haemorrhoids (page 50). The veins in the legs contain one-way valves that allow blood to flow back up towards the heart. If the calf muscles weaken, for example after prolonged standing, or the valves start to work less efficiently from other causes such as pregnancy, obesity or poor nutrition, then blood collects in the veins, and they swell.

AROMATHERAPY

All the natural therapies are likely to recommend both periods of rest, especially with the feet raised above the level of the thigh to let gravity assist venous return, and exercise to improve muscle tone.

Massage, above the area of varicosed veins and in an upwards direction towards the heart, will reduce the congestion. Essential oils of prime use here are Cypress, Chamomile and perhaps Juniper; use diluted at 2 per cent in vegetable oil.

HERBALISM

Externally, apply tinctures (see page 14) of Marigold *(Calendula officinalis)* or Witch Hazel *(Hamamelis virginiana)*, diluted 50:50 with water, 2 or 3 times a day. Internally, a cup daily of an infusion (see page 12) of Lime Blossom *(Tilia europaea)*, can help to improve peripheral circulation. Horse Chestnut *(Aesculus hippocastanum)* has a strengthening effect on the blood vessels; it may be taken in tablets as directed, or as the tincture at the rate of 30 drops twice daily.

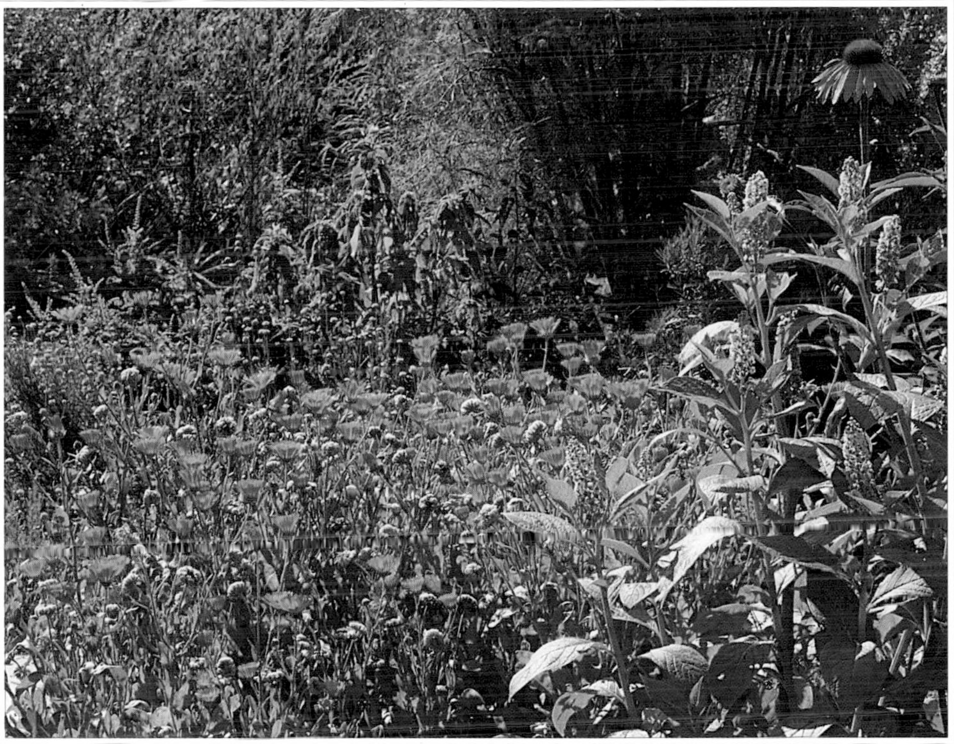

MARIGOLD *(Calendula officinalis)*

HOMEOPATHY

CARBO VEG: for a sluggish circulation leading to blueness of the skin, cold extremities and painful varicose veins.

HAMAMELIS: for swollen, congested veins with a purplish blotching under the skin and tired, aching legs; may also have piles.

PULSATILLA: for painful veins, blue in colour; may be associated with pregnancy; pains in legs eased with walking about and in cool, fresh air.

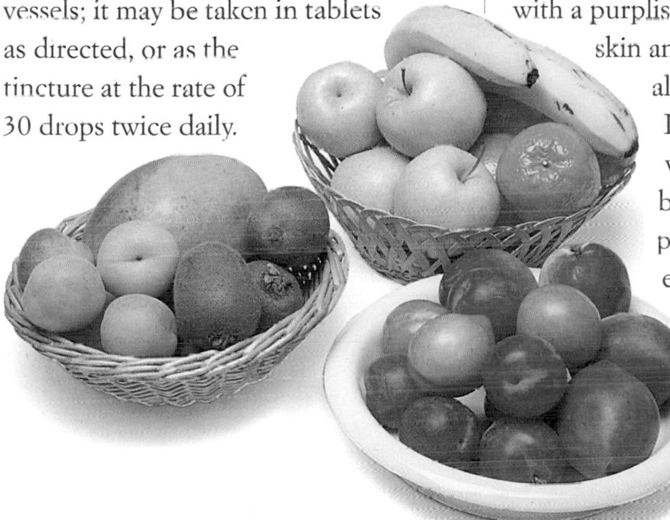

Plenty of fresh fruit is essential in any diet.

NATUROPATHY

Use hot and cold bathing of legs, or spray cool water up the legs at the end of a shower. Walk more; also look at yoga and swimming as good forms of exercise. Reduce alcohol intake; if very overweight try to lose weight steadily.

A supplement of Vitamin E (up to 400 iu daily), together with 5 ml (1 tsp) Lecithin granules daily, can ease the swelling and pains by improving the elasticity of the blood vessels; another helpful substance is Vitamin C (up to 500 mg). In the long term just take plenty of fresh fruit and vegetables and keep fats to a lower level.

THE DIGESTIVE SYSTEM

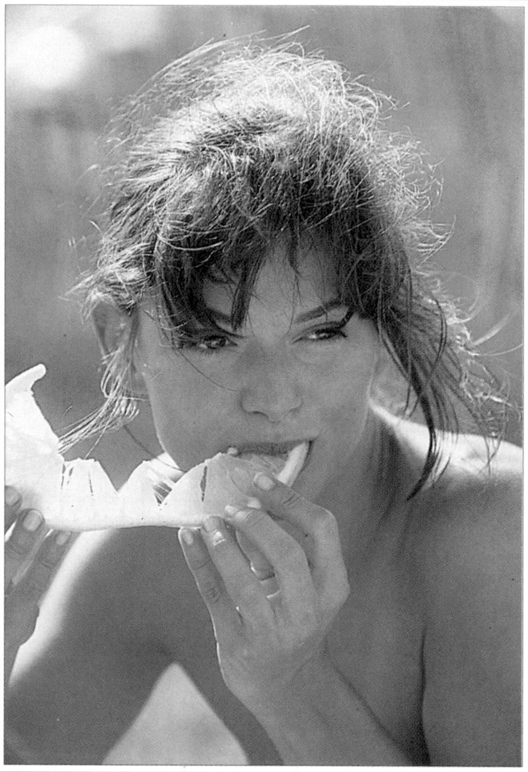

In many respects the digestive system is the most important set of organs in the body, for it is here that we absorb all the nutrients we need in order for all our cells to function and hence for us to survive. The old adage "we are what we eat" has a lot of validity, since poor nutrition can lead not only to problems such as constipation, flatulence or diarrhoea but also to more general ailments like headache, chronic tiredness, poor concentration and memory.

The digestive system is also an integral part of our immune defences, recognizing potentially toxic substances and either breaking them down into safer compounds or else eliminating them. Western dietary and lifestyle habits have created their own disorders, from gastric ulcers to constipation and irritable bowel syndrome; this last condition has become something of a "waste-basket diagnosis" – if nothing else shows up, then that is what you have! Treatment for this should really be individual, as stress, diet, posture and exercise all play a part in each person's symptoms.

ABOVE: Eating fresh fruit is a good way of increasing dietary fibre intake.

ACIDITY AND HEARTBURN

Many people get occasional bouts of acid dyspepsia, usually related to a temporary problem such as having eaten rich, spicy foods or having eaten too quickly when feeling rushed and stressed. If the symptoms happen very regularly, you may need to look more carefully at what you eat and how fast you eat it. If there is persistent discomfort, seek professional treatment; see also Flatulence and Indigestion (pages 59 and 61).

AROMATHERAPY

Using hot or warm compresses (see page 15) over the abdomen, with up to 10 drops of oils such as Chamomile or Lavender in a small bowl of water, can give relief from the inflammation and spasm that accompany excess acidity. These oils, diluted at 2 per cent in a base oil, can also be gently massaged into the abdomen if the discomfort is not too great.

HEARTBURN SYMPTOMS

When excess acid leaks back up into the gullet, this inflames and irritates the lining of the oesophagus and the feeling of heartburn is produced. Taking antacid tablets regularly may not only mask underlying problems, but can also be counter-productive as the stomach tries to compensate by creating more acid.

SLIPPERY ELM *(Ulmus fulva)*

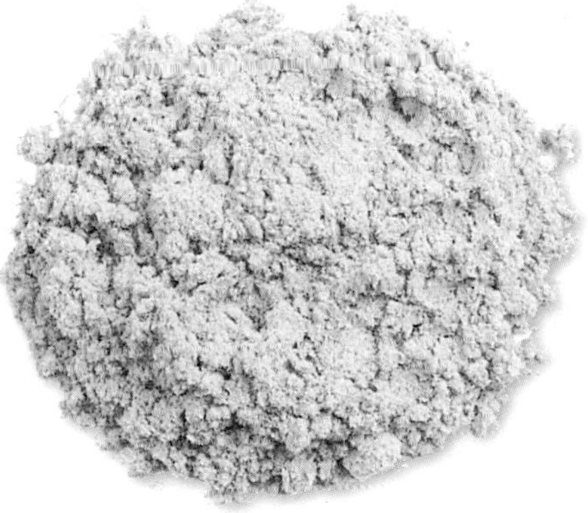

HERBALISM

Digestive disturbances generally respond very well indeed to herbal treatment, and acid dyspepsia can be improved considerably. For a temporary problem choose from the suggested herbs and use as warm teas; for repeated acid/heartburn symptoms use stronger, as infusions (see page 12) or as otherwise directed.

CHAMOMILE (*Chamomilla recutita*): a relaxant and anti-inflammatory remedy that helps the whole digestive tract; if acid symptoms are related to stress and/or over-eating of rich foods, this herb makes an excellent choice.

LEMON BALM *(Melissa officinalis)*: another excellent herb where the condition is caused by stress; if available use the fresh leaves for a much finer flavour.

MEADOWSWEET *(Filipendula ulmaria)*: although chemically related to aspirin, Meadowsweet is soothing for an inflamed stomach (but may need to be avoided if there is a hypersensitivity to salicylates such as aspirin) and reduces acidity.

SLIPPERY ELM *(Ulmus fulva)*: this is highly soothing to the inflamed gullet or stomach, and may be taken before meals, either as tablets or by mixing 5 ml (1 tsp) of the pure powder in a little warm water – it lives up to its name as it goes down, coating and soothing the membranes.

HOMEOPATHY

As usual, individual characteristics will determine proper prescribing of remedies, but initially choose from:

CARBO VEG: for a burning feeling in the stomach, and acid reflux with waterbrash (gas being brought up into the mouth with acidic fluid) and sometimes nausea; symptoms often caused by over-eating or drinking.

LYCOPODIUM: for definite heartburn, much wind and a feeling of fullness after only a little food.

NUX VOMICA: when taken too much rich food, alcohol and coffee leading to nausea and acidity but also an empty, hungry feeling in the stomach.

NATUROPATHY

Often a glass of milk is suggested as a temporary measure, to neutralize the acid. This is not always suitable, and certainly not on a regular basis, as dairy produce can create its own digestive problems. It may be helpful to avoid solids for up to 24 hours after a bad bout of acid heartburn. Using a hot compress over the abdomen can relieve pains. Avoid coffee, alcohol, tobacco, chocolate, pastries or spicy foods for at least a couple of days, and if prone to this complaint, then try to slowly cut them out.

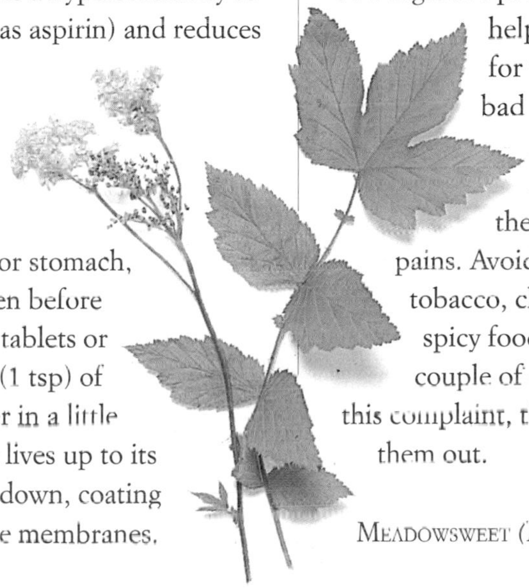

MEADOWSWEET *(Filipendula ulmaria)*

COLIC

Colic is the term used to describe spasmodic bouts of cramping pains, especially in the bowel which often associated with trapped gas; see Flatulence (page 59). Colic is especially common in babies. The symptom may be related to tension generally, but if there are other digestive disturbances, do seek professional advice. It is always a sensible precaution to seek medical advice where babies are concerned.

Abdomen Massage

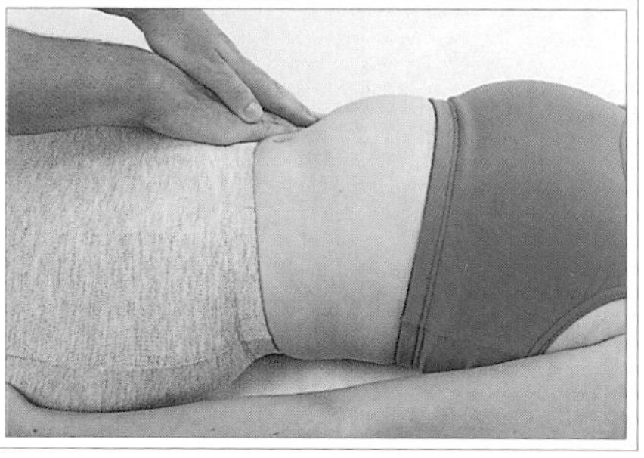

1 Starting in the lower right hand corner, steadily but firmly press in with both hands.

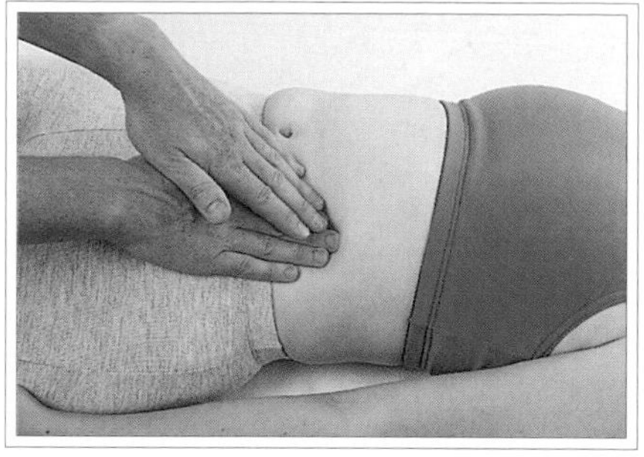

2 Slowly move hands in a clockwise direction around the abdomen, using small circles to massage the colon.

AROMATHERAPY

Gentle massage of the abdomen, in a clockwise direction, using oils of Chamomile, Fennel or Peppermint will help – dilute the oils at the ratio of 3-4 drops per 5 ml (1 tsp) of base oil.

HERBALISM

For an occasional attack of colic, use hot teas of Catmint *(Nepeta cataria)*, Chamomile *(Chamomilla recutita)*, Fennel *(Foeniculum vulgare)*, Ginger *(Zingiber officinalis)* or Peppermint *(Mentha piperita)*. Using aromatic seeds like Aniseed *(Pimpinella anisum)*, Caraway *(Carum carvi)*, Dill *(Anethum graveolens)* or Fennel *(Foeniculum vulgare)* in food, or simply chewing a few of the seeds after a meal can help a lot if you are prone to colic after eating. If the problem is frequent, get professional treatment.

HOMEOPATHY

BRYONIA: if the spasms are made worse by any movement, or by local heat, better by lying still with bent knees.

CHAMOMILLA: especially good for colicky babies, or teething infants; the bloated abdomen tends to be improved by local warmth, such as a hot water bottle.

MAGNESIA PHOSPHORICA: if warmth, pressure over the abdomen and walking about ease the discomfort, but burping does not.

NUX VOMICA: for colic brought on by over-eating or drinking alcohol; symptoms eased by sitting or lying down, and worse if upright.

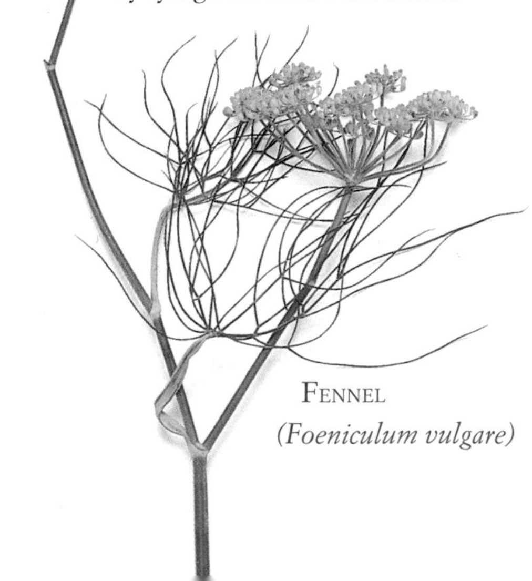

FENNEL
(Foeniculum vulgare)

NATUROPATHY

In most cases local warmth over the lower abdomen helps; a hot-water bottle is the easiest method. Internally, herbal teas, as detailed above, will give the best relief, as they not only reduce spasm but aid digestion too. It may well be necessary to look at and treat other digestive problems; see also entries for Constipation, Diarrhoea and Gall-Bladder Problems (pages 57, 58 and 60). If frequent colic occurs, do look at how fast you eat, whether you curl up into a comfortable chair after a meal, or if your diet has a lot of fatty, spicy foods or dairy produce. If any of these apply, try to change that pattern and see if the colic improves without needing other treatment; if not get advice. Often it is most helpful simply to eat meals in a more relaxed way, rather than gulping food down while "on the run".

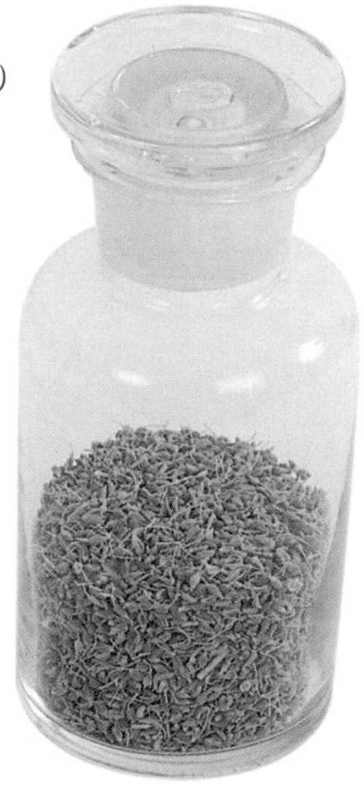

ANISEED
(Pimpinella anisum)

CONSTIPATION

This is a problem that is largely confined to a typical Western diet and lifestyle. Inadequate amounts of dietary fibre, and perhaps a lack of exercise, lead to the slow passage of faeces through the bowel and this in turn allows water to be re-absorbed, leaving hardened, rabbit-like stools. The frequency of bowel movements is less important than the harder consistency; straining can cause piles (see Haemorrhoids, page 50).

AROMATHERAPY

One of the most effective methods of self-help is daily clockwise massage of the lower abdomen (see page 50), and this can be performed using 2 drops of oils of Lavender, Marjoram or Rosemary in 5 ml (1 tsp) of base oil. Lavender and Marjoram are more relaxing, if tension is a factor, while Rosemary has a more tonic effect.

HERBALISM

Always start with gentle laxatives, or aperients, which increase bowel tone without giving griping. One of the best is Dandelion Root *(Taraxacum officinale)*, ideally taken as a decoction (see page 12) – although you may get a gentle action from one of the Dandelion coffee drinks on the market. Another simple herb to use is Liquorice *(Glycyrrhiza glabra)*; either chew one of the liquorice sticks that you can buy from a health food shop or add it to the Dandelion Root for the decoction. If constipation persists, switch to trying another herb that works in quite a different way. Linseed *(Linum usitatissimum)* absorbs liquid and creates a soft bulk internally that aids the peristaltic wave movements that propel faeces through the bowel. Take 10 ml (2 tsp) at breakfast, with at least 300 ml (½ pt/1¼ cups) of water. Ideally soak the Linseed overnight in a little water to start the swelling process. It may look like frog-spawn but it can relieve tense constipation! Make sure you take plenty of liquids however.

TYPES OF CONSTIPATION

There are essentially two types of constipation. Where there is inadequate fibre and a sluggish digestive system, treatment should be aimed at toning up the bowel; when the constipation is linked to high levels of stress and spasm, see Colic (page 56), treatment may need to focus on relaxation and even reducing excessive fibre such as bran. If in doubt seek professional treatment, as the regular use of laxatives may be completely counter-productive. Given that approaching $500 million are spent in the United States each year on self-prescribed laxatives, there are good reasons to look at more natural ways!

HOMEOPATHY

As usual, try to match the symptom pattern to the person.

BRYONIA: for hard, dry stools with much thirst and a dry mouth too. The stools can look a very dark brown colour.

NUX VOMICA: for a bloated abdomen; after a bowel movement there is a definite feeling that the bowel has not been properly emptied. Often due to a history of over-eating and chronic use of laxatives.

SULPHUR: for dark, hard stools which are moved only with pain and straining and may cause a burning sensation. Sometimes there is a pattern of alternating constipation and looseness.

NATUROPATHY

In most instances, increase dietary fibre by eating more fresh vegetables and fruit, whole grains and beans or pulses. Bran is a somewhat excessive form of fibre when taken on its own rather than as part of a wholefood meal, so take only small amounts of it, if at all. Ensure that you increase exercise, particularly for the abdominal muscles, and regularly do deeper breathing exercises to encourage the diaphragm to move up and down; this acts internally to massage part of the colon and aid peristalsis.

If constipation occurs after antibiotic treatment, the normal intestinal bacteria can be stimulated by taking a Vitamin B complex supplement, and also with *Lactobacillus acidophilus*. This is the bacteria that turns milk into yoghurt. Taking a little plain, *live* yoghurt daily may do the trick; if this is not enough or if sensitive to dairy foods try one of the proprietary acidophilus supplements.

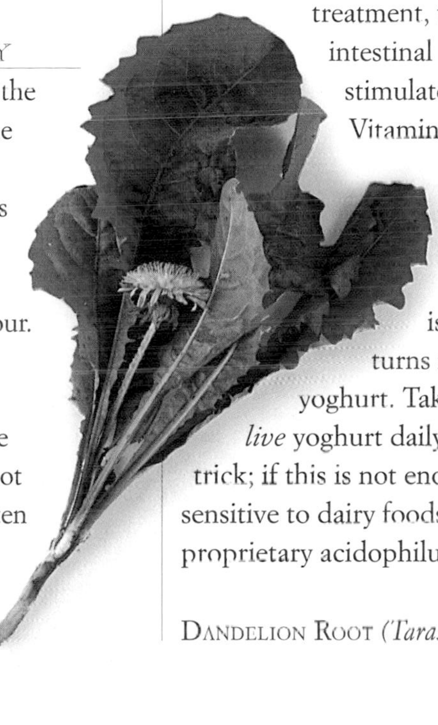

DANDELION ROOT *(Taraxacum officinale)*

DIARRHOEA

Loose, frequent bowel movements can happen as a short-term reaction to infection, inflammation or food poisoning, and as such are quite a positive, cleansing action. A common experience is holiday diarrhoea, and this is usually a response to exposure to unfamiliar bacteria.

AROMATHERAPY

Massage of the abdomen (see page 56) with antiseptic and relaxing oils like Chamomile, Lavender and Neroli can ease diarrhoea caused by minor upsets and also by anxiety and nervousness. Eucalyptus can be used in the same way if an infection is definitely suspected as the cause. Add Fennel or Ginger if there are griping pains with the diarrhoea. For all these oils, dilute to 3 per cent in a base oil.

HERBALISM

If mild food poisoning or infection has upset the bowels, as well as a choice of infusions (see page 12) listed below, try eating garlic as a natural gut disinfectant.

AGRIMONY *(Agrimonia eupatoria)*: astringent and healing to the inflamed and swollen membrane lining the gut, helpful in mild gastro-enteritis.

CHAMOMILE *(Chamomilla recutita)*: calming and anti-inflammatory, reduces the impact of tension on the digestive tract. This is one of the first herbs to think of in many digestive disorders.

MEADOWSWEET *(Filipendula ulmaria)*: this will help to settle an acidic stomach, see Acidity and Heartburn (page 55), as well as being mildly astringent.

RIBWORT *(Plantago lanceolata)*: this has excellent toning, soothing and healing properties for use in diarrhoea from many causes, where there is inflammation.

THYME *(Thymus vulgaris)*: this will fight infections and improve digestion generally, settling churning, loose bowels and killing harmful bacteria.

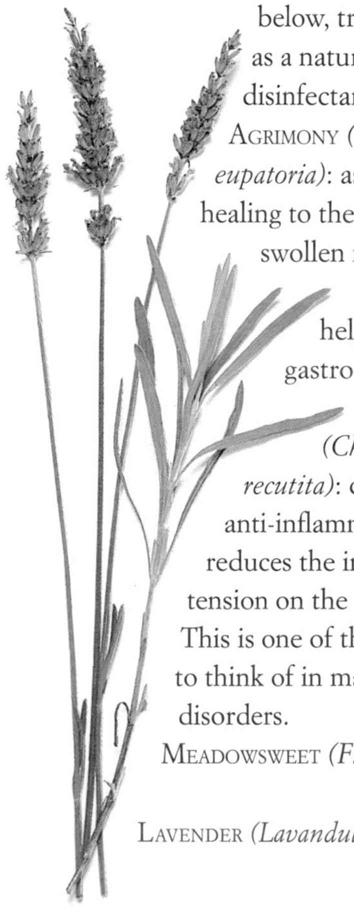

LAVENDER *(Lavandula angustifolia)*

CAUSES OF DIARRHOEA

Some foods have a laxative effect naturally, for instance prunes or figs, so over-indulgence will give temporary diarrhoea. Stress and anxiety often increase peristalsis and hurry bowel contents through. Repeated diarrhoea may indicate more complex digestive problems and should be treated professionally. Prolonged diarrhoea, especially in young children, can be quite serious as it causes dehydration; ensure adequate fluid intake and seek professional advice. A simple yet dramatically effective rehydration drink can be made by dissolving 5 ml (1 tsp) salt and 15 ml (1 tbsp) sugar in 600 ml (1 pt/ 2 1/2 cups) of boiled water. Keep in the refrigerator in a screw-topped bottle and give small amounts frequently. Use for a short time only.

HOMEOPATHY

Many homeopathic remedies feature diarrhoea in their symptom "picture"; three generally useful remedies are:

ARSENICUM ALBUM: typically for diarrhoea from food infected with bacteria; the stools tend to be burning to the skin, dark, greenish brown and smelly.

NUX VOMICA: diarrhoea alternating with constipation, due to over-rich foods, alcohol and so on. Worse after a large meal, any discomfort is relieved by bowel movement.

PULSATILLA: rich, fatty meals, or foods like onions, or excessive nervousness are common triggers for the diarrhoea. The stools are very variable. (Pulsatilla people tend to be gentle, shy, pale and prone to being weepy if ill.)

NATUROPATHY

Try not to use treatments to stem diarrhoea for at least 24 hours, to allow any natural cleansing process to take place. Take plenty of fluids, especially mineral water or herb teas if warm drinks are desired. Moving on to easily assimilated foods such as soups, fruit or vegetable juices helps replace lost nutrients, speeds up recovery and lets the inflamed bowel settle. Plain boiled rice is one of the best first solids, or possibly dry toast.

It may be useful to consider a multi-mineral supplement if diarrhoea was intense, to replenish the minerals lost. Fruit and vegetables can soon be returned to the diet as well.

FLATULENCE

The accumulation of gas in the stomach or intestines can occur as an isolated event, for instance after a meal containing particularly wind-producing foods, or can be a constant, chronic sign of a digestive problem. In the latter case, it may indicate a condition such as diverticulitis or irritable bowel syndrome, and these will need to be addressed in order to sort out the causes of the flatulence.

AROMATHERAPY

Many essential oils have a carminative action, which means that they help to shift gas out of the digestive system (up or down, depending where it is!) and also reduce bloating and spasm that can go with the wind. It may be most appropriate, however, to use the aromatic herbs from which the oils are extracted (see Herbalism entry below). Oils such as Caraway, Chamomile, Fennel, Marjoram and Peppermint could also be used as a warm compress (see page 15) over the abdomen to help relieve the symptoms; use up to 5 drops in a small bowl of warm water.

HERBALISM

A number of herbal teas are excellent at relieving flatulence, but do remember that if this is a major problem to get professional herbal treatment. Choose from Catmint *(Nepeta cataria)*, Chamomile *(Chamomilla recutita)*, Lemon Balm *(Melissa officinalis)* or Peppermint *(Mentha piperita)* if the problem is in the stomach; any of these plus Dill *(Anethum graveolens)* or Fennel *(Foeniculum vulgare)* if the small intestines seem to be affected, and Ginger *(Zingiber officinalis)* or Peppermint *(Mentha piperita)* for bowel flatulence, although there are several others that may be useful depending on the problem (see other entries in this section).

Eating Habits

A useful starting point for self-treatment of flatulence is to look at eating habits; are you eating very quickly, while tense, or grabbing a bite to eat "on the run"? This is likely to lead to swallowing gas with the food; inadequate digestive enzymes may be produced and the meal can ferment in the intestines rather than be properly digested. This leads to more gas being created and flatulence gets worse. Also, take care not to do a lot of bending, or sitting curled up on a low sofa, immediately after a meal, as this encourages a gas build-up with bloating and collicky pains.

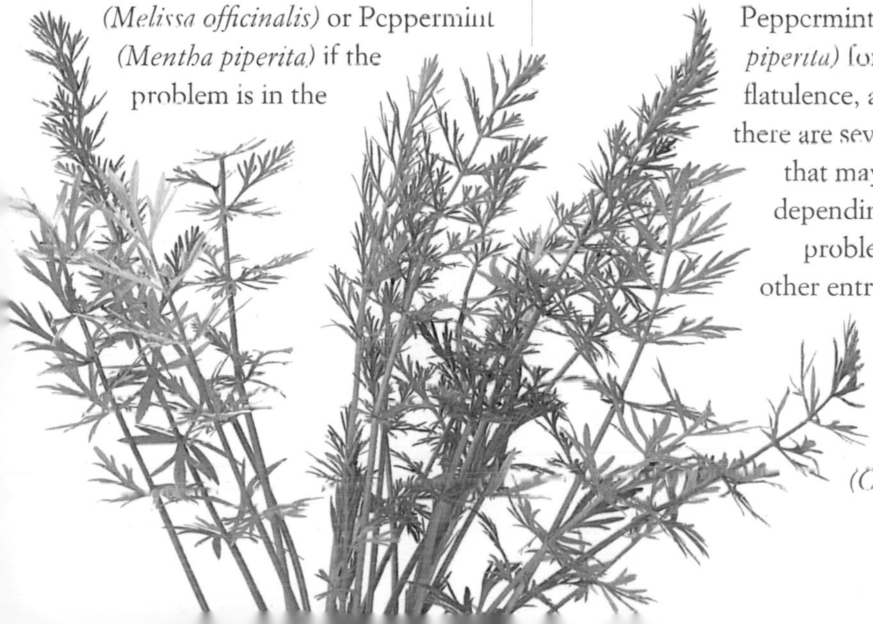

Caraway *(Carum carvi)*

HOMEOPATHY

Several remedies featured elsewhere in this section may help; try to look beyond the flatulence to deeper causes and seek the remedy for those. Initially, pick from Chamomilla, Carbo veg, Nux vomica or Pulsatilla, for flatulence brought on by eating too rich or too big a meal.

NATUROPATHY

Often flatulence can be caused by eating too heavy a mixture of foods – consider reducing the fat content of your diet, and restricting the combinations of proteins and carbohydrates you eat. If this helps a lot, then you might want to consider exploring the Hay system of eating.

One reason for flatulence can be after administration of antibiotics, as the intestinal bacteria have been decimated; these can be encouraged to multiply by taking plain "live" yoghurt, or possibly more concentrated supplements such as *acidophilus* tablets/powders. A high-fibre, raw-food diet is often recommended for general health; this is in itself likely to give you more gas, especially if you switch over suddenly to this kind of diet. The increase in bacteria needed to cope with the fibre creates a lot of wind. Some flatulence is therefore quite natural, if not exactly sociable! It is often better to change the diet more gradually to ease the problem.

GALL-BLADDER PROBLEMS

Gallstones may steadily grow in size or number with very few symptoms for a long time, except perhaps increased indigestion or flatulence, but may cause acute colic if the gall-bladder gets inflamed. Gallstones need professional treatment, and sometimes surgery, but there is much that can be done to ease the discomfort alongside qualified medical help.

AROMATHERAPY

Not really a first-choice discipline, but warm compresses (see page 15) over the right side of the abdomen, using diluted oils of Lavender, Marjoram or Rosemary, may relieve spasm and colic.

HERBALISM

Start with the most gentle herbs. If gallstones are definitely present, a scan is needed to establish their size before any treatment is prescribed.
CHAMOMILE *(Chamomilla recutita)* tea is both anti-inflammatory and anti-spasmodic, and gently stimulates the whole digestive process.
DANDELION ROOT *(Taraxacum officinale)* is an excellent mild liver tonic; ideally make a decoction (see page 12) and take a small cupful twice a day. Look also at the herbs listed for Colic and for Flatulence (pages 56 and 59); they are likely in most cases to aid digestion and relieve congestion in the liver and gall-bladder.

MARJORAM *(Origanum majorana)*

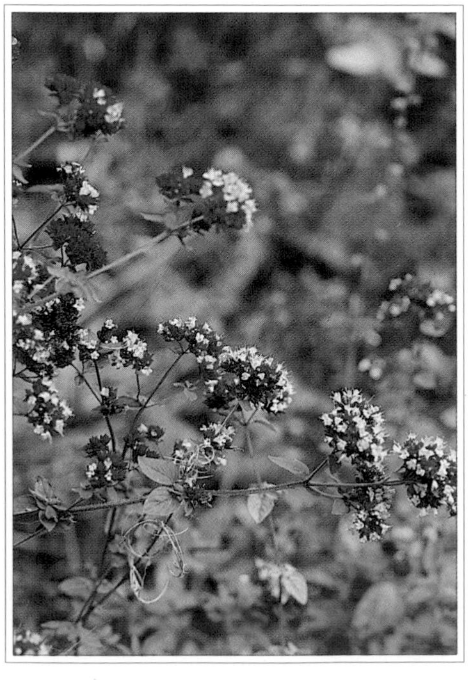

DANDELION DECOCTION

Although dandelion leaves can be made into a tea, a stronger medicine can be made from the roots by making a decoction.

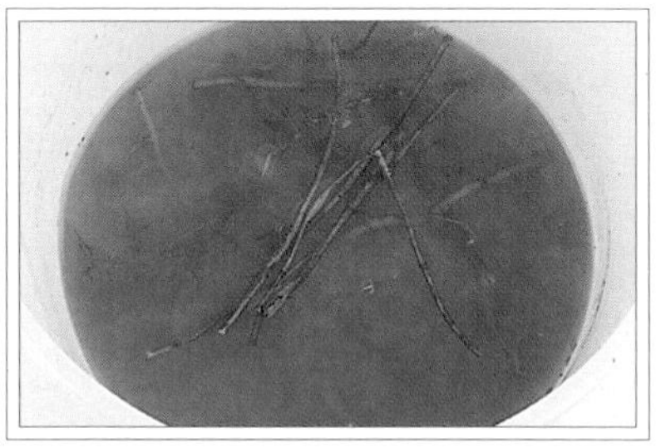

1 Simmer 50 g (2 oz) clean, chopped root in water.

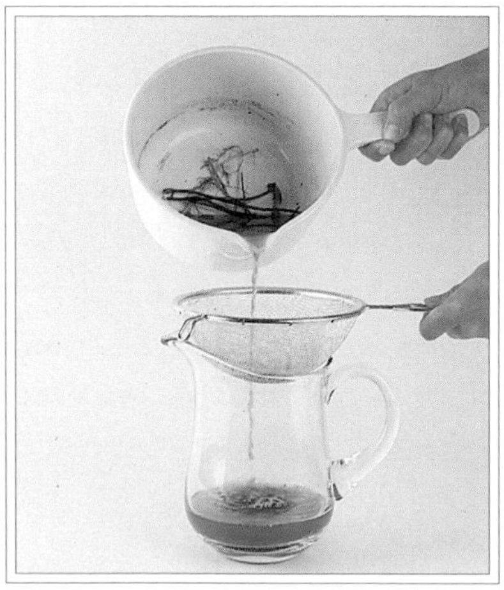

2 Strain through a sieve and store in the fridge. Give in doses of 5-20 ml (1 tsp-1½ tbsp), 3 times a day. It will keep for 3 days.

ROSEMARY *(Rosmarinus officinalis)*

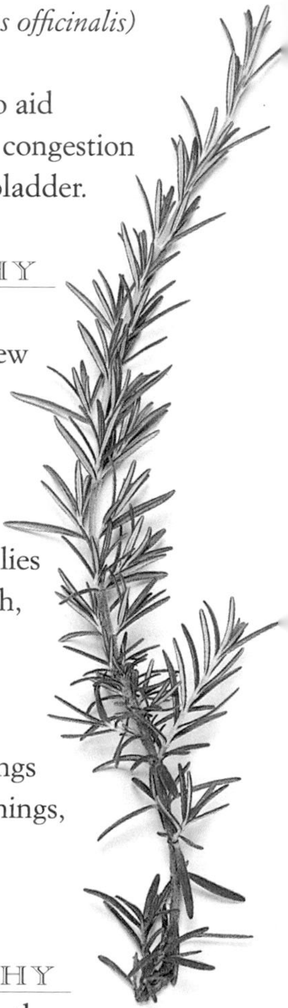

HOMEOPATHY

As a short-term measure, try a few doses of either of these before consulting a qualified practitioner:
BRYONIA: where food lies heavily in the stomach, there may be nausea, biliousness and headache.
NUX VOMICA: for feelings of nausea in the mornings, if brought on by rich meals.

NATUROPATHY

Disturbances in the gall-bladder, with or without gallstones, will affect how well fats are digested, so the first step is to restrict animal fats and dairy produce, while increasing vegetables and fruit. To encourage bile production and flow, eat vegetables such as artichokes and bitter salads such as endive and chicory, as well as taking plenty of garlic and fruit to reduce cholesterol (lemon juice is powerful in this respect). Use smaller amounts of light oils such as Olive, Sunflower and Safflower in dressings.

INDIGESTION

Indigestion is a general term for discomfort, often accompanied by bloating, acidity, heartburn, nausea or bowel disturbances (see other entries in this section). Usually it is a temporary problem, brought about by eating too much or the wrong kind of food, excess alcohol or from stress. Longer-term digestive pains may be caused among other reasons by taking aspirin-related drugs, by heavy smoking or other digestive ailments.

AROMATHERAPY

A warm compress (see page 15) including Chamomile or Lavender oils may give some relief, or try gently massaging a 2 per cent dilution of one of them into the abdomen if indigestion is milder.

HERBALISM

Herbal teas in the first place may well sort out the immediate indigestion, choose from:

CHAMOMILE *(Chamomilla recutita)*: for the effects of over-eating, also if in a stressed state.

LEMON BALM *(Melissa officinalis)*: for nervous indigestion; related to meals or not, settles a churning stomach.

MEADOWSWEET *(Filipendula ulmaria)*: for acid indigestion, especially if accompanied by some looseness in the bowels.

LEMON BALM *(Melissa officinalis)*

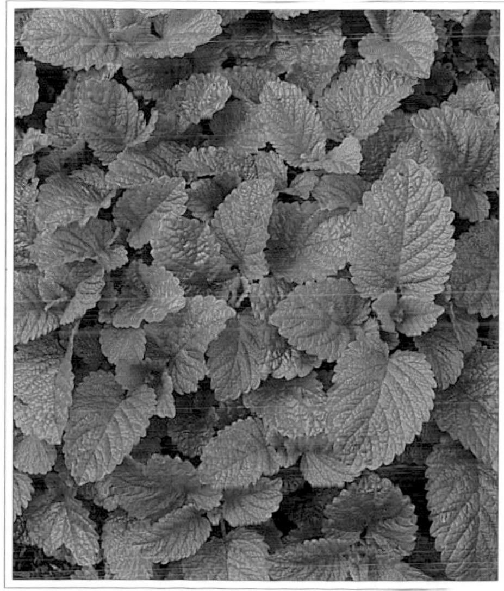

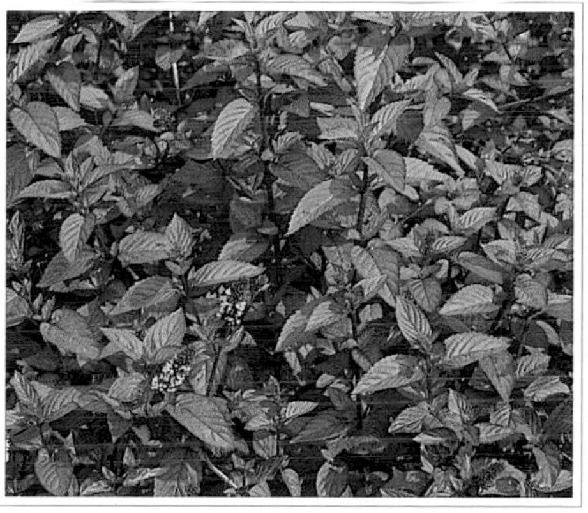

PEPPERMINT *(Mentha piperita)*

PEPPERMINT *(Mentha piperita)*: for indigestion with plenty of flatulence and bloated abdomen, or even nausea. Also think of taking Slippery Elm *(Ulmus fulva)* if indigestion pains are persistent, either 5 ml (1 tsp) of the powder blended in a cupful of water, or the pure tablets, with one or more meals, to soothe the stomach.

HOMEOPATHY

For an occasional bout of indigestion, try a couple of doses (see page 10) of:

ARGENT NIT: where there is a lot of wind, with belching and possibly heartburn, a craving for sweet or fatty foods which tend to upset the digestion and give diarrhoea.

LYCOPODIUM: for pains and wind; if hungry but can only take small amounts of food, worse with cold foods or drink.

NUX VOMICA: useful for the effects of eating and drinking too much, causing pain, heartburn and even vomiting.

NATUROPATHY

If indigestion is quite bad, cut out solid food for 24 hours if possible, taking only herb teas or fruit juices (particularly pineapple which contains digestive enzymes), and reintroduce foods gently, starting with something light like soup or puréed apple. If indigestion is repetitive, try taking a Vitamin B complex supplement as a digestive stimulant, or else look at a digestive enzyme supplement such as Pepsin in the short term, but it may be better to get professional treatment. Avoid drinking lots of fluid at mealtimes, as this will dilute your natural digestive juices.

Chamomile tea is a relaxing aid to the digestive system.

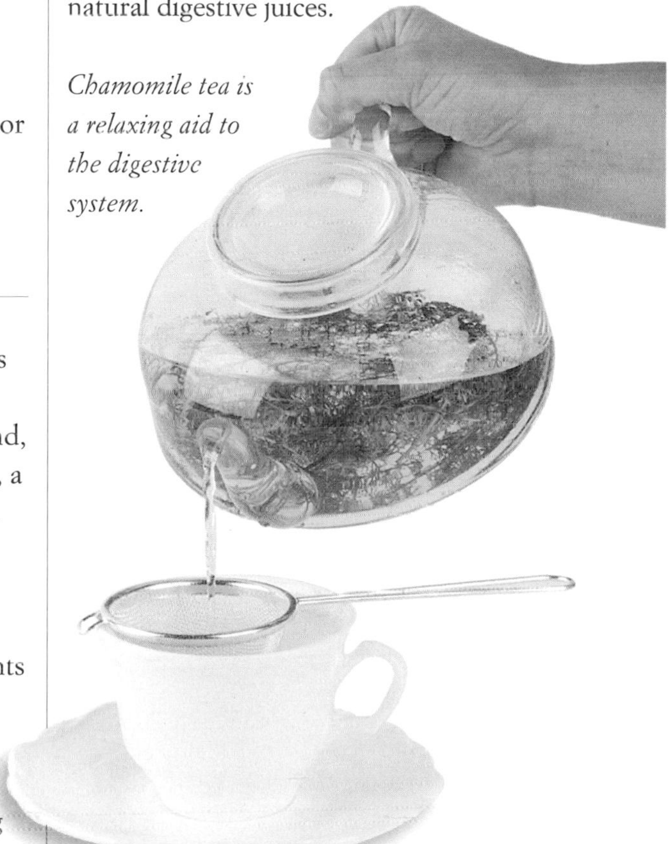

MOUTH ULCERS

These small ulcers, that can occur on the tongue, gums or the lining of the mouth, are sometimes due to local trauma, for instance biting your cheek or wearing ill-fitting dentures, but often they reflect a state of generally being run-down. Recurrent "crops" of mouth ulcers may therefore need more overall treatment; see Stress (pages 28-9) as well as anything directed locally.

AROMATHERAPY

The essential oil of choice for treating mouth ulcers is undoubtedly Myrrh. This is not only astringent and healing but also has an anti-fungal property; one of the reasons for mouth ulcers can be fungal infection, for example *Candida albicans* (the cause of thrush). Myrrh is best used in tincture form (see Herbalism below); you can make your own in small amounts by dissolving the essential oil in alcohol – use 5 drops in 5 ml (1 tsp) of a spirit such as vodka or brandy. This can be applied neat right on to the ulcers, or use 2.5 ml (½ tsp) in a little water as a mouthwash. You can add 1 drop of oil of Fennel to make it taste better, dissolving it thoroughly.

HERBALISM

Local treatment is by means of herbal tinctures (see page 14), to stimulate healing and reduce the inflammation. The strongest, although worst tasting, is Myrrh *(Commiphora molmol)*; others to choose from are Marigold *(Calendula officinalis)*, Sage *(Salvia officinalis)* and Thyme *(Thymus vulgaris)*. Pay attention to general health, and seek professional treatment if the ulcers are persistent or recurring. Cone Flower *(Echinacea angustifolia* or *E. purpurea)* may be a useful herb to take; it boosts the immune system and is widely obtainable in tablet form, or a tincture of the fresh plant is also available – take 10 drops in water 3 times a day.

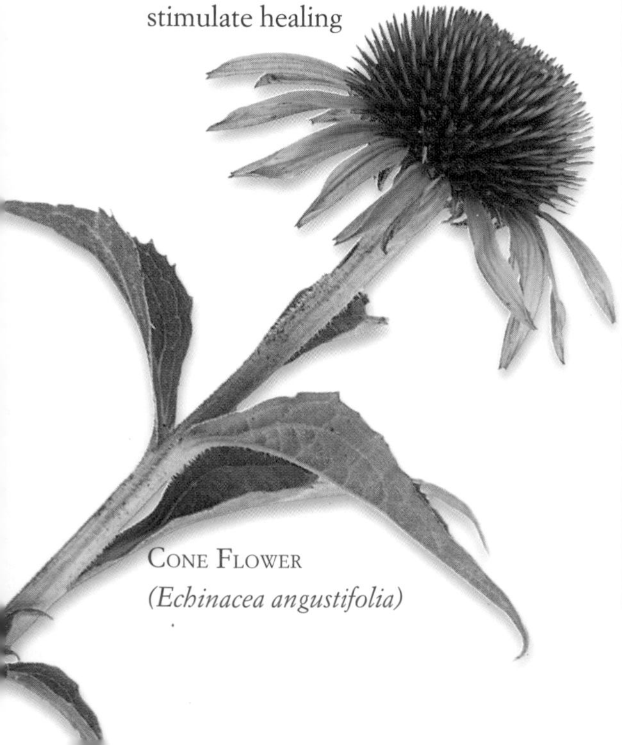

Cone Flower *(Echinacea angustifolia)*

HOMEOPATHY

Remedies are more likely to be of benefit if they are chosen for the background causes, but some examples of those remedies that are of value for the ulcers are:

Borax: for painful small ulcers that feel hot in the mouth and may even bleed, when eating for instance.

Merc sol: when there is an unpleasant, metallic taste in the mouth, with larger, almost greyish ulcers and perhaps bleeding gums; good for oral thrush.

Nat sulph: for very painfully sensitive ulcers which may look like blisters, the discomfort is relieved by something cold such as an ice cube.

NATUROPATHY

Recurrent mouth ulcers can often indicate a poor diet, or nutritional deficiencies. Nutrients most likely to be lacking, and consequently of most benefit in treating the problem, are Vitamin B2, Vitamin C and zinc, and supplements of these may be needed in the short term until the diet can be improved to give sufficient amounts – increase green leafy vegetables, fresh fruit, whole grain bread (including the wheatgerm) and for non-vegetarians eat some meat and fish.

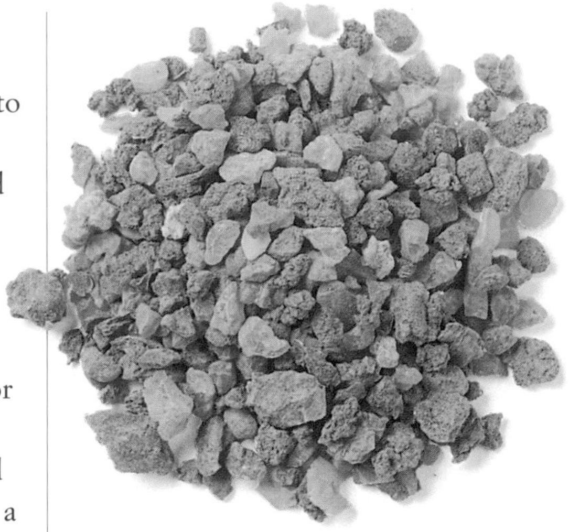

Myrrh *(Commiphora molmol)*

Mouth ulcers most often occur at times of stress or when the immune system is lowered in some way, so it is generally advisable to look at ways of reducing the impact of stress (see pages 28-9) if ulcers are recurring frequently.

For direct local treatment, try applying pure wheatgerm oil, for example by piercing a natural, oil-based Vitamin E capsule, and dabbing a little on to the ulcer. If there are foods, for instance vinegar, that do aggravate the ulcers, obviously leave them out of the diet for a while.

NAUSEA AND VOMITING

There are a great many reasons for feelings of nausea, or actual vomiting. Often this is a temporary reaction, for example to over-eating or drinking, food poisoning, a gastric infection, violent coughing, travel sickness, or associated with a migraine; if nausea or vomiting is persistent, then professional help is essential. Children in particular can easily become dehydrated from repeatedly vomiting.

AROMATHERAPY

Warm compresses (see page 15) over the stomach may be of help. Choose from oils of Chamomile, Lavender or Peppermint, up to 5 drops in a small bowl of water. Taking 1 drop *only* of oil of Cloves or Peppermint, on a sugar lump, may help to directly settle the stomach. A useful oil to spray around the sick room is Lemon, this is not only helpful to allay feelings of nausea but also is much fresher smelling and less sickly than some oils, so will be generally appreciated by the household!

HERBALISM

The remedy of first choice is probably Ginger *(Zingiber officinalis)*; either take frequent sips of a weak tea, or of 10 drops of tincture (see page14) in a little water, or chew a small piece of fresh ginger. Another possibility – say, for travel sickness – is to chew a little crystallized ginger, or drink flat ginger ale.

Other potentially useful herbs to settle the stomach are Chamomile *(Chamomilla recutita)*, Lemon Balm *(Melissa officinalis)* and Peppermint *(Mentha piperita)*; try weakish herb teas. All these herbs aid digestion generally, and ease flatulence, so can help to sort out the causes of nausea as well as the symptoms themselves.

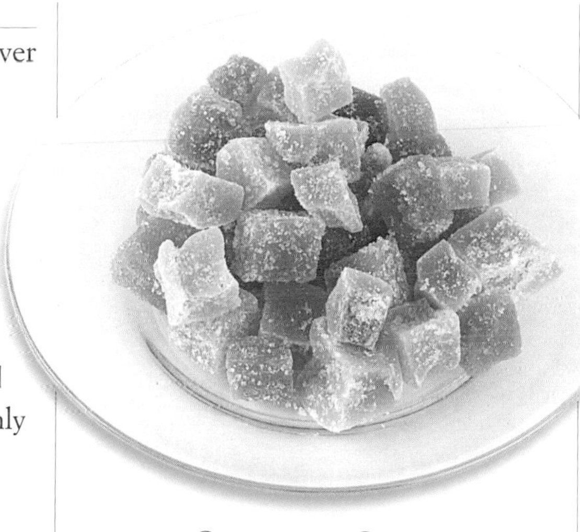

CRYSTALLIZED GINGER

CAUSES OF NAUSEA

Nausea or vomiting can usually be linked to a specific situation eating too much rich food, or drinking too much alcohol, anxiety or travel are common triggers. Continual feelings of nausea indicate a greater disturbance; again this may be obvious as in morning sickness of pregnancy. Where the cause is not obvious, and if symptoms are not quickly cleared up with self-help, get medical advice as soon as possible.

HOMEOPATHY

As ever, try to establish the causes and the overall pattern. In the meantime, useful remedies include:

ARSENICUM ALBUM: for severe nausea, perhaps associated with diarrhoea, and a great thirst but unable to take more than a few sips at a time.

IPECACUANHA: for sudden and persistent nausea or vomiting, with much watery saliva and frequent belching; symptoms are made worse by cold drinks.

NUX VOMICA: following over-indulgence or excessive drinking, nausea may come on soon after the meal, with waterbrash and food coming back into the mouth.

NATUROPATHY

Obviously keep off solids in the short term, but do keep up fluid intake, either warm or cool drinks depending on preference. When the sickness has subsided, re-introduce light, easily assimilated foods such as clear soup, then slightly more solid dishes like plain whole grain toast, boiled brown rice and cooked vegetables. Gradually return to your normal diet over a couple of days. Smaller meals will be helpful. If anxiety is producing the nausea, then relaxation exercises will help; see Anxiety and Stress (pages 19 and 28-9).

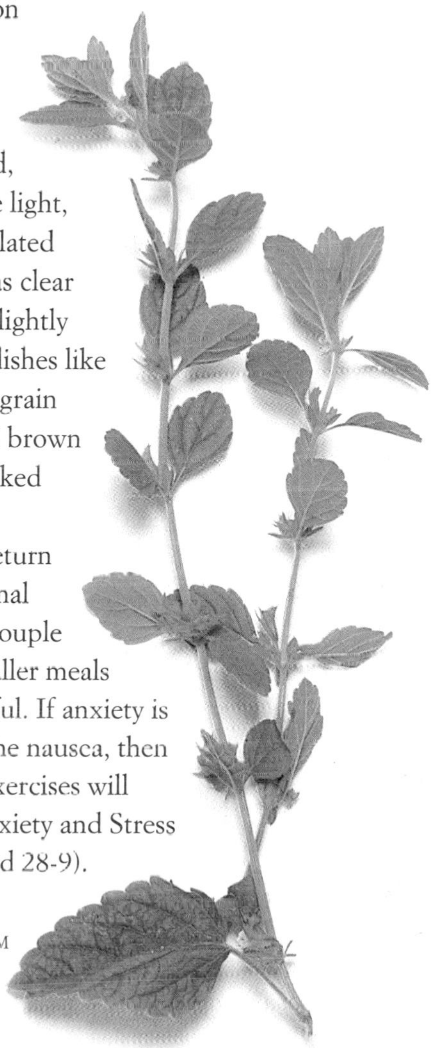

LEMON BALM *(Melissa officinalis)*

MORNING SICKNESS

At least half of all pregnant women experience nausea or vomiting during the first 12 weeks or so of their pregnancy; only in rare circumstances does this become so severe as to warrant drugs or hospital treatment. There seems to be good reason to link the sickness, which may actually occur at any time of day or night, with a lowered blood sugar level, and it is often very useful to eat regularly to maintain a more even state.

AROMATHERAPY

Essential oils can be of some use in this condition – their concentration and powerful effects, however, mean that caution is needed during pregnancy with all oils (see page 64 for further advice). For nausea, simply try smelling a drop of Ginger or Peppermint oil on a paper tissue.

HERBALISM

The prime remedy for nausea, including morning sickness, is Ginger *(Zingiber officinalis)*. This can be taken in various ways; try chewing a piece of crystallized ginger, or even a piece of peeled fresh ginger, or making ginger tea and sipping frequently. A very useful method is to eat biscuits (cookies) made with fresh ginger, nibbling one as and when the need arises – this temporarily raises the body's sugar level as well as providing the effect of the ginger itself. Other useful herbs are Chamomile *(Chamomilla recutita)* and Peppermint *(Mentha piperita)* taken as teas; as a practitioner I have found that in pregnancy the smell of the former often seems to be more off-putting than any benefit from the herb, but see for yourself.

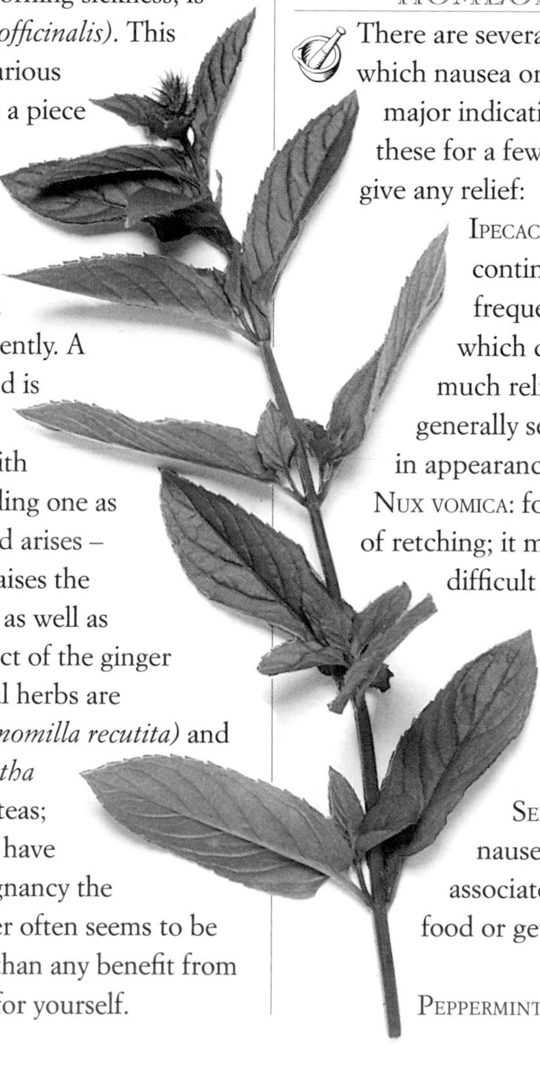

PEPPERMINT *(Mentha piperita)*

CAUTION

While the suggestions made here are all well-tried and safe, it is not advisable to self-treat during pregnancy. This book is not a substitute for seeking professional or medical advice, this is especially true for ailments during pregnancy.

HOMEOPATHY

There are several remedies in which nausea or vomiting are major indications; try one of these for a few days to see if they give any relief:

IPECACUANHA: for continual nausea, and frequent vomiting, which does not give much relief. The tongue generally seems quite clean in appearance.

NUX VOMICA: for nausea and a lot of retching; it may be more difficult to vomit but it does help ease the nausea. The tongue is coated and may look almost brown.

SEPIA: mostly just for nausea, especially associated with smelling food or getting chilled; or when the symptom is relieved with warm drinks or possibly a warm application to the stomach.

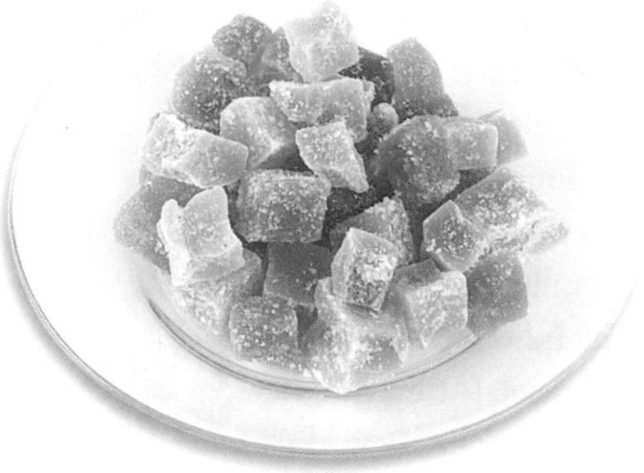

GINGER *(Zingiber officinalis)*

NATUROPATHY

The fact that early morning is a particularly bad time for getting the nausea confirms the importance of the blood-sugar levels; try keeping some whole grain biscuits by the bed to nibble if you feel empty and nauseous on waking. In general avoid greasy or fatty foods and cut down on coffee and alcohol. A diet with plenty of whole grains, pulses and vegetables will help to keep blood-sugar levels more constant, as will eating at regular times during the day.

Eating a piece of fruit when hungry can help keep nausea at bay.

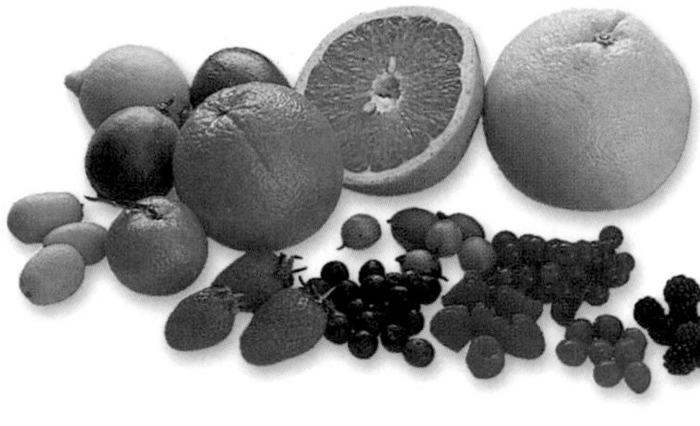

PRE-MENSTRUAL SYMPTOMS

There are a number of symptoms that can occur in the second half of the menstrual cycle, i.e. leading up to the period, due mostly to imbalances in hormone production. These symptoms tend to be lumped together by the medical profession into pre-menstrual syndrome (PMS), but not all women experience them in the same combination or in the same way.

AROMATHERAPY

Essential oils can be helpful in reducing fluid retention; this is most effectively done by using them with lymphatic drainage massage, so do see a professional aromatherapist if this is a major part of your symptoms. Using oils such as Geranium, Grapefruit, Juniper or Rosemary in the bath, and also doing skin-brushing, frequently stroking your limbs up from the extremities towards the heart, are good methods of self-help.

HERBALISM

Probably the most valuable herb for disturbances of the second half of the menstrual cycle is Chaste Tree *(Vitex agnus castus)*. The berries are used, and they help to normalize hormone function, particularly in lifting progesterone levels – lowered progesterone is most often the trigger for the symptoms. They can be obtained in tablet form. In very large amounts Chaste Tree can give an irritating sensation under the skin; if this occurs simply stop taking it.

Herbs which have diuretic effects may be useful in giving some relief; try infusions (see page 12) of either Cleavers *(Galium aparine)* or Couch Grass *(Agropyron repens)* – yes, this scourge of gardeners does have important medicinal properties! Two other helpful herbs are Chamomile *(Chamomilla recutita)*, both as a diuretic and gentle relaxant, and Lemon Balm *(Melissa officinalis)* which eases the emotional

Common PMS Symptoms

Symptoms include mood changes, with irritability and/or weepiness, headaches and sometimes migraines, fluid retention, tender breasts, and deep aching in the low abdomen or thighs before and at the start of the period. This half of the cycle can also be when creativity and energy, including sexual energy, can be higher so do not automatically assume that the pre-period phase has to be awful.

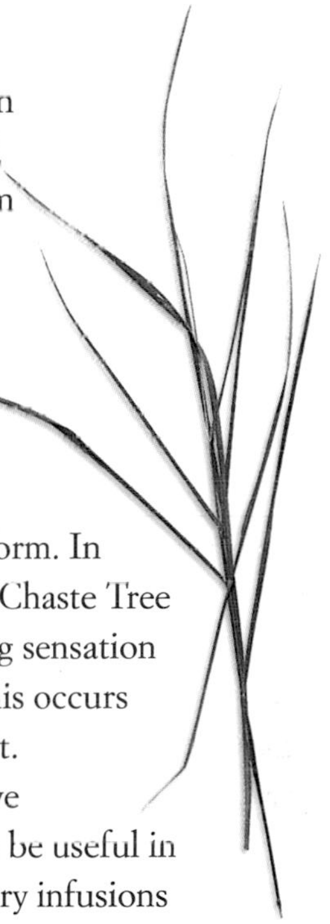

Couch Grass
(Agropyron repens)

Skin Brushing

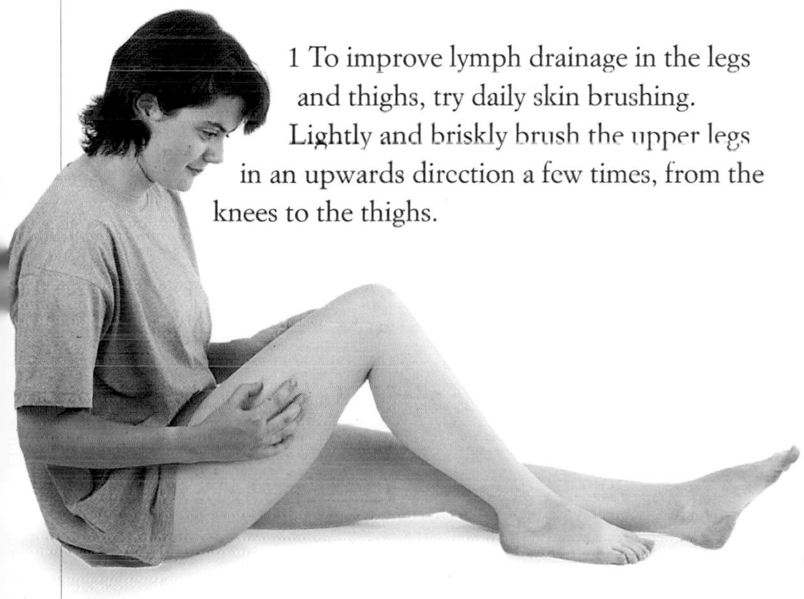

1 To improve lymph drainage in the legs and thighs, try daily skin brushing. Lightly and briskly brush the upper legs in an upwards direction a few times, from the knees to the thighs.

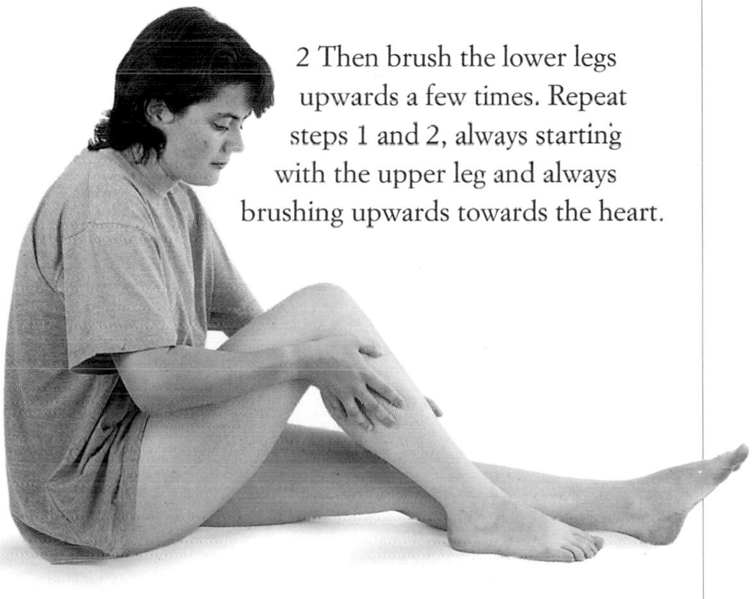

2 Then brush the lower legs upwards a few times. Repeat steps 1 and 2, always starting with the upper leg and always brushing upwards towards the heart.

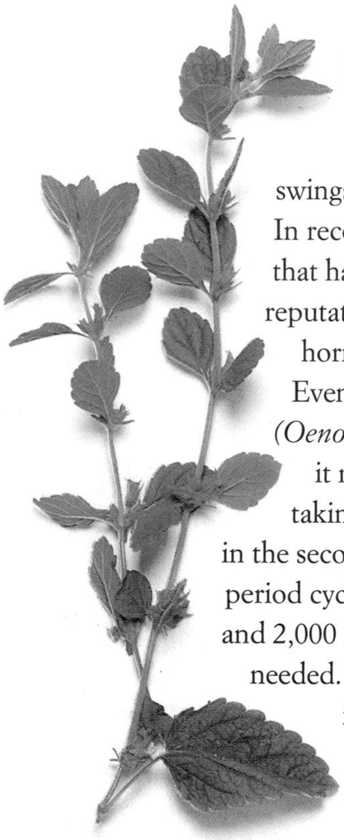

Lemon Balm
(Melissa officinalis)

swings that may happen. In recent times one herb that has gained a high reputation for balancing hormonal swings is Evening Primrose *(Oenothera biennis)*, and it may be worth taking capsules of this in the second half of the period cycle, between 1,000 and 2,000 mg are usually needed. Any improvement in symptoms may take 3-6 months to appear.

HOMEOPATHY

Some possible remedies are:

Calc carb: for overweight people who feel the cold easily if only during this phase, and have clammy hands and feet; may also experience tension and low abdominal pains.

Calc phos: for cold but drier extremities, pains and cramping, with pre-menstrual bloating.

Women for whom either of the above remedies are suited will probably get relief from pre-menstrual discomfort by taking a warm bath or using a hot-water bottle.

Lycopodium: this may be appropriate when there is a good deal of pre-period irritability and tension, which quickly ease when the period starts. Abdominal pain associated with this tension is the major physical symptom.

Stress and PMS

It can be easy to label all physical and emotional upsets as PMS (men tend to this very often), and overlook other causes of problems. Try to keep a check on whether symptoms definitely occur in monthly cycles. A good way of doing this is to keep a diary to keep a record of mood swings and general discomfort. Tension and irritability can be due to over-stress, or genuine relationship problems, which need to be sorted out. Trying to relax can also help if in a stressful situation (see also Stress, pages 28-9).

NATUROPATHY

Both diet and exercise can help tremendously in minimizing pre-menstrual problems. Cut down on alcohol and coffee during this part of the cycle at least, as they both affect fluid balance, and drink plenty of water to encourage kidney function. There has been a lot of evidence that Vitamin B6 can reduce symptoms; this is probably best taken as a supplement (up to 50 mg) as part of a whole Vitamin B complex, maybe with the addition of magnesium (200 mg). Evening Primrose oil has already been discussed earlier; for both this and Vitamin B6 it may be easier to take half the suggested doses throughout the whole of the month.

Regular exercise such as walking, cycling, swimming and running can help reduce the pelvic congestion that may accompany PMS; similarly, splashing hot and cold water around the lower abdomen regularly will improve circulation (see also Menstrual Problems, pages 68-9).

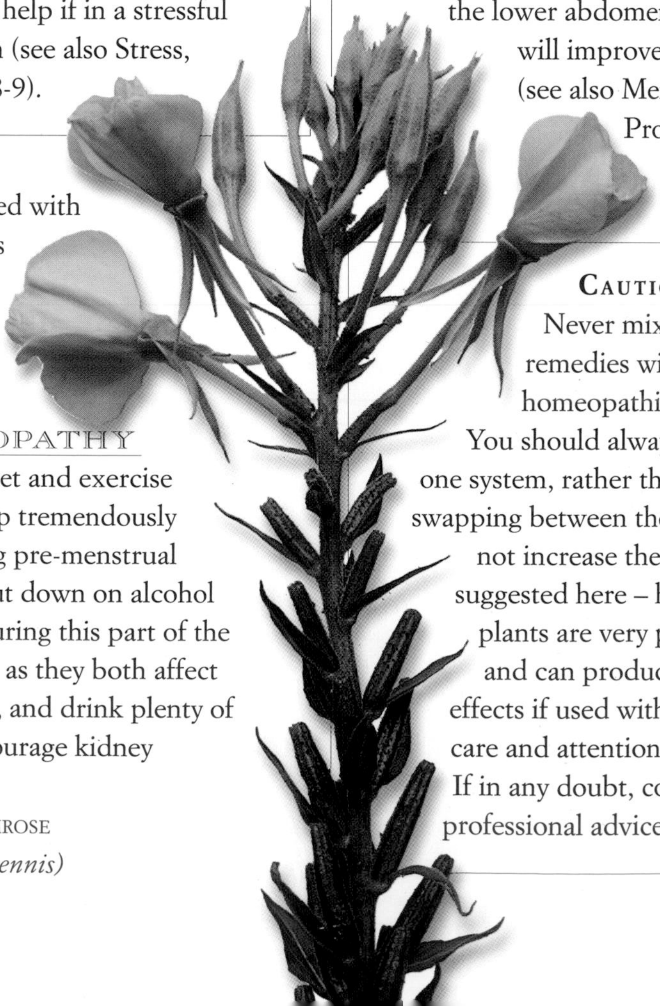

Evening Primrose
(Oenothera biennis)

Caution

Never mix herbal remedies with homeopathic ones. You should always keep to one system, rather than swapping between the two. Do not increase the dosages suggested here – herbs and plants are very powerful and can produce adverse effects if used without due care and attention. If in any doubt, consult professional advice.

PROSTATE PROBLEMS

The prostate gland is situated at the base of the bladder, and produces part of the seminal fluid. It surrounds the urethra, but normally causes no problems for urine flow. It is roughly the size of a walnut, but a common condition as men get older is a benign enlargement. This leads the prostate to compress the urethra, and perhaps even the bladder, and urine flow becomes slower to start and/or stop, with some dribbling.

AROMATHERAPY

To be used only as an adjunct to seeking professional treatment. Where there is benign prostate enlargement causing some difficulty in passing urine, placing a hot compress (see page 15) using a few drops of oils of Chamomile, Juniper or Pine over the low abdomen can quickly ease the pressure and get the urine to flow better. If the prostate is inflamed, oil of Chamomile should be included due to its anti-inflammatory effect.

HERBALISM

For an enlarged prostate, an infusion (see page 12) of one or both of the following remedies can help a good deal:

HORSETAIL *(Equisetum arvense)*: a strong diuretic, increasing urine flow and helping the bladder to empty itself completely – failure to do so can lead to cystitis. It is also astringent and anti-inflammatory, toning the swollen membranes.

WHITE DEADNETTLE *(Lamium album)*: another astringent remedy, which seems to have a regulatory effect on blood flow through the pelvic area, and so can reduce excess swelling of the prostate.

These two herbs combined can soothe the membranes and improve urine flow.

Benign prostate enlargement is often associated with lowered testosterone levels, and Saw Palmetto *(Serenoa serrulata)* is a very useful herb in this context. The berries not only have a diuretic and urinary antiseptic effect, but they also have a hormonal action to address the underlying problem. A decoction (see page 12) is strongest, but the berries could be taken with one or both the other suggested herbs in infusion form.

SCOTS PINE *(Pinus sylvestris)*

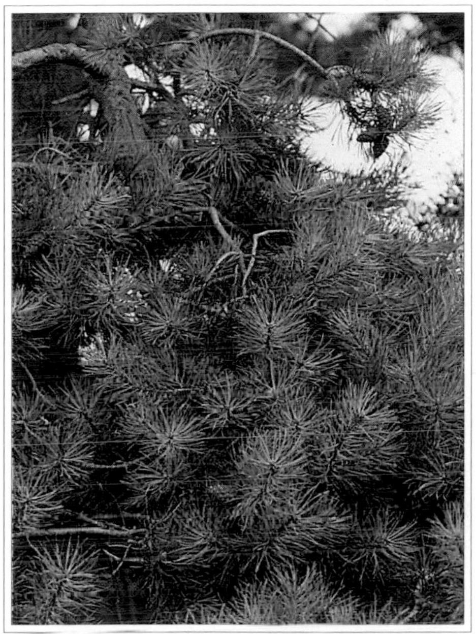

INFLAMMATION OF THE PROSTATE

Another problem can be prostatitis, or inflammation of the prostate, possibly due to a low-grade infection, and this can produce frequent, uncomfortable urination and tenderness of the gland itself. More rarely, although important to bear in mind in older men, prostate cancer can occur. This is, of course, outside the scope of self-treatment; it may be symptomless for some time, until the swollen gland restricts urine flow.

HOMEOPATHY

Some possible remedies are:

APIS MEL: when there is inflammation, probably with some enlargement, so that there is a frequent desire to pass water, but with only small amounts of stinging, burning urine.

BELLADONNA: when urination is also painful and difficult; the pressure causes some involuntary dribbling of urine when standing or moving around.

PULSATILLA: for frequent, urgent need to pass water, slight dribbling, or incontinence with any movement such as coughing, laughing or sneezing.

NATUROPATHY

Stick to a varied wholefood diet, with plenty of fluids during the day to keep urine moving through the bladder, but reduce coffee, tea or alcohol which can all irritate. Zinc is of special benefit to the prostate. Pumpkin seeds are a good food source and a supplement (up to 20 mg) may be needed daily for a while if symptoms of enlarged prostate develop.

Hydrotherapy treatment is a valuable aid; use alternating hot and cold water for the low abdomen (3 minutes hot and maximum 1 minute cold), either using a shower or splashes in the bath. The ideal method is using Sitz baths, as in hydrotherapy spa clinics.

THRUSH

Thrush is the common name for a fungal infection of the mucous membranes by the yeast *Candida albicans*. It can affect the mouth, and this is sometimes seen in tiny babies, or around the anus or on the penis, but most commonly it is a vaginal infection. A number of things can trigger off an attack of thrush; one of the major causes is often a course of antibiotics, which seriously destroy our helpful, defensive bacteria.

AROMATHERAPY

One of the most significant natural anti-fungal agents is essential oil of Tea Tree. This is available in pessary (insertable) form in some countries, but the oil can be used in the bath or in more concentrated form in a hand-basin of water; use 6 drops in warm water and bathe the vaginal area with it. Although Tea Tree oil is much more soothing than most anti-fungal drugs, do use it well diluted at first in case of any irritation. Other useful oils to use in this way are Lavender and Myrrh, and they could be blended with Tea Tree to help speed up healing.

HERBALISM

Herbalists will probably give much of the advice discussed under Naturopathy below, and are equally likely to recommend the above oils for local use; other herbs that have healing, soothing and anti-fungal effects include Marigold *(Calendula officinalis)* and Cone Flower *(Echinacea angustifolia* or *E. purpurea)*. These are best used in tincture form (see page 14); dilute at the rate of 5 ml (1 tsp) to 600 ml (1 pt/2½ cups) of warm water, and use as a local wash. For oral thrush in babies apply a little with a cotton bud (swab), and in adults use 5 ml (1 tsp) of the tincture in a little water as a mouthwash. A powerful internal anti-fungal remedy is garlic, and if thrush recurs frequently, taking either fresh garlic or garlic capsules daily can help to combat general yeast infection. It can also be used locally, although it may irritate the vaginal membranes if they are very inflamed – peel a clove of garlic, dip it in olive oil (you may want to tie a piece of cotton thread around it, so you don't lose it inside!), insert in the vagina and leave overnight.

Other Possible Causes of Thrush

Quite often a vicious circle can be set up by an infection: cystitis – treated by antibiotics – leading to thrush. Other factors can be the contraceptive pill, frequent digestive infections, a diet high in sugars, or generally being over-stressed and run-down. Conventional treatment involves the use of anti-fungal creams, or pessaries; both of these treatments may be irritating to the membranes, and self-help measures can often be the best route to avoid repetition of the infection.

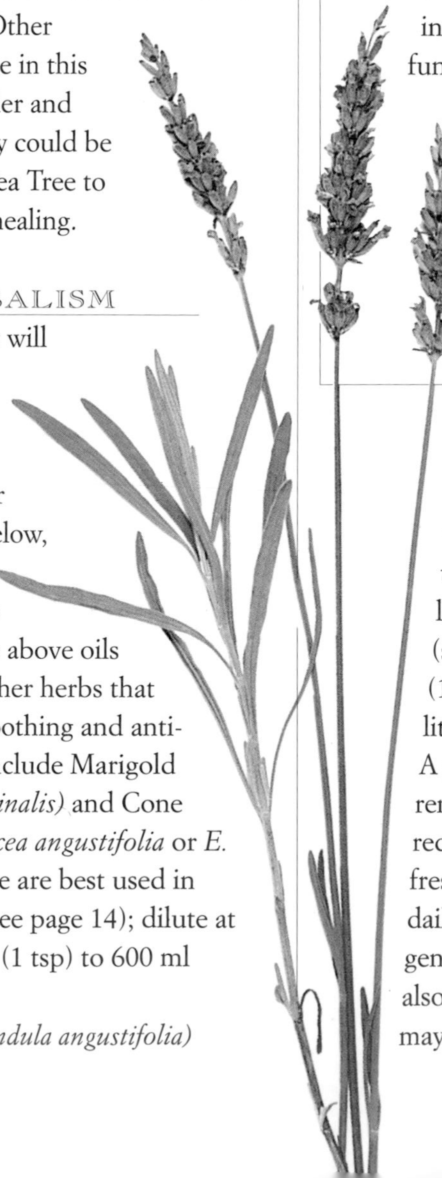

Lavender *(Lavandula angustifolia)*

HOMEOPATHY

Treatment will focus on internal remedies, backed up by local self-help measures (see next page). Practitioners may even prescribe homeopathic doses of *Candida* itself, but some other possible remedies are:

Merc sol: for reddish patches, especially if oral thrush when there may be blisters on the mucous membranes, with thick, slimy discharge and some mould-like odour.

Nat mur: for white spots, less of a discharge but more painful irritation; in oral thrush

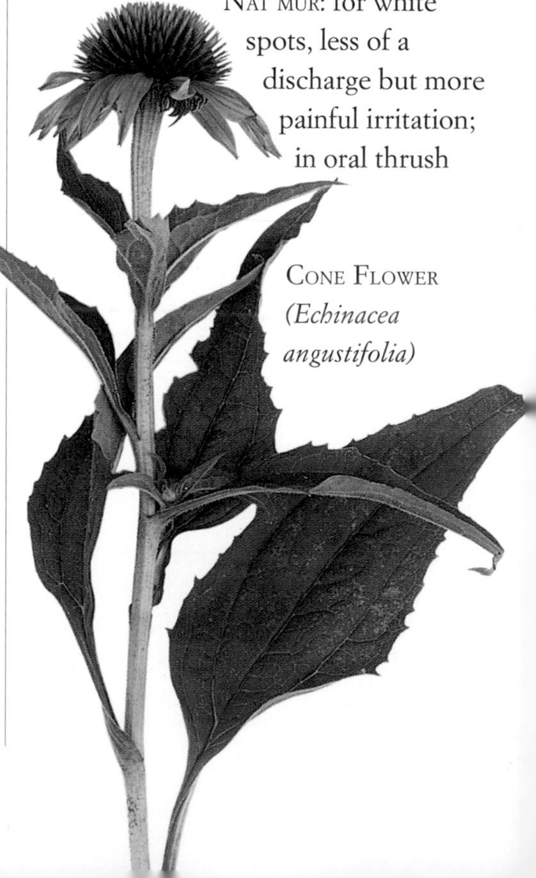

Cone Flower *(Echinacea angustifolia)*

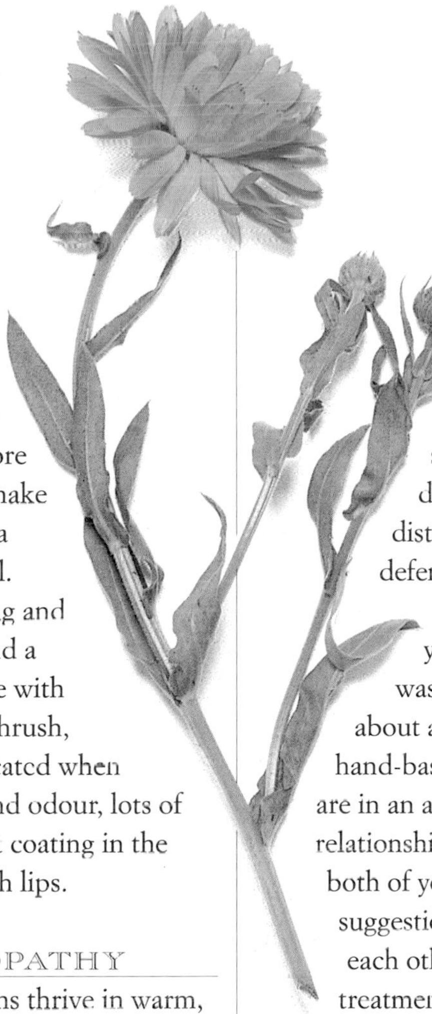

MARIGOLD
(Calendula officinalis)

there may be painful blisters on the lips or tongue. Drier and more inflamed symptoms make this more suitable as a remedy than Merc sol.
SULPHUR: for an itching and burning sensation, and a thick, white discharge with some odour. In oral thrush, Sulphur may be indicated when there is a foul taste and odour, lots of white blisters or yeast coating in the mouth, and dry, rough lips.

NATUROPATHY

Fungal infections thrive in warm, damp environments, so it is important to keep the vaginal area cool and dry, and let it "breathe" more freely – only use cotton underwear, and avoid tights or tight jeans. Do not use bubble baths or strong vaginal deodorants as they can disturb your normal defences. Apart from the oils or herbs to use locally, you may find it helpful to wash with salt water – use about a handful of salt in a hand-basin of warm water. If you are in an active sexual relationship, it is important for both of you to look at these suggestions, as you may re-infect each other without joint treatments. Live, natural (plain) yoghurt can also be used locally, on a sanitary towel (napkin) or tampon; this helps to encourage the defensive bacteria to multiply. If a recent course of antibiotics seem to be the cause, then eating live yoghurt will aid the defensive flora in the gut too.

Since yeasts will flourish on sugars, reduce all concentrated sugar and refined carbohydrates in the diet, and also severely restrict alcohol. Eat plenty of vegetables and whole grains, and use a fair amount of olive oil for any salad dressings, as this has a natural anti-fungal effect (it may be applied sparingly locally too, especially if the area is dry and inflamed). As a supplement, *Lactobacillus acidophilus* has a significant effect on suppressing yeast invasion and encouraging the gut flora; it is the bacteria which converts milk into yoghurt, but occurs in much higher concentrations in the capsules or powder that are quite widely available. If diarrhoea develops, then stop taking it immediately.

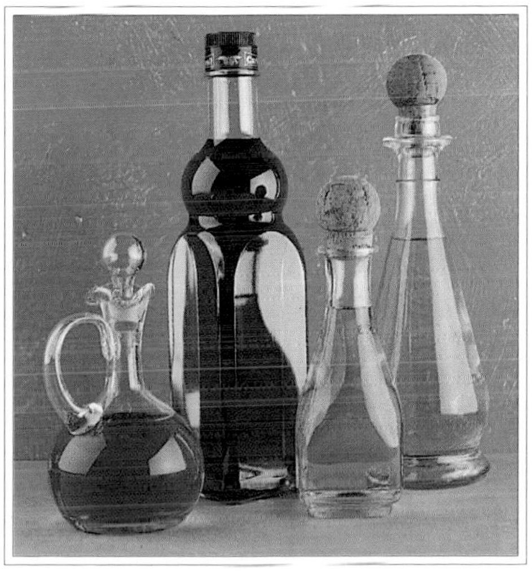

Pure Olive oil, as used in salads, has a natural anti-fungal effect.

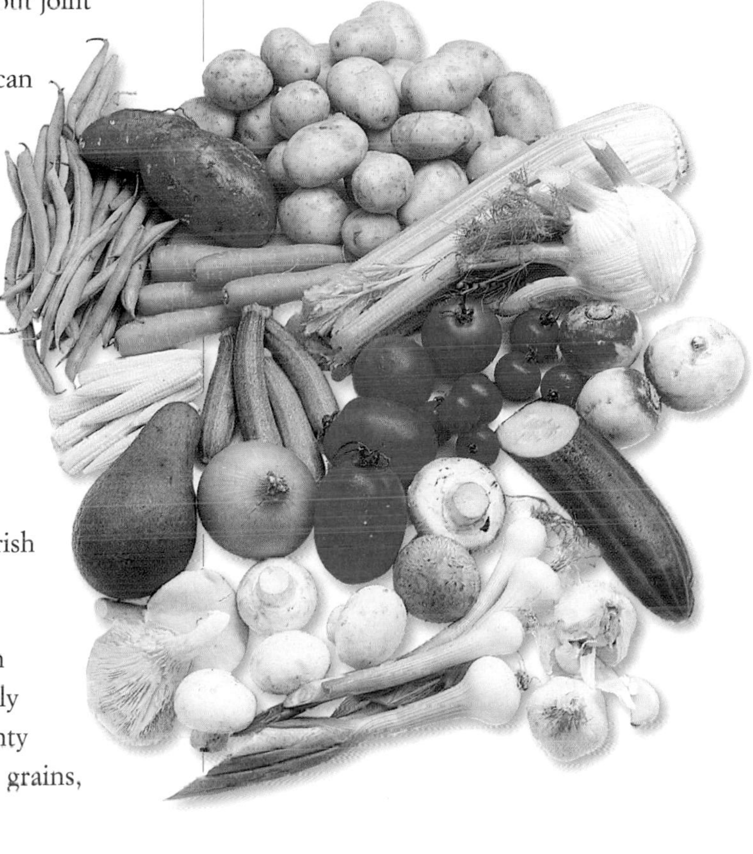

A diet high in fresh vegetables, and low in refined sugars, helps to prevent recurrent thrush.

THE URINARY SYSTEM

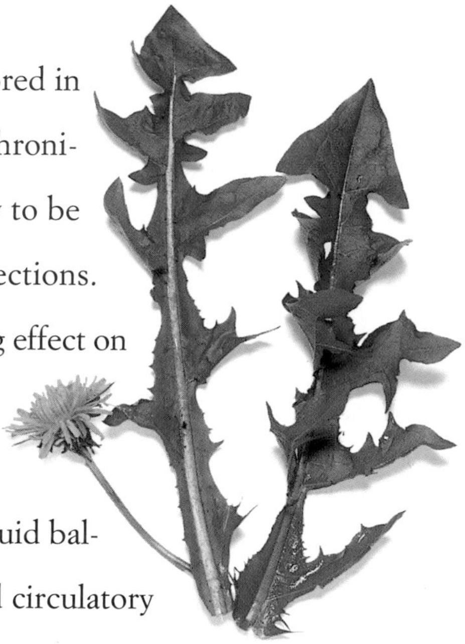

Our general health and vitality are often mirrored in the health of our urinary system. If we are chronically stressed or run-down, we are much more likely to be prone to recurrent cystitis or other urinary infections. Conversely, disorders of our kidneys have a weakening effect on our energy overall, and need to be treated by professional practitioners.

The urinary system is essential in maintaining the fluid balance within the body, and together with the heart and circulatory system it controls blood pressure. Equally importantly the kidneys keep our electrolytes, or fluid-soluble minerals, in balance and aid in removing toxins. Problems of urination can arise not only from infection or serious illness, but are affected by hormonal changes and in men the functioning of the prostate (see The Reproductive System, page 64), and by stress. Muscle tone is also important, especially as people get older and the bladder tends to shrink, or atrophy, and exercises can be helpful for maintaining control of bladder function.

*ABOVE: Dandelion (*Taraxacum officinale*) is a highly effective diuretic. It is also rich in potassium, thereby counteracting any loss of potassium that occurs through urination.*

CYSTITIS

Cystitis is an acute infection of the bladder, which may often recur and become a chronic condition. It is more common in girls and women than in boys or men, due to the much shorter length of the urethra in women; in many women it can be triggered off by irritation during sexual intercourse, and useful advice can include emptying the bladder before sex (if pre-meditated enough!) and certainly afterwards.

AROMATHERAPY

Essential oils have quite powerful antiseptic properties, and should be used at the earliest possible stage of cystitis. A useful way to use them is to add them to the bath, up to 10 drops in total added just before getting into the water. Some of the most suitable oils are Bergamot, Chamomile, Lemon (perhaps only use 5 drops if this oil is chosen), and Sandalwood. A warm compress (see page 15), with 3-5 drops of Chamomile or Lavender oils added, can be placed over the lower abdomen if there is a lot of discomfort.

CYSTITIS SYMPTOMS

Symptoms of cystitis can include frequent urging to pass water, accompanied generally by a sharp pain – in women this is usually felt in the urethra, and there is usually inflammation (urethritis) here too, while men tend to experience pain in the penis. The urine may look cloudy or strongly coloured and may have a strong smell. Sometimes there is pain just before or just after urination, perhaps with a feeling of needing to pass water again as fresh urine trickles into the inflamed and irritated bladder.

HERBALISM

There are many herbs which have specific effects on the urinary tract, so if the cystitis persists or recurs, do seek professional treatment. In the first instance, drink plenty of fluid, especially water or infusions (see page 12) chosen from the following herbs. In mild cases simply drinking plenty of herb teas such as Chamomile *(Chamomilla recutita),* or Meadowsweet *(Filipendula ulmaria)* may reduce the inflammation sufficiently to solve the problem. These two herbs can of course also be taken as stronger infusions in acute attacks. Buchu *(Barosma betulina)* is a particularly useful herb, not only acting as a urinary antiseptic but soothing the inflamed membranes too, and helping to escape the cycle of cystitis-antibiotics-cystitis which can easily occur with conventional treatment. Bearberry *(Arctostaphylos uva-ursi)* is another strong antiseptic remedy, most helpful when the urine is acidic and sharply burning. To these herbs can be added Celery Seed *(Apium graveolens)*, which has a very alkaline effect on the urine, Agrimony *(Agrimonia eupatoria)* to tone and astringe the swollen tissues, and/or Marshmallow *(Althea officinalis)* (ideally the root, but the leaf is also good) for its pure soothing properties. It is generally recommended to take plenty of garlic internally to fight infection and to cleanse the tissues for some time after the attack has subsided.

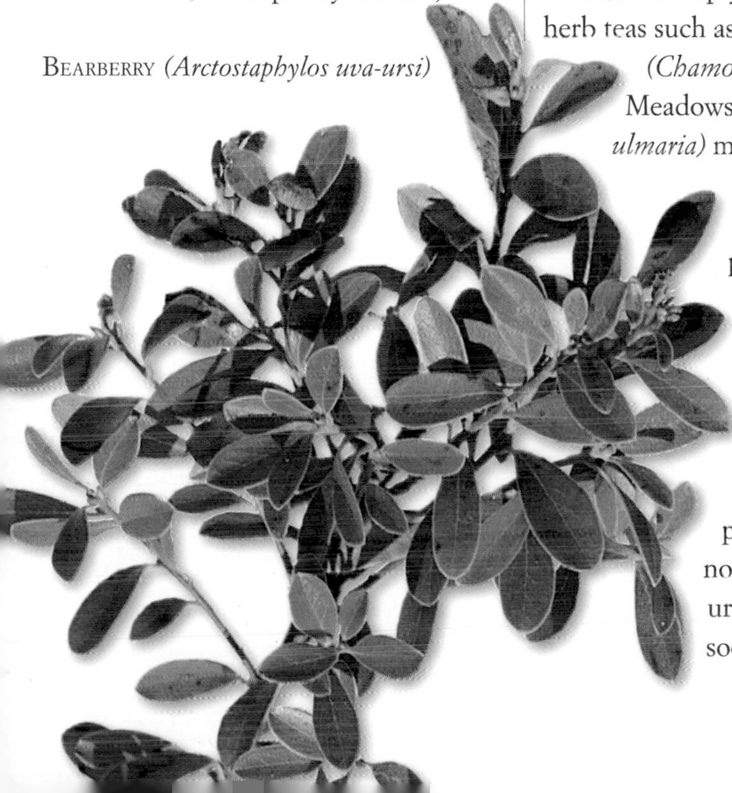

BEARBERRY *(Arctostaphylos uva-ursi)*

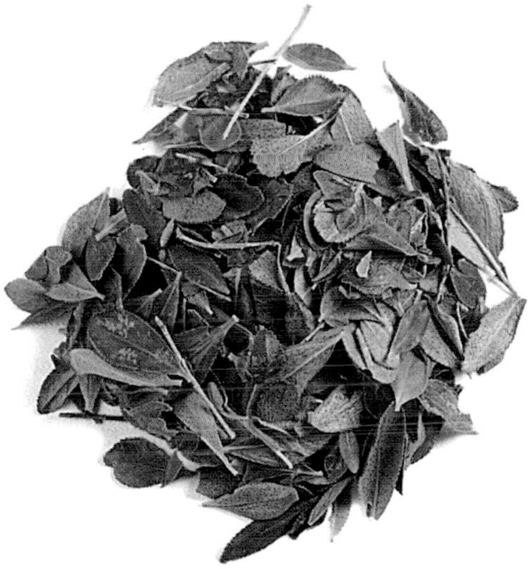

BUCHU *(Barosma betulina)*

HOMEOPATHY

Symptoms of discomfort when passing urine are a feature of the "remedy picture" (see Introduction to

Making Barley Water

Home-made lemon barley water is a nutritious drink to take in place of tea and coffee when suffering from cystitis.

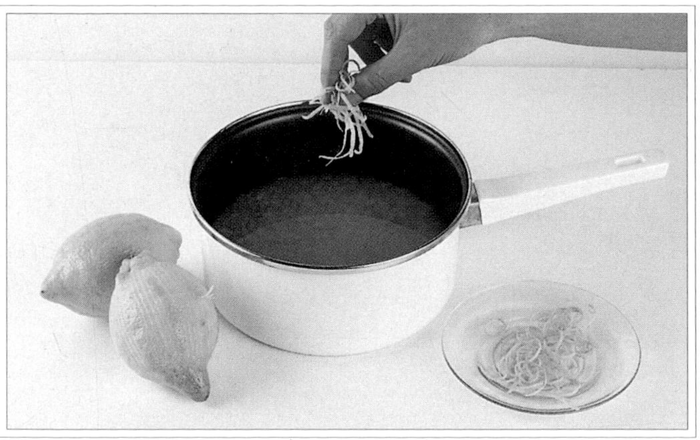

1 Cover 100 g (4 oz) of pearl barley in a little water and bring to the boil, strain and throw away this water. Pour 600 ml (1 pt/2½ cups) of boiling water over the barley (or ideally simmer the barley in 750 ml (1¼ pt/3⅔ cups) of water for 5 minutes, to extract the full benefit.)

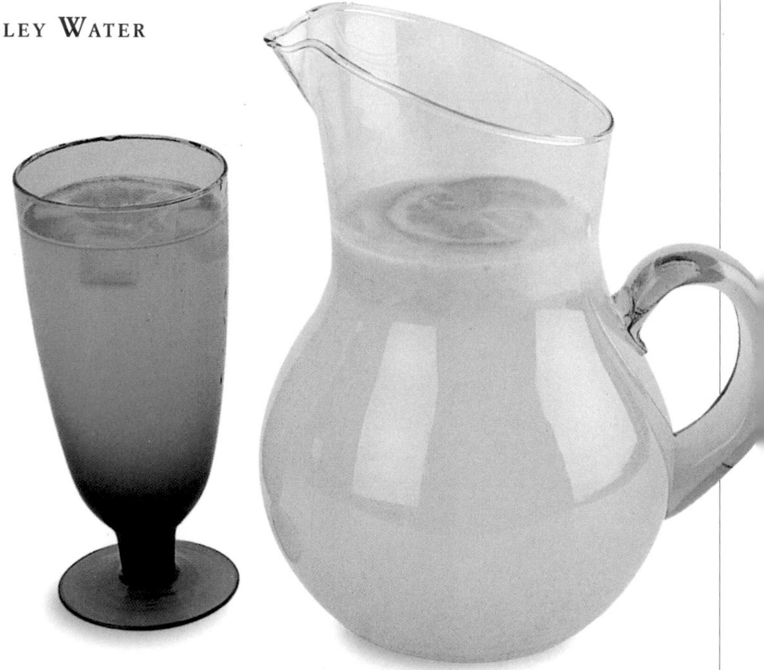

2 Add the zest of a lemon and leave to cool. Strain and keep the liquid in the fridge. Drink often.

Homeopathy, page 10) for a large number of homeopathic medicines, so the professional practitioner has a wide choice. For self-treatment, choose initially from:

CANTHARIS: for the classical symptoms of cystitis, burning pains with passing water, which comes only slowly, and also a frequent urge to urinate.

PULSATILLA: for a great urge, and urgency to urinate, causing some pains and distress. Urine may easily dribble out, when coughing or laughing.

STAPHYSAGRIA: when the vulval area is sore or bruised – often given for "honeymoon cystitis".

NATUROPATHY

In the first place, as soon as you feel the twinges of cystitis coming on, drink plenty of water, or herb teas. Avoid alcohol, or strong tea and coffee, which can irritate the bladder lining further. Sometimes it can be helpful to add a pinch of bicarbonate of soda to water to make it alkaline. Avoid obviously acidic foods such as vinegar, unripe fruit or ones like gooseberries, plums, rhubarb or tomatoes.

Many people tend to suffer periodically with cystitis, and for recurrent problems, look at things such as not wearing tight jeans or trousers, avoid vaginal deodorants and be careful to rinse underwear thoroughly (biological washing powders or detergents can leave irritant traces). If you have had antibiotics, it is very helpful to take plenty of live yoghurt afterwards to repopulate the defensive gut bacteria; a little can also be applied to the vaginal and urethral openings for local effect, especially if you are prone to cystitis.

This helps to alter the local acidity, which encourages the body's natural defences to multiply, and it is also quite cool and soothing to the irritated and inflamed surface.

FLUID RETENTION

Excess fluid in the tissues, or oedema, can happen in a variety of ways. Local, temporary swelling will occur with an injury, for instance a sprained ankle or a large bruise (see First Aid, page 104, for treatment). Fluid retention in the thighs and hips in women is often associated with a build-up of toxins, as in cellulite, and a general detoxifying programme of diet, exercise and massage will be most effective.

AROMATHERAPY

For problems such as fluid retention linked to cellulite, or temporary ankle swelling due to heat or long flights, massage the legs and thighs in an upwards sweeping movement, with a 1-2 per cent dilution of essential oils in a base oil (see page 17). Beneficial oils are Geranium, Grapefruit, Lemon and Rosemary; Juniper has an even stronger diuretic effect, stimulating the kidneys to excrete excess fluid, but do not use if there is any kidney problem or in pregnancy. Another essential oil of value is Fennel, but this has a mild oestrogenic action too, so be careful not to use for long if oedema is hormone-related.

Pregnancy is a time when ankles might swell, but use essential oils sparingly (less than 1 per cent), if at all, and get professional advice if you are unsure. Do not use Fennel or Juniper, and only use Rosemary later on, from the fifth month of the pregnancy, if ankle oedema is a problem.

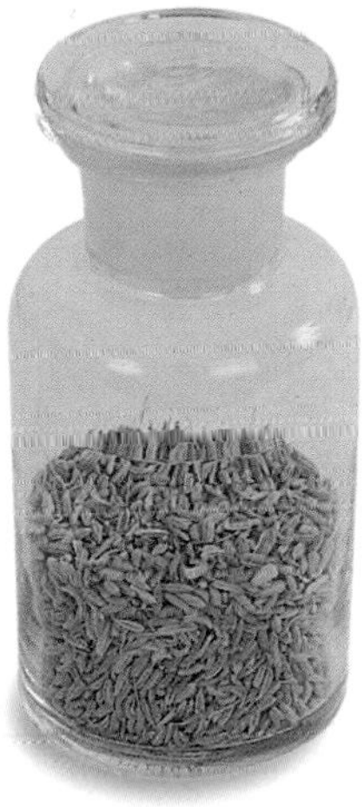

FENNEL
(Foeniculum vulgare)

OTHER CAUSES OF FLUID RETENTION

Fluid retention is often aggravated during the pre-period phase (see also Pre-Menstrual Problems, page 71), especially in the breasts and abdomen. In hot weather most people find that they have some fluid retention, and ankles tend to swell during long plane flights – drink plenty of fluid (but *not* alcohol), and move about the plane as much as possible.

Severe leg and ankle oedema is often a sign of kidney and/or heart malfunction, and should be treated professionally, without delay, as should any unexplained or prolonged fluid retention.

HERBALISM

In order to encourage the removal of fluid, the simplest approach is to use herb teas which have a diuretic effect. Do not use for more than a week at a time; long-term stimulation of the

THIGH AND LEG MASSAGE

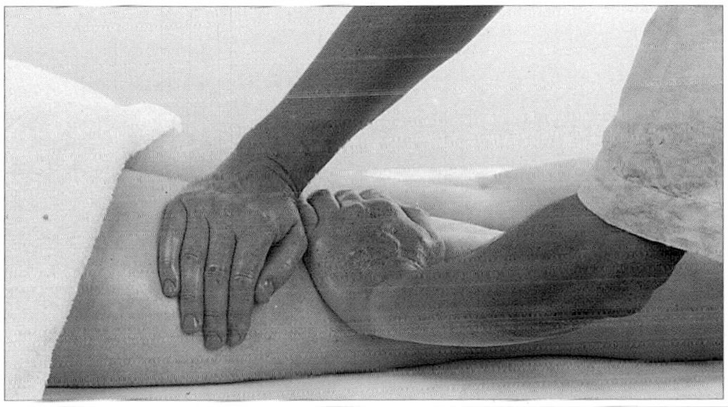

1 To improve circulation in the legs, firstly oil the legs. Place hands on the thigh and stroke upwards to the buttock a few times, with light but steady sweeping movements, hand-over-hand.

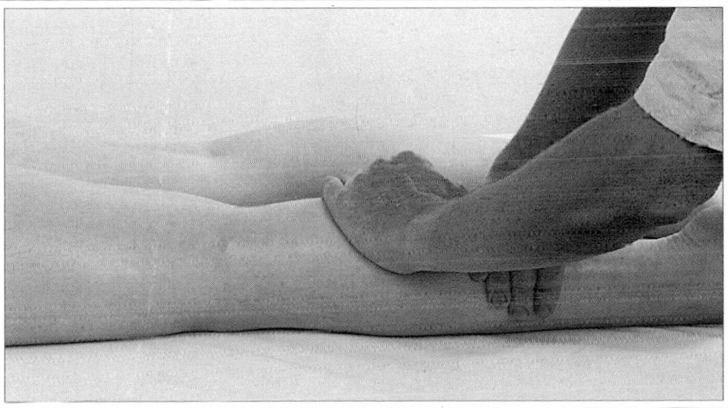

2 Move hands down to the lower leg and stroke up to the back of the knee a few times. Repeat steps 1 and 2; always start this movement on the upper leg, and always stroke up towards the heart.

urinary system can be tiring and if the swelling has not subsided within a short period, qualified advice and treatment may be necessary.

One of the best herbal diuretics is Dandelion Leaf *(Taraxacum officinale)*, indeed its common name in many languages translates as "Wet-the-bed"! When you pass urine, potassium is lost in the fluid, and with some prescribed diuretics this can lead to a potassium deficiency, which is itself a serious condition. Dandelions are so rich in potassium that this loss is counteracted. Make a tea and drink three cupfuls a day initially.

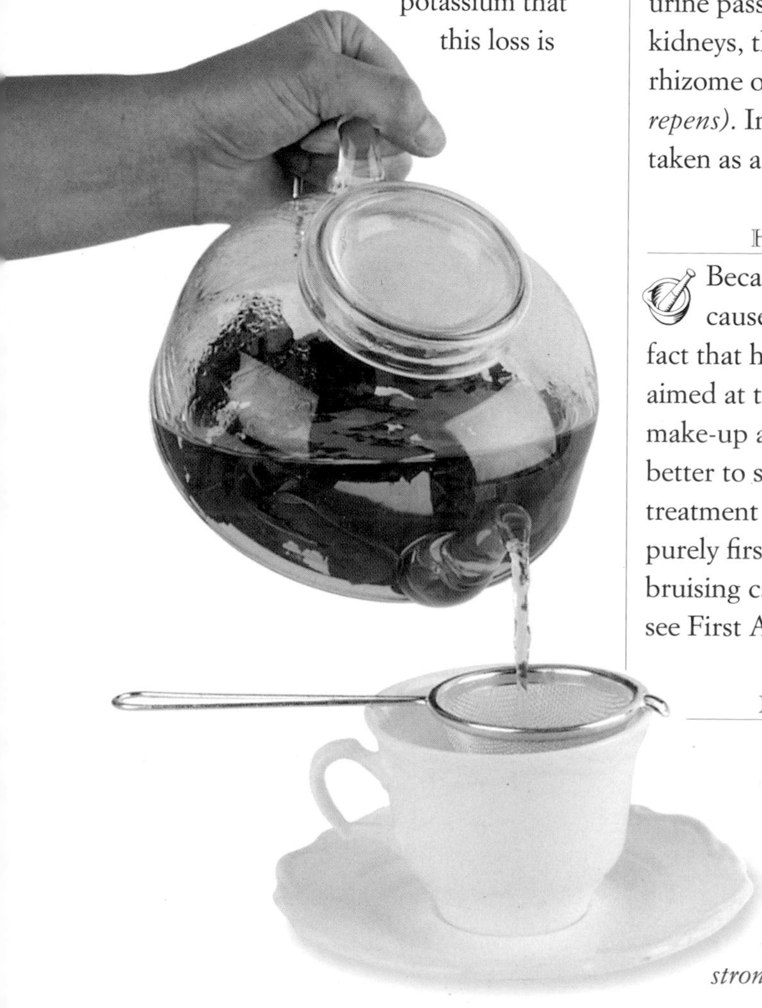

Dandelion leaves can make a strongly diuretic tea.

Other common and useful herbs are Chamomile *(Chamomilla recutita)*, Fennel *(Foeniculum vulgare)* (but see Aromatherapy section earlier), Meadowsweet *(Filipendula ulmaria)* and Yarrow *(Achillea millefolium)*, all of which are diuretic among their other properties.

For just increasing the amount of urine passed, without strain on the kidneys, the best herb is the creeping rhizome of Couch Grass *(Agropyron repens)*. In the short term this can be taken as a decoction (see page 12).

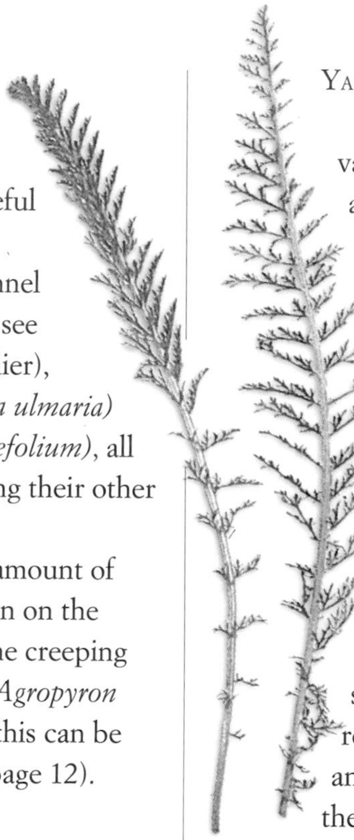

Yarrow *(Achillea millefolium)*

HOMEOPATHY

Because of the complexity of the causes of fluid retention, and the fact that homeopathic remedies are aimed at the person's constitutional make-up as far as possible, it is much better to seek professional homeopathic treatment for any water retention. For purely first aid problems such as bruising causing some local swelling, see First Aid, page 104.

NATUROPATHY

Since fluid retention in the ankles and legs is often associated with circulatory problems like varicose veins, all the general advice given under that section (see page 53) will be useful. Exercise is vital to improve the blood flow, and hence speed up the removal of fluid. Look at the diet, and in particular at salt intake; in most cases it will be very beneficial to reduce salt intake, since excessive amounts of sodium encourage fluid retention and also place an undue burden on the kidneys.

Massage is most helpful, especially gentle lymph drainage techniques – for self-massage, lightly and repeatedly stroke the affected areas in movements directed towards the heart. If the swelling is in the legs for instance, stroke the upper legs first in an upwards direction, before repeating the action to the lower legs, so that the fluid has somewhere to drain into from the ankles.

Try to have the legs raised, supported on something soft such as a cushion, to allow gravity to assist in draining fluid back towards the heart. In a similar way, swelling of the wrist can be eased by raising the arm or supporting it in a sling. Continued swelling, in any part of the body, requires medical attention.

URINARY INCONTINENCE

The inability to control the bladder and prevent dribbling of urine, or bed-wetting, is something that can affect people at both ends of life in particular. Children may get into problems with involuntary bed-wetting through something simple such as a chill or shock, or from a deeper upsetting worry, or just because they sleep too deeply (see Children's Ailments, page 112).

AROMATHERAPY

Alongside any self-help measures such as pelvic floor exercises, an excellent essential oil to use is Cypress, which is astringent, toning up the tissues and encouraging efficient excretion of fluid. Use it in the bath, about 6 drops, or make a compress with 2 drops in a small bowl of warm water and wring out a small towel in the liquid, placing it over the low abdomen. For daily use it may be easier to use a diluted oil, 2 per cent dilution (about 50 drops in 100 ml (3½ fl oz/½ cup) of base oil), and massage a little into the lower abdomen each day. Another oil that may help in this way is Pine, but use 1 per cent of this only. In either case do not use daily for more than 10 days at a time.

HERBALISM

Probably the foremost herb for this condition is Horsetail *(Equisetum arvense)*, which is quite a strong diuretic, but more significantly it contains appreciable amounts of silica. This has an astringent and toning effect on the bladder tissues, encouraging it to empty efficiently and regain some of the lost muscle tone. Horsetail is perhaps best taken as the fresh juice, available in some countries, take 10 ml (2 tsp) twice a day; otherwise a decoction may be taken (see page 12). If emotional upset is a part of the problem, then also taking St John's Wort *(Hypericum perforatum)* may help a good deal – use the juice at the same rate or take an infusion (see page 12) for a week or two (take care not to overdo this remedy if going out in strong sunlight, as it can increase sun sensitivity). For individualized treatment get professional help.

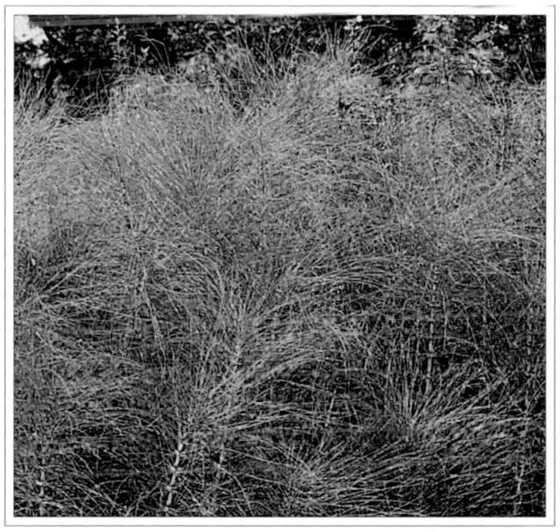

HORSETAIL *(Equisetum arvense)*

HOMEOPATHY

Several possibilities exist within homeopathy for treating this condition, some suggestions with a brief "snapshot" of the symptom picture for each remedy are:

ARGENT NIT: with incontinence at night in particular, although also possible in the day, brought on by nervousness, restlessness and anxiety. This remedy is useful for older people who may easily get anxious, perhaps over a move or travelling, and hence become incontinent; the urine may burn a little when passed.

BELLADONNA: with a constant urge to pass water when awake; there may be some involuntary dribbling when standing, and also during sleep.

PULSATILLA: this remedy is often appropriate for shy, sensitive people who are prone to crying. It is helpful if they experience bed-wetting at night, whether children or older people; there may be an easy tendency to dribble in the daytime too, with difficulty in retaining urine.

NATUROPATHY

One of the first things to look at is the muscle tone within the pelvic basin generally. Exercises such as alternately tightening and relaxing the buttocks can help to regain control of the bladder and urethra. Another exercise that may be useful is to try and stop in midstream while actually urinating, and hold for a couple of seconds before restarting to pass water. If done regularly, this can be a great aid in tightening and strengthening the muscles of the bladder.

Another approach is to employ hot and cold water applications to the lower abdomen and back. This can be via alternating hot/cold compresses, around 3-4 minutes hot and 1 minute cold, repeated once or twice. A simpler method is to have a fairly warm bath, followed by a short splash of cool water around the waist and bladder, or else when finishing a shower turn the temperature down to cool and use on this area for a minute. These methods will help to stimulate pelvic circulation, which in turn will encourage better muscular control.

THE MUSCULO-SKELETAL SYSTEM

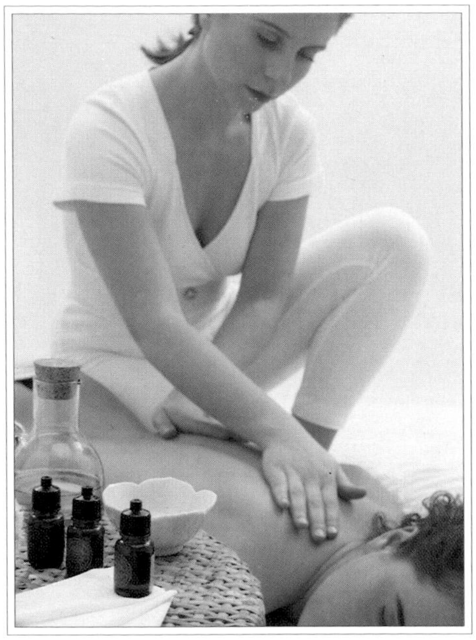

Problems of the muscular and/or skeletal systems are for most of us simply a fact of life, ranging from simple aches and pains after unaccustomed exercise or effort, to the inevitable wear and tear on our bodies as we get older. In the great majority of cases these problems represent "everything that we don't die of", yet their impact on our health, vitality and mobility can be enormous, causing great problems. Back pain alone is the major cause of time lost from work in most industrialized countries, and the often crippling discomfort of chronic arthritis reduces the quality of life for sufferers by a considerable amount.

While it is true that wear and tear are a part of living, their effects *can* be lessened and much greater levels of comfort and mobility are possible. It is perhaps a sobering thought that much of our predisposition to problems with skeletal disorders in later life is established in the first few years of childhood; prevention, especially in terms of diet, is an important part of the equation therefore, and very hard to achieve when adult. Changes to lifestyle later on can make differences however, together with some of the suggestions under the sections that follow.

ABOVE: Massaging with aromatherapy oils is a wonderful and natural way to ease the body.

ARTHRITIS

Although specialists identify up to 200 divisions of arthritic conditions, it is useful to think of arthritis falling into two categories: osteoarthritis (OA) and rheumatoid arthritis (RA). Osteoarthritis is the natural wear and tear of the joints that occurs with ageing, as the cartilage surrounding the bones becomes thinner and the surface becomes rougher. This leads to friction and degeneration occurs as the joint gets deformed.

AROMATHERAPY

The two principles of many natural approaches to arthritis, namely detoxification and improving circulation around the joints, are the main aims of aromatherapy treatment. Essential oils which aid tissue cleansing include Cypress, Juniper and Lemon, and these can be used as bath oils (see page 8) regularly. Juniper also has an anti-inflammatory and mildly analgesic effect; similar properties are found in Chamomile, Lavender and Rosemary oils. These may all be used either in the bath or diluted in a base oil and gently massaged into the affected areas. If this is painful or difficult to do, they may be used in a hot compress (see page 15); try combining any two of these oils for greater effect, varying them to avoid overuse of any one oil. To stimulate the circulation, use oils such as Black Pepper, Ginger, Marjoram and Rosemary in any of the above ways. As you can see, some oils have overlapping effects and can help with relieving arthritic discomfort in many ways.

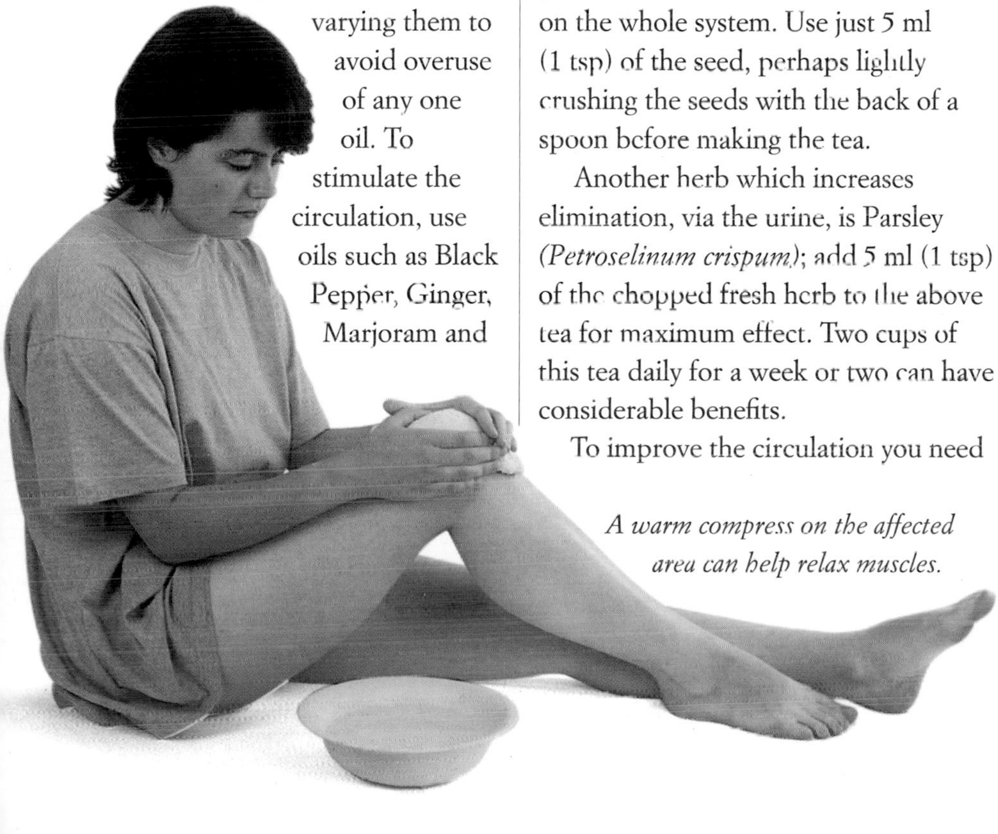

A warm compress on the affected area can help relax muscles.

HERBALISM

The herbal pharmacopoeia are full of herbs that can be of benefit in treating arthritis; as mentioned above, it is useful to think of treatments in terms of detoxifying and stimulating the circulation, thus removing the need for local inflammation, as much as any simply pain-relieving action. For self-help treatment, apart from the dietary advice discussed below, an initial cleansing programme can be adopted. In order to remove acidic toxins, make a tea from Celery Seed *(Apium graveolens)*, which has an alkaline effect on the whole system. Use just 5 ml (1 tsp) of the seed, perhaps lightly crushing the seeds with the back of a spoon before making the tea.

Another herb which increases elimination, via the urine, is Parsley *(Petroselinum crispum)*; add 5 ml (1 tsp) of the chopped fresh herb to the above tea for maximum effect. Two cups of this tea daily for a week or two can have considerable benefits.

To improve the circulation you need look no further than Ginger *(Zingiber officinalis)*; chop up a small piece and make a tea from it, or add to the mixture above. For a more direct anti-inflammatory action, a couple of suggestions are Meadowsweet

Other Causes of Arthritis

Other factors include previous injuries and occupations – high amounts of some sports, or physical jobs such as farming can lead to greater wear on certain joints. Since it is sometimes associated with an excess of acid waste matter in the body accumulating around the joints, diet is important too.

Rheumatoid Arthritis

Rheumatoid arthritis is a different problem altogether. It is an inflammatory process that seems to be what is called an auto-immune disorder, meaning the body's defences for some unknown reason start to attack its own cells. In RA, not only are the synovial membranes lining the joints inflamed and thickened, but the bone underneath is steadily destroyed, leading to painful and often badly deformed joints. People are quite likely to feel ill in themselves as a result of this disorder, and professional treatment is essential to try to deal with the underlying condition.

(Filipendula ulmaria) and Feverfew *(Chrysanthemum parthenium)*. An infusion (see page 12) of Meadowsweet may be taken twice daily, while Feverfew may be taken in tablet form. The fresh leaves of Feverfew can also be chewed and eaten instead; just three leaves a day is a medicinal dose, but occasionally they can give mouth ulcers.

HOMEOPATHY

As a first treatment of arthritis, try one of these remedies:

BRYONIA: this is applicable for hot joints, when the pains are worse with warmth or with movements, and seem to be eased by the use of cold applications or compresses (see page 15).

PULSATILLA: if the pains and inflammation seem to move rapidly from one joint to another, with a quick change in symptoms. A pulsatilla-type of person usually feels much better in the fresh air, and this remedy seems to suit women better.

RHUS TOX: this is often the first remedy to be thought of in many rheumatic conditions; symptoms are better with warmth and after some movement, while the person is likely to feel stiff and painful after some time of resting. Cold, damp weather also makes the symptoms worse.

NATUROPATHY

Attention to the diet is an important part of treatment, and ideally this should be adapted individually by a practitioner. In most instances, it is essential to eat plenty of fresh vegetables, raw or cooked, and also fresh fruit – although citrus fruits are often to be avoided by sufferers. Other foods to reduce include red meats, cheeses, sugary foods and excessive coffee or tea.

An approach that has found some popularity is the Hay diet, named after its originator Dr Hay. The diet essentially involves avoiding combinations of proteins and carbohydrates at any one meal; this is beyond the scope of this section, but has been written about in other books.

To relieve stiffness, especially in winter in cooler, less sunny climates, there is a lot of value in taking cod liver oil capsules, one or two a day. The occasional use of a bath containing Epsom salts is also excellent to ease stiffness and discomfort; dissolve 60 ml (4 tbsp) of the salts in a hot bath and soak for 15 minutes. In an acute inflammatory stage of arthritis, with very hot joints, try using an ice-pack or cold compress. Often in chronic conditions, with cold, stiff joints, a warm compress is better (see page 15).

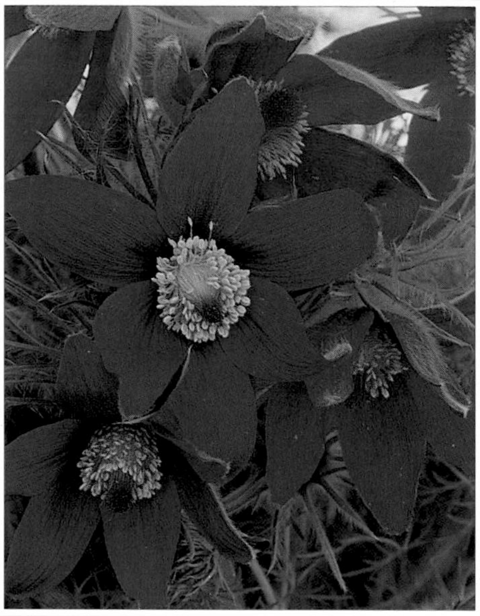

PASQUE FLOWER *(Pulsatilla vulgaris)*

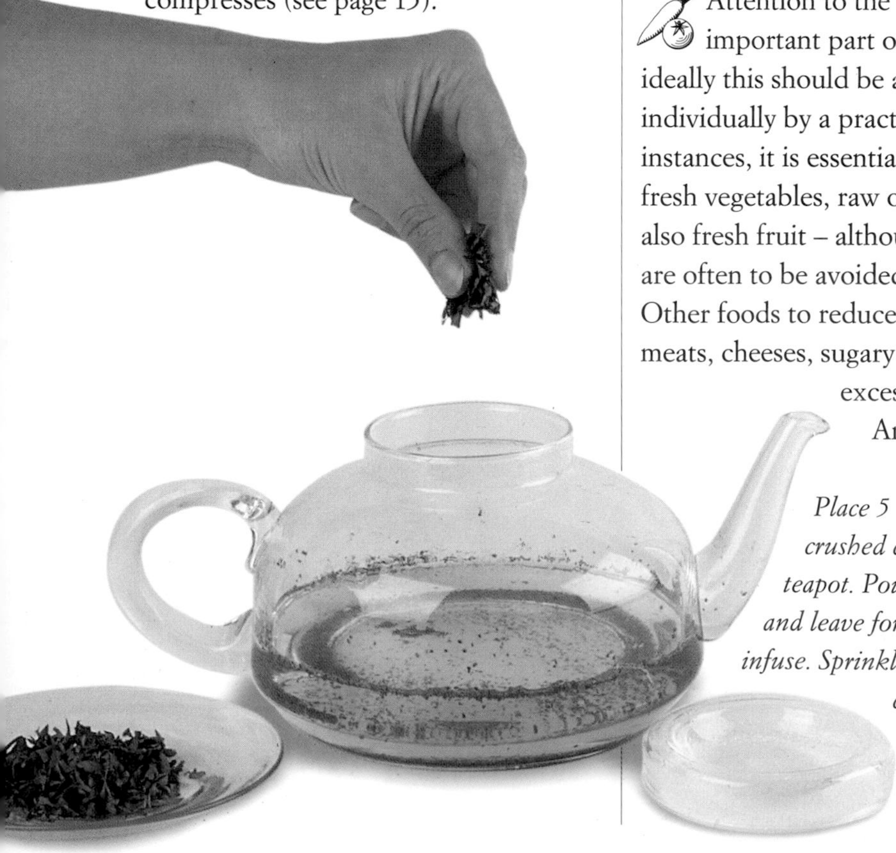

Place 5 ml (1 tsp) of lightly crushed celery seeds in a teapot. Pour on boiling water and leave for 5 minutes to infuse. Sprinkle 5 ml (1 tsp) chopped fresh parsley on top of the tea, strain and drink a cupful.

CRAMP

Acute and very painful contractions of muscles produce the feelings of cramp. It is probably most common in the calves, but can occur in any large muscles, for instance in the thighs, back, neck or abdomen. It can occur suddenly, often without warning and can be frightening for children the first time it occurs.

AROMATHERAPY

In order to improve the local circulation and so bring in more blood and oxygen to the muscles, massaging the area is often very beneficial. Firm effleurage, or stroking movements, are particular helpful, always done in a direction towards the heart. To aid this action, diluted essential oils like Juniper, Lavender, Marjoram, Rosemary or even Black Pepper should be used. These are all rubefacient, meaning they dilate the local blood vessels and encourage increased blood flow. The muscles become warmed and relaxed. For frequent leg cramps for instance, regular massage of the legs and thighs with one or more of these oils can help a good deal.

CAUSES OF CRAMP

A major factor is inadequate circulation to the muscles, especially if cramp comes on with exercise or effort (see also Poor Circulation, page 51); with athletes or people doing hard physical work there may also be a problem of salt deficiency from excessive sweating.

Repetitive movements, such as typing, can provoke cramping and lead on to inflammation – repetitive strain injury is a potential consequence of overuse of a set of muscles in this way. Night cramps are probably due to a combination of reduced circulation, tiredness and stress, and the whole person needs to be treated.

HERBALISM

One of the most effective treatments for cramp is the aptly named Cramp Bark (European Cranberry Bush) *(Viburnum opulus)*, better known to gardeners as the guelder rose. The bark is made into a tincture (see page 14) that is almost a specific remedy for muscle spasms, both internally in instances of, say, period pains or abdominal cramps, and used locally for leg cramps. Either make a warm compress using the tincture diluted about 1:4 with hot water, or incorporate it into a cream (see page 16) and massage into the affected areas. Internally, take 5 ml (1 tsp) once or twice daily, ideally in a little hot water. It is very effective, but unpleasant! For reduced circulation leading to cramping sensations, you may also find it helpful to drink Ginger *(Zingiber officinalis)* tea, especially in the evening for helping night cramps.

To ease stiff, aching arm muscles, oil the arm and then massage deeply down the length of the arm with the thumbs.

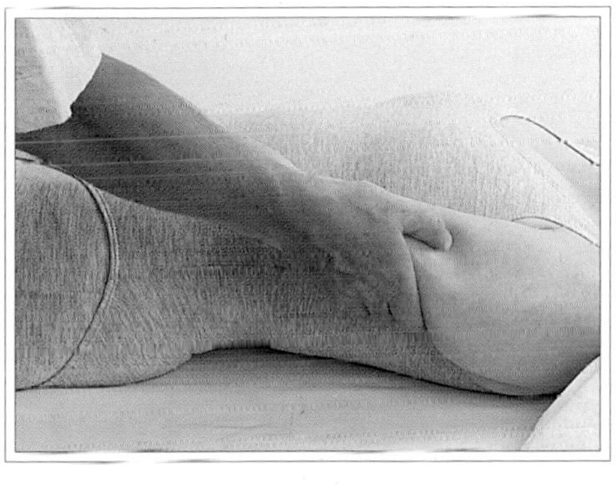

HOMEOPATHY

Some possible remedies are:

COLCHICUM: for cramps usually in the soles of the feet.

CUPRUM MET: for severe cramps, often starting in the toes or fingers and spreading up the limb; symptoms are aggravated by cold winds, and often come on in the evening.

GELSEMIUM: for writer's cramp, especially if associated with mental exhaustion or tension.

NUX VOMICA: this is most often used for digestive problems due to over-eating, but can be helpful for night cramps.

NATUROPATHY

When a cramp occurs, the first self-help action needs to be to stretch the affected muscle; for example if the calf muscle has gone into spasm, it can be relieved by pushing down with the heel to elongate the muscle again, even though this initially feels very painful! If taking hard physical exercise in very hot weather, there may be a case for ensuring you have more salt in the diet, although this should be temporary and not overdone.

Using alternate hot and cold compresses on the affected areas is another way to improve local circulation in cases of repeated cramps. For long-term problems look at one of the many relaxation techniques around.

FIBROSITIS

This is inflammation of the muscle fibres, often a chronic condition which can lead to the formation of hard nodules within the muscle. Fibrositis particularly affects the large muscles of the back, neck and shoulders, and sometimes into the buttocks. It may occur as a result of an injury, but is equally likely to arise from chronic stress and tension or poor posture. It needs to be differentiated from arthritis or other causes of pain.

AROMATHERAPY

Massage of the affected area is one of the most effective forms of treatment, and professional massage may well be needed to get deep into the tight muscles. At home, stroking and kneading the muscles with an oil containing essential oils of Eucalyptus, Lavender, Marjoram, Pine or Rosemary will help to warm and relax the affected fibres, stimulating the local circulation.

HERBALISM

Any anti-inflammatory herbs that might be taken internally can often be used in conjunction with local agents, for instance the oils suggested above. Furthermore, since stress is often a factor, look at herbs for easing tension generally (see Stress, pages 28-9). A couple of herbs that may be appropriate to take are Meadowsweet *(Filipendula ulmaria)* as an infusion, or Willow Bark *(Salix alba)* taken as a decoction (see page 12), unless tablets are available. Both these plants contain substances that are related chemically to aspirin; indeed this was first synthesized from extracts of Willow, and was named after an older Latin name for Meadowsweet, *Spiraea*. They are, however, much safer for the stomach, notably Meadowsweet, but seek advice before using if you are allergic to aspirin.

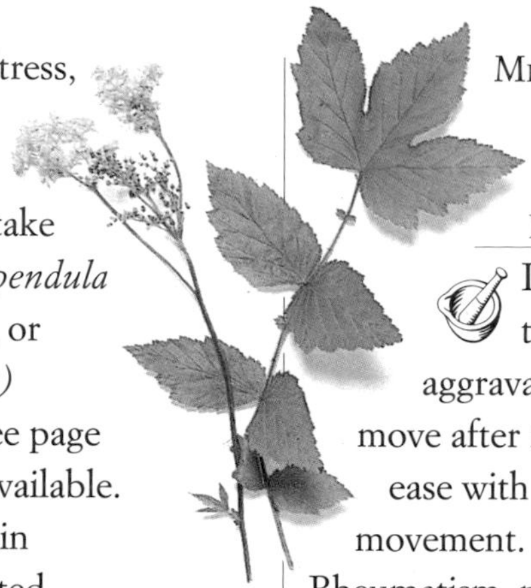

MEADOWSWEET *(Filipendula ulmaria)*

HOMEOPATHY

In the first place try Rhus tox if the pains are aggravated when first starting to move after resting, but gradually ease with continued steady movement. For other suggestions see Rheumatism, pages 88-9.

NATUROPATHY

Massage, stretching exercises and attention to posture will all help greatly, as will proper rest and relaxation. See a Naturopathy therapist for the best advice which will suit your own health and lifestyle.

MASSAGE FOR FIBROSITIS

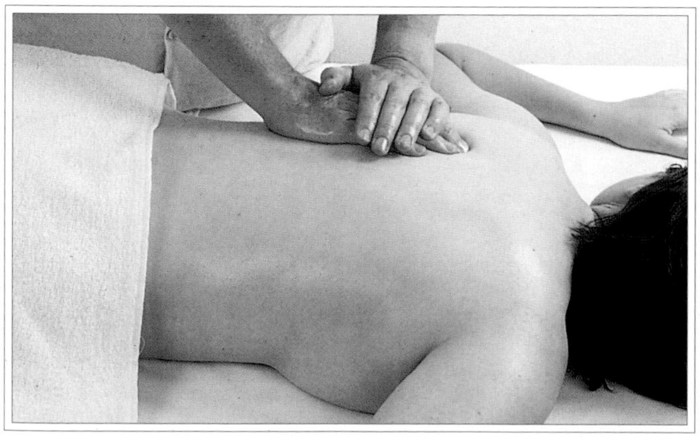

1 To ease stiff muscles in the shoulder, oil the back, using a base oil and essential oils as recommended. Place fingers just inside the shoulder blade, supporting with the other hand. Keep a relaxed but firm pressure.

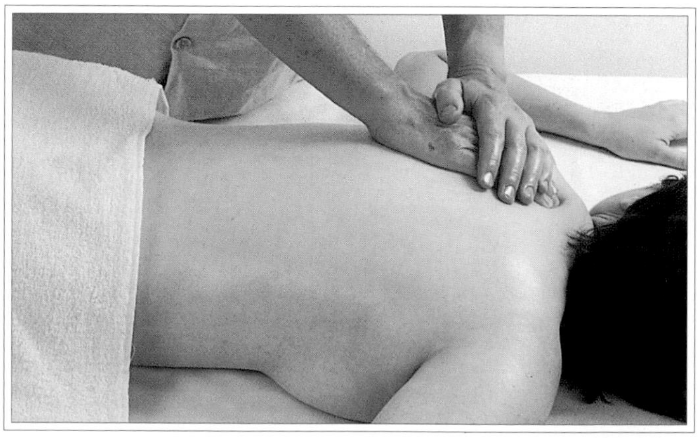

2 Move fingers steadily around the shoulder blade, pressing in firmly but within comfort limits. Repeat several times. Ease the pressure if too uncomfortable. Try this massage daily for a week.

GOUT

This condition occurs when there is an excess of uric acid in the body, and the kidneys cannot get rid of it effectively. The acid crystallizes into tiny sharp deposits like miniature needles; these collect in joints, often in the toes or feet but sometimes elsewhere such as the earlobes, causing intense pain and inflammation. The first signs of an attack may in fact be a feverish feeling, before the joint swells.

AROMATHERAPY

In an acute attack it is definitely not appropriate to massage the affected area – there is too much inflammation. Instead, use oils in cool or cold compresses to reduce the discomfort. For a detoxifying effect, try Cypress, Fennel, Juniper, Lemon or Pine oils. These may also be used in the bath. As the swelling and inflammation reduce, perhaps switch to oils such as Lavender or Rosemary for inducing local warmth and flushing toxins out of the joints.

HERBALISM

The classic herb is undoubtedly Celery Seed *(Apium graveolens)*; this may be taken in tablet form or by making a tea from 5 ml (1 tsp) of the seeds, lightly crushed with the back of a spoon, in 300 ml (½ pt/1¼ cups) of boiling water. Take 2 to 3 cupfuls a day for acute attacks of gout, to encourage strongly the excretion of uric acid. More directly anti-inflammatory herbs such as Meadowsweet *(Filipendula ulmaria)*, Willow Bark *(Salix alba)* or Devil's Claw *(Harpagophytum procumbens)* may be taken alongside the Celery Seed.

CELERY SEED *(Apium graveolens)*

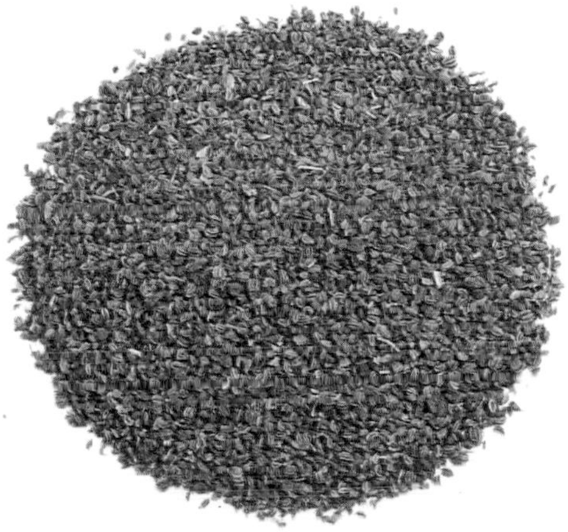

SELF-HELP FOR GOUT

Uric acid may accumulate within the kidneys themselves, leading to kidney stones, which may have to be surgically removed. Generally speaking, all the advice for Arthritis (see pages 83-4), will be applicable to gout.

An acute attack of gout is extremely painful and may require medical treatment. Try reducing food to a minimum but make sure to drink plenty of water, which will encourage removal of uric acid from the body.

The first two are described under Fibrositis (see page 86) while Devil's Claw is widely available in tablets or capsules, which are probably the easiest method in which to take it, up to 3 g per day. A general cleansing herb which is excellent to use regularly for chronic gout is Nettle *(Urtica dioca)* – simply drink it as a tea, 1 or 2 cups a day for a month or so.

HOMEOPATHY

A couple of remedies that often give some relief are:

ARNICA: for repeated attacks of gout, especially affecting the big toe, with hot, painful and very tender joints.

RHUS TOX: a versatile remedy for most rheumatic or arthritic problems; suitable for hard, painful swelling of the joints – these can be mistaken in mild attacks for a bunion.

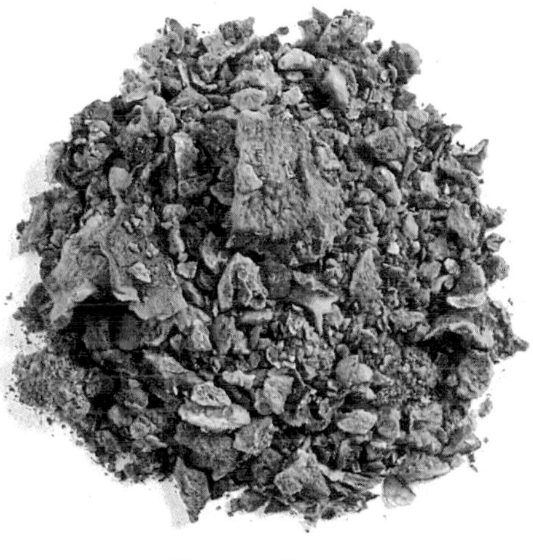

DEVIL'S CLAW
(Harpagophytum procumbens)

NATUROPATHY

Use cold compresses (see page 15) to reduce the swelling, switching to hot/cold applications in the longer term to encourage better circulation around the joint. Increase vegetable intake, especially raw or juiced, for a more alkaline intake, and cut out cheese, red wine (in the short term all alcohol), red meats, coffee and strong tea. When the swelling and inflammation has subsided, increase exercise to maintain joint mobility.

Drink plenty of mineral or spring water to encourage kidney action. Pain can be eased with some of the herbs discussed above.

RHEUMATISM

This is a general term which covers any inflammatory process in the muscles or joints; here its meaning will be limited to muscular rheumatism as Arthritis has already been covered (see pages 83-4). Much of the advice for Fibrositis (see page 86) is also relevant here as this is sometimes simply placed under the heading of rheumatism.

AROMATHERAPY

To aid the cleansing of the tissues, essential oils are probably best used in the bath (see page 8); appropriate oils are Cypress, Juniper, Pine and Rosemary, while Lavender may be added for greater muscle relaxation. Lavender and Rosemary are in addition quite analgesic in effect, giving some welcome relief from the pains and stiffness. If not too uncomfortable, massaging in a choice from these two, or else Juniper or Marjoram, diluted to 2 per cent in a base vegetable oil, speeds up the removal of toxins and improves blood supply to the affected muscles, and can be done regularly.

RHEUMATISM

As a rule, the emphasis of natural treatments is placed even more on detoxifying the system than is the case with joint problems, removing waste matter that congests and irritates the muscles to allow greater freedom of movement. A combination of dietary changes, exercise within limits of comfort, and other natural methods outlined in this section can dramatically improve rheumatic disorders over time.

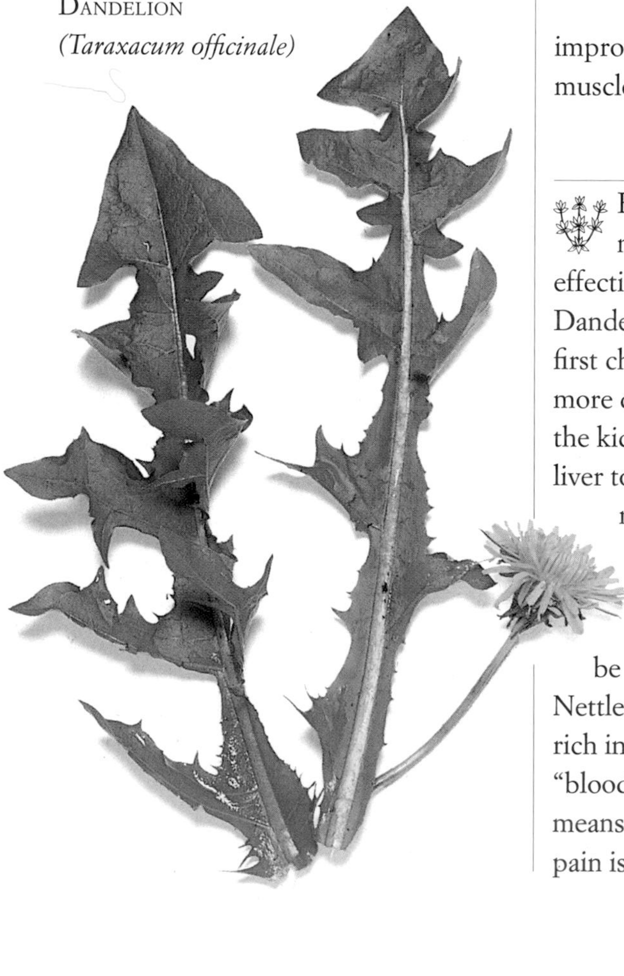

DANDELION *(Taraxacum officinale)*

HERBALISM

Elimination of irritant waste materials can be encouraged very effectively by herbal remedies. Try Dandelion *(Taraxacum officinale)* as a first choice for home use; the leaf is more diuretic, increasing output from the kidneys, while the root is a gentle liver tonic and mild laxative. For maximum benefit, make the leaf as an infusion and the root as a decoction (see page 12), and take each for a week. They can be combined with a herb such as Nettle *(Urtica dioica)*, which is not only rich in various minerals but acts as a "blood cleanser", helping to provide the means for tissue repair and renewal. If pain is a significant factor, a remedy like Meadowsweet *(Filipendula ulmaria)* can be very useful. These last two herbs can be used as infusions for a couple of weeks; for persistent discomfort get professional treatment.

If the circulation is definitely restricted, and the aching and stiffness are made worse by damp, cold weather, add a small amount of fresh Ginger *(Zingiber officinalis)* to any infusion. Ginger root is a strong circulatory stimulant and has a large part to play in treating many rheumatic/arthritic disorders.

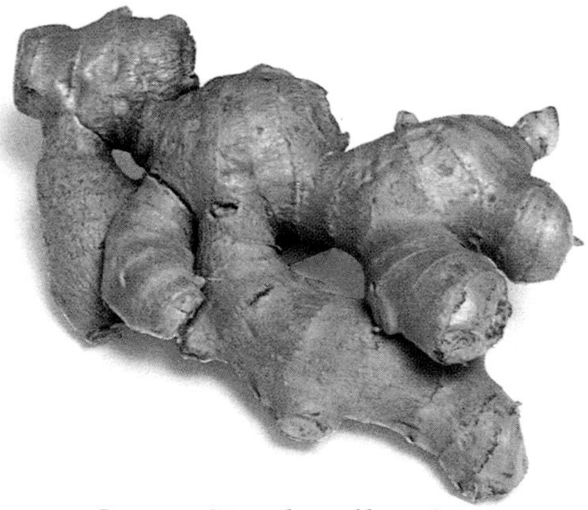

GINGER *(Zingiber officinalis)*

HOMEOPATHY

Here are a few potentially helpful remedies; also compare with the suggestions for other conditions in this section which may be appropriate.

ACTAEA RAC: particularly good for painful, stiff muscles in the back and neck; also good for aching muscles after exercise or for neuralgic pains.

ARNICA: for general aching of limbs, with a feeling of being bruised (see also First Aid section, page 102).

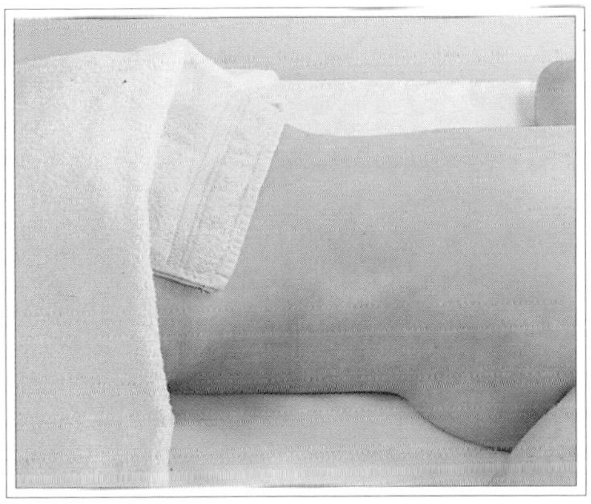

Compresses can stimulate circulation and reduce inflammation.

BRYONIA: for stiffness and swelling, for instance of the hands and arms; if the joints feel uncomfortable and "crack" with movement, this remedy may well be very useful too.

RHUS TOX: for the typical stiffness pattern of rheumatic disorders, aggravated after resting and improving after some movements. The remedy for lumbago, with low back pains on rising or after long periods of sitting.

RUTA GRAV: for pains felt in the tendons and muscles, and joints such as wrists, knees and ankles. May also be helpful in relieving sciatic pains (see page 25).

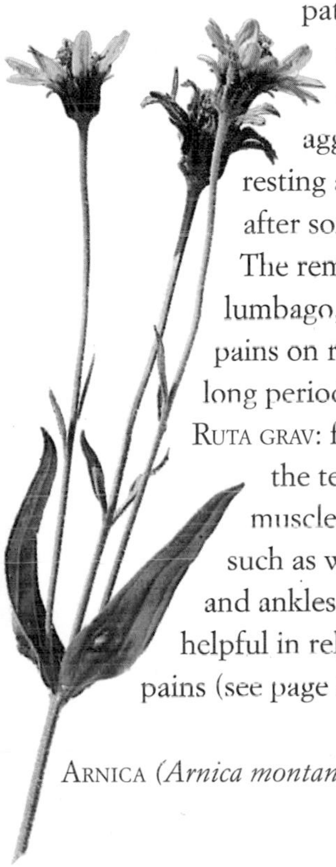

ARNICA *(Arnica montana)*

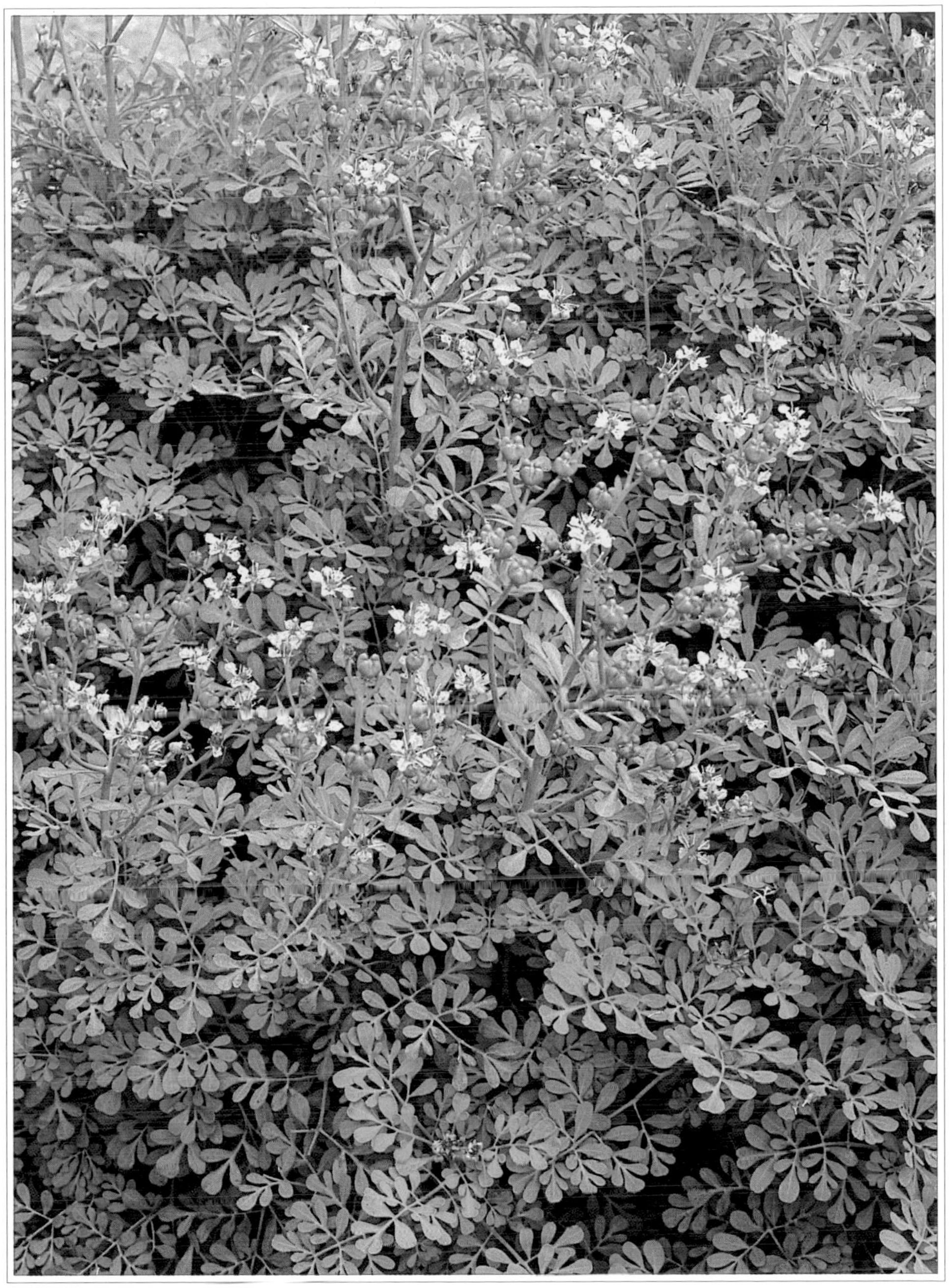

RUE *(Ruta graveolens)*

NATUROPATHY

Often a good soak in a hot bath (perhaps with a handful of Epsom salts) eases the stiffness and aching of muscular rheumatism, but too frequent a use of hot applications may produce too much congestion, so try alternating hot/cold compresses, if you can, in order to stimulate blood flow. A brisk rub with a thick, coarse towel will certainly aid this process. It is important to keep active as far as possible, so exercise is to be encouraged within individual limits of ability. Diet should be aimed at reducing acid waste matter, with plenty of vegetables and fresh fruit (with the probable exception of oranges) and very little refined carbohydrates or sugary foods. A supplement may be useful: take a multi-vitamin and mineral tablet once a day, or else initially just take a Vitamin B supplement. In winter, especially in cooler climates, taking a fish oil supplement such as cod liver oil capsules may ease stiffness.

THE SKIN

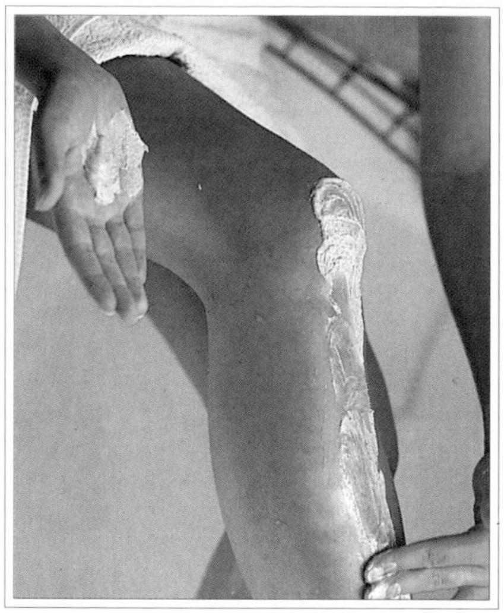

The natural approach to skin problems starts by taking the view that most disorders of the skin reflect inner imbalance, and that the whole person needs to be treated for truly effective results. This is especially so in conditions such as eczema or psoriasis, which can be highly complex disorders requiring professional treatment on an individual basis. Chronic or persistent problems should be referred to a practitioner. Given the potential negative effects of orthodox treatments such as steroid cream for eczema, there is much to be gained by looking at natural therapies.

The traditional treatment of many skin problems involves considerable attention being paid to the cleansing of the whole body. Both Western and Eastern (for example, Chinese or Indian) systems of herbal medicine have developed successful strategies for treating the skin. The role of other factors such as hormone balance, stress and lowered vitality also needs to be considered; for self-help other sections of this book may therefore be very useful.

As with all the conditions discussed in this book, do not overdo any of the self-help treatments suggested; if any skin problems get worse or continue for more than a short time, then stop the treatment and/or get professional help. Do not mix therapies; this is particularly true of homeopathy since the pattern of individual symptoms will be affected by other treatments, making the choice of homeopathic remedy more difficult. Small is beautiful in all the therapies – if a dose of something is helpful, do not think that doubling the dose will have double the benefit; quite often it is the opposite!

ABOVE: Herbal creams and ointments can bring relief to problem skin sufferers.

ABSCESS

An abscess is a localized inflamed swelling, containing pus. Abscesses can develop externally on the skin, but also internally in the mouth or on other mucous membranes – these should be referred for qualified medical treatment. Treatments locally on the skin will generally involve hot compresses or poultices to draw out the toxic waste matter; recurrent abscesses often indicate a weakened immune system. See also Boils, page 95.

AROMATHERAPY

Apply a hot compress (see page 15) to the area, by adding 5-6 drops of essential oil to a bowl of water as hot as you can bear, and soaking a piece of absorbent material in it. Suitable materials include lint, a clean handkerchief, or a face flannel. Fold over a couple of times for a thicker pad, and place on the abscess, covering with a bandage or piece of cling film (plastic-wrap) to hold in position. Renew when cooling to body temperature, and keep on for at least 30 minutes.

Appropriate essential oils for this process are Bergamot, Chamomile, Lavender and Tea Tree, either separately or in a combination such as Bergamot for its antiseptic properties, together with Lavender (also antiseptic) for a greater anti-inflammatory effect. (Remember that the number of drops suggested is the *total* amount used, not the number for each herb.)

HERBALISM

Make a hot poultice (see page 15) from a herb such as Marshmallow *(Althea officinalis)* for external treatment of the area. Either pour boiling water on to some fresh leaves, or mix the powdered root with hot water to make a paste. It may be helpful to use a little oil on the skin first to stop the poultice sticking, then place the herb on the abscess and cover with a clean gauze or strips of cotton, holding in position as above. Such a poultice can be kept on for several hours, but

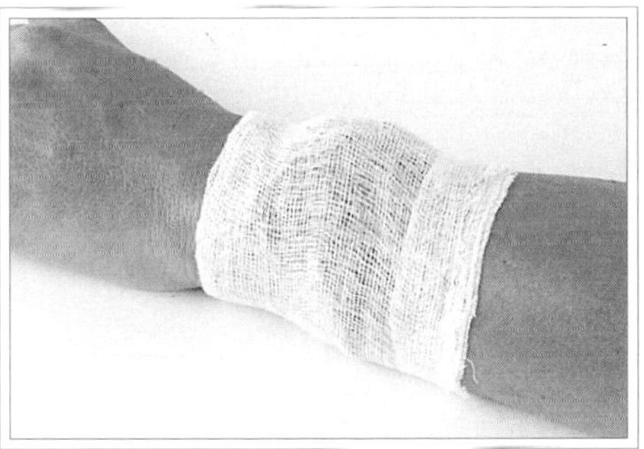

Apply a hot poultice on to the affected area, applying a little base oil to the skin first so that the poultice does not stick.

may need replacing every couple of hours. Another excellent herb to help draw out pus is Slippery Elm *(Ulmus fulva)*; use the powdered inner bark as for the Marshmallow root above.

For mouth abscesses, it may be appropriate simply to place a hot compress, made with an infusion of Chamomile (*Chamomilla recutita*), on the cheek over the area until a doctor or dentist can be seen. Internal treatment, as described under Boils (see page 95), will be most helpful in cleansing the system as a whole and boosting immunity.

HOMEOPATHY

Hot compresses are likely to be suggested by practitioners here too, perhaps using tinctures of Hypericum or Calendula. Pour 15 ml (1 tbsp) of hot water on to 2 drops of either remedy, and soak a piece of gauze in it. Place on the area and cover, renewing when cooling down.

Internally, take a few doses of either Hepar sulph if the abscess is hot, throbs with pain and is very tender to the touch, or else Silica if the abscess, although equally painful, feels cold to the touch, and the discharge is slow to clear up. These two remedies are very good for suppurating (oozing) skin conditions generally, given their different symptom pictures.

NATUROPATHY

If nothing else is available, use just hot water to make a compress, or put a hot water bottle over the affected area. You can use cabbage leaves from the garden with excellent results; take a few of the outer leaves, cut out the central rib and coarsely chop the leaves, pour on boiling water and make a poultice as outlined above. This is very soothing and helps to draw out infection. You may obtain Kaolin from a pharmacist to make a poultice, spread on a dressing and use over the area. When an abscess bursts, cover with a sterile dry dressing. For repeated problems a programme of dietary reform will be most helpful; for further information, see Boils, page 95.

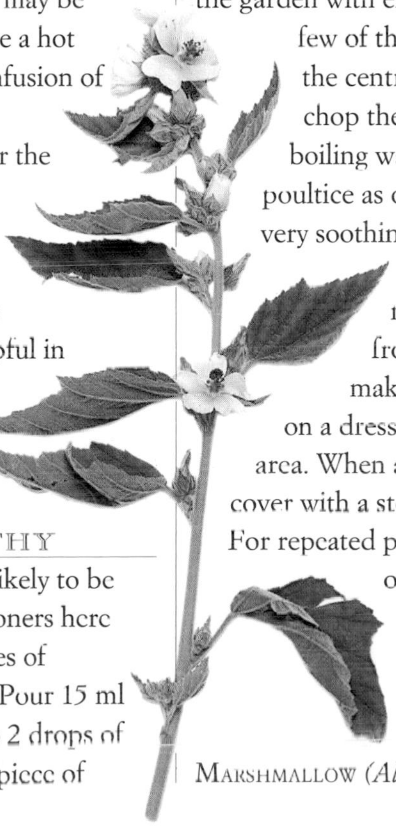

MARSHMALLOW *(Althea officinalis)*

ACNE

This is a very common skin condition during puberty, although it may continue into later life for some people. Increasing levels of hormones during adolescence lead to greater activity of the skin's sebaceous glands, and if this becomes too great, excessive amounts of sebum, our natural oily skin lubricant, are produced. This in turn can cause the glands and hair follicles to become blocked and infected.

AROMATHERAPY

Many essential oils are not only antiseptic but also promote healing or generation of new healthy skin cells. Some of the best are Bergamot, Geranium, Lavender and Lemon; these may need to be used in varying combinations depending on the state of the skin and the person as a whole. Bergamot, for instance, is an effective antidepressant, and this emotional quality may be helpful at times as acne can understandably make the sufferer feel low (adolescence is a time of fluctuating self-esteem at the best of times), and as an astringent, antiseptic oil it is excellent for greasy, infected skin. Do not, however, overuse this oil as it increases the skin's sensitivity to the sun; moderate amounts of sunlight are generally good for drying and healing the skin too.

These oils may be used in a light carrier vegetable oil such as Grapeseed, which has a slight astringency of its own, or Coconut, or else mixed into gentle cleansing creams for regular use on the affected areas. Another base might be a toning lotion such as triple-distilled Rosewater, Orange Blossom water or perhaps distilled Witch Hazel for extra astringency. Use 1-2 per cent of essential oils in any of these base carriers. If there is much evidence of scarring after the condition has improved, use the essential oils in a carrier which includes 10 per cent Wheatgerm oil to promote skin elasticity and healing.

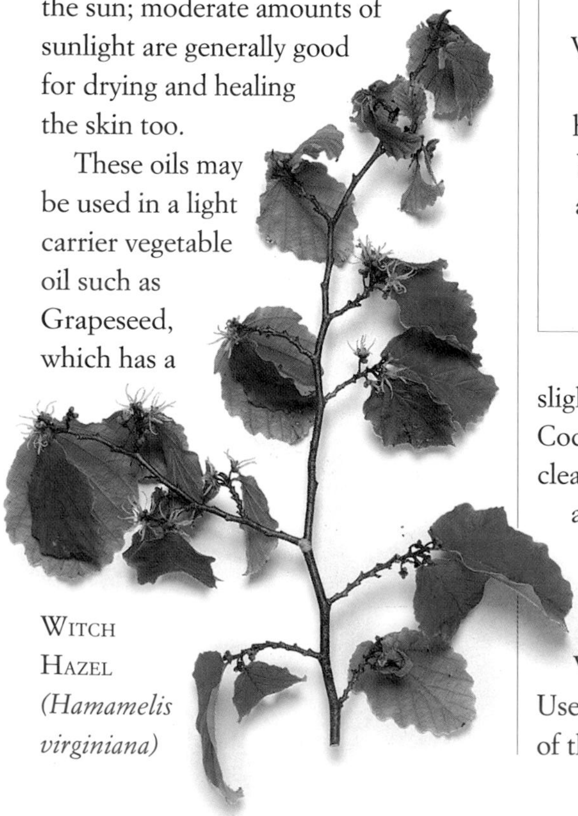

Witch Hazel *(Hamamelis virginiana)*

Self-help for Acne

The most common reaction of most people is to squeeze the spots; this almost always serves to spread the infection into surrounding tissues, and if done repeatedly can damage the local skin areas, producing scarring. Any programme of treatment therefore needs to include a lot of self-help to be successful. The natural therapies offer the most successful and safest ways to improve the condition and rebalance of the skin.

The best approach is to combine local, external cleansing with internal treatment; all therapies are likely to emphasize the importance of diet in treating acne.

Where acne persists for years after adolescence, there may well be a hormonal imbalance that needs to be addressed, and again there are appropriate natural remedies that may be used – seek professional treatment if needed.

HERBALISM

Initial treatment should be firmly geared towards cleansing of the skin and of the whole system. Locally, any of the essential oils described above may be used, or else cleanse the skin with an infusion of herbs (see page 12) such as Elderflower *(Sambucus nigra)*, Lavender *(Lavandula vera)* or Marigold *(Calendula officinalis)*; adding 5 ml (1 tsp) of distilled Witch Hazel *(Hamamelis virginiana)* to 300 ml (½ pt/1¼ cups) of the infusion will gently increase the astringency if needed.

The main use of herbal remedies though will be internally: choose a mixture of the following herbs:

Burdock *(Arctium lappa)*: a powerful tissue cleanser, encouraging the removal of waste matter from the skin via the blood supply, and equally helping the transport of nutrients to the skin. The root is more powerful, and a decoction should be used (see page 12), the leaf is made into an infusion.

Start by taking small amounts of this herb (about 45 ml (3 tbsp), 3 times a day) as it can initially stir things up and the skin seems to get worse.

Cone Flower *(Echinacea angustifolia* or *E. purpurea)*: the best all-purpose immune stimulant, aiding resistance

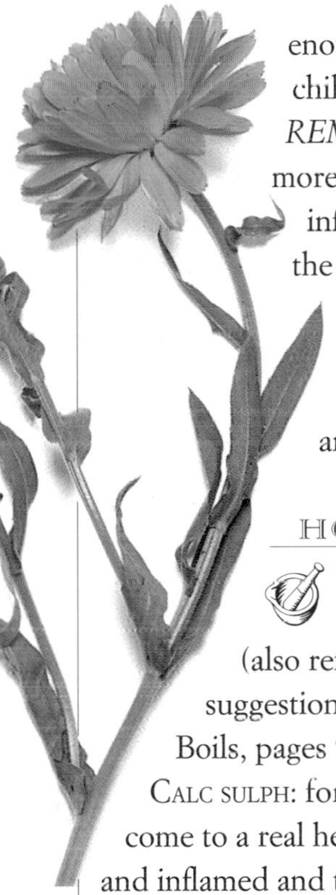

MARIGOLD *(Calendula officinalis)*

and speeding up our reactions to infection. Used together with the above herbs, this creates a strong detoxification process.

DANDELION *(Taraxacum officinale)*: the root in particular is helpful in improving the detoxifying action of the liver, and also as a gentle laxative, taking pressure away from the skin as an organ of elimination.

RED CLOVER *(Trifolium pratense)*: another excellent blood and tissue cleanser, the infusion can also be used externally to carefully bathe inflamed spots and is gentle enough to use on children in this way.

REMEMBER: if using more than one herb in an infusion or a decoction, the amount of each herb included is reduced to maintain the given overall maximum amounts.

> **ACNE AND THE ADOLESCENT**
>
> Acne can be a major blight on adolescence, causing much emotional upset and even relationship difficulties, so it is important that familes and all concerned do not exaggerate the condition. Concern and practical help are better then either dismissing the problem or worst still, making negative comments. Gentle, but regular, cleansing of the skin, attention to hygiene and diet will all help keep acne to a minimum, so encouragement of these activities is useful, even if met with opposition!

HOMEOPATHY

In the short term try one of these remedies (also refer to the remedy suggestions for Abscesses and Boils, pages 91 and 95).

CALC SULPH: for spots that never come to a real head, but get tender and inflamed and then seem to subside after a while (suitable for "blind boils").

HEPAR SULPH: for lots of pus-filled spots, which feel hot and tender to the touch, and generally unhealthy-looking skin.

SILICA: for slow-healing of the skin, spots that develop pus which is slow to clear; this remedy is particularly good for helping the healing of scarring.

NATUROPATHY

The first basic principle of the naturopathic approach (as with all the other natural therapies) is to overhaul the diet, as far as is possible given teenage fads! A reduction of sugary, fatty foods is essential, shifting the balance towards fresh fruit and vegetables, whole grains and lean forms of protein. It is often desirable to reduce dairy products for a while, especially milk or strong cheeses. Taking plenty of fluids regularly is important, *not* fizzy drinks or tea and coffee, but water or fruit juices. Alcohol should also be reduced.

Stimulating the circulation, either by self-massage or using hydrotherapy – for instance, by briskly rubbing the trunk and limbs with a loofah dipped in cool water – is a helpful aid to cleansing of the skin. Allow the skin to breathe by wearing cool clothes, and pay strict attention to hygiene. Sunshine is usually helpful, although be careful not to stay in the sun too long, and take adequate sun-protection measures.

Supplementation of the diet can speed up the cleansing/healing processes initially; important vitamins are A (around 2,500 iu daily), B complex and C (up to 300 mg daily), while one of the most useful minerals is zinc (up to 15 mg daily). Evening Primrose oil has been found to be of benefit in some cases; take up to 1,500 mg daily.

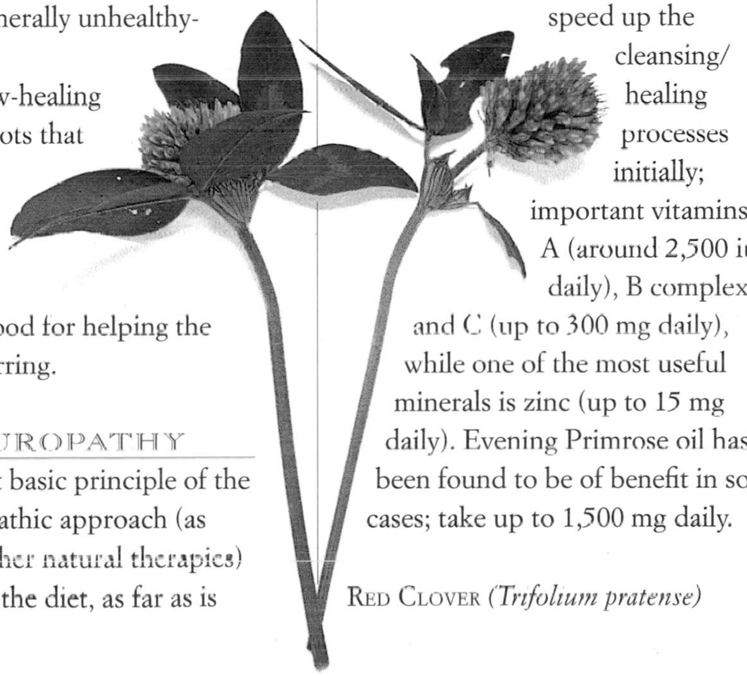

RED CLOVER *(Trifolium pratense)*

ATHLETE'S FOOT

This fungal skin condition can be produced by a number of different microscopic fungal growths, causing inflammation and itching. Despite its name, it is neither confined to the feet nor only restricted to athletes!

AROMATHERAPY

The most suitable anti-fungal essential oils to use are Lavender, Myrrh and Tea Tree, all of which not only tackle the infection directly but are also soothing and healing. Initially they may be best applied dissolved in a little neat alcohol, at 2-3 per cent dilution, or even used sparingly on their own on the moist, infected skin; when the skin is drier, they might then be incorporated into a cream base, up to 3 per cent dilution (see page 16).

Another useful base is Olive oil, which in itself seems to have some anti-fungal activity (see also Thrush, pages 74-5). Oil of Calendula, or the Old English Marigold, has very helpful healing properties and may be used as a base too. It may be helpful in the beginning to use a footbath, with 10 drops of one of the essential oils mentioned, but it is essential that the feet are dried thoroughly afterwards, and kept aired as often as possible.

MARIGOLD *(Calendula officinalis)*

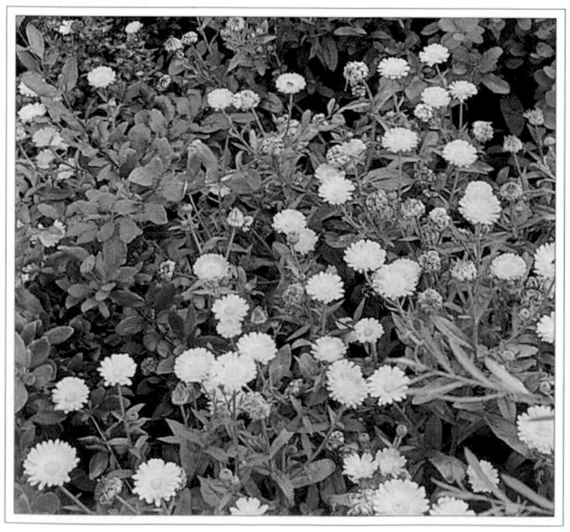

SELF-HELP MEASURES

The commonest sites are where the skin gets moist and hot, such as between the toes or in the groin, and on the scalp where it may take the form of ringworm. The most important self-help measures involve keeping the affected area cool and dry, and paying scrupulous attention to hygiene as the fungus can accumulate under the nails causing infection between the fingers or simply spreading by contact.

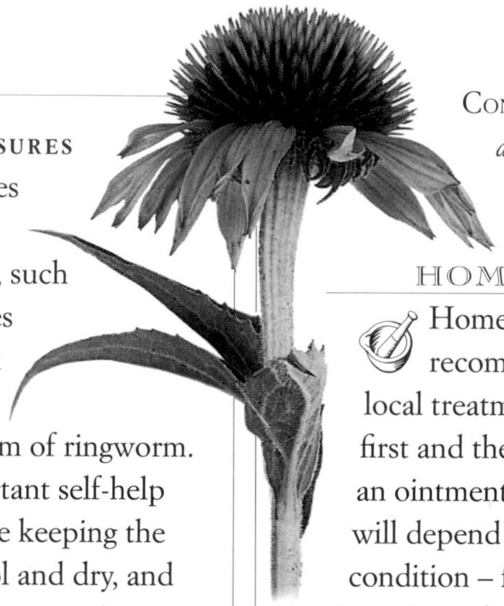

CONE FLOWER *(Echinacea angustifolia)*

HERBALISM

External applications of tinctures of either Marigold *(Calendula officinalis)* or Myrrh *(Commiphora molmol)* are powerfully anti-fungal; leave the application to dry out on the skin. If the skin is very moist, these two herbs may be applied in powder form if available, either neat or by mixing with unperfumed talcum powder.

Widespread or recurrent infection may also require internal remedies to bolster the immune system – take Garlic *(Allium sativum)* regularly, either in food or perhaps as a capsule; a short course of Cone Flower *(Echinacea angustifolia* or *E. purpurea)*, as an infusion, tincture (see pages 12 and 14 respectively) or in tablets (around 1,500 mg per day) may help.

HOMEOPATHY

Homeopaths may well also recommend Calendula as a local treatment, the tincture at first and then perhaps the oil or an ointment. Internal remedies will depend on the nature of the condition – for instance, if the area is moist and suppurating, a choice may be made from Hepar sulph, Merc sol, Silica or Sulphur, among others, so it is most advisable to seek a qualified practitioner.

NATUROPATHY

The first action to take is to ensure that the affected area keeps as dry and well-ventilated as possible, as the fungi responsible love hot, damp conditions. Use cotton socks and underwear, changing the garments daily. Ideally avoid wearing trainers and use leather shoes. Wash feet and other affected areas at least once a day, drying very thoroughly by patting dry rather than rubbing and chafing the skin. Use talcum powder to help keep the feet dry. Wash underwear in very hot water; the fungi may survive a low temperature wash cycle. Do not share towels or flannels as the infection may be passed on through physical contact. Footbaths can have 10-20 ml (2-4 tsp) of cider vinegar added, for a stronger anti-fungal effect.

BOILS

A boil is an acute inflamed and infected area on the skin, often in a blocked hair follicle. If a number of boils occur together, they may produce a large inflamed lump with several pus-filled "heads", and are termed a carbuncle (the medical term for a boil is a furuncle; if they are recurring, you are suffering from furunculosis). A stye is effectively a boil occurring in the base of an eyelash.

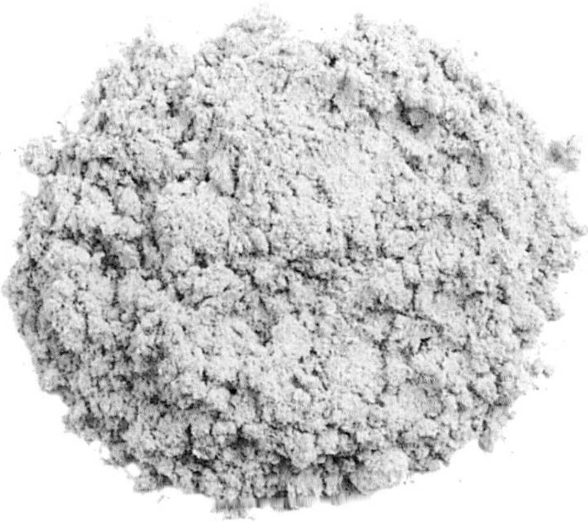

Slippery Elm *(Ulmus fulva)*

AROMATHERAPY

In order to keep the tissues surrounding the boil clean and free from bacterial infection, it is very useful to wash the area 2 to 4 times a day with a 2 per cent dilution of essential oil of Lavender in cooled, boiled water, using sterile cotton wool (cotton pad) if possible. For drawing out the boil, a hot compress (see page 15) with oils such as Bergamot, Chamomile, Lavender or Tea Tree will be useful. These are variously antiseptic, anti-inflammatory and speed up healing; they may additionally be used in the bath as more general detoxifying remedies. The oil of choice would probably be Lavender; this is the most versatile oil to have for home use.

Causes of Boils

Boils tend to occur when people are run-down, either by stress or through poor diet and hygiene, but can be more frequent in some other illnesses, such as diabetes when the higher blood sugar levels provide food for bacteria (see also treatment suggestions for Abscess and Acne, pages 91 and 92-3). Generally, treatments are geared initially towards bringing the boil to a head and allowing it to burst and discharge the pus. It is important that all external applications are as clean as possible – for example, use sterile dressings for applying any poultices. In the medium to longer term, the natural therapies are ideally suited to cleansing the system as a whole, building up immunity to further outbreaks and restoring health and vitality.

Deeper causes of lowered vitality, such as prolonged stress, will need attention too, and oils may be used in the bath or in massage to help restore normal functioning. For additional help with stress, see pages 28-9.

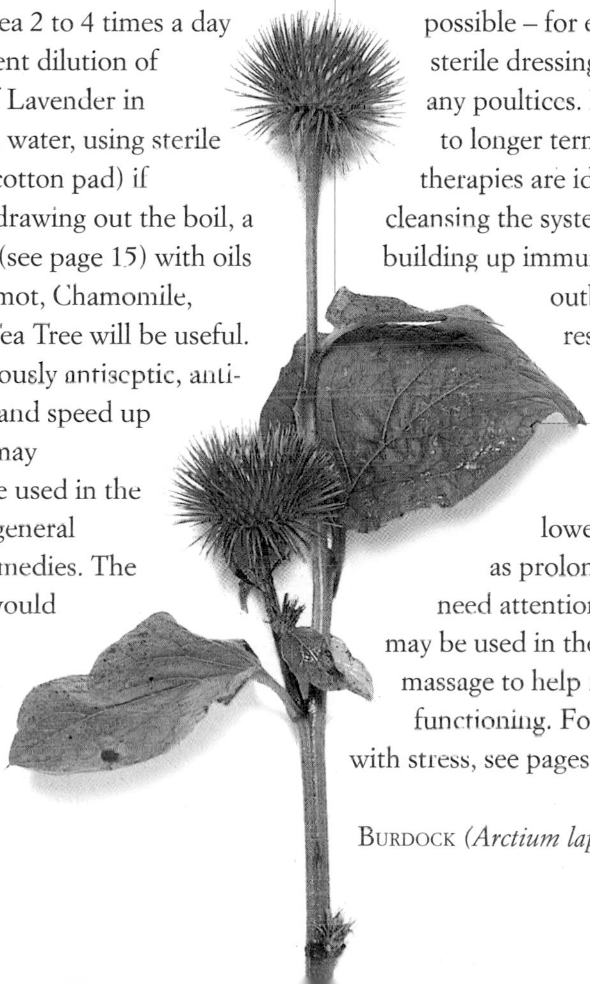

Burdock *(Arctium lappa)*

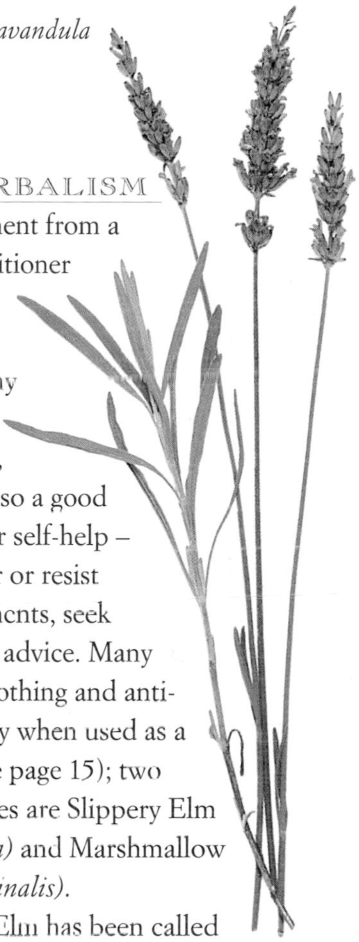

Lavender *(Lavandula angustifolia)*

HERBALISM

Treatment from a herbal practitioner will focus internally as well as on any local applications, and this is also a good approach for self-help – if boils recur or resist home treatments, seek professional advice. Many herbs are soothing and anti-inflammatory when used as a poultice (see page 15); two excellent ones are Slippery Elm *(Ulmus fulva)* and Marshmallow *(Althea officinalis)*.

Slippery Elm has been called the "herbalists' knife" for its ability to bring a boil to bursting point; simply thicken the powder with a little boiling water and apply as a paste, as hot as you can bear. Powdered Marshmallow root can also be used, or else the fresh leaves can be softened with boiling water and applied as a hot poultice. When the boil has burst, wash the area with cooled Lavender *(Lavandula vera)* tea or else keep using Slippery Elm as a cool poultice to speed up healing. If no other herbs are available, use fresh Garlic *(Allium sativum)* on the inflamed area, gently rubbing a cut clove over the skin.

Internally, Garlic may also be helpful, as a powerful antibiotic and immune-booster. Blood-cleansing herbal remedies include Burdock *(Arctium lappa)*, Yellow Dock *(Rumex crispus)* and/or Dandelion Root *(Taraxacum officinale)*, all most effectively taken as decoctions (see page 12), and Cleavers *(Galium aparine)* or Red Clover *(Trifolium pratense)* made as infusions (see page 12). It may be valuable to take Cone Flower *(Echinacea angustifolia* or *E. purpurea)* tablets or drops for a couple of weeks afterwards to help restore natural immune function.

HOMEOPATHY

Remedies to choose from are:
BELLADONNA: for very reddened skin probably in the earlier stages of developing a boil when it is throbbing and feels burningly hot to the touch.
HEPAR SULPH: for a hot, pus-filled boil which is coming to a head; this remedy will help it to mature and burst.
SILICA: this remedy is appropriate when the boil, although painful, feels if anything cold to the touch. This remedy and the previous one, with their differing symptom patterns, can be thought of as the "homeopath's knife", helping the boil to discharge.

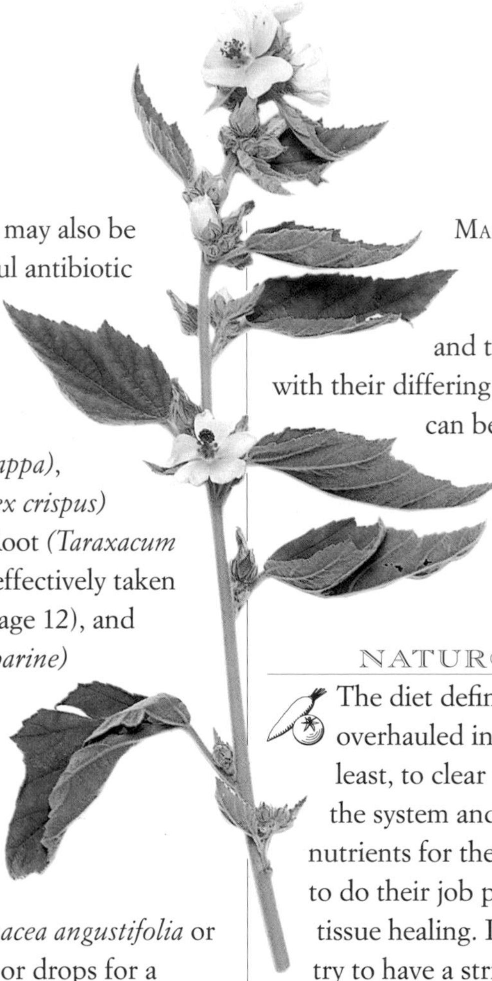

MARSHMALLOW *(Althea officinalis)*

NATUROPATHY

The diet definitely needs to be overhauled in the short term at least, to clear waste matter out of the system and provide essential nutrients for the immune defences to do their job properly and to aid tissue healing. If possible, try to have a strict diet for a week, cutting out all sugar, refined carbohydrates, tea, coffee, alcohol, cheese and fried foods; eat plenty of fresh vegetables, raw or cooked fresh fruit, whole grains and a little lean protein.

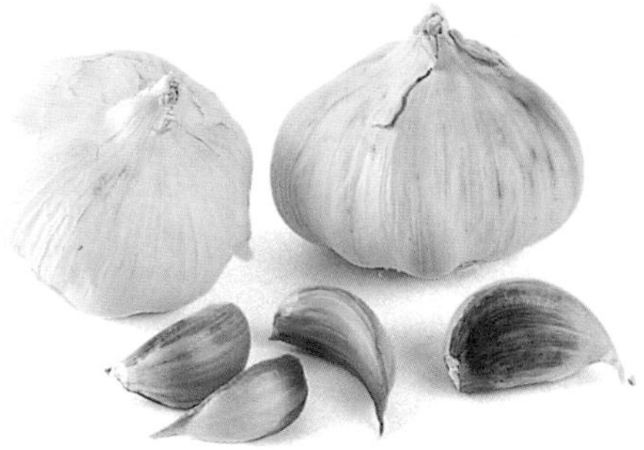

GARLIC *(Allium sativum)*

Fluids should mostly be water, especially spring water, or else fruit juices (diluted in hot weather) or herbal teas. Alcohol should be avoided if at all possible.

There may be a case for taking extra nutrients in the form of a supplement: if the diet has been poor for a while, take a high quality multi-vitamin and mineral supplement, or else try taking zinc, up to 25 mg daily for a week and then 15 mg daily for another month.

Locally, bathing the boil in hot water may bring it to a head, or use a hot poultice (see page 15) made from the outer leaves of a cabbage, roughly chopped.

If boils recur, or continue, then seek professional help.

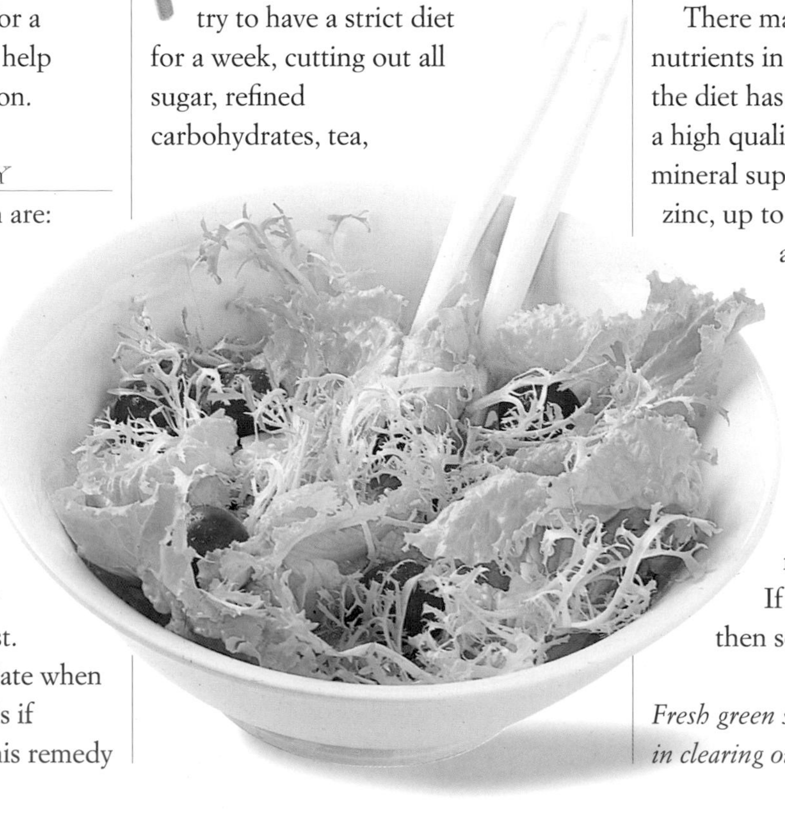

Fresh green salad leaves can greatly assist in clearing out the system.

COLD SORES

These are caused by the virus herpes simplex, another strain of which produces genital herpes (although it may be the same virus behaving differently). This virus is able to lie dormant in our tissues almost indefinitely until conditions trigger off an attack; it is probable that nearly everybody has acquired this virus at an early age from another person, so the key factor is what allows the virus to multiply and erupt.

AROMATHERAPY

Some essential oils are excellent for local use, and at the earliest stage possible of an outbreak are probably the most effective treatment for cold sores. Particularly good are Bergamot, Eucalyptus, Lavender, Lemon and Tea Tree. These may be applied neat, using just 1 drop on a cotton bud (swab), but may be better if diluted in a little alcohol; for home use a spirit such as vodka will do very well: add 5 drops of essential oil to 5 ml (1 tsp) of alcohol and dab on frequently. Neat Lavender oil may be dabbed on a little later to speed up healing.

HERBALISM

Local applications of herbs are most effective when they are used in tincture form (see page 14), dabbed on to the cold sores frequently to dry and heal the area. Some of the best are Lavender *(Lavandula vera)*, Marigold *(Calendula officinalis)*, Myrrh *(Commiphora molmol)*, Wild Indigo *(Baptisia tinctoria)* and Witch Hazel *(Hamamelis virginiana)*.

Where the appearance of cold sores indicates overall exhaustion, the herb St John's Wort *(Hypericum perforatum)* is an excellent choice; the tincture can be used locally as above, and may be taken internally as a calming restorative for the nervous system, 20 drops 3 times a day. *CAUTION*: this herb increases sensitivity to sunlight, so avoid prolonged exposure to strong, bright sunshine while taking internally.

ATTACK TRIGGERS

One of the most common predisposing factors is the ordinary cold, hence the name, but any respiratory infection can trigger an attack, as can being generally run-down. Extremes of temperature, or exposure to strong sunshine are other possible causes.

When an attack does occur, small blisters come out on the lips or at the corner of the mouth. These form a crust and remain moist underneath for up to 10 days or so before drying out. They are highly infectious during all the moist, weeping stages.

HOMEOPATHY

For a first-time eruption, try one of the following remedies, for up to 5 days at 30c potency (see Introduction, page 10, for explanation of potencies). If cold sores persist or recur, see a homeopath.

NAT MUR: for cold sores associated with a swelling of the lip, possibly even causing a deep crack, the sores forming several blisters.

RHUS TOX: for when the corners of the mouth get sore and there is a burning sensation; the eruptions may also spread out on to the chin, and the remedy "picture" often includes a red tip to the tongue as part of the overall symptoms.

NATUROPATHY

A simple yet highly effective home remedy is to apply freshly squeezed lemon juice to the cold sore, at the first signs of the problem (since the zest contains the essential oil, there is an obvious connection with Aromatherapy treatment). For a drying effect, you may find good quality eau-de-Cologne dabbed on and left to dry can be useful. It is often helpful to take a short course of a Vitamin B complex supplement, backed up by zinc (10-15 mg daily), and Vitamin C (500 mg daily). This is especially true when cold sores are recurring frequently, since these nutrients help to boost the immune system generally, as well as enhancing our ability to cope with chronic stress.

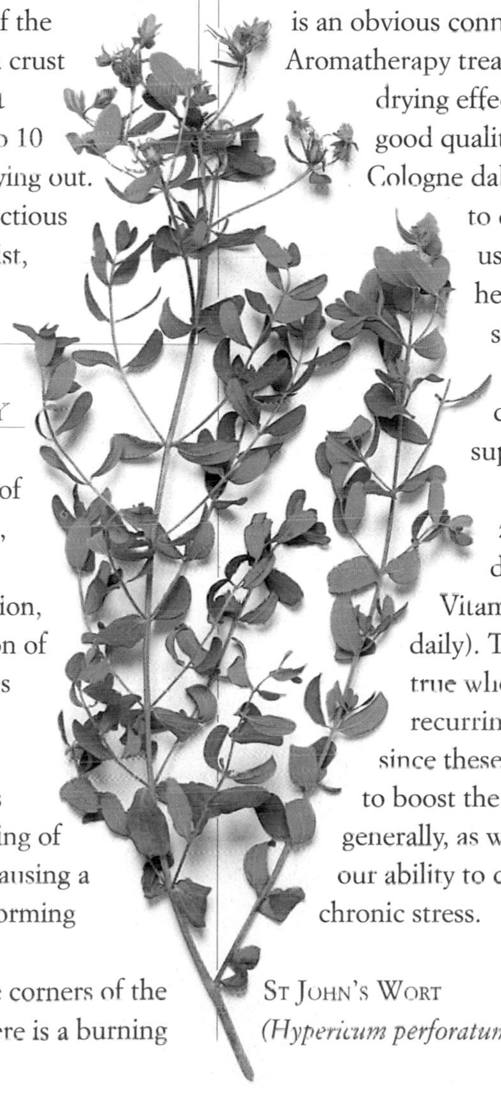

ST JOHN'S WORT
(Hypericum perforatum)

ECZEMA

This is a complex skin condition, and in most instances will need professional treatment. The natural therapies have an extremely good record in treating people with eczema, and given the problems associated with the long-term, regular use of steroid creams, there is a lot to be said for looking at other options.

AROMATHERAPY

The most important thing to remember when trying to help ease eczema is to be as flexible as possible. You may well need to vary the oils, and change the way you use them, since the nature of the condition can be due to so many factors, and the skin can get better for a while with one oil and then may need something different as the symptoms change.

Some of the most useful oils to use on the skin are Chamomile, Geranium, Lavender, Lemon Balm (often listed as Melissa, the first part of its Latin name) and perhaps Rose. They should be used in at most a 1 per cent dilution initially, and can be incorporated in a light aqueous cream, or perhaps use a thicker cream, ointment or pure vegetable oil base if the skin is extremely dry or weakened (see page 16 for how to make creams and ointments). Try these oils one at a time at first, to see whether the skin reacts to any of them.

Chamomile
(Chamomilla recutita)

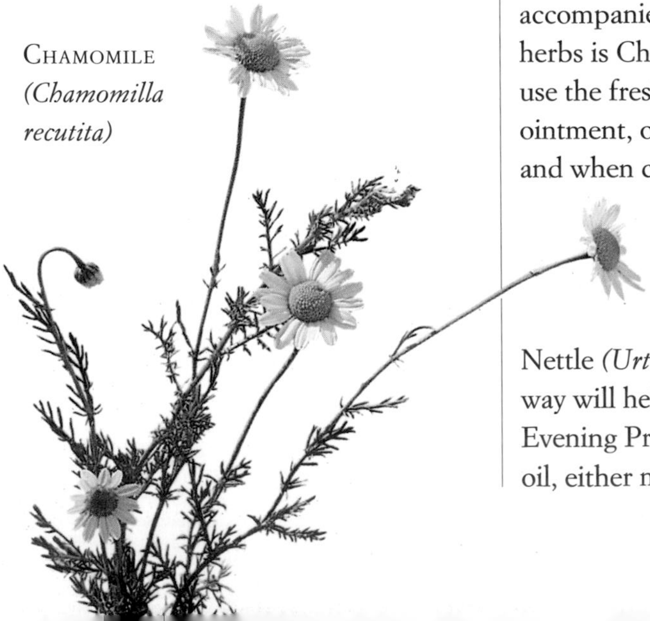

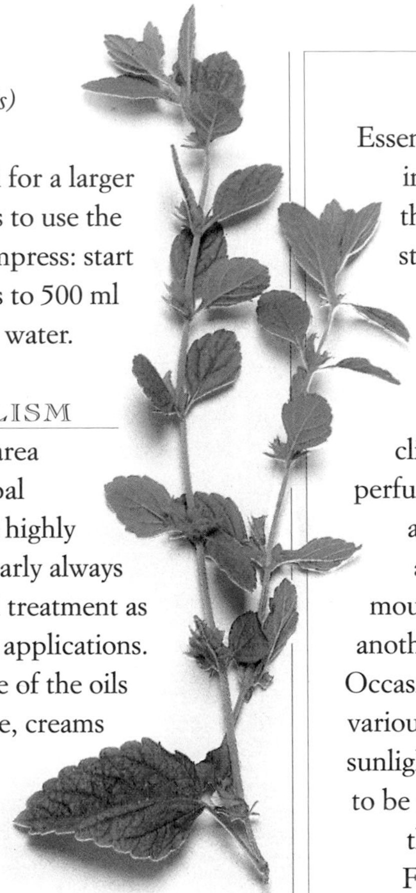

Lemon Balm
(Melissa officinalis)

Another method for a larger area of eczema is to use the oils in a cool compress: start with just 5 drops to 500 ml (16 fl oz/2 cups) water.

HERBALISM

This is an area where herbal medicine can be highly effective, and nearly always involves internal treatment as well as any local applications. Apart from some of the oils mentioned above, creams or ointments made with Comfrey *(Symphytum officinale)* or Marigold *(Calendula officinalis)* can help to reduce inflammation and speed up healing. For the intense itching that often accompanies eczema one of the best herbs is Chickweed *(Stellaria media)*; use the fresh herb to make a cream or ointment, or simply make an infusion and when cooled apply as a compress.

If the skin is weeping, then infusions of Heartsease *(Viola tricolor)*, Red Clover *(Trifolium pratense)* or even Nettle *(Urtica dioica)* used in a similar way will help to dry the area. Applying Evening Primrose *(Oenothera biennis)* oil, either neat or in a cream base, can

Causes of Eczema

Essentially, eczema is an allergic inflammation and irritation of the skin. There may be a fairly straightforward external cause – for instance, a reaction to nickel which is often found in cheaper jewellery, watch straps, zips (zippers), clips and so on. Cosmetics, perfumes and hair colourings are another source of potential allergens, and fur, feathers, mould spores or dust make up another major group of irritants. Occasionally people react badly to various plants, especially in bright sunlight, and keen gardeners need to be aware of possible dangers if they have sensitive skin.

For many eczema sufferers, however, any external irritants are secondary to inner factors. In what is termed atopic eczema, there is often a family history of eczema, asthma or hay fever (all similarly over-reactive disorders), and problem areas such as emotional upsets, stress and food intolerance play a bigger part in the individual's eczema pattern. Unravelling the particular combination of factors for each person is often a detective story, which is where seeking treatment from a qualified natural therapist can be so valuable, with their focus on the whole person.

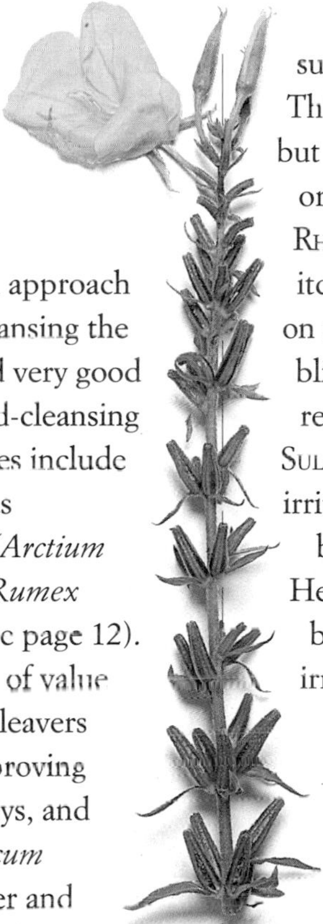

EVENING PRIMROSE *(Oenothera biennis)*

be very soothing and healing.

The traditional herbal approach to eczema focuses on cleansing the tissues, and this can yield very good results. Herbs with blood-cleansing or "alternative" properties include Red Clover and Nettle, as infusions, and Burdock *(Arctium lappa)* or Yellow Dock *(Rumex crispus)* as decoctions (see page 12). Two other herbs that are of value in removing toxins are Cleavers *(Galium aparine)* for improving elimination via the kidneys, and Dandelion Root *(Taraxacum officinale)* to tone the liver and gently open the bowels. The former should be used as an infusion and the latter as a decoction. Mixtures may be made from the above herbs. Do not use for more than 3 weeks and if the skin gets worse, reduce the dosage by half.

HOMEOPATHY

Since eczema can initially flare up with treatment, take just one dose of a 30c potency (see page 10) per week, selecting from the following remedies (if there is no improvement within a month, consult a qualified practitioner):

GRAPHITES: for a moist, weeping skin which forms scabs that easily break off. The discharge is sticky, and the exposed surface of the skin may also bleed. This condition may be anywhere, but typical areas are behind the ears or on the face.

RHUS TOX: for a dry, very intensely itching eczema, such as might occur on the hands and wrists. Often little blisters form in the patches of redness.

SULPHUR: for hot, dry and burningly irritating skin. There is acute itching, but scratching makes it very sore. Heat of any kind (for instance, hot baths or lying in bed) makes the irritation much worse.

NATUROPATHY

Given the importance of stress in aggravating many kinds of eczema, looking at relaxation techniques may be valuable (see also Stress, pages 28-9). With regard to diet, many foods can be potential problems, most notably dairy foods. Where eczema has been around from infancy, it is often very beneficial to try eliminating cow's milk, cheese and other dairy products from the diet for up to three weeks. Reducing sugar, spicy foods, coffee, tea and alcohol, and keeping food additives to a minimum are other potentially useful approaches. Taking a supplement of Vitamin B complex can help, and sometimes Vitamin A (up to 5,000 iu for a month) is needed. Evening Primrose oil can be taken internally as well as used locally; to boost the essential fatty acids within the body, take up to 1,500 mg daily.

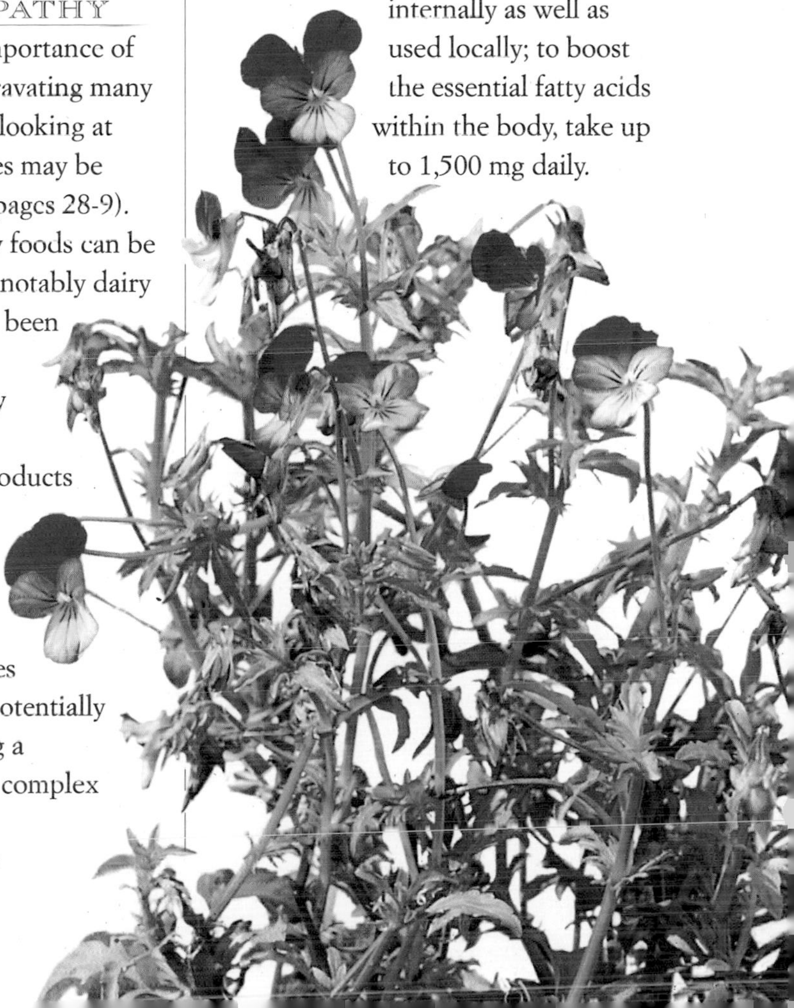

HEARTSEASE *(Viola tricolor)*

DIETARY ADVICE

Specific dietary advice will obviously require professional consultation, as there may be particular foods which provoke or aggravate an individual's eczema. If the suggestions in the Naturopathy section do not radically improve the skin with 6-8 weeks, get professional advice.

PSORIASIS

This is a skin disease where the skin cells start to grow too rapidly; the immature cells over-produce but fail to mature into proper keratin. The new cells grow more rapidly than the old dead layers can be shed and so thick, reddened patches form which are covered with a silvery scale. They can appear in patches almost anywhere, often on the outer surfaces of the elbows or knees, and in severe cases can cover the whole body.

AROMATHERAPY

Essential oils which help to reduce inflammation may help locally (see Eczema, pages 98-9), but it may be just as helpful to concentrate on lowering the stress levels. Thus oils may be added to the bath: choose from Bergamot, Chamomile, Geranium, Jasmine, Lavender, Neroli or Rose for their relaxing and/or uplifting qualities. Change the oils around depending on the emotional state, and be prepared for limited success and slow improvements in the skin! Do not despair, psoriasis is notoriously difficult to treat, and sufferers carry the possibility of a recurrence even after the skin has cleared.

SELF-HELP TREATMENT

Psoriasis can run in families, and is a very complex condition with no simple treatment. It is frequently aggravated by stress and by being run-down, and seems to be an example of an auto-immune disorder, that is, when the body's immune system fails to recognize its own cells and starts to react against itself. In nearly every case exposure to sunlight is helpful, and often the condition will disappear on a summer holiday, when sun and relaxation are combined.

HERBALISM

Traditionally, psoriasis was linked to liver sluggishness as well as stress, and so herbal liver tonics and tissue cleansers form an initial part of treatment. Look at the herbs discussed under Eczema, particularly Yellow Dock *(Rumex crispus)* and Dandelion Root *(Taraxacum officinale)*. These may be combined and made as a decoction (see page 12), to stimulate bile flow and clear toxins out of the whole system. Nettle *(Urtica dioica)* is also valuable as a cleanser; ideally take the juice (available in some countries) or else combine in an infusion (see page 12), with Cleavers *(Galium aparine)* for added effect. Topically, the thickened skin can be encouraged to slough off by rubbing with moistened fine oatmeal. Marigold *(Calendula officinalis)* can be used in a cream or ointment to reduce the inflammation, or else Red Clover *(Trifolium pratense)* may be tried in similar fashion. If stress is an obvious factor, taking teas of gentle relaxants such as Chamomile *(Chamomilla recutita)*, Lavender *(Lavandula vera)*, Lemon Balm *(Melissa officinalis)* or Lime Blossom *(Tilia europaea)* over a period of time may help to restore balance.

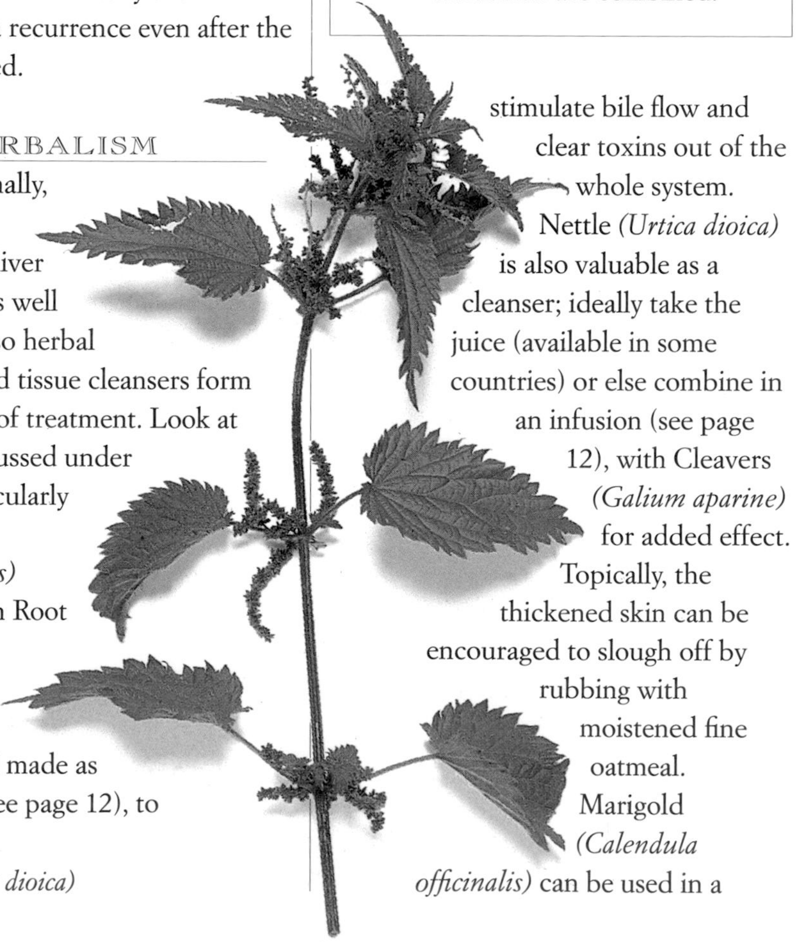

NETTLE *(Urtica dioica)*

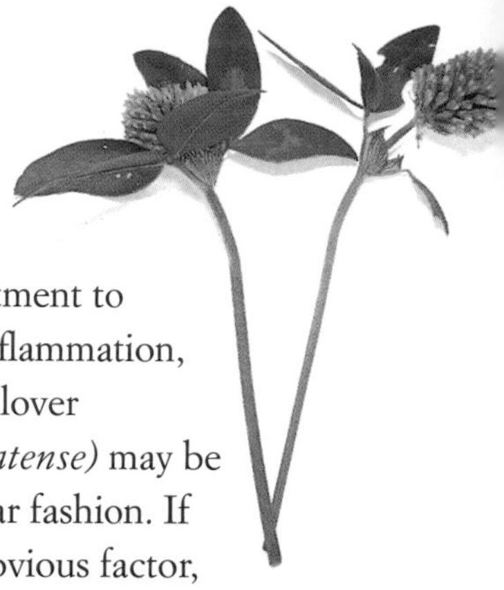

RED CLOVER *(Trifolium pratense)*

HOMEOPATHY

Some short-term suggestions are:

ARSEN ALB: for roughened, scaly skin that may have a burning sensation, although often cold to the touch. The skin is exceptionally dry.

GRAPHITES: for when the skin dries out and cracks, producing a thick, sticky discharge. The cracked areas may also bleed, and the skin itches considerably.

SULPHUR: for hot, dry and itchy skin which is made worse by heat (although not necessarily the sun). Scratching gives very temporary relief, but then causes soreness and burning.

NATUROPATHY

Much of the dietary advice echoes that given under Eczema (see pages 98-9); there may be a case for looking at wheat as a source of food intolerance too; try eliminating suspected foods on a rotation basis, a couple of weeks or so off each food group. For a short while Vitamin A may be taken in quite high doses (up to 7,500 iu daily for 2-3 weeks), but this is stored in the liver and can be toxic in over-large amounts. A multi-vitamin supplement may give a gentler but safer effect over a long period of time.

Sunshine is most likely to benefit, but do not get sunburnt! It is still necessary to take sun-protection measures when exposing skin to sunlight for any prolonged period of time (see pages 110-11). The Dead Sea is famous as a treatment area for psoriasis, using the mineral salts from

Natural creams and oils can be gently massaged into affected areas of skin.

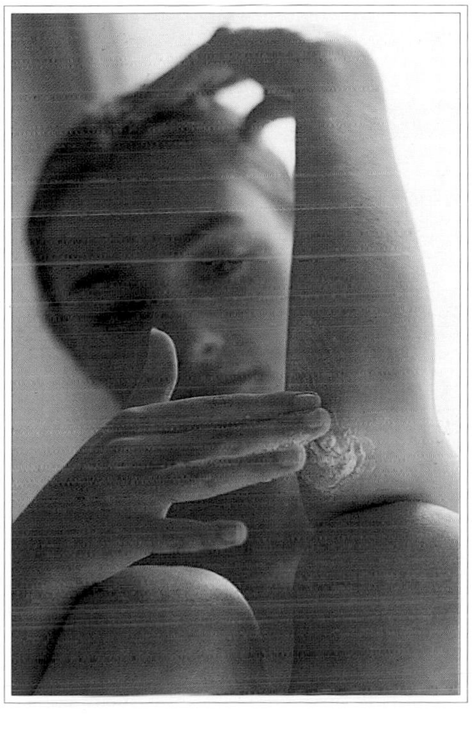

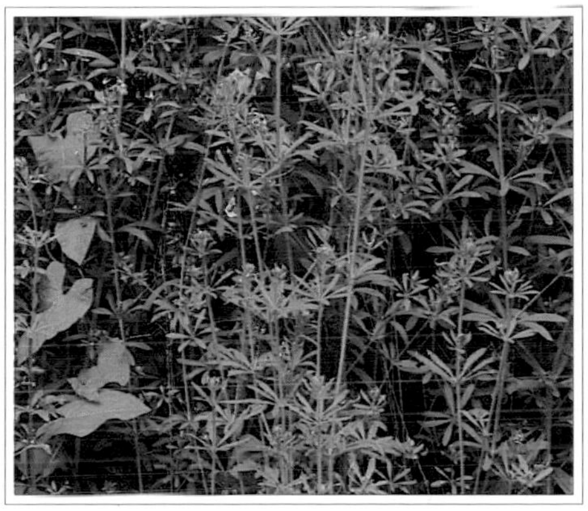

Cleavers *(Galium aparine)*

the sea together with sunbathing. These salts are now available in many countries, and can be added to the bath or a wash basin to bathe smaller areas of skin. Evening Primrose oil may be of help, both locally and internally (take up to 1,500 mg daily). Relaxation techniques or classes can be important parts of self-help, learning how to cope with stress and not internalize it.

Due to the complexity of factors involved, psoriasis is not easily treated with self-help, and professional treatment may be the best course of action. It can be associated with other disorders, such as digestive problems, and may lead on to a specific form of arthritis, so read the suggestions under these headings (see pages 61 and 83-4) to see how the natural therapies can work on the whole person, and to suit your own condition.

Lime Blossom (Tilia europaea) *tea can help reduce stress levels.*

Improving the Condition

One cannot really say that psoriasis can be cured, but natural treatments can greatly improve the condition for long periods of time.

As psoriasis sufferers often have a tendency towards tense, insular personalities, the following Bach Flower Remedies (see page 102) can sometimes help: Agrimony, Crab Apple, Water Violet or Willow.

Whatever treatment is used, patience is required as visible improvement can take a while to show through.

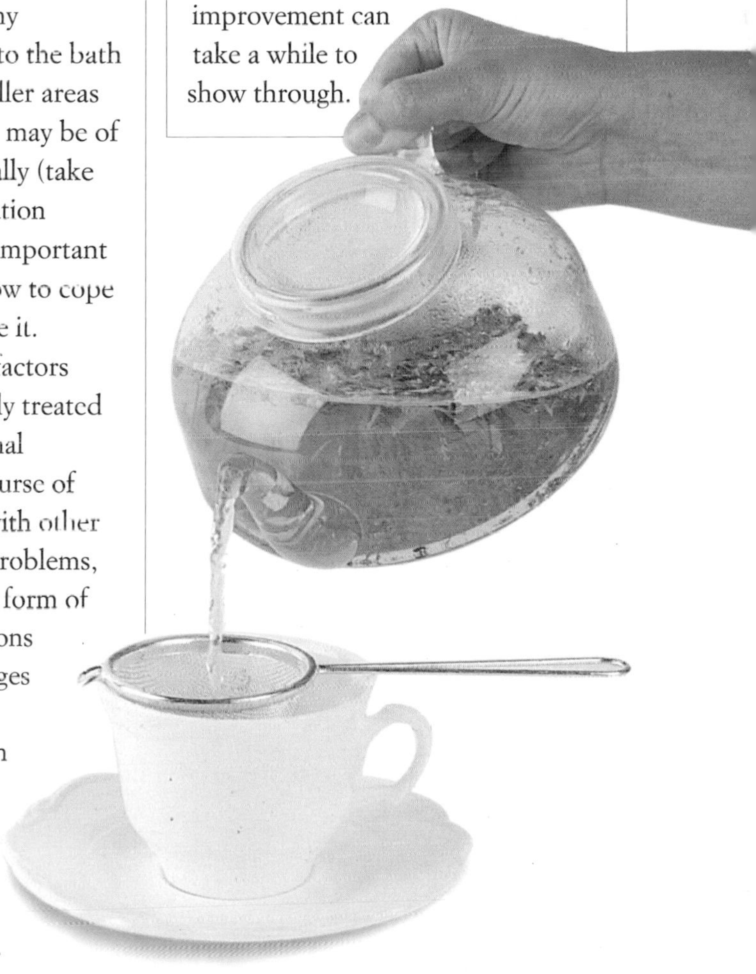

First Aid

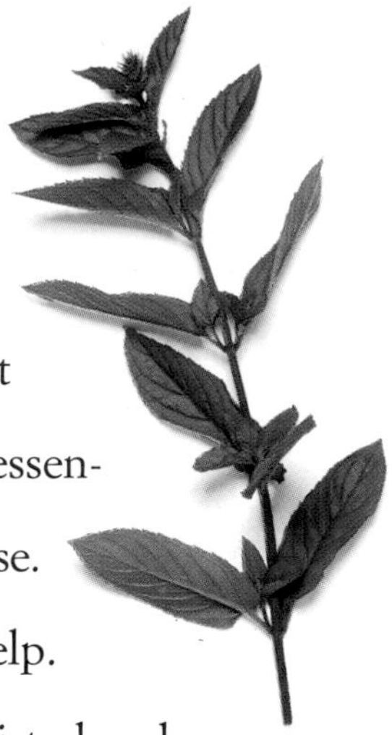

There are a number of instances when natural remedies can be used for first-aid treatment, and you may find it useful to build up a natural first-aid kit, to go alongside items such as plasters, bandages and so on. The important feature to remember is that situations needing first-aid treatment are acute, so prompt help is essential, and also they should be limited in duration anyway, such as a bruise.

If symptoms get worse or persist, despite first aid, seek medical help. In this section some of the common problems that might arise are listed and possible forms of treatment identified.

A choice of items for a natural first-aid kit is up to each individual, but some excellent remedies are Comfrey ointment for bruises, sprains and strains; Lavender essential oil for burns, bruises, sprains and strains; Calendula cream (herbal or homeopathic) for cuts and grazes; homeopathic Arnica tablets at 6c or 30c potency for bruises and shock; and Rescue Remedy for all types of shock. The last is not technically part of mainstream herbalism, but is one of Dr Edward Bach's Flower Remedies. These are a series of gentle plant remedies which are intended to treat various emotional states, regardless of the physical disorder. For practical purposes, the Rescue Remedy is the finest treatment available for alleviating symptoms of shock.

Above: The distinctive smell of peppermint is highly effective when used as a smelling salt.

BITES AND STINGS

Bites and stings can occur from any number of insects, some being much more painful than others. In any situation where a bite or sting affects the mouth or even the throat, and also if there are signs of an allergic reaction, with distress and/or difficulty in breathing, get medical help immediately.

AROMATHERAPY

A drop of Lavender or Tea Tree oils may be applied to the area, ideally in a little iced water. This may be repeated every 10 minutes or so until the pain and irritation has subsided, or it can be made into a cold compress (see page 15) and left on for a couple of hours.

HERBALISM

A cold dressing made from an infusion (see page 12) of Chamomile *(Chamomilla recutita)*, Elderflower *(Sambucus nigra)*, Lavender *(Lavandula vera)* or Red Clover *(Trifolium pratense)* can be used over the area. Other herbal help can be to use fresh leaves of plants such as Lemon Balm *(Melissa officinalis)* or Plantain *(Plantago major* or *P. lanceolata)*, or Yellow Dock *(Rumex crispus)* leaves – famous for treating nettle stings – directly on to the skin. Fresh onion may give quick relief from insect stings, placed over the area. For continued irritation, apply a cream (see page 16) made with Chickweed *(Stellaria media)* or perhaps Marigold *(Calendula officinalis)*. For bites, Marigold, Myrrh *(Commiphora molmol)* or St John's Wort *(Hypericum perforatum)* tinctures (see page 14) can help – use a drop or two neat on the bite or dilute 5 ml (1 tsp) into 15 ml (1 tbsp) of water for a cold dressing.

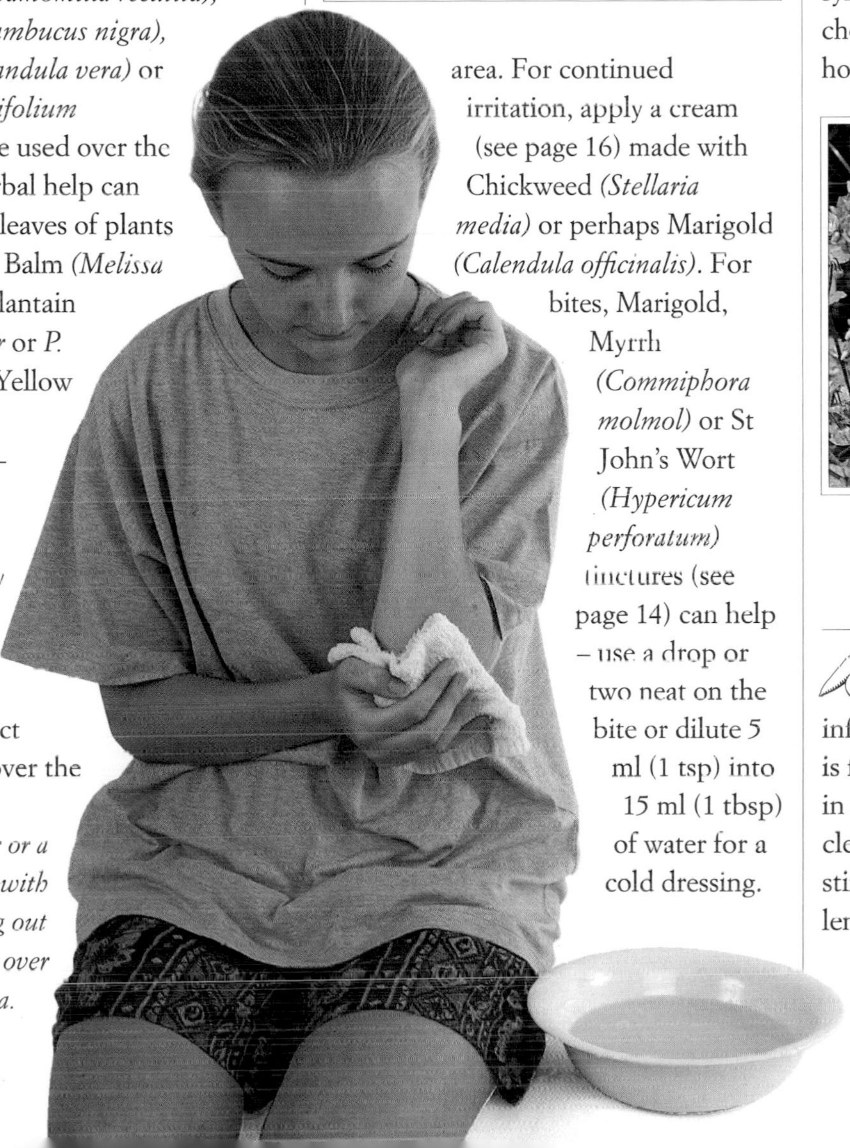

Use either water or a herbal infusion, with ice added. Wring out a cloth and hold over the inflamed area.

REMOVING A STING

Some stings, for instance from bees, result in the sting being left behind in the skin, and this should be carefully removed first. This is probably best done by flicking the sting out with a sharp knife; tweezers may be used, but these can result in squeezing the poison sac of the sting and thereby sending more toxin into the puncture hole.

HOMEOPATHY

Two classic remedies are Ledum, the remedy of choice for puncture wounds generally, or else Apis mel when there is much redness and swelling around the sting. Use 30c potency (see page 10), and take a dose every 20 minutes until the symptoms are much relieved. If there is a rash around the sting, apply a cold dressing using 2 drops of Urtica urens tincture to 15 ml (1 tbsp) of water. If there are symptoms of shock, the remedy to choose is Arnica, 1 dose per hour for 4 hours if needed.

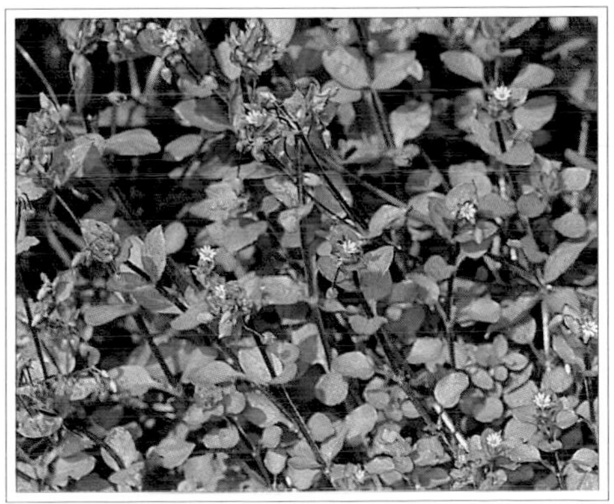

CHICKWEED *(Stellaria media)*

NATUROPATHY

If possible, apply ice to the area as soon as possible to reduce inflammation and swelling. If the sting is from a bee, there may be some value in using diluted bicarbonate of soda to clean the area; conversely, if it is a wasp sting, it may be helpful to use diluted lemon juice or vinegar for the same purpose. Bites should be thoroughly cleaned before any treatment.

BRUISES

Bruises can happen for several reasons; a knock, crushed finger or toe, sprain or other injury are the normal causes. However, if bruising is severe, frequent and without obvious cause, then it may indicate a lack of Vitamin K, or even be a sign of diabetes or kidney disease; get professional advice if dietary changes (see below) do not help.

AROMATHERAPY

Immediate use of oil of Lavender, in an ice-cold compress, can be the most effective treatment to avoid swelling and widespread bruising. If a bruise has developed, at a later stage when it is changing colour and resolving, use Rosemary essential oil diluted in a vegetable oil base to massage gently into the tissues to increase local circulation and speed up the healing process.

HERBALISM

Ice-cold compresses can be made with distilled Witch Hazel *(Hamamelis virginiana);* either dilute 15 ml (1 tbsp) in 300 ml (½ pt/1¼ cups) of cold water and apply on a dressing, or else be prepared beforehand and keep some ice-cubes made with the Witch Hazel in a separately labelled bag in the freezer (this is a useful policy if you have children!). An infusion of Comfrey *(Symphytum officinale),* chilled with ice-cubes, can also be used for a cold compress. For aftercare, Comfrey oil or ointment (see page 16) is ideal, quickly healing the damaged tissues.

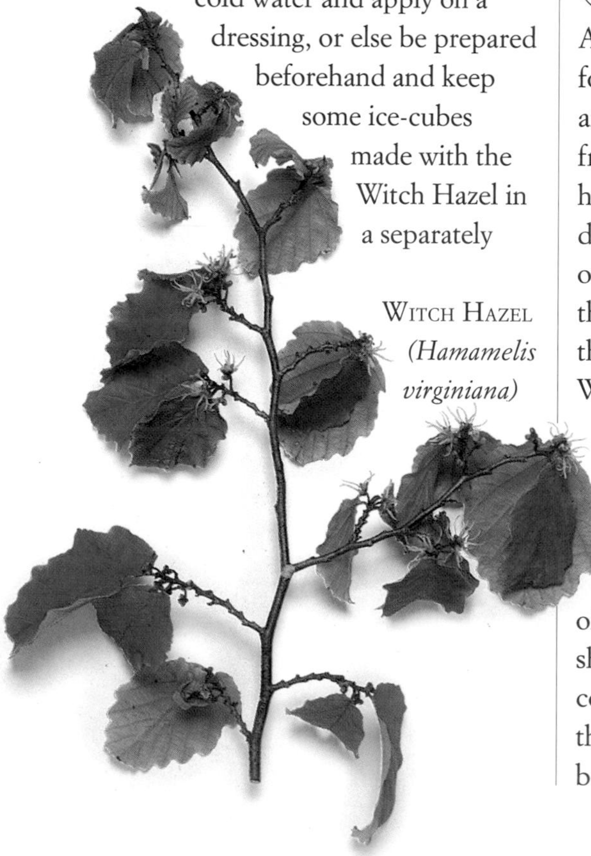

Witch Hazel *(Hamamelis virginiana)*

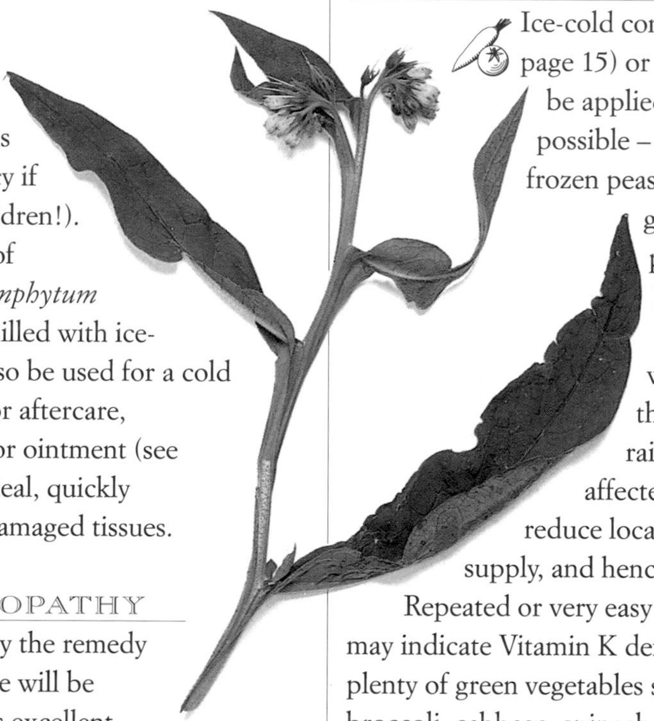

Comfrey *(Symphytum officinale)*

HOMEOPATHY

Probably the remedy of choice will be Arnica; this is excellent for any physical (or emotional) trauma and shock, and will help with bruising from a blow or injury. Take every 2 hours for up to 6 doses, then 3 times a day for 3 days, if needed. Keep an eye on symptoms; as they improve, reduce the frequency of dosage or stop taking the remedy altogether if much better. When the skin is unbroken, Arnica ointment may be applied to the bruised area; if there is damage to the skin, then Hypericum or Calendula ointments should be used instead. All the above ointments are available in most health shops. Other remedies for internal use could be Ruta grav or Rhus tox when the muscles, tendons or bones have been injured, for example in a sprain.

NATUROPATHY

Ice-cold compresses (see page 15) or packs should be applied as soon as possible – a bag of frozen peas makes a good temporary pack. If the bruise is severe or widespread, then try to raise the affected area to reduce local blood supply, and hence swelling.

Repeated or very easy bruising may indicate Vitamin K deficiency; eat plenty of green vegetables such as broccoli, cabbage, spinach and so on, and also try taking plenty of live yoghurt to stimulate the gut flora that make this vitamin. To encourage dispersal of bruises, eat fresh pineapple, or drink the juice; it contains enzymes which aid this process. If bruises linger, it may be additionally helpful to take Vitamin C (500 mg daily for a few days).

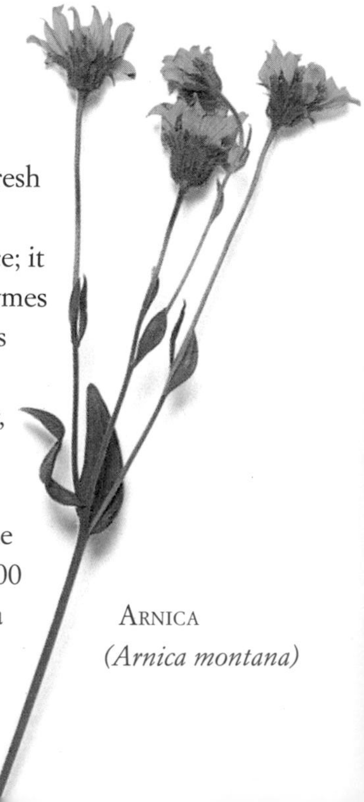

Arnica *(Arnica montana)*

BURNS

Severe burns require urgent medical assistance; do not delay in getting treatment, especially for children and babies. The immediate treatment should be to apply cold water for up to 10 minutes if necessary, to reduce the heat. If the burn is from a chemical, remove any clothing that might have been affected. However, if there is burnt clothing stuck in the burn, then generally do not remove as this might do more damage.

AROMATHERAPY

Essential oil of Lavender is almost a specific treatment for burns; it is anti-inflammatory and analgesic, and promotes healing of the tissues. If applied quickly it can prevent scarring in many instances (I speak from personal experience). For a larger area put on to sterile gauze or smooth lint; otherwise drop on neat.

HERBALISM

In herbal practice Lavender *(Lavandula vera)* oil will most likely be used, as described above; another option for minor burns is Tea Tree *(Melaleuca alternifolia)* oil, a couple of drops applied to prevent blistering. If available, fresh Aloe vera gel is an excellent first-aid treatment for burns and scalds. Break open a leaf and spread the thick gel directly on to the burn – again, this can produce completely scar-free healing if done as soon as possible. Other possibilities are infusions of Chamomile *(Chamomilla recutita)* or Marigold *(Calendula officinalis),* applied on a smooth dressing. Marigold cream (see page 16) may be used after some time has elapsed to ease continuing inflammation and soreness.

LAVENDER *(Lavandula vera)*

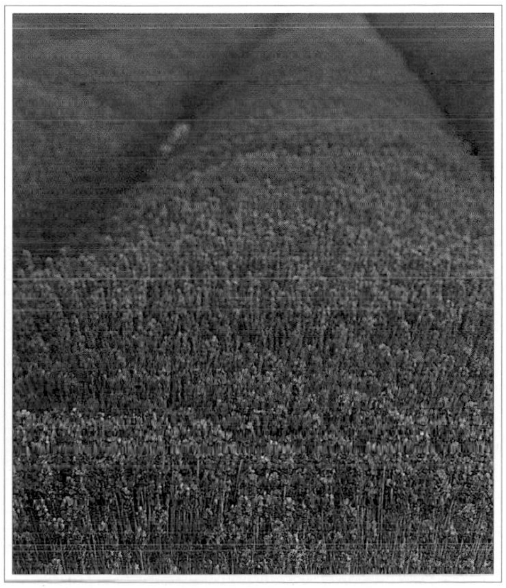

HOMEOPATHY

Probably the most-used homeopathic remedy for the first-aid treatment of burns is Arnica, followed by Cantharis; this helps to remove the burning pains that accompany blistering of the skin. For very minor burns Urtica urens may be suitable; probably only a couple of doses will be needed in this case. Urtica is also available as an ointment and is very effective for soothing superficial burns. Alternatively, after cooling of the skin it may be appropriate to use a commercial cream on a small burn.

CAUTION

Burns larger than the palm of your hand should be seen by a doctor immediately, regardless of any self-help treatment that has been advised here. All burns are painful and should be touched as little as possible.

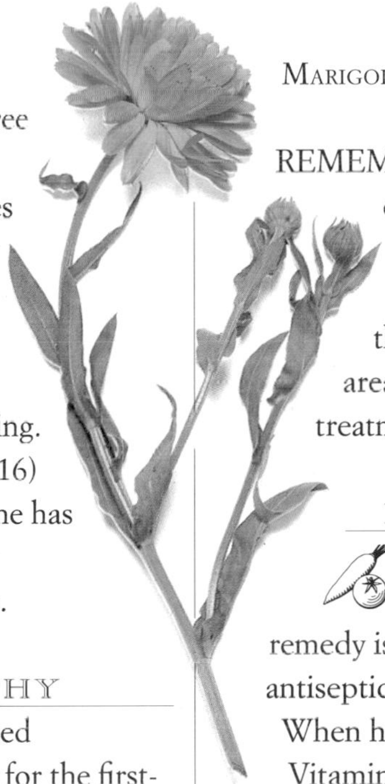

MARIGOLD *(Calendula officinalis)*

REMEMBER, do not use greasy ointments, butter or other fats on new burns as all this does is simply fry the skin. Always cool the area thoroughly as the first treatment.

NATUROPATHY

Once the skin has been cooled, a valuable home remedy is honey; this is both antiseptic and promotes healing. When healing has started, a Vitamin E cream can aid restoration of tissue elasticity and reduce scarring. Do not give hot drinks to someone who has a burn; frequent small sips of cool water can help to replace lost fluids in more serious cases.

CHAMOMILE *(Chamomilla recutita)*

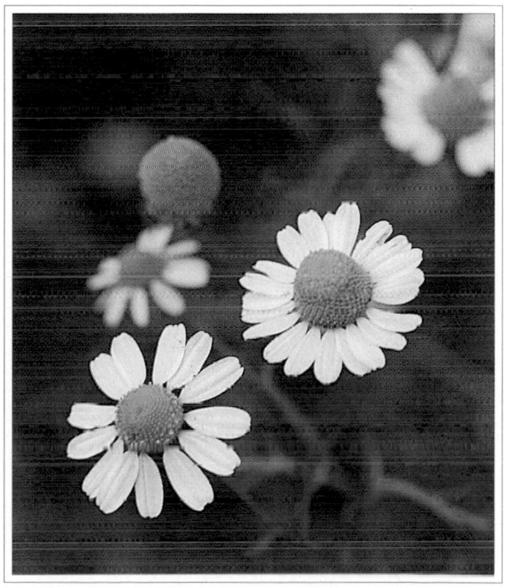

CUTS AND GRAZES

The first priority is to clean the area gently but thoroughly to remove any dirt. If the wound is deep, needing stitches, cover with a dry dressing and get medical help. It may be a sensible precaution to consider a tetanus jab (shot) if the cut has been from a dirty object or an animal, especially if there is a puncture wound.

AROMATHERAPY

The two oils of choice are probably Lavender and Tea Tree. These may be used neat on small cuts and scratches; they will sting temporarily but this soon passes. They can be added to a bowl of water for bathing (see page 8) and cleaning the affected area initially, or a couple of drops may be placed on a plaster or other clean dressing and applied over the site of the injury. Both these oils fight any infection as well as stimulating healing, and are generally very safe to use neat in this way.

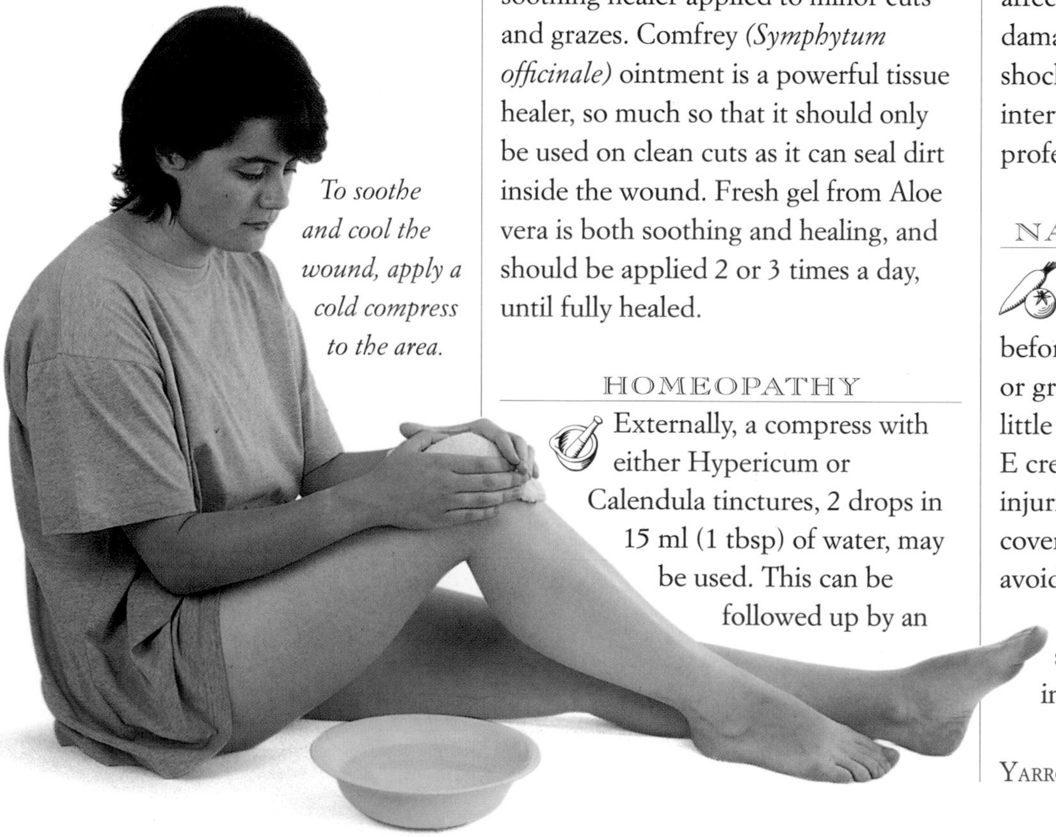

To soothe and cool the wound, apply a cold compress to the area.

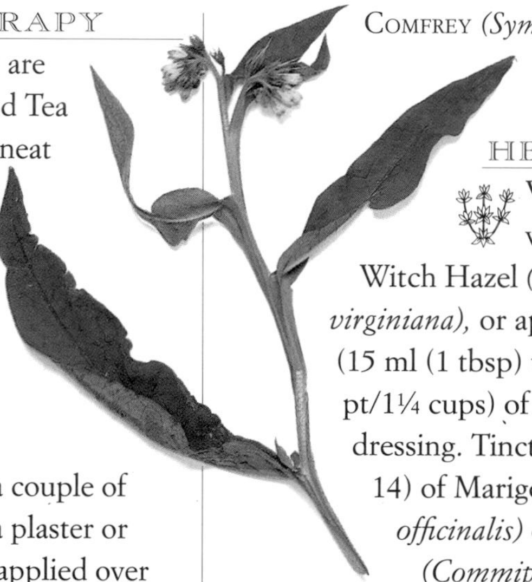

Comfrey *(Symphytum officinale)*

HERBALISM

Wash the area with distilled Witch Hazel *(Hamamelis virginiana),* or apply it diluted (15 ml (1 tbsp) to 300 ml (½ pt/1¼ cups) of water) on a dressing. Tinctures (see page 14) of Marigold *(Calendula officinalis)* or Myrrh *(Commiphora molmol),* similarly diluted, are alternatives for use on a dressing, or use an infusion (see page 12) of Yarrow *(Achillea millefolium).* Marigold cream is an ideal soothing healer applied to minor cuts and grazes. Comfrey *(Symphytum officinale)* ointment is a powerful tissue healer, so much so that it should only be used on clean cuts as it can seal dirt inside the wound. Fresh gel from Aloe vera is both soothing and healing, and should be applied 2 or 3 times a day, until fully healed.

HOMEOPATHY

Externally, a compress with either Hypericum or Calendula tinctures, 2 drops in 15 ml (1 tbsp) of water, may be used. This can be followed up by an ointment from either of these (or any commercial cream made from both). Internally, take up to 4 doses of either Hypericum, especially if the injury has affected the fingers or toes and damaged local nerves, or Arnica for the shock of the injury, at 4-hourly intervals. For anything more serious get professional treatment.

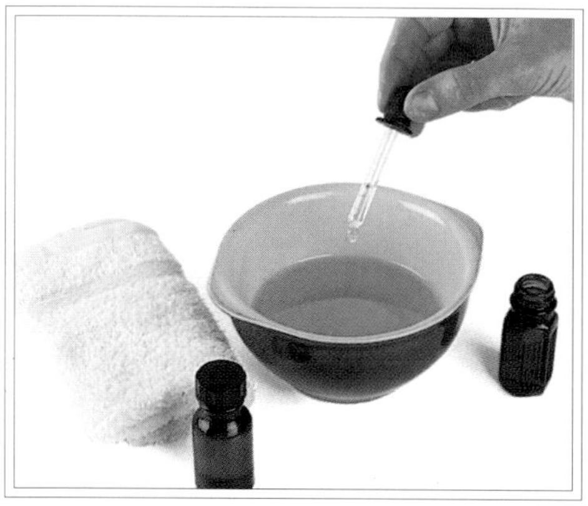

Add 2-3 drops of Lavender oil to a cold compress as a powerful antiseptic.

NATUROPATHY

Clean your own hands thoroughly before cleaning the cut or graze, and apply a little honey or a Vitamin E cream on minor injuries. Keep the area covered if possible to avoid infection, and watch out for any swelling or inflammation.

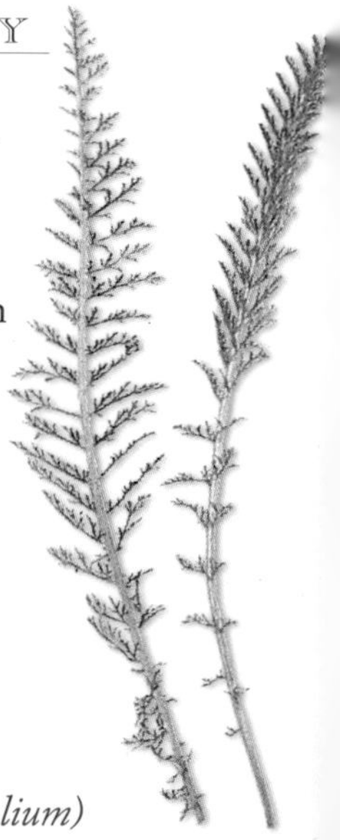

Yarrow *(Achillea millefolium)*

FAINTING

Feeling faint, or actually blacking out, is due to a temporary lack of blood to the brain, and an isolated incident can be due to a number of immediate causes, such as excess heat or cold, fear, emotional upset, sight of blood, needles or something else that the person considers unpleasant.

AROMATHERAPY

For someone feeling faint, use one of the following oils like smelling salts, holding the bottle under the nose or else putting a couple of drops on a tissue and getting the person to breathe the aroma. Peppermint is particularly good, also Lavender, Neroli, Petitgrain and Rosemary. A drop gently massaged into the temples can be useful – a good commercial product for this use is Tiger Balm, which contains menthol and eucalyptol.

HERBALISM

Generally, any strong-smelling substance tends to stimulate the brain and relieve feelings of faintness. If available, tinctures (see page 14) of Lavender *(Lavandula vera)* or Peppermint *(Mentha piperita)* are pleasant and effective when used as smelling salts. One of the best remedies, especially when shock or upset has caused the faint feeling, is Rescue Remedy. If the person is conscious, put 4 drops under the tongue; if not, then moisten the lips with a couple of drops, and give 4 drops under the tongue when he or she comes round; repeat in half an hour if still feeling woozy.

HOMEOPATHY

Apart from the usual first-aid approach of making the person comfortable, if there is an obvious cause for the fainting, then a single dose of one of the following remedies may be called for.

ACONITE: for the effects of fright.
ARNICA: for faintness due to an accident, injury or shock.
IGNATIA: for over-excitement, or even feelings of hysteria.
NUX VOMICA: for faint feelings associated with seeing blood, or from strong smells, or after a rich meal.
PULSATILLA: for the effects of being in a hot, stuffy atmosphere.

Finally, if the person has fainted, and on coming round feels chilly but desires fresh air, try a dose of Carbo veg – sometimes called the corpse reviver!

POSTURAL HYPERTENSION

One of the commonest causes of fainting is postural hypotension (that is, a sudden change in position, such as standing up quickly), which lowers the blood pressure to the brain. Repeated fainting attacks call for expert investigation into the causes, which may range from low blood pressure or anaemia to changes in blood sugar levels. When someone has fainted, do not try to lift them up; falling down brings the head level with the heart and helps to bring blood to the brain more easily.

NATUROPATHY

Use basic first aid, such as ensuring there is enough fresh air if possible, helping the blood flow by sitting the person down and placing their head down between the knees, or else assisting them to lie down with their legs slightly raised. When recovering, give a few sips of water or better still warm peppermint tea.

FEELING FAINT

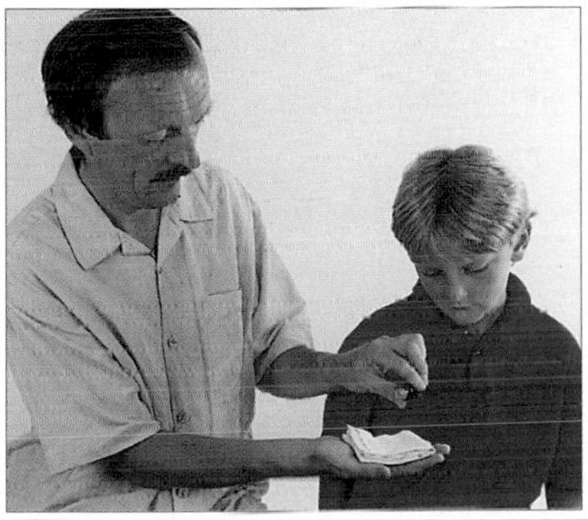

1 Put a couple of drops of essential oil on to a tissue.

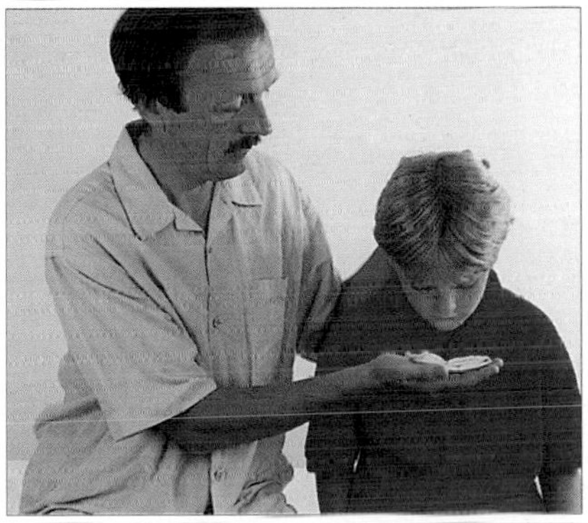

2 Hold the tissue under the nose and lean the head slightly forward.

NOSEBLEED

This is most often due to a blow on the nose, rupturing some of the tiny blood vessels, and can be quite common in children. Occasionally a nosebleed is sparked off by very hot, humid weather, or by excitement, and if they occur frequently, professional treatment should be sought.

AROMATHERAPY

Soak a pad of cotton wool in cold, or even iced water with a couple of drops of Lemon oil added, and place firmly across the bridge of the nose. A more effective method is to place a small piece of this as a plug in the affected nostril. The essential oil helps to speed up clotting. Sometimes placing a cold compress on the back of the neck can be helpful in reducing the local blood flow too.

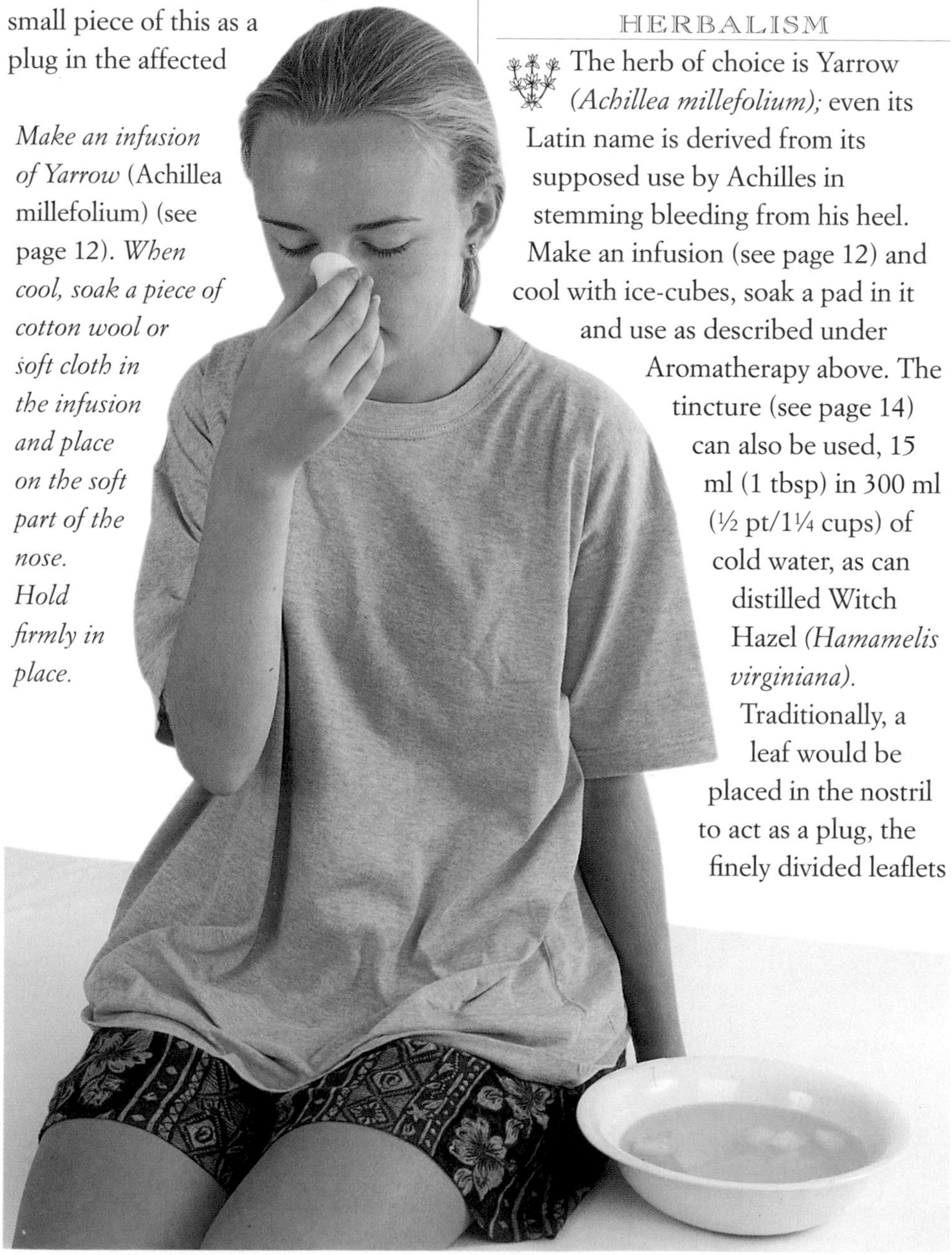

Make an infusion of Yarrow (Achillea millefolium) (see page 12). *When cool, soak a piece of cotton wool or soft cloth in the infusion and place on the soft part of the nose. Hold firmly in place.*

HERBALISM

The herb of choice is Yarrow *(Achillea millefolium);* even its Latin name is derived from its supposed use by Achilles in stemming bleeding from his heel. Make an infusion (see page 12) and cool with ice-cubes, soak a pad in it and use as described under Aromatherapy above. The tincture (see page 14) can also be used, 15 ml (1 tbsp) in 300 ml (½ pt/1¼ cups) of cold water, as can distilled Witch Hazel *(Hamamelis virginiana).* Traditionally, a leaf would be placed in the nostril to act as a plug, the finely divided leaflets acting as a mesh for the blood platelets to produce a clot; however, removing this leaf often starts the nosebleed off again, so it is not particularly recommended.

HOMEOPATHY

Some useful remedies are:

FERRUM PHOS: for the results of a minor injury, or else from a head cold; a good remedy for childhood knocks.

HAMAMELIS: for profuse bleeding, with a feeling of pressure in the nose and sinus areas which is relieved by the blood loss to some extent.

PHOSPHORUS: for a heavy nosebleed associated with blowing the nose violently or sneezing, especially if occurring in the evening.

NATUROPATHY

In the first instance, get the person to sit down and lean forward slightly, pinching the soft part of the nose firmly between forefinger and thumb for several minutes. An ice-cube, or better still a pad of cotton wool soaked in iced water, can be held in place over this area too, to astringe the swollen blood vessels further.

CAUTION

In rare instances, conditions such as high blood pressure may be the reason behind the nosebleeds. Any unexplained or very heavy bleeds need immediate medical attention.

SPRAINS AND STRAINS

A sprain is an injury affecting a joint, with the tendons that attach muscles to the bones being overstretched and often torn. A strain is an injury to the muscles themselves, usually due to excessive or inappropriate exercise, lifting heavy weights and so on. The first treatment is a cold application (see Naturopathy entry below); massage of the area is not helpful at this stage, but can be used if the after-effects linger on.

AROMATHERAPY

The most useful essential oil is Lavender; use 5 drops to 15 ml (1 tbsp) of iced water for a compress. Chamomile oil may be used in the same way; where there is a sprain, try to keep the affected joint as still as possible initially to reduce internal bleeding and to allow healing to start as quickly as possible, ideally with the limb raised.

HERBALISM

Make an infusion of Comfrey leaves *(Symphytum officinale)* and apply as a cold compress (see page 15), or use diluted tinctures (see page 14) of Comfrey or Marigold *(Calendula officinalis)*, 15 ml (1 tbsp) to 300 ml (½ pt/1¼ cups) of cold water. When the swelling has subsided, gently rub in Comfrey ointment to speed up healing of the damaged fibres. If muscles ache through over-exercise, this ointment is a good home treatment with massage of the surrounding area twice a day.

When treating a strain, the colder the water for the compress, the more effective it will be for the strain.

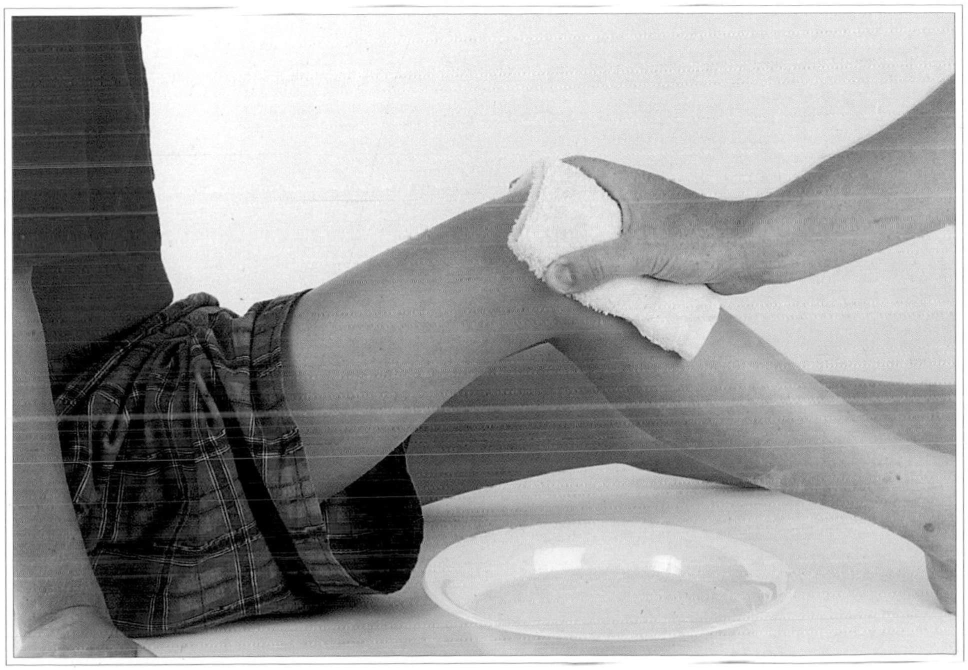

HOMEOPATHY

Choose from these remedies:

ARNICA: for the results of a fall or accident, with soreness and also a feeling of shock.

RHUS TOX: for muscular strains, from lifting heavy weights for instance, with pain, stiffness and swelling.

RUTA GRAV: for torn ligaments or tendons, especially in sprains of the ankles or wrists, with a feeling of bruising in the bones.

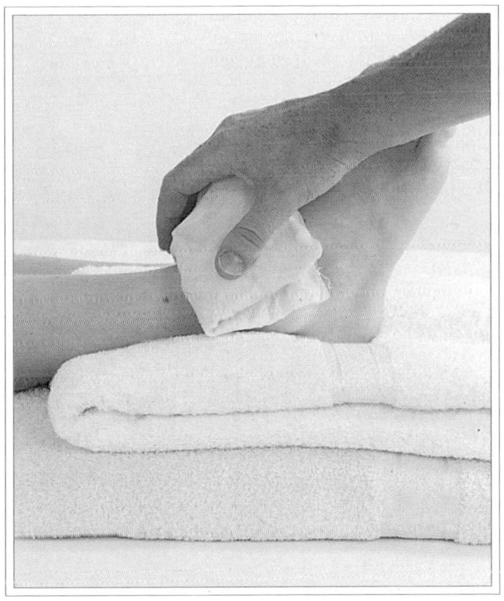

Raise the leg and support the ankle on something soft. Place an ice pack (a bag of frozen peas is a quick substitute) over the area and hold firmly in place.

NATUROPATHY

The immediate treatment is to apply the ICE approach : ice, compression and elevation. For example, a pack of frozen peas, held firmly around a sprained ankle, with the leg raised and supported, will help a good deal in reducing internal bleeding and joint swelling.

After the symptoms have subsided, there may be a case for using alternate hot and cold compresses (3 minutes hot followed by 1 minute cold, repeated for about 15 minutes) to improve local circulation to the relevant muscles, and later treatment may include massage to relieve muscular aches. Diluted oil of Lavender (about 2 per cent in a base oil) is helpful here.

SUNBURN

In most respects sunburn should be treated as for Burns (see page 105). The first thing to do is to avoid further exposure to the sun until symptoms have been cleared. Severe sunburn can produce bad blistering, dehydration and sunstroke, and occasionally people have an allergic reaction to the sun's ultraviolet rays.

AROMATHERAPY

For mild, widespread sunburn use Chamomile oil, either in a bath, or add 5 drops to a small bowl of water and carefully dab on to unbroken skin. With children, essential oils for the bath should ideally be pre-diluted in 5 ml (1 tsp) of Sweet Almond or similar oil. If the sunburn is more severe, use Lavender oil in similar ways, or apply neat on to any blistered areas.

As aftercare for the dry, leathery-looking skin, use essential oils of Chamomile, Lavender, Rose or Sandalwood diluted at 2 per cent in a base oil such as Sweet Almond and gently massaged in twice daily. Very dry skin may benefit from the use of

Elderflower *(Sambucus nigra)*

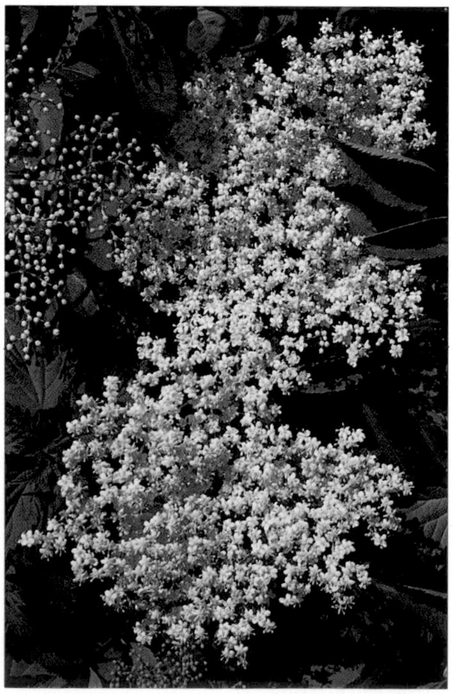

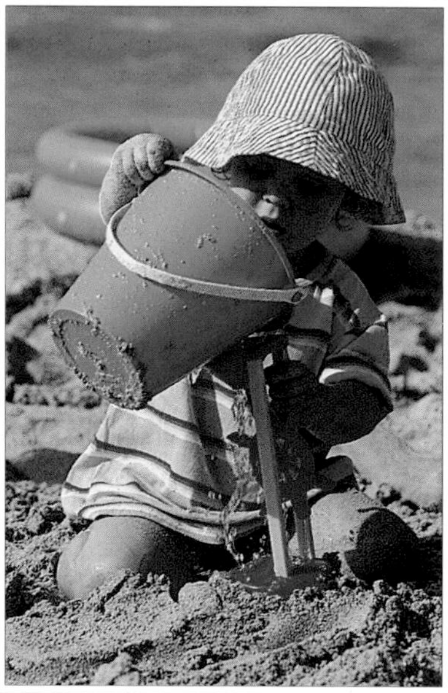

The Risk of Skin Cancer

An increasingly frequent sequel to excessive exposure to the sun is skin cancer, and reductions in the Earth's ozone layer make this likely to become dramatically more common in future years, even in countries some distance away from the Equator.

In any case, the sun has an ageing effect on the skin, so enjoy it but use good suntan creams and after-sun moisturizing creams, and keep out of the midday sun if possible.

REMEMBER: sunbeds do not protect against sunburn so you still need to take it carefully when out in hot sunshine, and use the appropriate sun protection factor (SPF) lotion.

French Lavender *(Lavandula stoechas)*

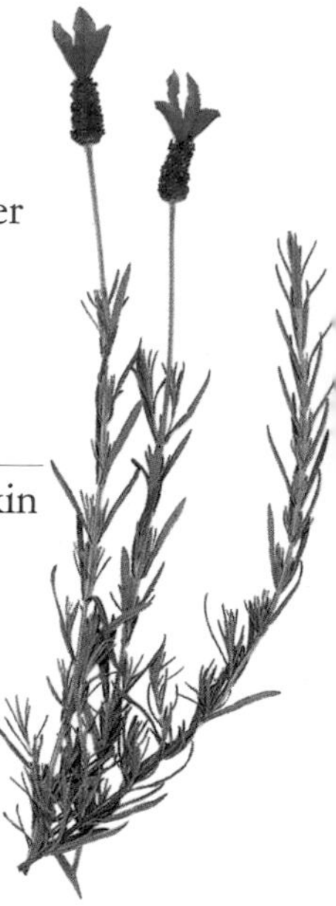

Wheatgerm oil at 10 per cent of the base oil for extra nourishment.

HERBALISM

Firstly cool the skin as for Burns (see page 105), or by applying a chilled infusion (see page 12) of either Chamomile *(Chamomilla recutita)*, Elderflower *(Sambucus nigra)* or Lavender *(Lavandula vera)* flowers. Marigold *(Calendula officinalis)* cream may be used afterwards, or else apply the blood-red oil of St John's Wort *(Hypericum perforatum)*, which

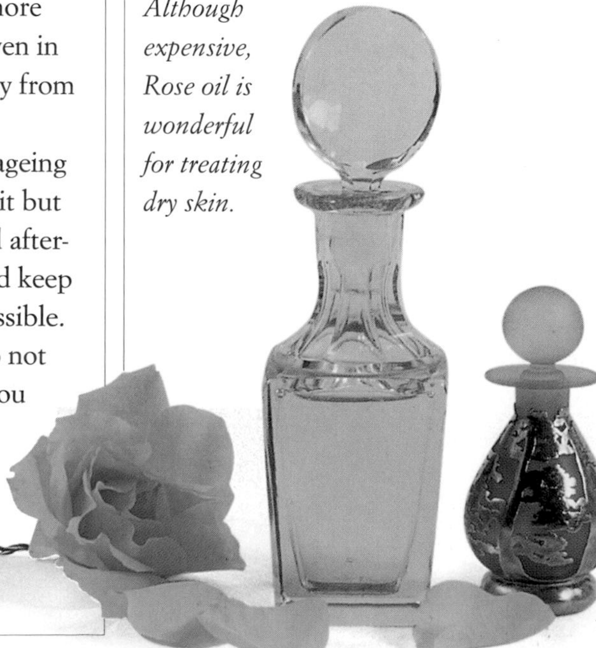

Although expensive, Rose oil is wonderful for treating dry skin.

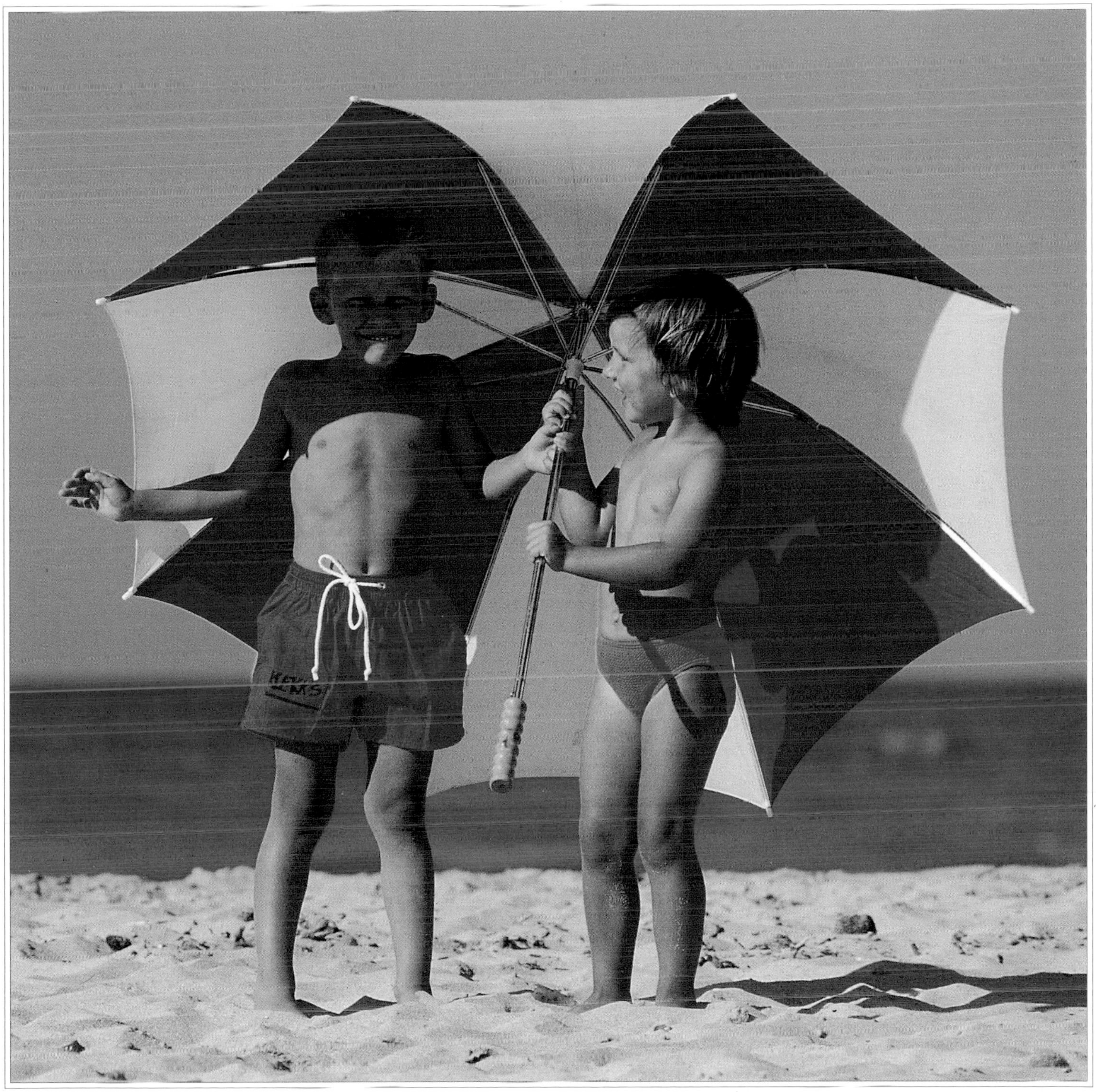

will take away much of the burning pain very quickly – it has been used to good effect on radiation burns. Pure Aloe vera juice is another highly soothing, cooling and healing herb.

HOMEOPATHY

Apply Cantharis, for when there is an intense burning sensation, before or after blisters have formed, and Urtica urens, for sunburn with an intense and persistent stinging sensation. For milder burns, then apply Hypericum and/or Calendula cream.

NATUROPATHY

After cooling the affected areas, apply Vitamin E cream, as well as taking Vitamin E internally (up to 500 iu daily) to improve healing and stop scarring. Widespread sunburn may heal more quickly if additional Vitamin C is taken (up to 1,000 mg daily for a few days). Sunburn is likely to mean dehydration, so take plenty of fluids (spring water and fruit juices, but not alcohol) in the short term.

Young children should always have plenty of sun-protection lotion on.

CHILDREN'S AILMENTS

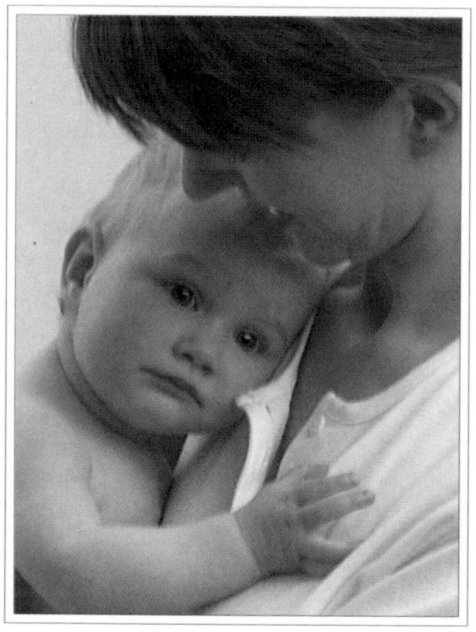

In general, children and adults are treated in the same way by the natural therapies, each person's health being considered individually and treatment given accordingly, and the same approach applies to self-help measures. There is of course the matter of dosage of remedies, and these should be reduced or adapted as explained below. There are a number of illnesses that tend to occur in childhood, such as chickenpox, German measles and measles, and children are also more prone to colds, coughs, ear infections and the like. As well as any specific treatment for such conditions, it is worth bearing in mind some general considerations.

Children usually react quickly to any illness, showing acute symptoms that can then often subside equally quickly (much to the amazement/relief/annoyance of parents!). Due to their high levels of energy and faster metabolism, children often show signs of illness through a high temperature, and this should be looked at as part of the ailment, not as the whole problem (see Fever, pages 48-9). Because of this, it is easier for children to become dehydrated, and an essential part of treatment is to give plenty of fluids – with vomiting and/or diarrhoea in infants this can be literally life-saving. Conversely, if a child is unwell, he or she can go off food for a while, and provided fluid intake is adequate, this is not normally a major problem in the short term.

REMEMBER: Keep all medicines and essential oils out of the reach of children.

Here are some comments about each of the therapies in relation to treating children, and some of the most useful remedies.

ABOVE: Self-help treatment may not always be appropriate for children. If in any doubt, seek medical advice.

AROMATHERAPY

All the various methods of using essential oils discussed through the book – baths, inhalations, massage oils, compresses and creams – can be used for children as well as adults, with a few safety provisos.

❦ Do not use any oil undiluted on a child, except for Lavender oil on small burns or bruises.

❦ Dilute essential oils in a base oil before adding them to a bath for a child; they tend to enjoy splashing around in the bath more than adults and could get the oils in their eyes otherwise. Reduce dosage too, to a maximum of 4 drops per bath. For young infants, perhaps simply make a tea, of Lavender flowers for example, and add that to the bath.

❦ In massage, use lower dilutions of essential oils: a maximum of 1 per cent for ages 12-16; ½ per cent for ages 8-12; and ¼ per cent for ages 4-8. Under 4-year-olds will need just a drop or two in 100 ml (4 fl oz/½ cup) of base oil.

❦ Never leave a young child alone with bottles of essential oils, and always supervise their use.

❦ Use steam inhalations only briefly, and not at all if breathing is affected. Sometimes it is better to put a drop or two into a wash-basin of steaming water and sit with the young child next to it, rather than bending over a bowl.

Although aromatherapy oils may appear harmless, they are very strong and should always be kept out of the reach of children.

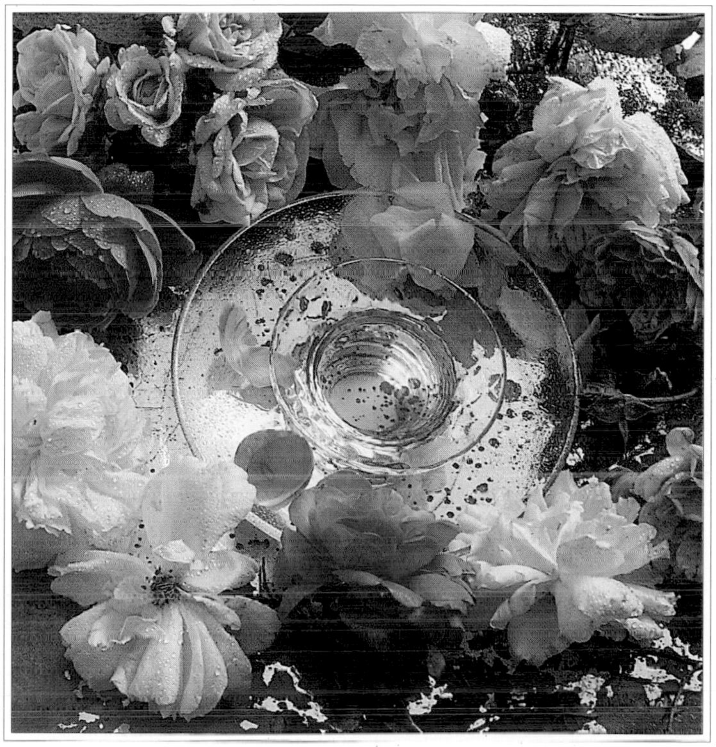

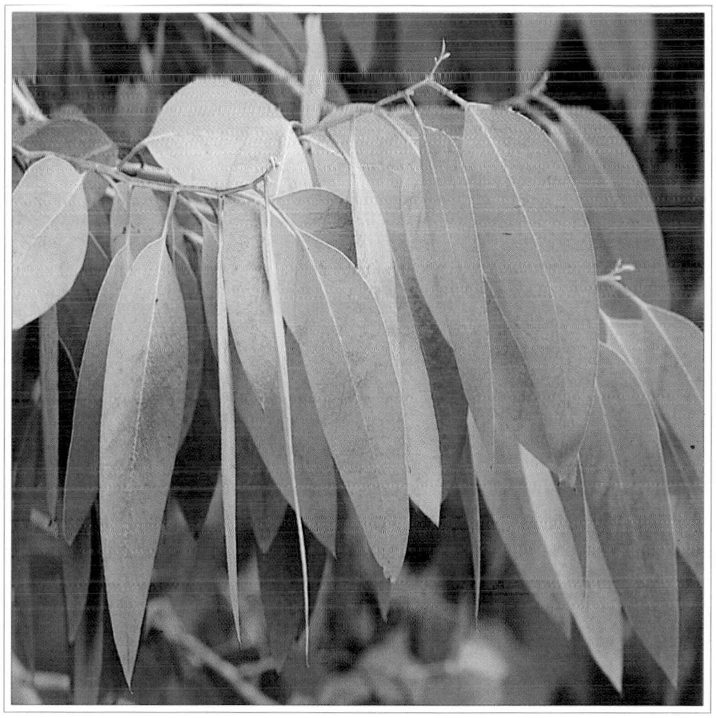

EUCALYPTUS *(Eucalyptus globulus)*

❦ A good way to help to fight infection, suitable for all ages, is to use a few drops in a plant spray, typically 600 ml (1 pt/ 2½ cups) capacity, fill with water, shake and spray the room at regular intervals. Use oils such as Lavender, Eucalyptus and Tea Tree.

Probably the two most suitable essential oils for use in childhood ailments are Chamomile and Lavender. They are both soothing, relaxing and anti-inflammatory, and help to calm the child as well as help to fight the illness. For instance, in a condition such as chickenpox, 2 drops of Lavender oil in 5 ml (1 tsp) of water can be dabbed on to the emerging spots to soothe the irritation and heal them at a much faster rate; Chamomile cream is very versatile, soothing many inflamed skin disorders. Additionally, the aroma of these oils helps to calm the child and give them a more restful sleep.

For colds and such like you may consider Benzoin, Frankincense and perhaps tiny amounts of Eucalyptus or Peppermint (also see other ailments).

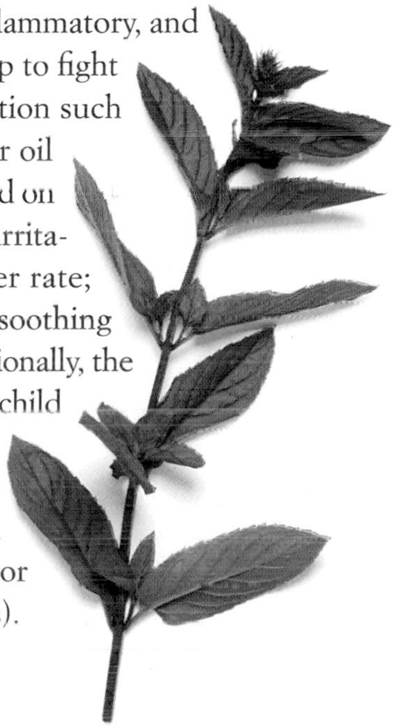

PEPPERMINT *(Mentha piperita)*

HERBALISM

Since children have a higher metabolic rate, and good underlying energy in most cases, herbs which stimulate the circulation are generally to be avoided. Herbal teas are one of the most suitable forms of treatment. With stronger preparations such as infusions and decoctions (see page 12), it is sensible to work on the principle of reaching an adult dose at age 16; hence, a child of 8 will be given half the dose, and at 4 only quarter the adult dose. This can be achieved either by reducing the amount of herb used in the preparation per given amount of water, or by reducing the amount of the preparation given to the child.

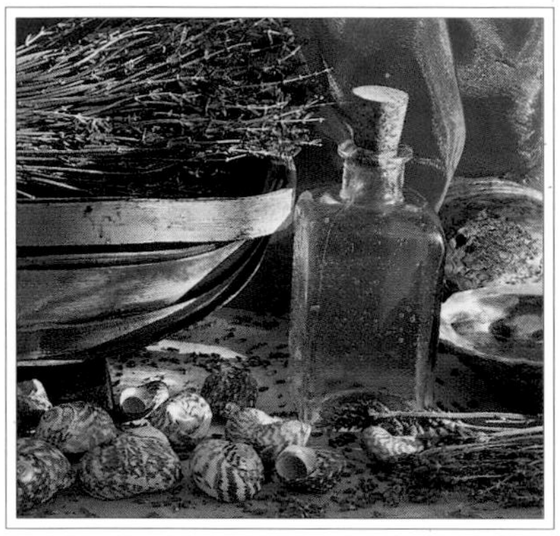

Actually preparing your own infusions can become part of the healing process.

Some of the most suitable remedies to give as teas to children are:

Catmint *(Nepeta cataria):* for nasal congestion and catarrh, repeated colds or blocked ears; of special benefit if there is a tendency to get feverish and restless with a respiratory infection or cararrh. Both this and Peppermint *(Mentha piperita)* have a slight underlying bitterness, which indicates their usefulness too in picking up the appetite after a feverish illness.

Chamomile *(Chamomilla recutita):* for most digestive upsets, from stomach pains to indigestion, the effects of overeating, flatulence and diarrhoea. As a mild relaxant, it is a valuable remedy for calming children who get irritable and cross when they are ill, or who find it difficult to get to sleep. Do not make a tea of Chamomile too strong, in the hope of knocking the child out at night, as it can have the opposite effect at an overdose level and make them more stimulated, or irritable!

Elderflower *(Sambucus nigra):* this is the best temperature regulator in feverish illnesses; give a hot tea when the child's temperature is too high and it will induce sweating, so cooling the system. It is very helpful in feverish colds and flu, and will help to relieve catarrh as well.

Lemon Balm *(Melissa officinalis):* this is a wonderful herb for gently aiding relaxation, at the same time acting as a digestive and nervous tonic. It is very helpful in convalescence,

Picking herbs can be fun for children too.

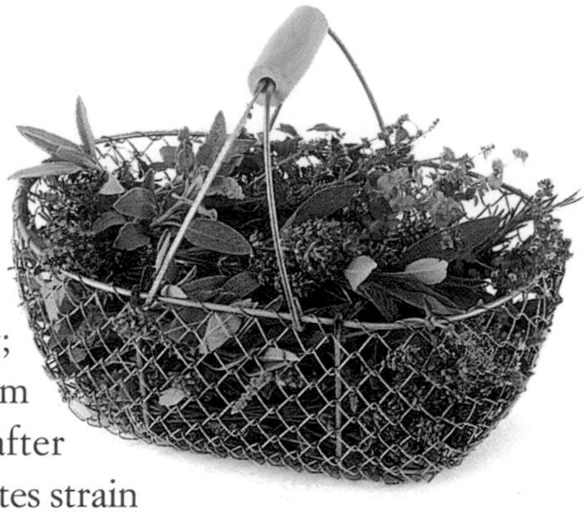

and makes a refreshing cold drink in summer; make a tea, ideally from the fresh leaves, and after infusing for a few minutes strain and keep in the refrigerator. It will keep for 2-3 days, and a slice or two of lemon can be added for extra flavour and additional benefit.

Lime Blossom *(Tilia europaea):* for tension headaches, mild digestive upsets and colds/flu with aching in the limbs. A tea of Lime Blossom at night can induce a calm and restful sleep.

Peppermint *(Mentha pip-erita):* this is one of the best remedies for trapped wind, nausea and indigestion from rich or heavy foods. Another area where Peppermint is excellent is in the early stages of a cold, with fluctuating temperatures and nasal congestion.

Many of these teas may be blended together (although Chamomile and Peppermint seem to be better kept apart) for extra benefit, and can be used, suitably diluted, for infants – sometimes it is best to add 5 ml (1 tsp) to a bottle of their normal juice or water.

A posy of fresh, sweet-smelling herbs was called a tussie-mussie or nosegay in Elizabethan times and was used to ward off foul odours and potential germs.

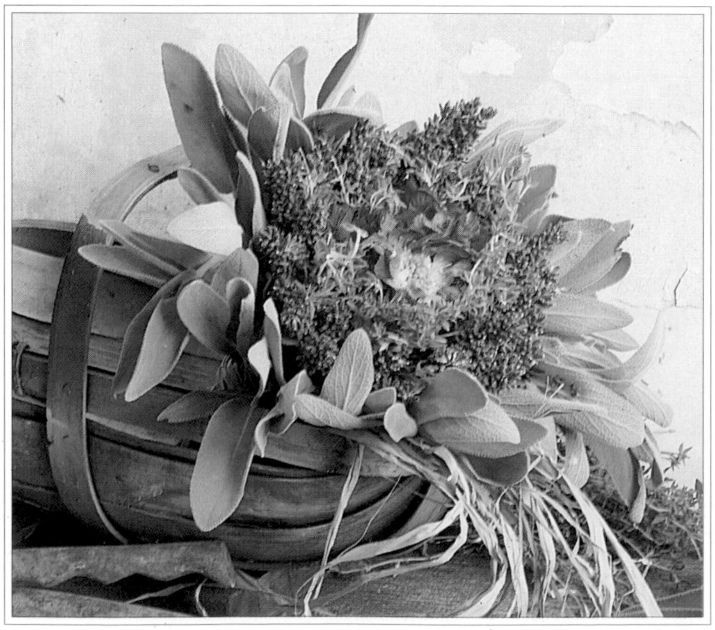

HOMEOPATHY

Since children react in general very quickly to treatment, any homeopathic remedies can usually be given in fewer doses than might be the case with an adult. If the symptoms are less acute, or in any case for young children, try the 6c potency (see page 10) first; in more acute circumstances give the 30c potency. As soon as the symptoms are less pronounced reduce the frequency of the medication, or stop it altogether. If in any doubt about the right potency, get professional advice. Homeopathy is a wonderful system of treatment for children, with no problems of taste to overcome, and the range of remedies is very wide.

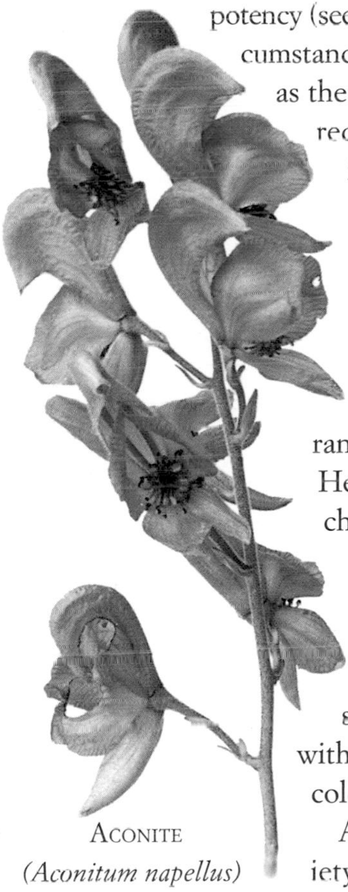

ACONITE
(Aconitum napellus)

Here are some typical remedies for childhood ailments:

ACONITE: give at the earliest onset of symptoms, very good for ailments brought on by catching a chill, getting wet and so on. The child may be upset, with a hot, dry skin and a thirst for cold water, and restless at night.

ARGENT NIT: for agitation and anxiety, perhaps when anticipating some event; the child is fidgety and restless. This remedy is strongly indicated if the child has a craving for sticky, sweet foods or ice-cream, but gets an upset stomach, nausea or even vomiting after eating.

ARNICA: this is the remedy for shock, given after any minor bump or fall. It can be excellent to give before, and after, a visit to the dentist, to reduce tissue damage or bruising, and to help the healing process.

ARSEN ALB: for the child who gets fractious after any exertion, easily gets a stomach upset or mild food poisoning, and wants to be carried. Usually, the picture for indicating this remedy is one where the child is peevish, wants to go from one person to another, and gets very thirsty, taking frequent, although small, sips of fluid.

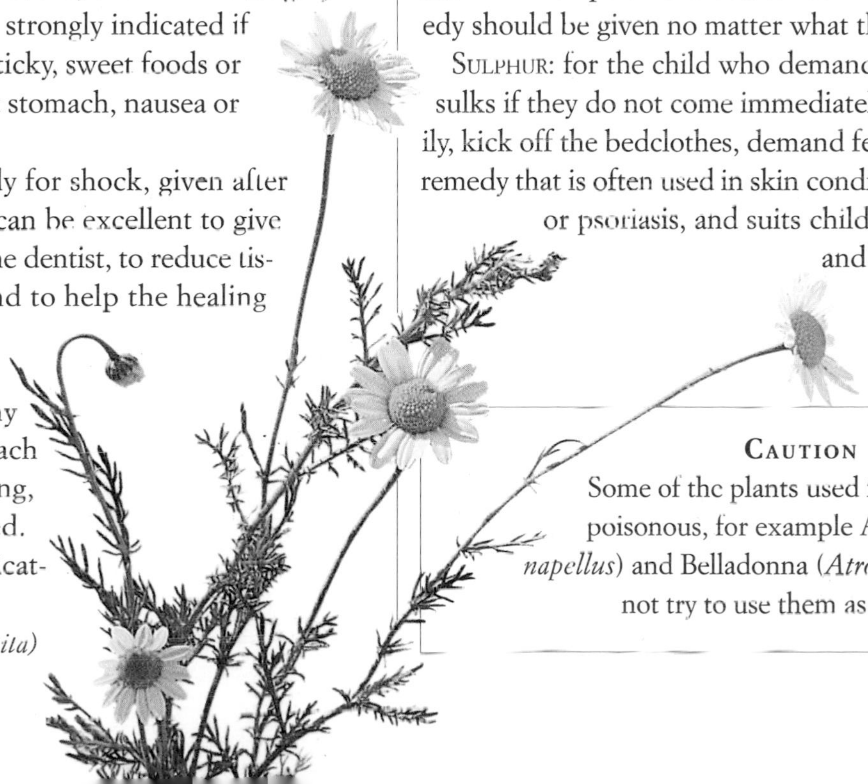

CHAMOMILE *(Chamomilla recutita)*

PASQUE FLOWER
(Pulsatilla vulgaris)

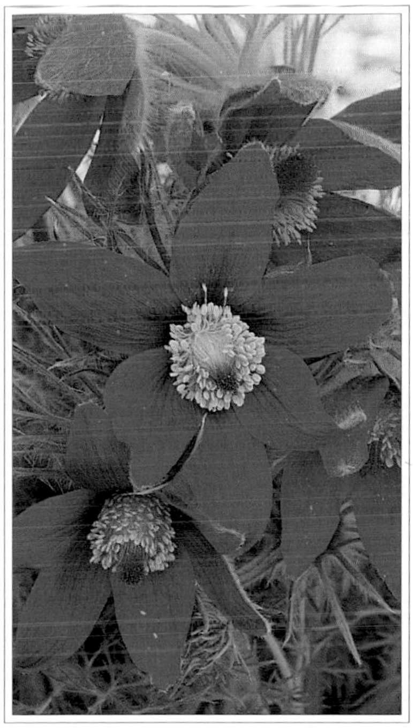

BELLADONNA: for sudden onset of symptoms, associated with great redness of the skin and face. All symptoms tend to be violently acute, there may be over-excitability or a bad headache. This is a good remedy to give a child who has had too much sun.

CHAMOMILLA: for whining, cross and irritable children who can only be calmed with constant soothing and attention. In granule form, often at a very low potency such as 3c (that is, diluted at one part in 1,000), this makes a highly useful remedy for infants who are teething.

PULSATILLA: for mild-natured children, who are easily moved to tears, yet can be obstinate. They often fear the dark, and generally liked to be fussed over and cuddled. If the child's temperament is suited to Pulsatilla, then this remedy should be given no matter what the physical ailment.

SULPHUR: for the child who demands things quickly, and sulks if they do not come immediately. Babies get hot easily, kick off the bedclothes, demand feeding often. This is a remedy that is often used in skin conditions, such as eczema or psoriasis, and suits children with rough, scaly and itchy skin.

CAUTION

Some of the plants used in homeopathy are poisonous, for example Aconite (*Aconitum napellus*) and Belladonna (*Atropa belladonna*). Do not try to use them as herbs!

NATUROPATHY

Probably the most significant time for having a healthy diet is in the first seven years of our lives, when we are most actively developing our body, and our whole system. This is unfortunately not the easiest time to get healthy food into children. The need for energy-giving foods is high, and the metabolic rate burns calories up very fast, so snacks of fruit, fresh or dried, can be given ad lib. Intake of vegetables by children is mostly too low; encouragement and a varied diet can help, and in winter, soups and stews can be a way of disguising vegetables.

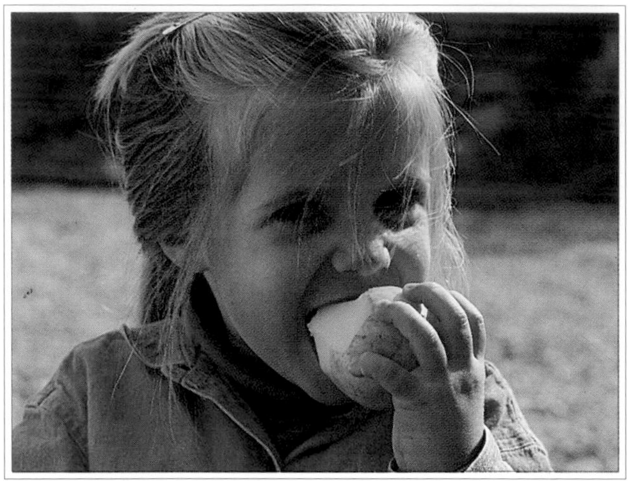

Although children love to eat sticky, chocolatey things, make sure their diet contains plenty of fresh fruit.

In acute, febrile illnesses such as chickenpox or influenza it is often helpful to allow a virtual fast for up to 48 hours (preferably check with your doctor first), but give plenty of fluids, especially fresh fruit juices. This stimulates a higher white blood cell count, improving the child's resistance to infection. Do not feed heavy stodgy foods in these illnesses; the appetite will nearly always come back with a vengeance after the acute stage has passed.

As for supplements, a multivitamin and mineral tablet can be useful, especially in winter. If the child is prone to colds, then Vitamin C is most important; dietary intake can be topped up with a supplement of 100 mg (1-3 times a day, depending on age and need). As girls move into puberty and menstruation starts, a multi-supplement containing a little iron can be a useful boost to the system.

The use of water applications, footbaths and so on, as described throughout the book, can be used quite effectively on children. For reducing fevers, sponge the face and/or upper body with water that is tepid, not cold, and allow to dry off naturally for a cooling effect. For dehydration, try a home-made rehydration preparation: dissolve 5 ml (1 tsp) of salt and 15 ml (1 tbsp) of sugar in 600 ml (1 pt/2½ cups) of freshly boiled water, leave to cool and keep in the refrigerator in a screw-topped bottle. Give 5 ml (1 tsp), up to 5 times a day if needed.

On the following pages are some suggestions for a few of the ailments that occur in childhood. Using the above information about the use of the natural therapies for children, and the other sections of the book, should help you treat most other common complaints. If in doubt get professional advice or treatment.

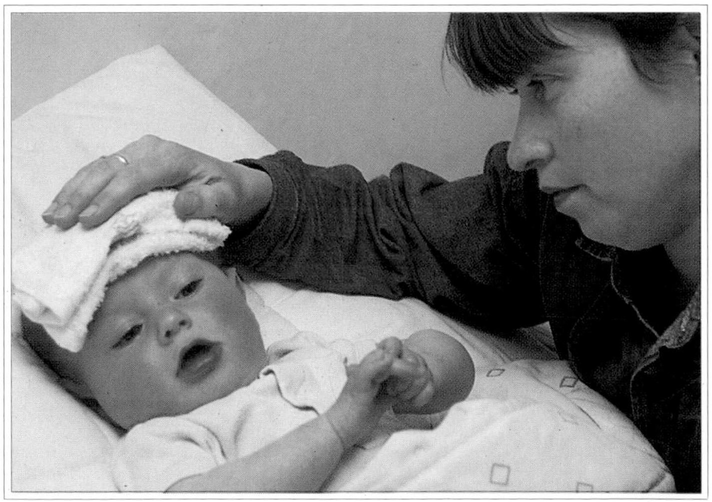

When a child is running a temperature, cool compresses can help calm and soothe the child and reduce body heat.

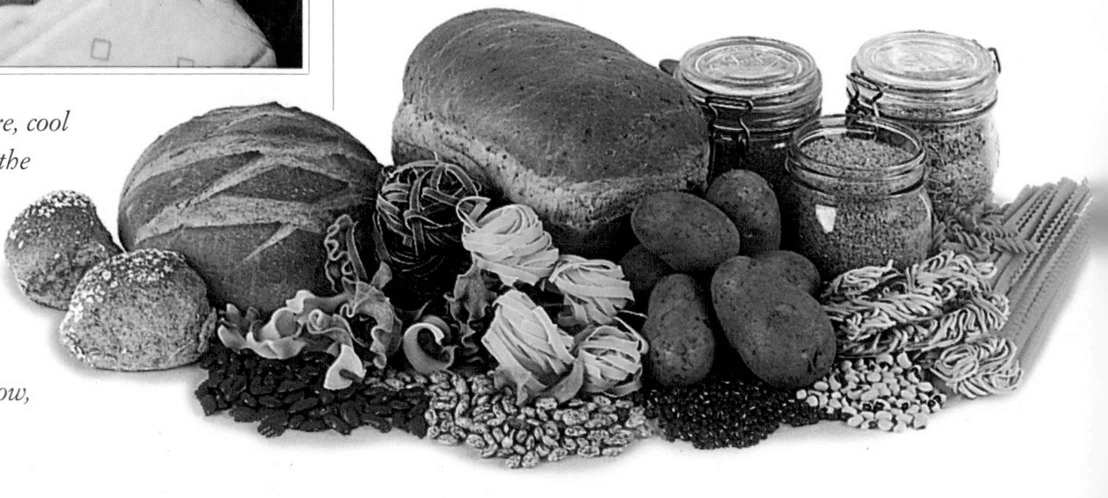

A well-balanced, sensible diet is the best start in life you can give to your child. Healthy eating habits, begun now, will reap rewards in later adult life.

CHICKENPOX

This is a highly infectious disease, not just restricted to childhood in fact, which is due to the same virus, herpes zoster, that gives adults shingles. It can be transmitted from an adult suffering from shingles, and in turn a child with chickenpox can give an adult shingles. The first signs may simply be a raised temperature and general feeling of malaise, and then a day later the spots appear, quickly developing into blisters containing a clear fluid. This is the most infectious stage, as the fluid contains the virus; after a few days the blisters dry up and form scabs which slowly drop off.

AROMATHERAPY

There are a few essential oils that are excellent for treating chickenpox, speeding up the drying and healing process and soothing the irritation. One of the best is Tea Tree oil. This can be made into a lotion to dab on to the spots – add 10 drops to 100 ml (4 fl oz/½ cup) water, or better still Rosewater, and shake. Since oils do not mix with water, you will need to shake before use each time. Add the oil to 50 ml (2 fl oz/¼ cup) distilled Witch Hazel for extra astringency and mix with 50 ml (2 fl oz/¼ cup) of Rosewater. To soothe the itching skin, add 5 drops of Chamomile oil as well, or else use 10 drops of Lavender oil with the Tea Tree to give the best healing results (use fewer drops for young children, see the Aromatherapy section, page 13 and 113). Other essential oils that are effective anti-viral agents are Bergamot and Eucalyptus: use 5 drops of each as above.

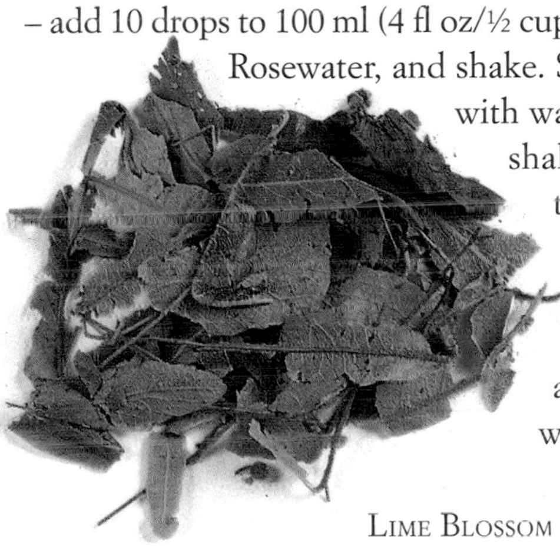

LIME BLOSSOM *(Tilia europaea)*

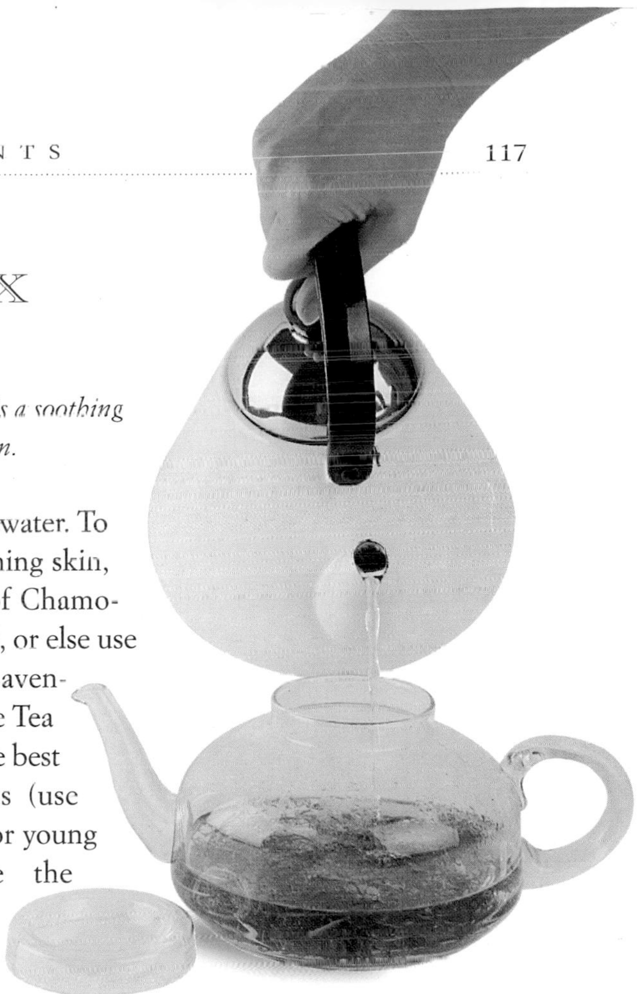

Chamomile tea is a soothing drink for children.

HERBALISM

If the child is a bit feverish, give teas of Chamomile *(Chamomilla recutita),* Yarrow *(Achillea millefolium)* or Lime Blossom *(Tilia europaea)* – or all 3 mixed – in 5 ml (1 tsp) doses (15 ml (1 tbsp) for over 3-year-olds) every 2 or 3 hours. Give plenty of fluids generally, and sponge with tepid water if the temperature is too high. To soothe itching on the skin, apply a little Aloe vera gel, which will also promote healing of the blisters.

COLIC

Colic in babies and infants is usually a sign of trapped wind (gas), but it is a problem that seems to affect bottle-fed babies more than breast-fed ones; this is partly due to the richness of cows' milk, and sometimes may indicate an intolerance to it. Colic, for this reason, can be noticed even in babies who are breast-fed, and may be due to the mother drinking a lot of cows' milk herself. If colicky symptoms are frequent then get advice.

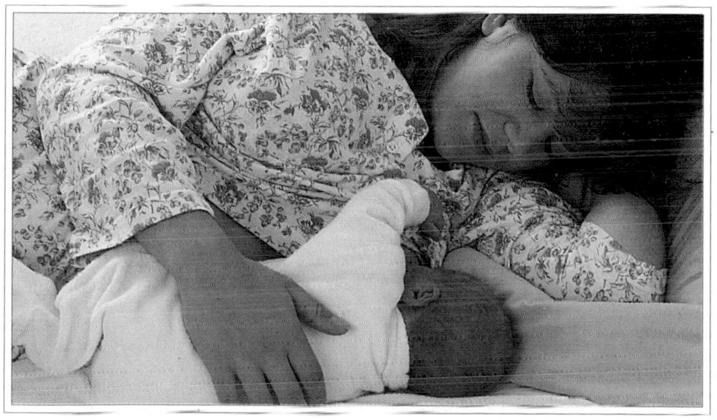

Colicky symptoms can cause anxiety and sleeplessness in both the parents and the child.

HERBALISM

Where babies are breast-feeding, and having problems with wind and colicky pains, it may be easier to give herb teas to the mother which will then work through into the milk. Some of the most effective herbs are Dill *(Anethum graveolens),* Fennel *(Foeniculum vulgare)* and Aniseed *(Pimpinella anisum);* a tea may be made by lightly crushing 5 ml (1 tsp) of the seeds and pouring about 300 ml (½ pt/1¼ cups) of boiling water over them. Leave to stand for a few minutes and strain. The mother should drink a couple of cups a day. For slightly older infants, make a tea in the same way and give in 5 ml (1 tsp) doses (10 ml (2 tsp) for children over 3 years) every couple of hours until the symptoms have gone. Another useful herb is Chamomile *(Chamomilla recutita),* given in the same way.

Peppermint *(Mentha piperita)* is another traditional herbal remedy for colic, taken as a tea; this tends to counteract a number of other homeopathic remedies, so do not mix therapies (homeopathy generally should be used on its own anyway, although there is a tradition in some countries of using combined herbal/homeopathic tablets in over-the-counter medicines). Peppermint *(Mentha piperita)* is better for slightly older children, say over 3-years-old; peppermint oil capsules are available, which dissolve lower down in the gut and so have a stronger effect on colon spasm; these should be kept for children over 8-years or so, and only used for a short time (up to 2 weeks maximum) before getting professional advice.

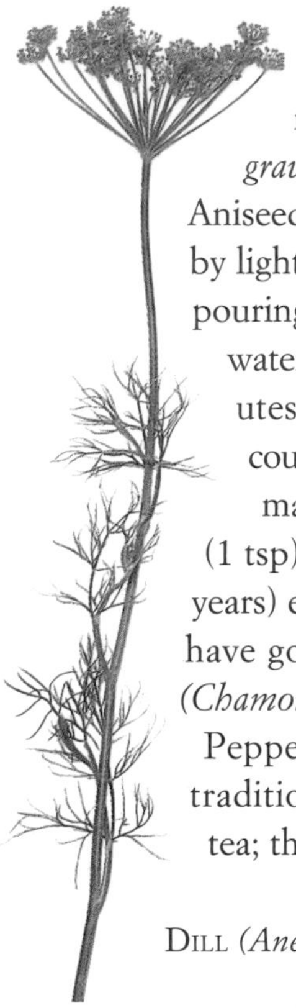

Dill *(Anethum graveolens)*

HOMEOPATHY

Chamomile is also a favourite homeopathic remedy for colic, given in 3c potency initially (see Homeopathy advice page 115) for infants. For children who have got colic after over-eating, or eating food that is too rich, give a dose of Nux vomica (6c potency probably will be appropriate).

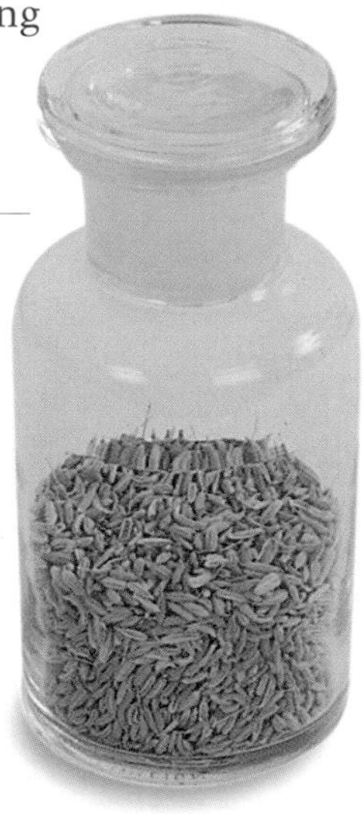

Fennel *(Foeniculum vulgare)*

HYPERACTIVITY

This is a difficult problem to identify, since the boundary between normal energetic behaviour and abnormal activity is a subjective one. There are a number of factors that may contribute towards hyperactivity, such as psychological disturbances or social pressures, and it may be the result of a brain disorder. In general, therefore, this problem needs careful assessment and qualified help.

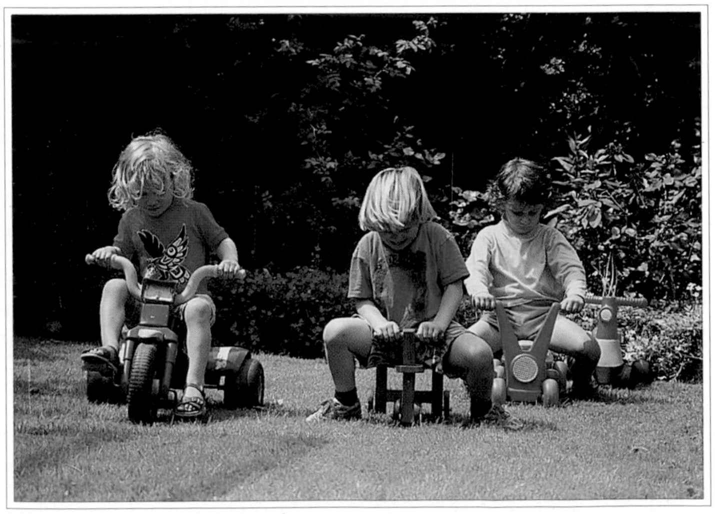

NATUROPATHY

One factor that had been overlooked in conventional medicine for some time is that of food intolerance. Studies have indicated that food additives in particular, especially some colourings and preservatives, can trigger off hyperactivity as well as other reactions; many of these additives have been steadily removed from foods as consumers have successfully protested at their use. If your child has a high proportion of foods containing colourings etc. then it may well be worth exploring a diet without such additives to see if this makes a difference. Changes in behaviour may take 3-4 weeks to be noticeable, although strong reactions to additives can be eased within a day or so.

Children naturally seem to have boundless energy and it can be difficult to spot the first signs of hyperactivity.

MEASLES

This is one of the more serious of childhood ailments, since there are possible secondary infections that can occur. These include middle-ear infections, bronchitis or even pneumonia. These complications are often more of a problem than measles itself, so preferably get professional advice. Initial symptoms are often those of a cold and cough, although a disliking of bright lights and sunlight is quite common at the outset. A clear diagnosis of measles can be made from the appearance of small white spots on the inside of the cheeks; 2-3 days later the rash appears, spreading from the face down the body to the legs. The red spots often join together to give a blotchy appearance, and the child normally has a fever, nasty cough and feels unwell. As the rash fades, it can leave a brownish stain that disappears by itself shortly afterwards, but can linger. The child starts to feel better as the rash spreads and then fades.

AROMATHERAPY

Since the immune system is temporarily lowered (hence the possibility of secondary infections) self-help measures to enhance this can be very helpful. Constant evaporation of essential oils like Tea Tree and Eucalyptus in the child's sick room can be important; use a burner or else add 20 drops of each oil to a 600 ml (1 pt/2½ cups) plant spray full of water. Shake and spray frequently into the air.

HERBALISM

For the fever, herb teas of Elderflower *(Sambucus nigra)*, Chamomile *(Chamomilla recutita)* and Lime Blossom *(Tilia europaea)* will help to induce sweating and cool the temperature; the last two herbs are additionally calming, helping to reduce the upset and aid sleep.

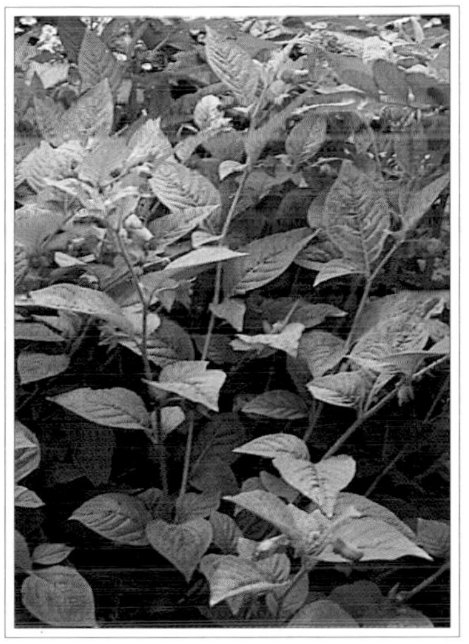

DEADLY NIGHTSHADE
(Atropa belladonna)

HOMEOPATHY

Suitable homeopathic remedies are:
BELLADONNA: for a bright red rash, sore/hot throat and overall heat, not helped by cold air or cold drinks.
EUPHRASIA: for the beginning of the ailment, with runny nose and eyes, and reaction to bright light and strong sunlight .
PULSATILLA: for itching and burning spots, causing the child to cry a lot; a dry throat and troublesome cough.

NATUROPATHY

Garlic capsules, and/or Echinacea tablets may be given as immune-stimulants. Vitamin C is valuable: give 100 mg per day for 4-8-year-olds, 300 mg per day for 8-12-year-olds, and 500-800 mg per day for over 12-year-olds, for the first week of symptoms. Half this dose may then be given until all symptoms have gone.

MUMPS

An acute viral infection, producing the typical swollen parotid (salivary) glands on either side of the jaw. It can affect one side only, in which case the other side can, although only rarely, be affected if exposed to the virus later in life. The most worrying complication for adults is a secondary swelling and inflammation of one or both testicles *(orchitis)*, but this only rarely causes any long-term problems. Alongside the swelling of the parotid gland(s) there is usually a fever, symptoms settling down in a week or so.

If there is difficulty in eating, give liquids or nourishing foods. Fluid is important because of the fever too, but avoid citrus juices which may increase saliva flow and add to the pains. A cold compress can be used to reduce the swelling; a drop of Lavender oil may be used in this, or perhaps use iced Lavender tea. Vitamin C may be given to boost the immune system, and herb teas taken to control the fever and act as general tonics (see Measles for suggestions).

Homeopathic remedies to look at include Belladonna where the face is red and burning hot, and Pulsatilla for a high temperature but a feeling of chill.

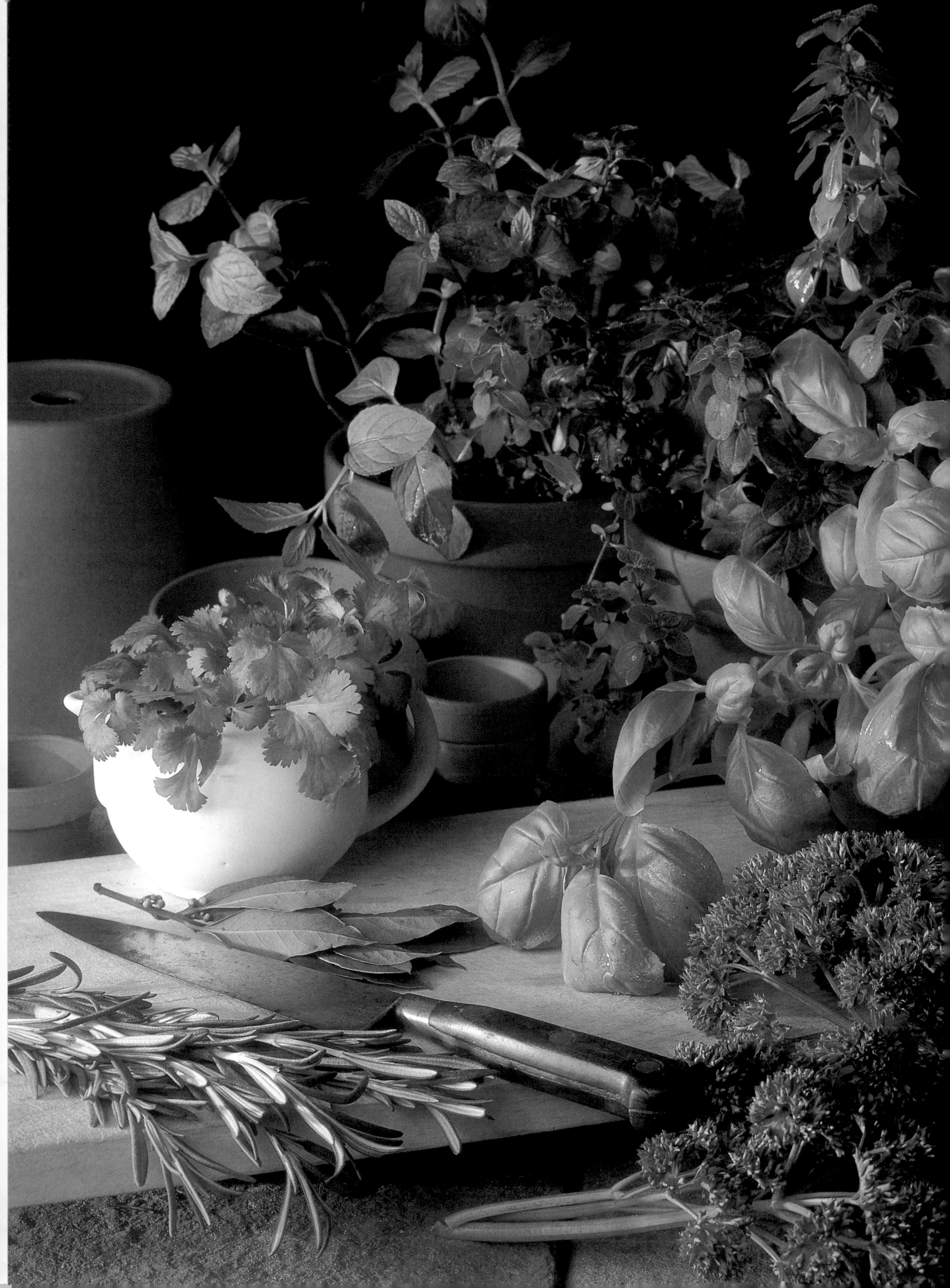

NATURAL THERAPIES

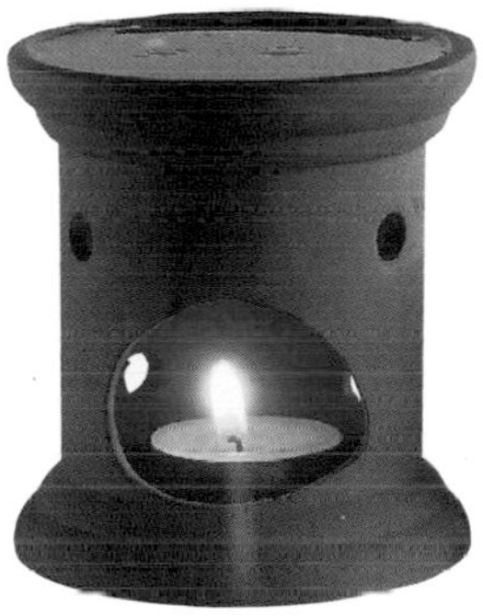

In a world of ever-increasing technology and machine-controlled medical interventions, people are beginning to feel the need for a human, individual touch; for a more natural approach to health that seeks to enhance life rather than dissect illness into more and more obscure diseases. Fortunately, there are a number of natural therapies which have just such a positive, holistic approach, and have also stood the test of time, to emerge as the most rational way to sustain our health into the twenty-first century. In the second section of this book the natural therapies are explored in five broad categories: Health from Plants covers herbal medicine, aromatherapy, the Bach Flower Remedies and Homeopathy; Naturopathy explores diet and exercise; Stress Management explains self-hypnotism and meditation as well as pyschotherapy, autogenics and healing; Bodywork offers detailed step-by-step routines in massage and reflexology, and the final category, Eastern approaches, covers shiatsu, makko ho, yoga and moxibustion with exercises that will introduce you to the benefits and theories of each discipline.

We have become accustomed to thinking of medicine as a crisis treatment for when we are sick, but one of the strengths of these therapies is their value in countering the effects of stress and helping to actually prevent illness. By reducing the impact of worries and stresses, many natural systems of treatment work to restore our vital energy and inner harmony. Eastern cultures have retained a strong tradition of therapies aimed at balancing energy, and in recent years these have gained increasing attention in the West. Our own traditional forms of treatment, such as herbalism and massage, have also undergone a resurgence in popularity, and there are the beginnings of major research projects to confirm their value. Natural therapies not only have a long history, they have a bright future.

HEALTH FROM PLANTS

The most basic and the most pervasive source of medicines throughout the world ever since time began has been the plant kingdom. From our earliest origins we can trace the use of plants for health; even today most people rely on herbal medicines for most of their primary health care.

In ancient cultures, diet and medicine were inextricably linked – let your food be your medicine, and your medicine be your food – and the importance of diet to health is discussed in another section, but plants provide an additional healthy element to our food. Herbs not only enhance the flavour of what we eat, but often contain useful trace elements and also help with the digestion of many foods. Herbal teas are low-caffeine drinks that carry many health benefits too.

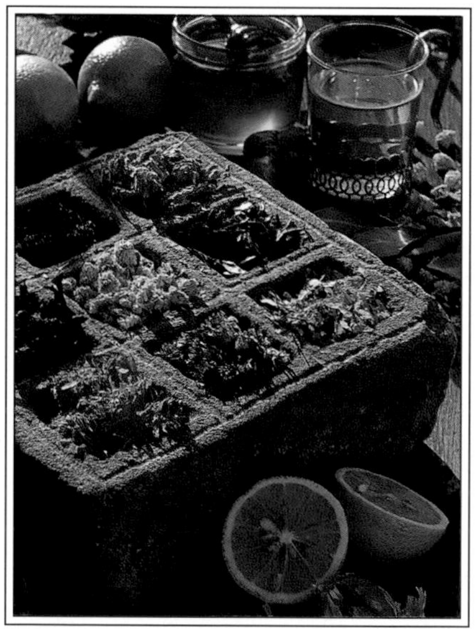

Professional herbal medicine may use plants with quite profound effects on our systems, while other therapies such as homoeopathy utilize the energetic qualities of plants, among other substances. In aromatherapy, the essential oils of plants are used to affect our emotional states, as well as for quite powerful anti-infective properties. As well as these therapies, requiring treatment from qualified practitioners, the plant world also offers many home remedies, and equally importantly plants can be used in many ways to maintain good health. This section shows some of these ways, and when to seek help.

ABOVE: A selection of herbs and dried flowers used in teas and tisanes.

OPPOSITE: A garden overflowing with plants used for centuries for their health-giving and medicinal qualities.

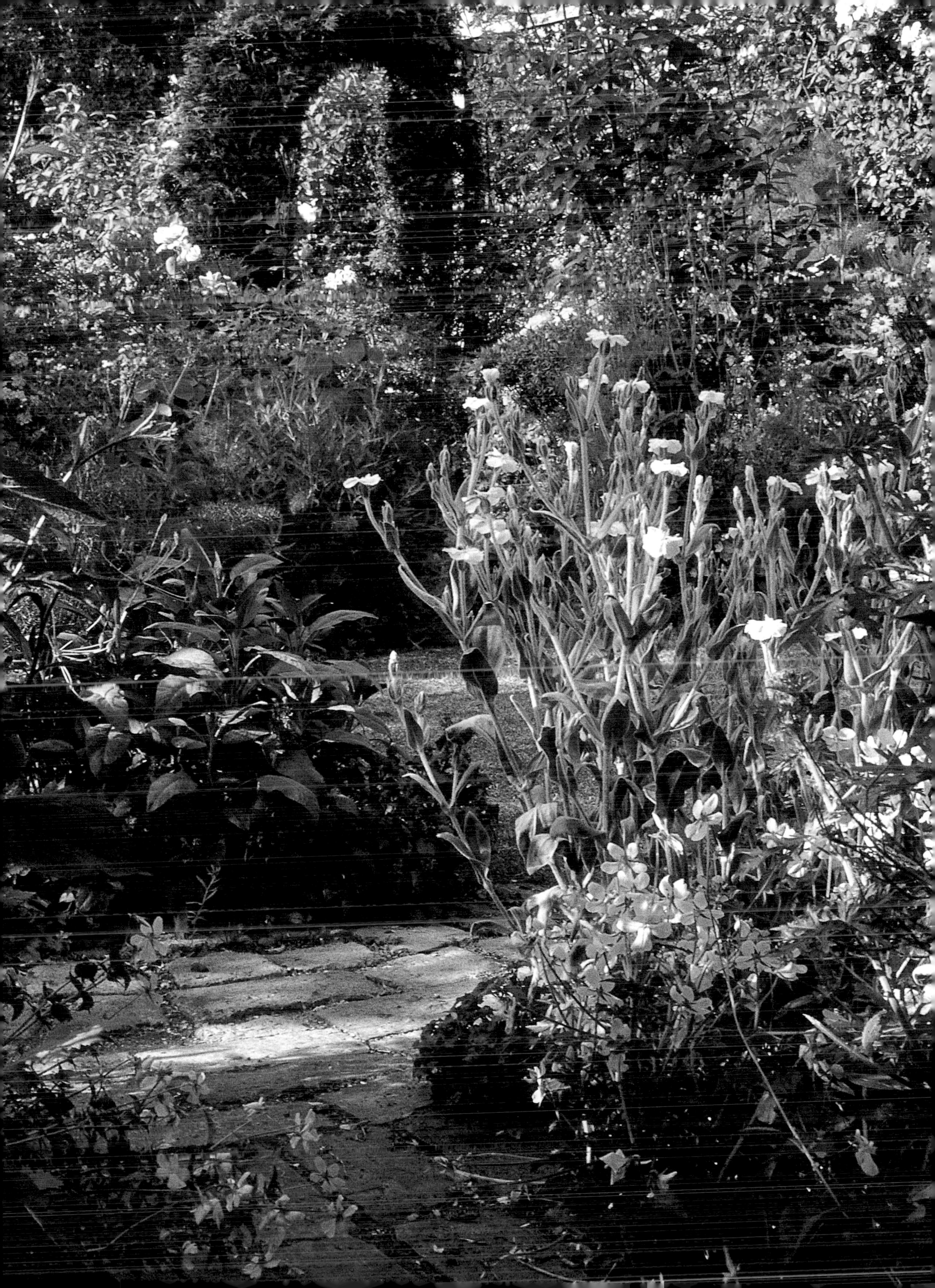

Herbal Medicine

History and Origins

The history of herbal medicine is really the history of humankind, for every culture throughout time has relied upon herbs for its medicines. Some cultures – for instance, in India and China – have maintained a strong, unbroken tradition of herbalism for several centuries, while in Europe and North America its popularity has soared and plunged periodically as Western medicine achieved greater prominence. Today, however, interest in herbal medicine has increased once more, with an appreciation of its safer, holistic approach.

Probably the first system of herbal medicine, apart from the almost instinctive use of plants for healing that existed from the dawn of history and is still practised by remote tribes, was developed in India well over 4,000 years ago.

From India, the use of plants probably travelled with migrating people into China; traditional Chinese medicine has developed a strong philosophical viewpoint on health and disease, with treatments ranging from herbal medicines to acupuncture, moxibustion and massage techniques.

Below: Although drying herbs alters their colour and flavour some, such as rosemary and thyme, keep many of their properties.

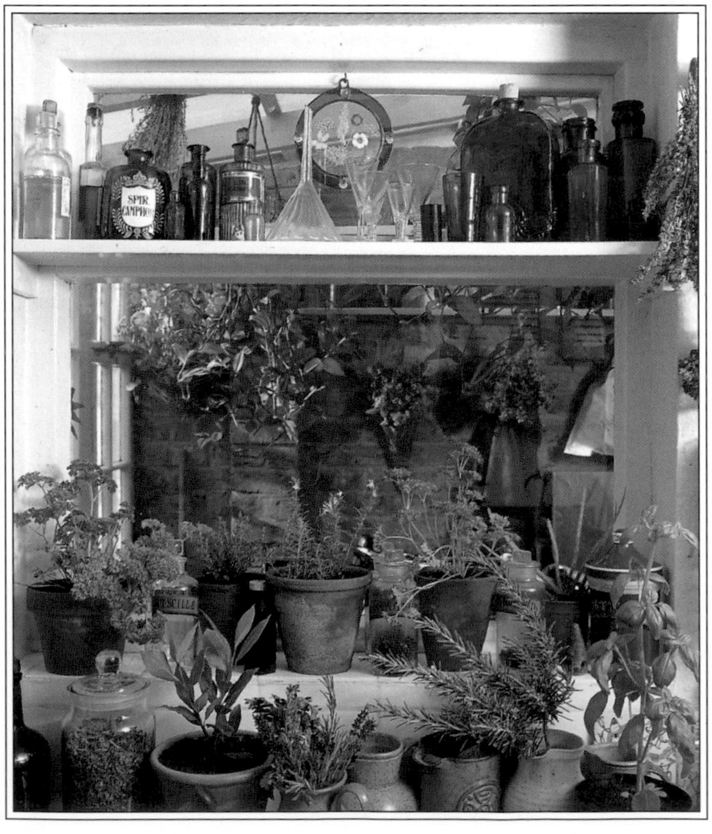

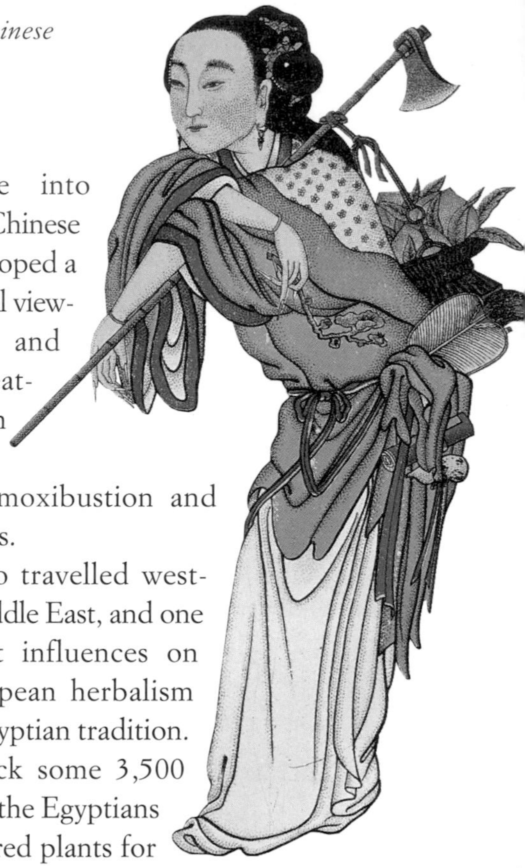

Right: Ma-Kou (a Chinese goddess) carrying her medicinal herbs.

Knowledge also travelled westwards, into the Middle East, and one of the significant influences on present-day European herbalism was the ancient Egyptian tradition. Papyri dating back some 3,500 years indicate that the Egyptians used several hundred plants for food and medicine. These two uses were inextricably linked for centuries, as one Greek writer put it: "Let your food be your medicine, and your medicine be your food."

As the ancient Greeks expanded their empire, so their knowledge and use of herbs was spread throughout the realm, and other plants were added to their *materia medica*. When the Romans superseded the Greeks, their army doctors carried herbs and herbal medicine all over the known world. A large number of Mediterranean herbs were thus spread through Europe and into Britain. During these two great civilizations, several major works were written on natural history and medicine which were to be fundamental to medical thought for centuries.

After the decline of the Roman Empire, much of its literature went eastwards to Byzantium and the Arabic cultures. Traditional medicine here has retained a good deal of this ancient philosophy, and some of it came back to Europe with the Moorish invasions.

After the printing press was invented, all the old Greek

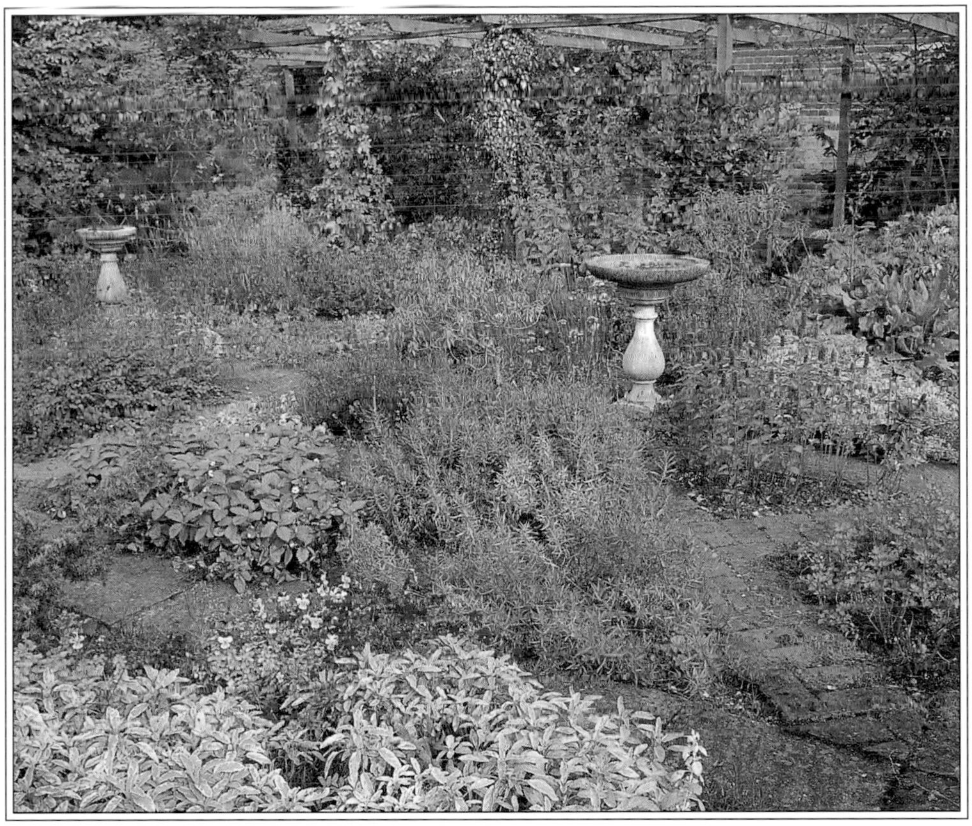

RIGHT: A traditional monastic layout is recreated in this twentieth-century garden, well stocked with a wide variety of herbs. Medieval monks kept physic gardens, growing herbs to make medicines for themselves and the local people, while the villagers would generally use simple plant treatments for all manner of ailments.

and Roman texts could be reproduced for a much wider readership. This coincided with the rapid expansion of towns and cities, and for the next three hundred years or so, knowledge and interest in herbs, in all areas of life, was greatly increased. By the sixteenth century, books about herbs were being published in the contemporary languages rather than Latin, and herbalism was an integral part of life. Books by authors such as Matthiolus, Turner, Gerard and Culpeper became bestsellers with practical advice on the uses of herbs; indeed Culpeper has never been out of print to this day, for over three hundred years.

Meanwhile, herbal medicines had been taken over by the settlers to America and used much as in Europe. It is possible to trace the spread of herbs along the eastern seaboard of the United States of America from early plantings by these settlers. Some of the more inquisitive migrants tried to learn from the Native Americans, since they were, before the importation of different diseases by the colonists, a healthy race.

The Native American system of health relied upon the use of herbs, simple yet nourishing food, fresh air and exercise. They also successfully used heat and water applications such as sweat lodges – teepees heated by a fire – with their physical and spiritual benefits.

The last ten to twenty years have seen another great resurgence in interest in natural medicine, and herbalism is both highly popular and increasingly respected as a safe and effective system of general medicine.

While today's professional practitioner of herbal medicine may see a wide range of people, often suffering from serious and chronic ill-health, the emphasis is always on the individual, looking at the whole picture of a person's health and not just any specific symptoms; this holistic approach is one good reason for its renewed popularity. Herbalism is also equally concerned with prevention or maintaining good health outside times of illness, and it is this aspect which attracts many people to use herbs in their daily lives.

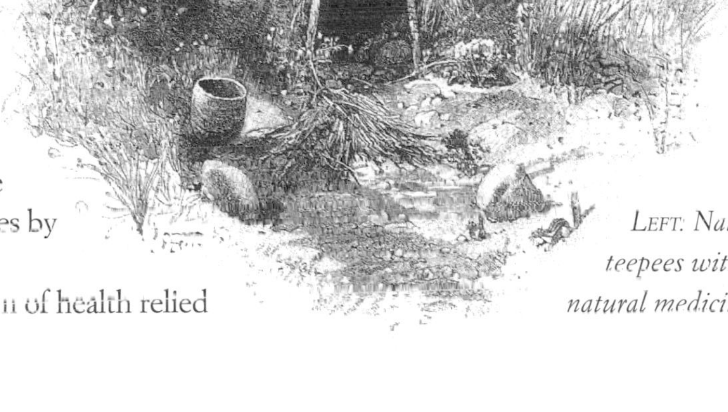

LEFT: Native Americans used sweat lodges – teepees with a fire inside – as part of their natural medicine treatments.

HERB TEAS

One of the most widespread methods of using herbs to maintain good health and ward off illnesses is by drinking herb teas, or tisanes as they are known in France. For medicinal purposes, when treating an actual ailment, stronger preparations such as infusions or decoctions are prescribed, but in general it is possible to make a simple tisane at home.

Herb teas can be used as everyday hot drinks, to replace tea and coffee and hence reduce the caffeine intake in the diet. As each herb differs greatly in taste and flavour, it is very much an individual choice. A couple that have some of the taste qualities of ordinary tea are rooibosch and maté. The former has long been the daily drink for many people in South Africa, and is now grown in several countries; it makes a very enjoyable, low-caffeine tea. Similarly, maté is well-known in South American countries for its refreshing effect, with a smoky flavour reminiscent of Lapsang Souchong tea.

In general, it is sensible to vary herb teas, not only to enjoy a variety of flavours but to ensure that their medicinal properties are not overdone. Some can, however, be drunk over some considerable time, to maintain health and prevent ailments. In winter, especially in cooler climates, rose-hips might be a good choice. These contain considerable amounts of Vitamin C, which is an excellent way to sustain resistance to colds, flu and so on. Vitamin C can have something of a laxative effect, but the tannin content of rose-hips helps to balance this out. Many of the early naturopathic clinics in Switzerland, such as that run by Dr Bircher-Benner, the creator of muesli, insisted that their clients drank a few cups of rose-hip tea daily. Tea bags are easily available in many countries and are very convenient to use, although quality varies.

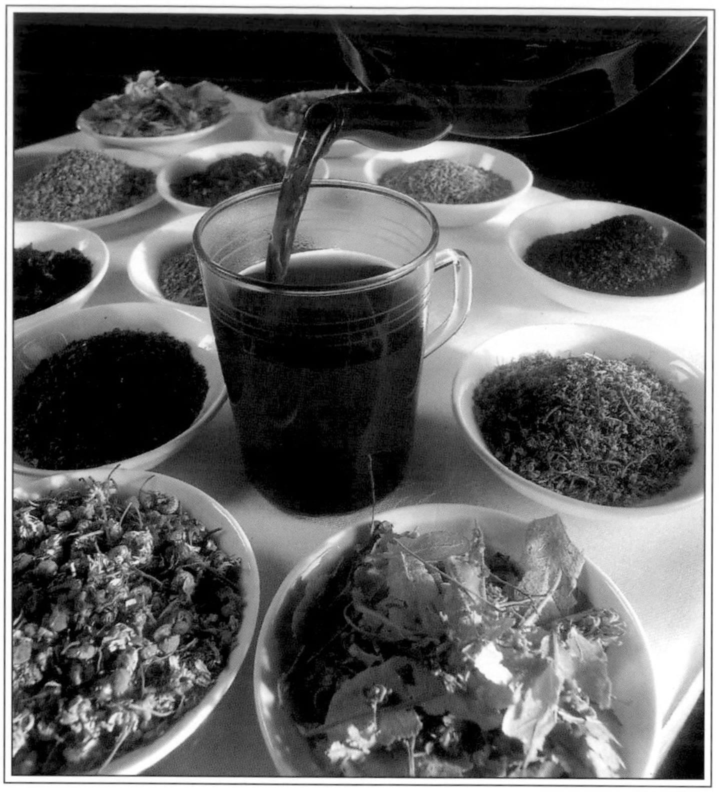

ABOVE: Most warm herbal teas have a comforting effect and are very easy to prepare.

A SIMPLE TISANE

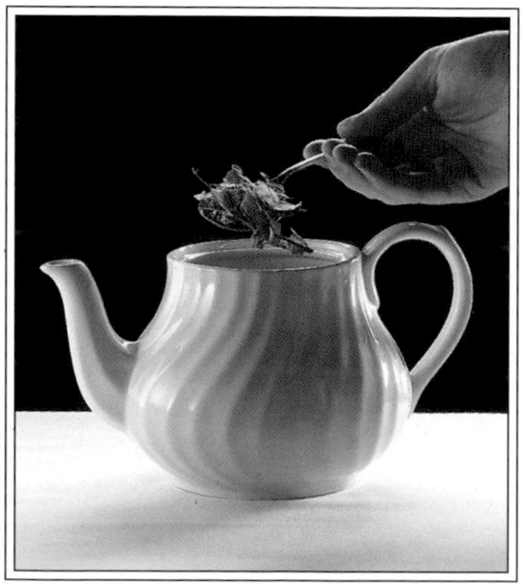

1 Warm a teapot and add one heaped teaspoonful of dried herb per person, or double for fresh herbs.

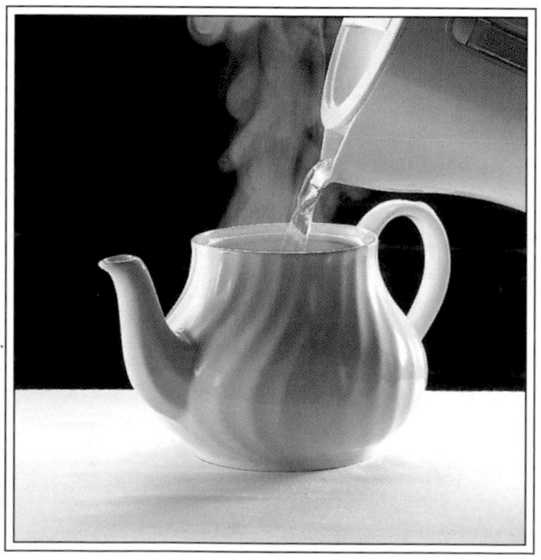

2 Pour on boiling water and allow to infuse for 2–3 minutes.

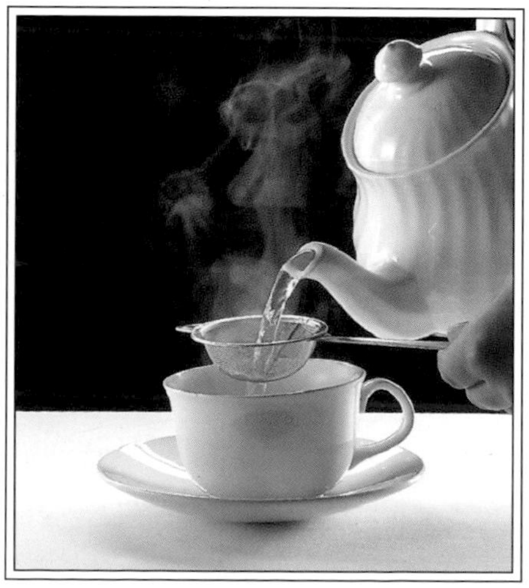

3 Strain and drink without milk or sugar (if you prefer a sweetener, use a little honey).

DANDELION TEA

Dandelions are a diuretic and can help to reduce water retention and bloated feelings. They can also help rheumatism. This tea acts as a mild laxative so should not be drunk in large quantities.

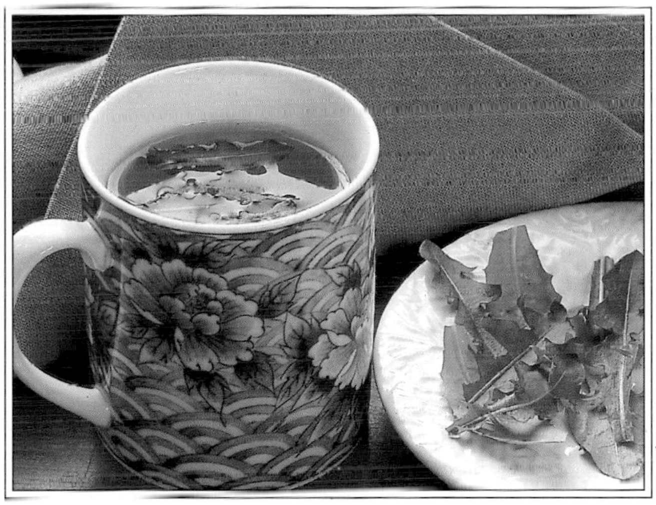

1 Remove any stems from the dandelion leaves. Tear them into strips and place in the bottom of a mug. Pour on enough boiling water to fill the mug and leave to stand for 5–10 minutes.

2 Strain, discard most of the dandelion leaves and drink. If you prefer a sweetener, add a small teaspoonful of honey.

A pleasant summer tea can be made from fresh lemon balm leaves: gather a few sprigs of the leaves, and make a tea, leaving it to stand for a few minutes. This herb reduces the impact of stress and anxiety on the system, especially where nervous indigestion is involved, and its balancing effects make it suitable for morning or evening drinking. The dried herb can be used too, but its flavour is inferior.

MINT *(Mentha x piperita)*

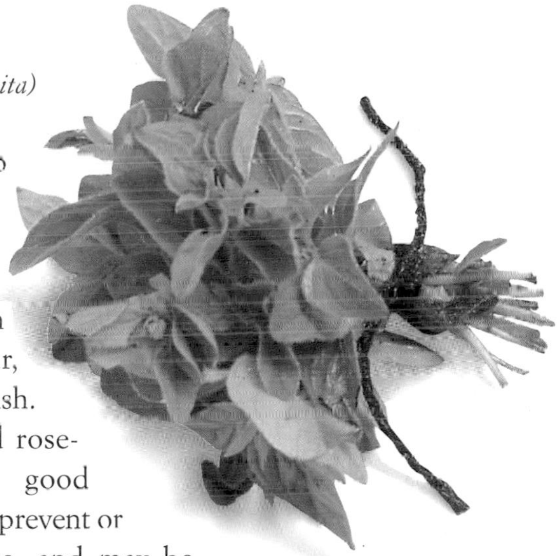

In hot weather, keep a jug of the tea in the refrigerator, perhaps with a slice or two of lemon for added flavour, and drink as you wish.

Peppermint and rosemary are both good pick-me-up teas, to prevent or overcome tiredness, and may be made from either fresh or dried leaves as a morning cup of tea – many blends of herbs in tea-bags are based upon the taste of peppermint. Peppermint tea is becoming more popular as a digestif drink to replace coffee after a heavy meal. Cinnamon and ginger make pleasantly warming drinks, separately or mixed together, for colder weather; just coarsely break a cinnamon stick into the teapot, while fresh ginger root may be sliced or grated. Chamomile flowers are one of the best digestive remedies, and the tea is often drunk in the evenings to aid restful sleep, or to soothe upset stomachs. Elderflowers make a thirst-quenching drink, with beneficial properties for warding off colds and catarrh, which is best made from dried flowerheads. All the above herbs can be used in combinations for extra flavour and medicinal effect.

Used regularly, herbal teas can make a significant contribution to a person's quality of health and wellbeing, not simply as replacements for stimulants such as tea or coffee, but for their general health-giving properties and specific medicinal benefits.

HERB TEA CHART

HERB	PROPERTY	BENEFIT
Chamomile	Relaxant, digestive, anti-inflammatory	Settles digestion, aids restful sleep
Cinnamon	Carminative, warming, diaphoretic	Improves digestion and good when cold/chilled
Elderflower	Expectorant, diaphoretic	Clears catarrh, reduces fevers by sweating
Lemon Balm	Relaxant, digestive, anti-depressant	Relieves nervous dyspepsia, good tonic
Lime Blossom	Relaxant, analgesic	Eases tension headaches or aching colds and flu
Peppermint	Antispasmodic and digestive	Reduces flatulence, is good for head colds too
Rosehip	Contains Vitamin C	Helps build resistance to colds and flu

HERB SUPPLEMENTS

All in all, therefore, herbs can play an essential role in maintaining one's health and vitality on a daily basis. They provide much more than extra flavouring to food, enjoyable though this may be, and their continued and universal popularity demonstrates how much people rely on them to keep well. Many herbs can be used as effective, powerful yet safe remedies for all kinds of ailments.

Herbs in other forms can also be used to maintain good health. Many people's experience of herbal medicines is in the form of tablets or capsules obtained from health stores or other outlets. Some of these extracts are more valuable in preventing ill-health than as medications; if you are actually ill, it may be better to consult a herbal practitioner since the principle of herbalism is based on individual treatment.

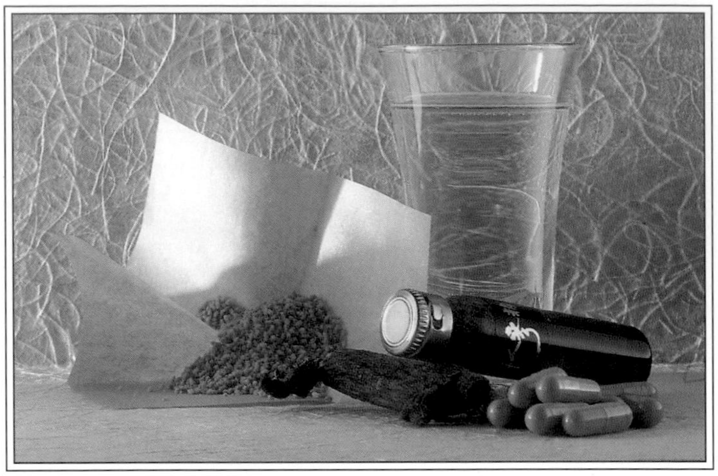

ABOVE: Ginseng, renowned in China as a powerful natural remedy for hundreds of years, is now used more and more in the West.

GARLIC

One of the most effective herbal remedies is garlic, which can help tremendously in building up resistance to respiratory infections, warding off colds, flu and so on. Garlic needs to be taken daily during the late autumn, winter and early spring months to sustain this resistance. Undoubtedly it is most effective when a fresh bulb is used, ideally raw, but as you can lose most of your friends if taking garlic this way every day, it may be more suitable to take one of the commercial garlic capsules that are easily found. These are less powerful, but should impart less odour to the breath – the reason for garlic's actions in resisting respiratory infections is that the (smelly) essential oil which gives it a powerful antiseptic property is 99 per cent excreted via the lungs.

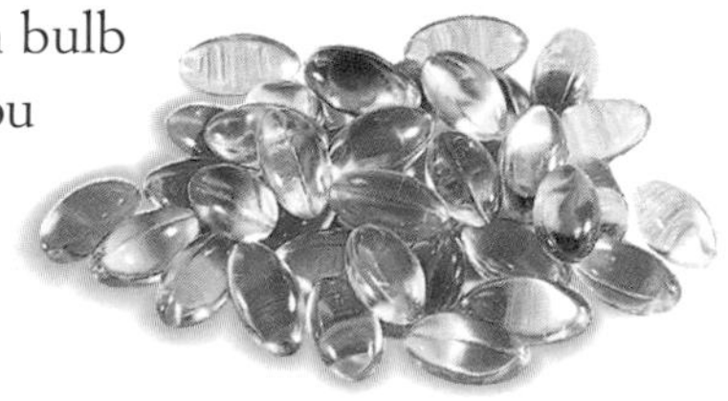

GARLIC TABLETS

ECHINACEA

Another herb with very useful properties is *Echinacea* (sometimes called purple coneflower). This stimulates the immune system, boosting general resistance to infection and illness. If vitality has been lowered, or if you simply wish to strengthen the immune response, *Echinacea* is available in either a liquid form or as tablets (sometimes it can be found combined with garlic), and a course may be taken for three or four weeks to raise immunity.

GINSENG

Chronic stress is one major source of impaired immunity, and it may well be useful before or during a time of increased stress, or indeed before the winter arrives in colder climates, to take a three-week course of herbs to improve your ability to cope with physical, emotional and mental stresses. The classic herbs for this are the various ginsengs. These are most suitable for waning energy and are to be used with caution (if at all) where people respond to stress with increased anxiety or tension and raised blood pressure. Korean, or Asiatic ginseng *(Panax schinseng)*, gives the most uplift, while American ginseng *(P. quinquefolium)* has a more relaxing effect. Siberian ginseng *(Eleutherococcus senticosus)* is a completely different plant, with similar effects to Korean ginseng in enhancing stamina. These are all available as tablets, and the two *Panax* species can often be found as the actual dried root, which may be chewed in small pieces or made into a tea.

EVENING PRIMROSE

A plant that has become very popular in recent years is the evening primrose; the oil extracted from the seeds is a potent source of essential fatty acids, particularly a substance called gamma-linoleic acid. Some people do not produce enough of this compound, which in turn can lead to a shortage of more complex compounds that have beneficial effects in a number of ailments, such as arthritis, eczema and even multiple sclerosis. Evening primrose oil, however, is perhaps best known and most widely used for its use in helping ease premenstrual problems or the symptoms of the menopause. Obviously, the full treatment of hormonal disorders requires professional attention, but

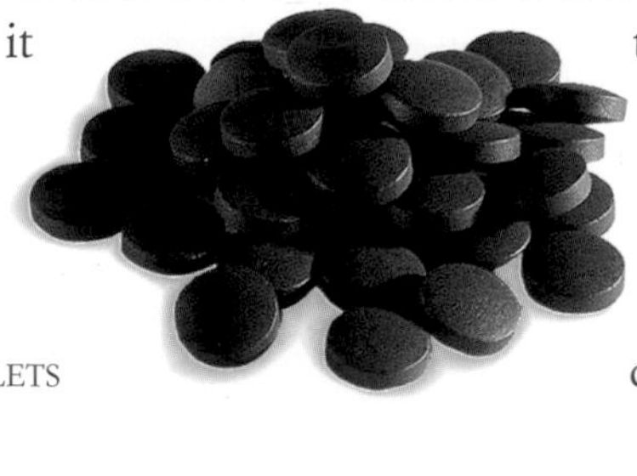

GINSENG TABLETS

there may be a case for taking evening primrose oil capsules daily (500–1500mg) as a preventive treatment in the early stages of the menopause.

Feverfew

Another good self-help herb to use in order to help prevent the occurrence, or recurrence, of ailment symptoms is feverfew. This is another plant which has gained in popularity, this time for its usefulness in warding off migraines. It is not to be thought of as a remedy to take when you have a migraine – the reasons for which can often be a detective story and need individual treatment – but as a preventive measure. The herb is now widely available in tablet form, daily dosage about 125mg, and as the fresh leaves taste very bitter and can occasionally cause mouth ulcers, the tablets are a convenient way to use feverfew.

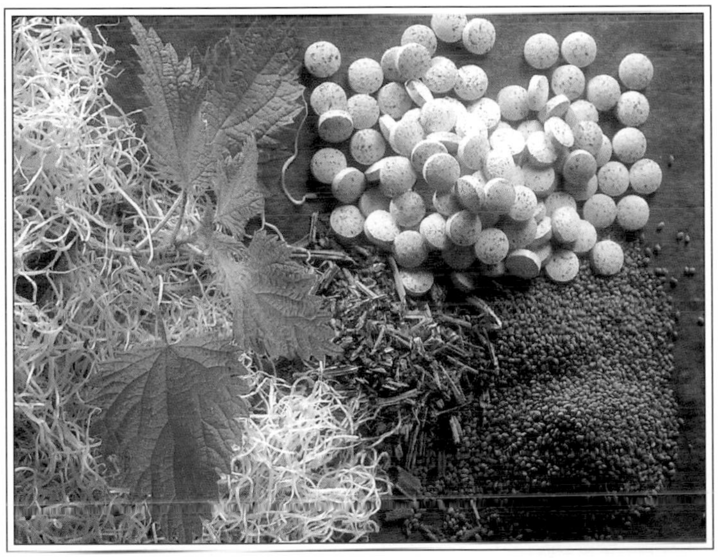

Above: Clockwise from top left: alfalfa sprouts, nettles, kelp tablets, alfalfa seeds and dried kelp.

Alfalfa and Kelp

Some herbs are sufficiently rich in nutrients to be thought of as food supplements, although it may be more appropriate to use them in different ways. Sprouted alfalfa, for instance, contains high amounts of several vitamins and minerals; this is best taken as part of the diet, eaten in salads where it gives a crunchy bite to the dish. Nettles are very rich in iron, together with some Vitamin C, and can make an energy-giving tea for people who are bordering on being anaemic. Kelp contains several minerals, notably iodine which acts as a tonic for the thyroid gland, and can aid those who have a sluggish metabolism; this herb should *not* be used by anyone taking thyroxine for an under-active thyroid gland – if in doubt, seek professional advice. Many seaweeds are used in cooking, especially in Japanese cuisine, and this is one way to take them; kelp is also easily found in tablet form, and this is a useful way to take a daily course for, say, four weeks to boost the system.

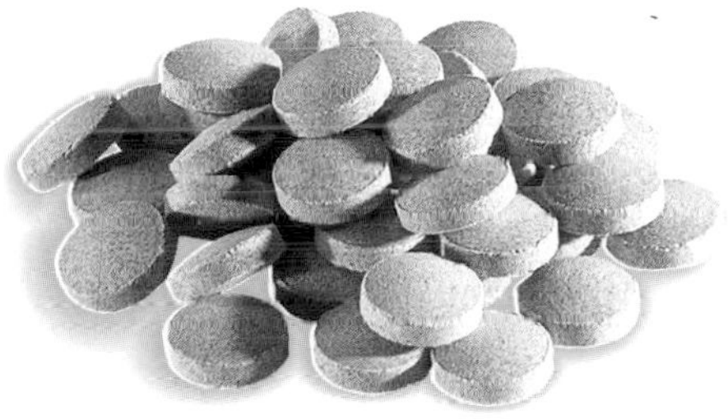

Kelp tablets

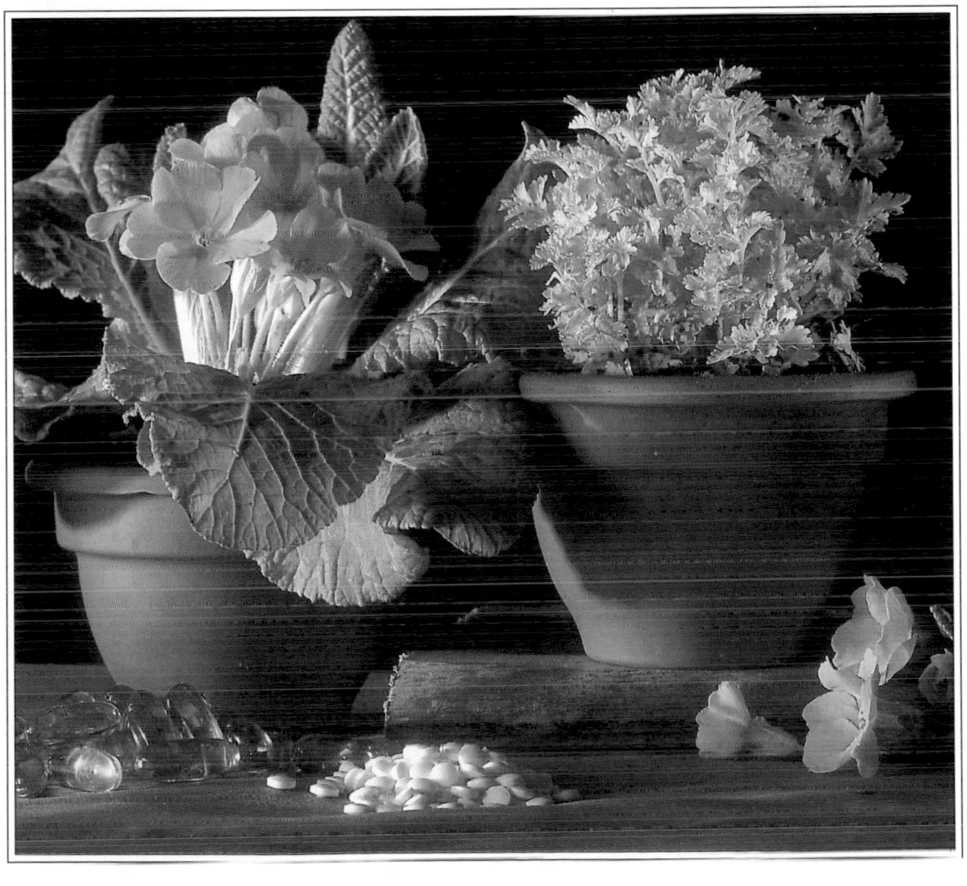

Right: Evening primrose is widely used to alleviate the side-effects of menstruation.

AROMATHERAPY

HISTORY

One of the most primitive forms of medicine involved burning aromatic plants in order to "smoke" illness out of a patient. This process was frequently interlinked with various rituals and religious practices, and sometimes plants with mind-altering properties were burnt too, to create a mystical, other-worldly experience as part of the healing ritual. The use of incense in the ceremonies of diverse religions through the centuries has perpetuated this aspect; many of the gums and resins that are used in incense have powerful therapeutic properties – for example, as respiratory antiseptics – as well as inducing a meditative, reflective state of mind in the worshippers.

Aromatic plants and extracts have been highly regarded by all the greater ancient civilizations, stretching through the Middle East from Babylonia and Persia to India and China. The oldest medical texts from these countries, dating back at least 3,000 years, list many aromatic plants and their uses. Some of the most detailed descriptions are to be found in ancient Egyptian writings; fragrant plants were employed in all aspects of life, from perfume and cosmetics to medicine and in the rituals for embalming the dead. Some of the ointment jars excavated from Tutankhamen's tomb contained

BELOW: Aromatherapy oils are now widely available and can be mixed with pure vegetable oils for use in massage.

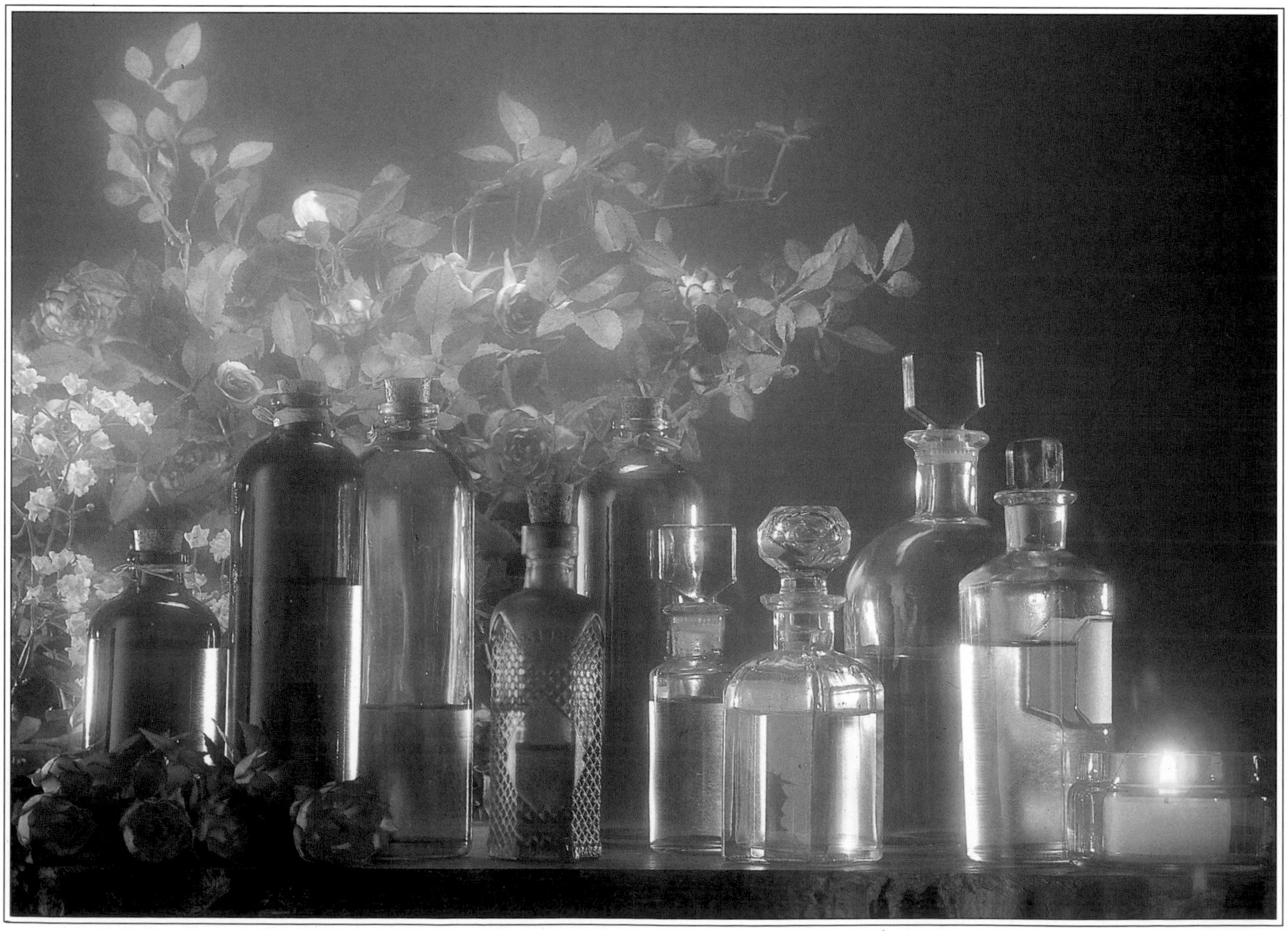

preservative resins such as frankincense which still had an odour after some 3,200 years.

The Egyptians were very aware of the value of fragrance in enhancing mood, and developed a reputation as masters of perfumery; Cleopatra may have owed something of her fabled attractiveness to Julius Caesar and Mark Antony from her use of vast amounts of rose petals to scent her living quarters. Interestingly, however, the Egyptians do not appear to have discovered the process of distilling the essential oils from plants, relying instead on infused oils and ointments. These were later widely used by the Greeks and Romans, both as medicine and as part of the daily ritual of public bathing, which the Romans in particular so enjoyed.

Many Greek physicians were employed by the Roman armies, and they carried the knowledge of aromatic, and other, plants across many countries. Galen, who rose to be the personal physician to the Emperor Marcus Aurelius, invented the original cold cream and was a great writer on all matters concerning health and medicines. His and other works formed the basis of medicine for many centuries, and with the decline of the Roman Empire much of this knowledge went eastwards into Byzantium. It was the Arabic countries that made the next great leap forwards in aromatherapy. By the ninth century, Baghdad was thriving partly due to being the centre of the rose industry, exporting rose water as far as India. The principle of distillation was first applied to roses and is generally credited to Abu Ali Ibn Sina, better known as Avicenna (980–1037), a philosopher and physician from Uzbekistan. Steam distillation enabled the pure essential oil to be extracted from many plants.

In the West, aromatic infused oils had continued to be used, and during the period of the Crusades, essential oils, or "perfumes of Arabia" as they were known, spread extensively throughout Europe. As the gums and resins of Asia were not easily available, native Mediterranean plants such as rosemary and lavender were used for making essential oils too. The French were particularly enthusiastic in adopting these oils, laying the foundations for today's perfumery industry as well as therapeutic uses.

Burning antiseptic herbs such as thyme and rosemary, to fumigate the air and ward off disease, was carried out in several French hospitals until well into the twentieth century. Indeed, it was a Frenchman, René Gattefosse, a chemist working in the perfumery industry, who coined the term aromatherapy some 50 years ago. He burned his hand badly in an accident in his laboratory. He used essential oil of lavender to cool the tissue and found it healed the burned flesh remarkably quickly, with no infection or scar. During both

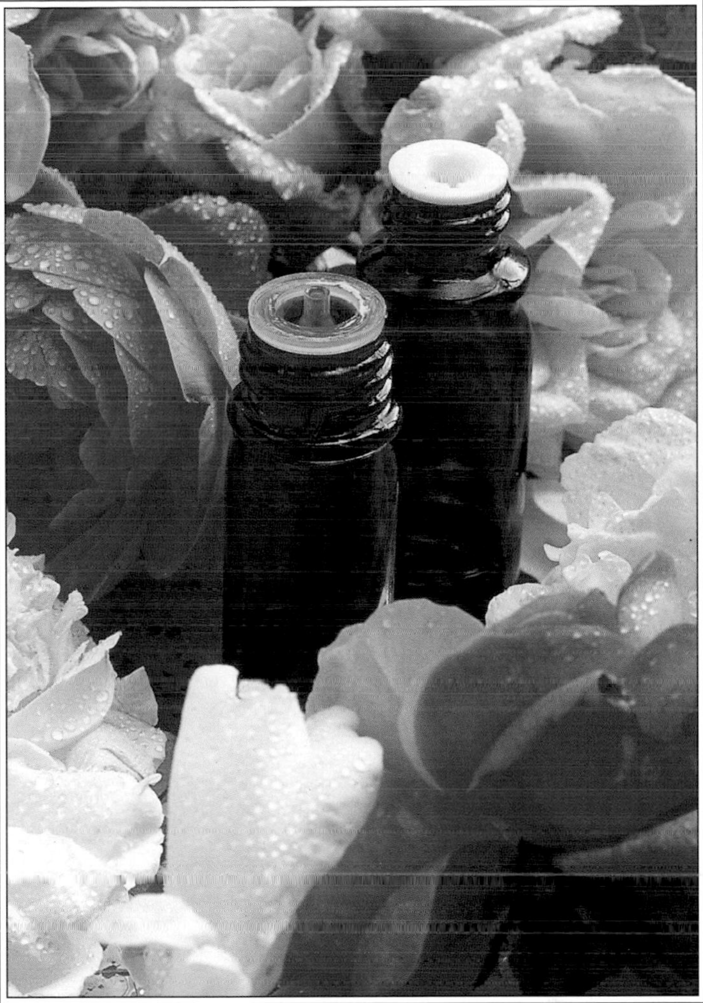

Above: Essential oils are highly concentrated; it can take 5,000 roses to produce just one teaspoonful of oil.

World Wars, essential oils were used to treat wounds and infections, and one of the pioneers of this work was Dr Jean Valnet, who published his findings in the late 1960s. Respected medical establishments in France are now looking at the medicinal aspects of essential oils.

It should not be forgotten, however, that the power of aromatic plants extends beyond antiseptic or anti inflammatory properties. It is well established that scent can evoke memories, change people's moods and make them feel good. Aromatherapy has developed in the UK, the US and many other countries in the last 20 years into a holistic system that tries to heal and balance the whole person. The oils are often incorporated into massage, or used in baths, or simply evaporated into the air in a burner to improve physical and emotional well-being. These methods would all be familiar to the ancients, and show a continuing tradition of usage of aroma in therapy. There are also more aromatherapy practitioners than ever before offering complete treatments.

OILS AND PREVENTION

Many of the beauty and cosmetic products now on the market contain essential oils, their popularity stemming both from their wonderful fragrance and the widespread interest in using as many natural ingredients as possible. Aromatic essential oils can also be used in a number of ways to maintain good health and prevent ailments; it should always be remembered, however, that self-help is not a substitute for seeking professional treatment for an illness or condition. Furthermore, the pure essential oils themselves are highly concentrated and should be treated with respect. For instance, it may have taken 5,000 roses to produce a teaspoonful of essential oil of rose!

A useful guideline when using essential oils at home – for instance, in the bath – is the 1–2 rule. Use only one or two oils together at any time; use one or two drops in the bath; and do not use any particular oil on a daily basis for more than one or at most two weeks.

Some essential oils have a stimulating effect on the uterine muscles and should therefore not be used if you are pregnant, or suspect you might be. The possibly problematic oils to be avoided during your pregnancy include basil, clary sage, fennel, hyssop, juniper, pennyroyal, peppermint, sage and thyme. Equally, if you ever get any skin irritation or allergic reaction to any oil, then you should of course stop using it. Many of these herbs are used in cooking and are quite safe for pregnant women in this form.

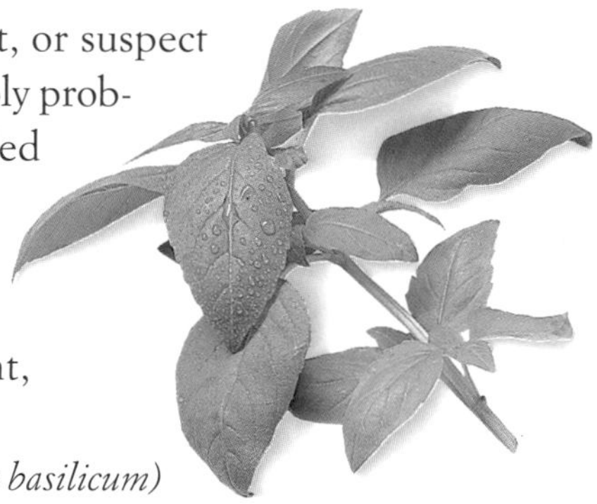

Basil (Ocimum basilicum)

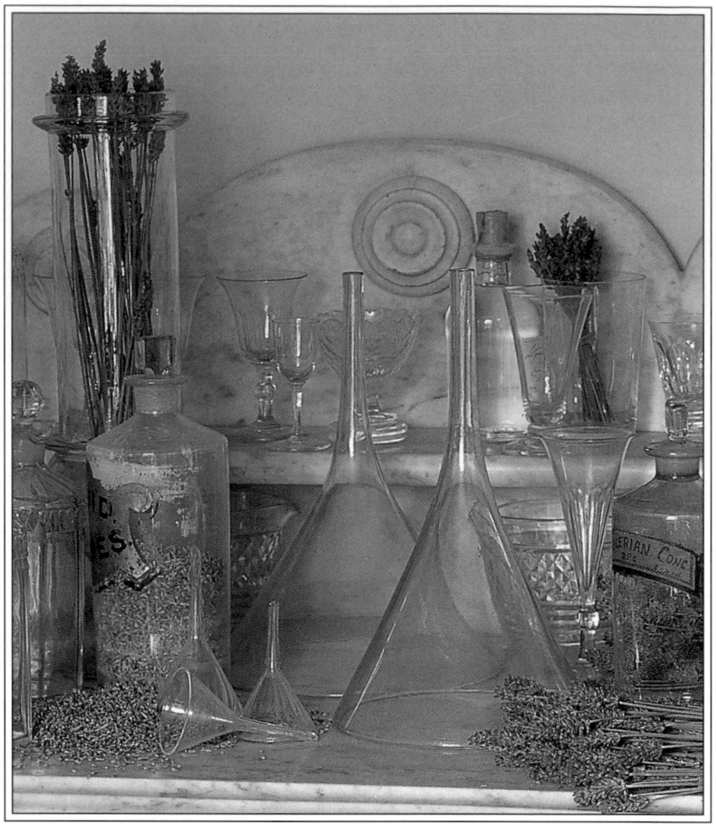

Above: Lavender is one of the most loved and well-known essential oils and has been distilled for centuries.

Essential Therapies

Aromatherapy Oil	Properties and Benefits
Lavender	Antiseptic, anti-depressant, healing; relieves stress and insomnia, soothes insect bites.
Rose	Anti-depressant, aphrodisiac, tonic; helpful for menstrual disorders; aids sleep.
Bergamot	Antiseptic, astringent, stimulative; helps to combat oily skin but can sensitize it to UV light.
Sandalwood	Healing, antiseptic; can relieve fluid retention, cystitis and insomnia.
Patchouli	Healing, soothing; helps combat dandruff and dry skin patches.
Ylang Ylang	Antiseptic, aphrodisiac, tonic.
Myrrh	Healing, antiseptic, calming; eases viral and fungal infections such as thrush (if added to a bath).
Juniper	Diuretic, antiseptic, cleansing, calming; avoid in first five months of pregnancy, not to be used by those with kidney disease.
Neroli	Calming; soothes nerves and upset stomachs; a good remedy for dry skin.
Chamomile, Roman	The most soothing oil; relieves anxiety, stress, allergies, and Pre-menstrual syndrome (PMS).
Basil	Reviving, decongestive.
Rosemary	Antiseptic, stimulating, balancing, diuretic, uplifting; not to be used in the first five months of pregnancy, or by those with high blood pressure.
Frankincense	Decongestive, relaxing; aids sleep.

OILS IN THE AIR

A widely used method of employing essential oils in the home is to fragrance the rooms by means of a vaporizer, or oil burner. Vaporizers are widely available, and range from the simple utilitarian version to the highly decorative, hand-crafted piece. Although they come in many forms, they all work on the same principle. The reservoir, or receptacle, is filled with water, to which are added drops of essential oil. The reservoir is then heated, causing the water to evaporate and the warm oil to release its perfume.

Choosing and Using a Vaporizer

When choosing a vaporizer there are two important points to consider. First, there should be a suitable distance between the source of the heat and the reservoir for oil and water. This will reduce the risk of completely evaporating the water and therefore burning the oil. Second, the vaporizer should be easy to clean, ready for use with a different oil.

The simplest type of vaporizer makes use of a candle as the heat source; a more efficient, but more expensive, type is the electric vaporizer. Under certain circumstances these are preferable to the type heated by a candle – for example in the reception area of an office, in a hospital ward, or at home, when you want to disperse oils for a long period of time without the necessity of frequent supervision. Some electric vaporizers have a silent fan that disperses the evaporating oils; others employ a heated ceramic dish. Either would be suitable for a child's bedroom, or a room occupied by someone who is bedridden.

Whenever you use a vaporizer of any kind, do make certain that you place the burner in a safe position, out of the reach of children and pets.

The number of drops of oil used in a burner depends on the size of the room: two to three drops for a small room, and as many as six to ten for a larger one. It is better to use fewer drops and refresh the burner more frequently, rather than use too many and saturate a room with scent. Remember too that your sensitivity to the scent will decrease, but this does not mean that the aroma is not still present and probably still quite strong.

If you do not have a vaporizer, or you feel the need for an instant aromatherapy treatment, try applying just a few drops of oil to a handkerchief or paper towel and gently inhaling the perfume. Placing the handkerchief on your pillow at night should ease breathing if you have a blocked nose; some oils will help promote a good night's sleep. It is not wise to take essential oils as a medicine except on the advice of a practitioner, but some people do use essential oils in tea, adding two or three drops of a suitable oil to a pot of black tea for digestive problems, urinary problems or stress.

These are just some of the ways in which aromatherapy can be used as a preventive healthcare system in the home. In general, start with just a few oils, find out about their properties and uses, and go from there. One of the best things about aromatherapy is the pleasure to be derived from the aromas; keeping healthy can be enjoyable and fun.

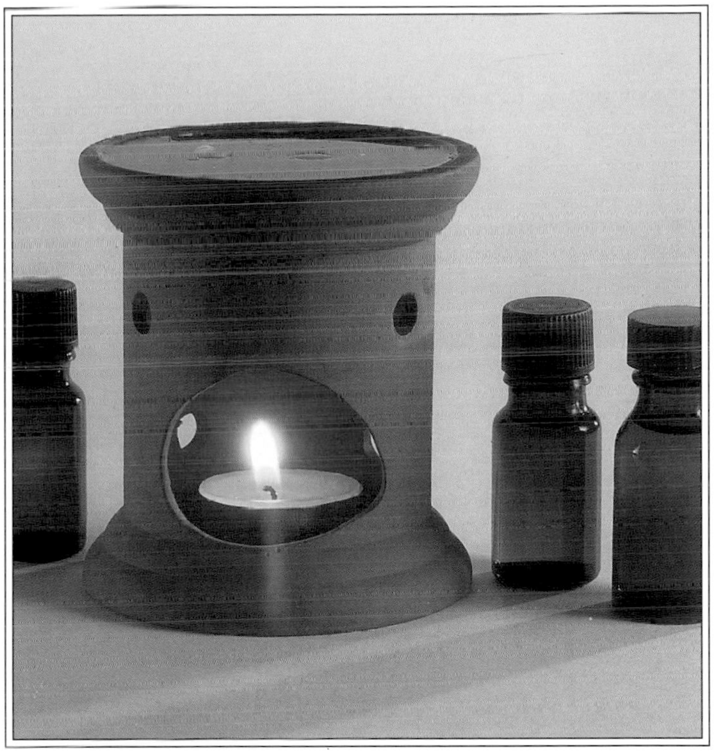

Above: A terracotta vaporizer makes a lovely, warm, friendly glow as it burns and is as much a pleasure to look at as to smell.

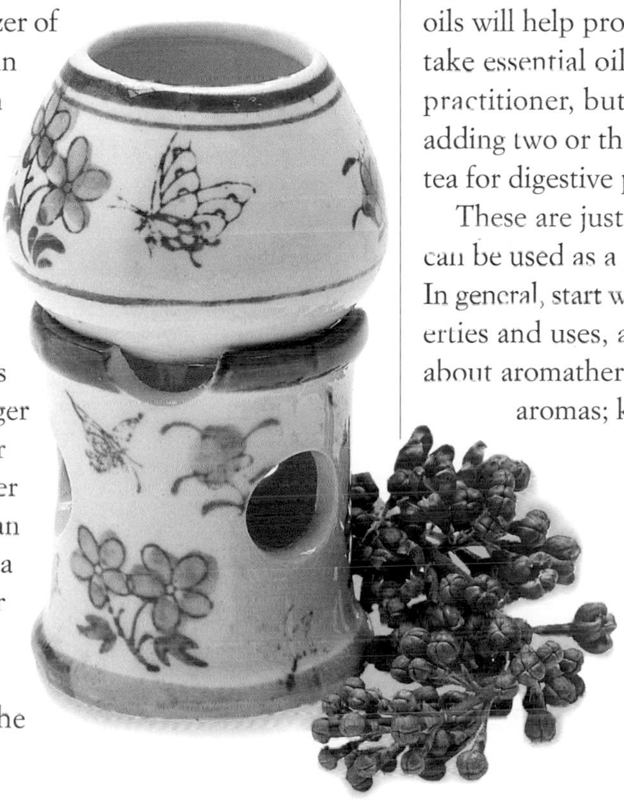

Left: A porcelain vaporizer; do not leave these burning unattended.

OIL IN WATER

One of the most pleasant ways of using aromatic oils is to put one or two drops into a bath just before you get in; they form a thin film over the surface of the water, which coats and penetrates the skin while you lie in the heady aroma. If you have very dry skin, try adding a couple of drops of your chosen essential oil to a teaspoonful of pure vegetable oil, such as sweet almond, and pour this into the bath.

To help ward off the effects of the cold in winter, try using oils that have a warming effect on the circulation, such as black pepper, ginger, marjoram or rosemary. These are especially good in the morning, to stimulate the whole system. Respiratory infections can be another problem of colder months, and using essential oils through the winter months can help to build resistance to colds, coughs and so on. Oils to consider here are benzoin, eucalyptus, frankincense, lavender, pine, tea-tree and thyme, as well as the circulatory stimulants mentioned above.

After the winter, many people can feel rather sluggish and perhaps be overweight. This can be a good time to use refreshing essential oils that also help to aid digestion. Among others, choose from fennel, geranium, grapefruit, lemon, mandarin and orange – most of these are citrus oils, which have an uplifting, stimulating quality.

On the emotional level, several essences have quite remarkable effects in helping to keep our moods in balance. The best anti-depressant oil is undoubtedly bergamot, and this can be used to ward off low vitality at times of stress and depression. A note of caution though – bergamot increases sensitivity to the sun, so do not overuse before exposure to bright sunlight.

Other mood-elevators are neroli (or orange blossom), jasmine, melissa and rose. All of these particular oils are very expensive to produce, and this in itself gives a feeling of luxurious pampering when using them.

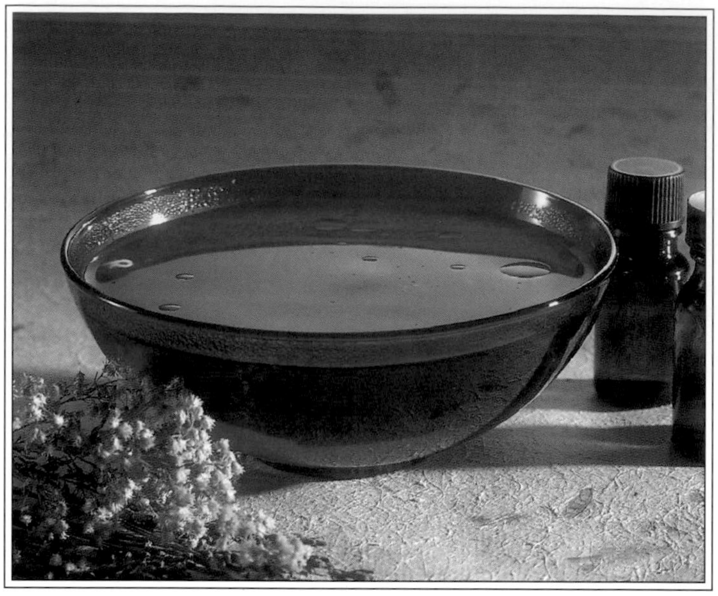

ABOVE: Essential oils have an ancient link with water and have been used since classical times as part of a bathing ritual.

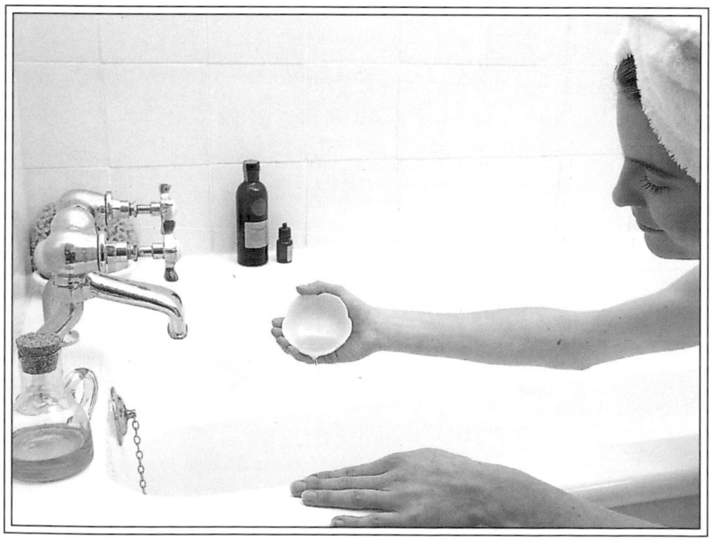

ABOVE: Add some pure vegetable oil and one to two drops of essential oil for a relaxing, steaming bath.

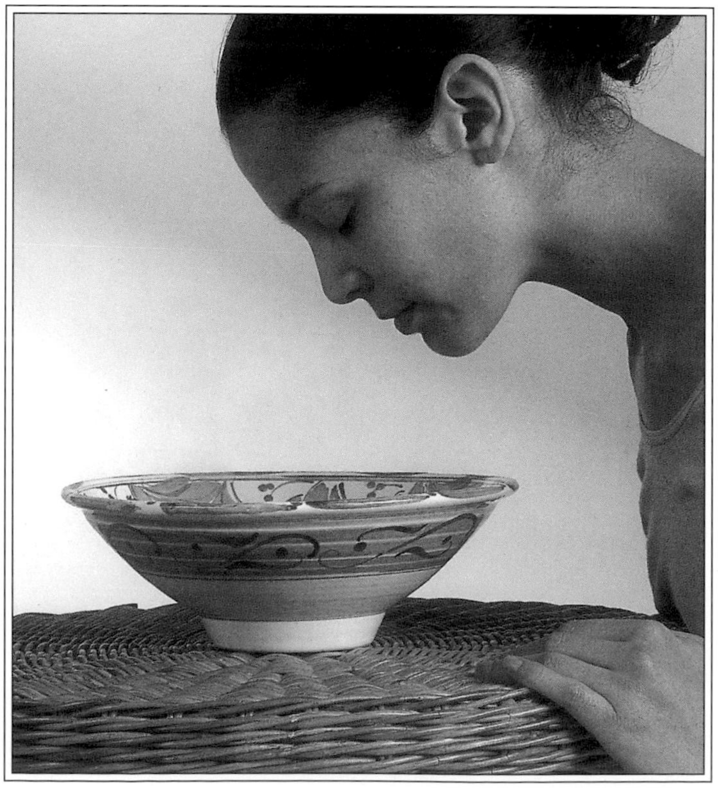

RIGHT: For a steam inhalation place ten drops of oil and a cup of hot water in a bowl. Inhale deeply through your nose.

OILS IN MASSAGE

For direct use on the skin, essential oils must be diluted. Use a good, pure vegetable oil as the base, such as coconut, apricot kernel, jojoba (actually a liquid wax) or sweet almond. If your skin tends to be very dry, add about ten per cent of avocado or wheatgerm oil to the blend – avoid the latter if you are allergic to wheat. The essential oils are added at one or two per cent; assuming 20 drops to 1ml, this means using one or two drops per 5ml (1 tsp) of base oil.

All the above suggestions for bath oils apply equally to aromatherapy massage. Another area of use is in skincare itself. Some essential oils have a balancing, healing effect on the skin; frankincense, lavender, neroli, rose and sandalwood in particular can all be massaged into the skin regularly. It may be easier to mix them, at the same dilution, into your favourite skin cream; make up small amounts at a time, and vary them after a while.

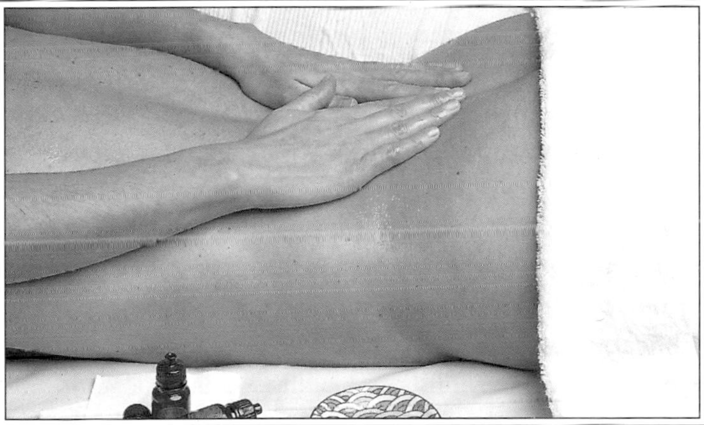

Diluting Oil for Massage

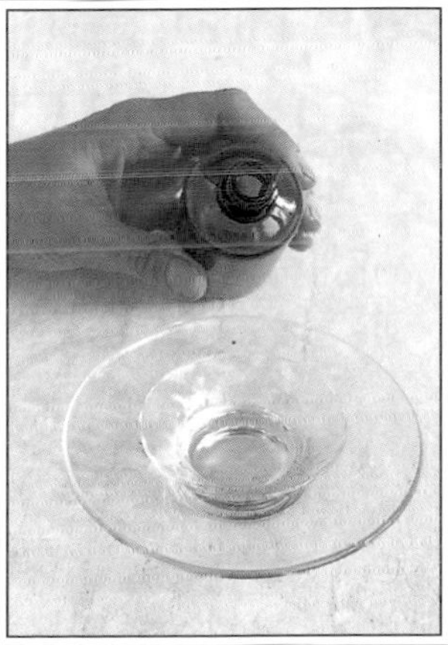

1 Pour the equivalent of two teaspoonsfuls of pure vegetable oil into a bowl.

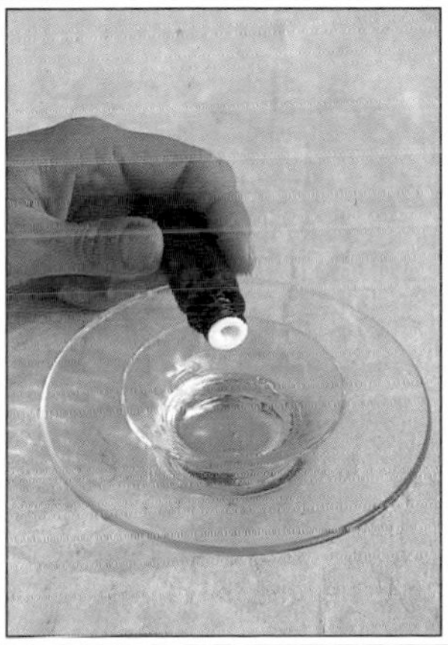

2 Very carefully add one or two drops of essential oil and mix together.

Sports Blends

The oils listed below are grouped according to their usefulness before and after sporting activities.

Before

- For stimulation: juniper, eucalyptus and rosemary.
- For supple, toned muscles: black pepper, ginger, rosemary, lavender, cypress, juniper, peppermint, grapefruit, orange.
- To aid a good strong respiratory system for aerobics: eucalyptus, peppermint, rosemary, geranium.
- To aid mental preparation before a competition: a blend of rosemary, lemon, lavender, chamomile.
- To promote good circulation: rose and palmarosa.

After

- To soothe and prevent aching muscles: eucalyptus, ginger and peppermint.
- To eliminate stress following a competition: lemon, nutmeg, clary sage, orange.

Left: Massaging with essential oils is a good way to appreciate their benefits.

Below: Remember to bring the oil to room temperature before you use it, to help release its precious aroma.

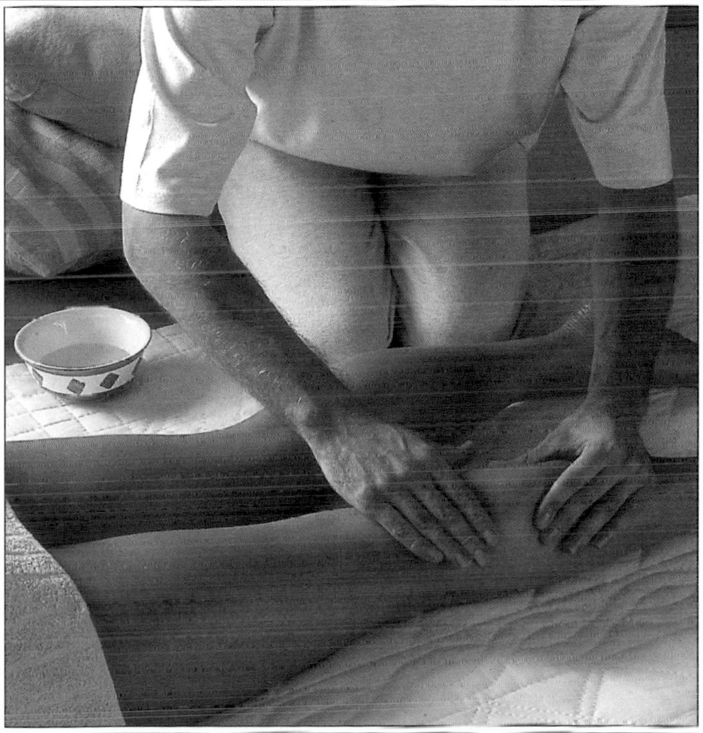

NATUROPATHY

This section is intended to cover those areas of self-help and professional therapies that do not fit into the other categories of this book. More than that, however, they comprise those approaches that focus on our natural healing abilities and try simply to enhance them. Iridology has been included here since it aims to diagnose imbalances by "reading" our own natural body signs, and treatment is often along naturopathic lines.

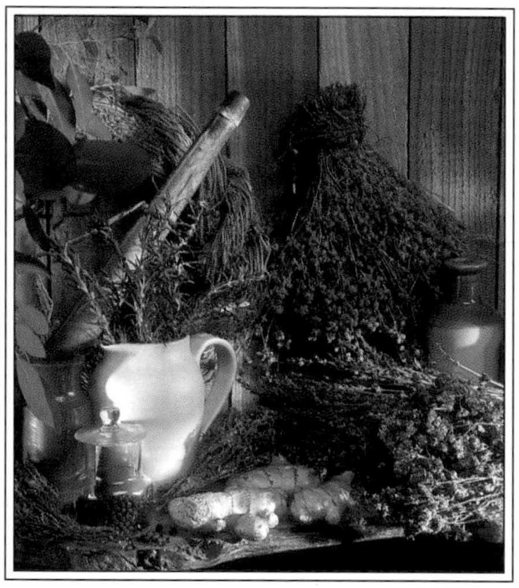

Naturopathy is itself a professional therapy, including diet, exercise, supplements and hydrotherapy within its field. Some traditions of naturopathic training also link with some of the hands-on professions such as osteopathy or chiropractic, and the practitioners of these latter disciplines may advocate other measures to help to restore full health. Hydrotherapy, or "water cure", has a strong tradition in Northern Europe, and is still carried out at centres in Germany, Austria, Switzerland and France. Increasingly it is also becoming more widespread in the US.

Both diet and exercise are vital elements in achieving and maintaining optimal health, and most of us can make adjustments in these areas. Some ideas for improvement are presented here; a key factor is to include exercises and dietary changes that you will enjoy, as a part of really appreciating life.

ABOVE: A selection of natural herbs and plants.

OPPOSITE: A balanced diet gives us a secure foundation for good health and vitality.

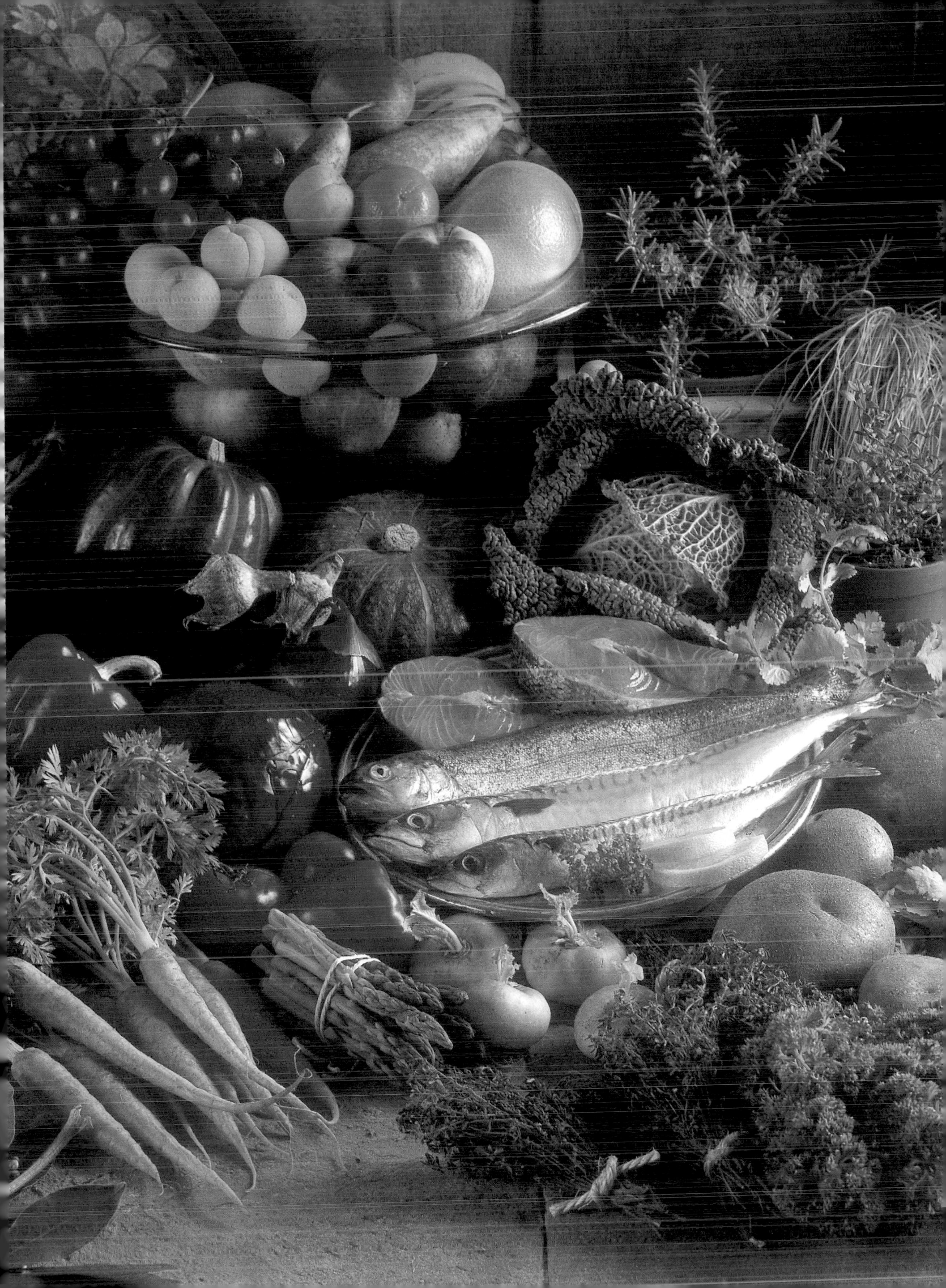

CARBOHYDRATES

Carbohydrates are our main source of energy, and need really to form the major bulk of our diet. They are broken down in the body into glucose, and used immediately for energy or else converted into glycogen for short-term storage in the liver. An excess of carbohydrates over time will be changed and stored as fat. This is a particular danger with refined carbohydrates or sugars, which do not take much processing in the body and provide large amounts of instant energy. Since they have less starchy bulk, refined carbohydrates do not make you as full, and therefore it is easier to eat too much of them, leading to fat storage and obesity.

The main sources of unrefined carbohydrates, providing dietary fibre and trace elements, are flour and grains, beans, peas and lentils, and potatoes. With grains, this is especially true when they are unprocessed, like wholegrain bread, whole oat cereals, muesli, wholewheat pasta, brown rice and so on which supply long-term energy supplies. For more immediate energy, fresh fruit, dried fruit or vegetables such as carrots or beetroot are high in fructose, or fruit sugar. This is easily broken down by the body for energy use, and since fructose metabolism does not require insulin, it can be an essential energy resource for diabetics.

There is almost complete accord among official governmental nutrition advisers and natural dietary therapists, that carbohydrates should be the chief element in our diet. In practical terms that means eating plenty of fresh vegetables and fruit, grains of all kinds (unless there are specific reasons for avoiding a particular grain, such as with a wheat allergy), potatoes, beans and lentils. A recent piece of advice from official organizations, for instance, has been to consume five portions of fruit or vegetables a day.

BELOW: Eat plenty of bread, wholemeal or granary if possible.

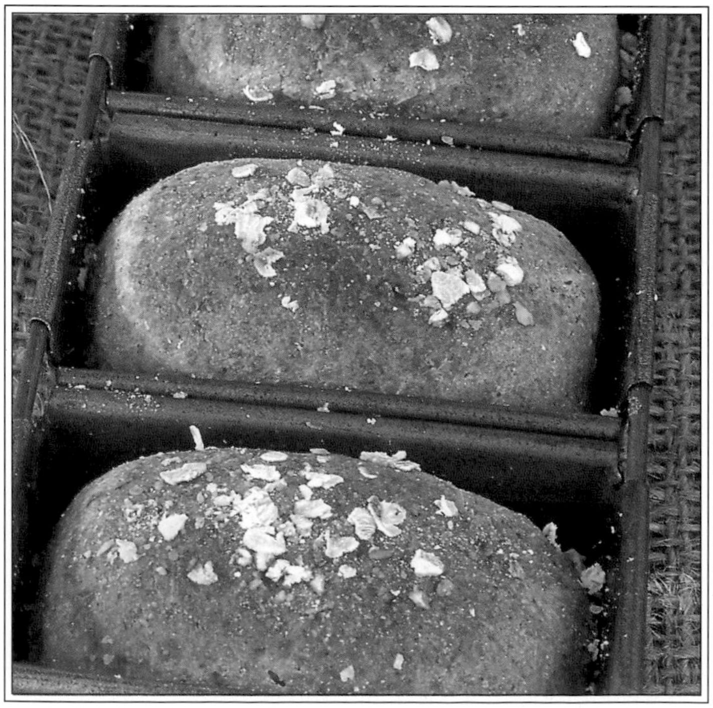

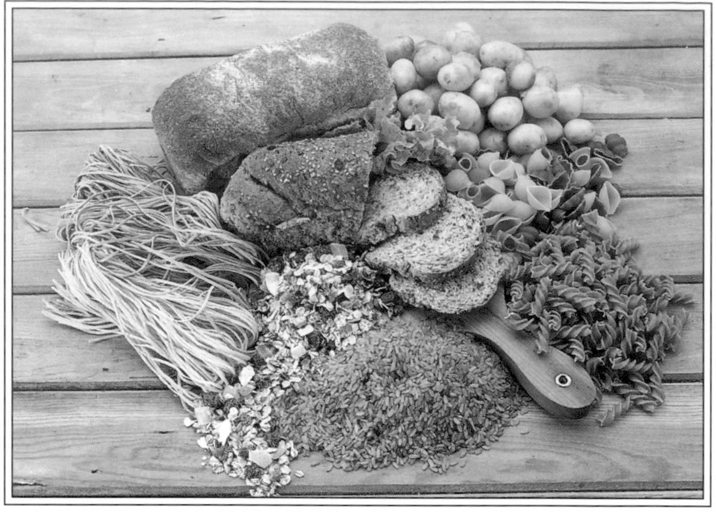

ABOVE: Bread, rice and pasta are important for the carbohydrates which give us vital energy.

FIBRE FACTS

Fibre is important to a healthy diet. Your body cannot digest it, so, in rather basic terms, it goes in and comes out, taking other waste with it. Fibrous foods include bread, rice, cereals, vegetables, fruit, and nuts. We should aim for about 30g (just over 1oz) of fibre a day. These are some examples of good fibre sources.

GOOD SOURCES	AVERAGE PORTION	GRAMS OF FIBRE
wholemeal pasta	75g/3oz (uncooked)	9
baked beans	125g/4oz	8
frozen peas	75g/3oz	8
bran flakes	50g/2oz	7
muesli	50g/2oz	4–5
raspberries	100g/3½oz	6
blackberries	100g/3½oz	6
banana	average fruit	3.5
baked jacket potato	150g/5oz	3.5
brown rice	50g/2oz	3
cabbage	100g/3½oz	3
red kidney beans	40g/1½oz	3
wholemeal bread	1 large slice	3
high-fibre white bread	1 large slice	2
stewed prunes	6 fruit	2

PROTEINS

Proteins are the essential body-builders, helping us to create muscles, bones, tendons, hair, skin and nails. They are also vital in most of our hormone and enzyme production. The first thing to say about protein is that in most developed countries people eat too much, so the problem is not so much increasing those foods that are high in protein but getting the balance right. An excess of high protein foods in the diet will be converted into glucose for energy use or else stored as fat.

Foods rich in protein include meat, fish, poultry, eggs, milk and other dairy products, nuts and seeds, beans and lentils, and grains (bread has a little under ten per cent protein). Human protein is made from a number of simple substances called amino-acids, and these need to be present in certain amounts or combinations in the protein in our diet for us to make use of them. Animal sources do contain the right amounts of these amino-acids, but also contain relatively high levels of fat. Plant sources of proteins often need to be combined in order to give adequate levels of amino-acids; this can be something as simple as beans on toast, or a spicy bean dish with rice, and generally means having a more varied, or even a more adventurous diet.

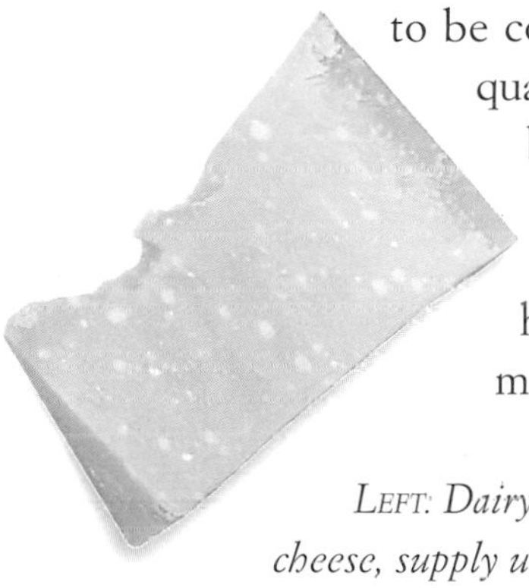

Left: Dairy products, such as milk, butter and cheese, supply us with not only protein but also fat.

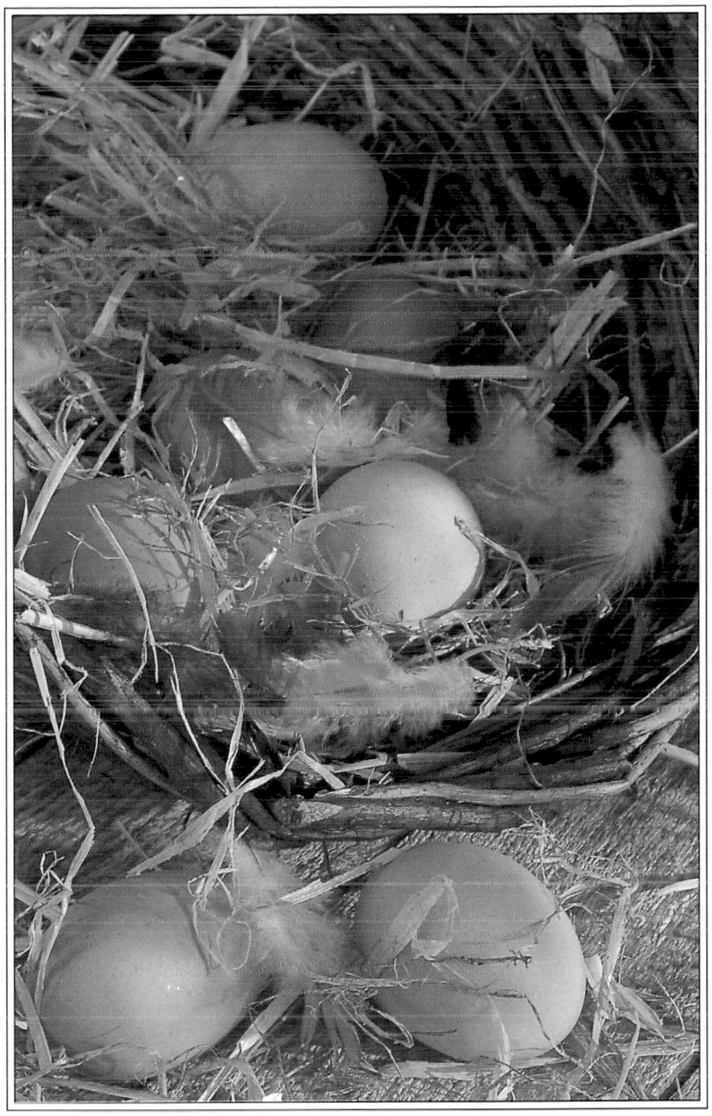

Above: Eggs are an important source of vitamins and protein but you should not eat more than two to three a week.

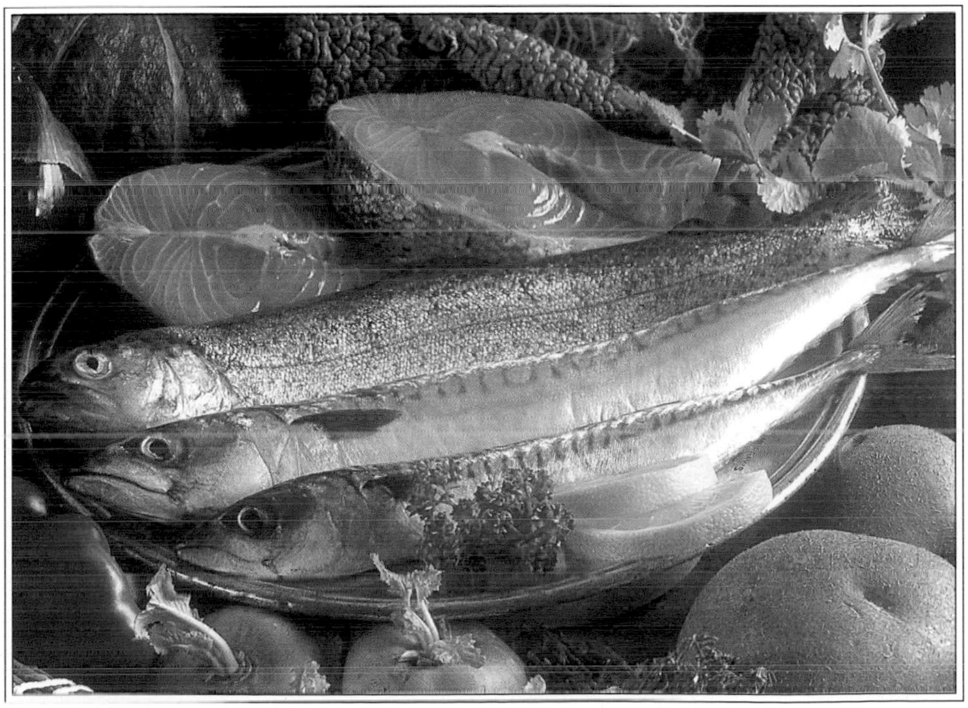

Left: One of the best sources of protein, fish is high in vitamins and minerals and is highly recommended by nutritionists.

Below: Eat unsalted nuts for their protein.

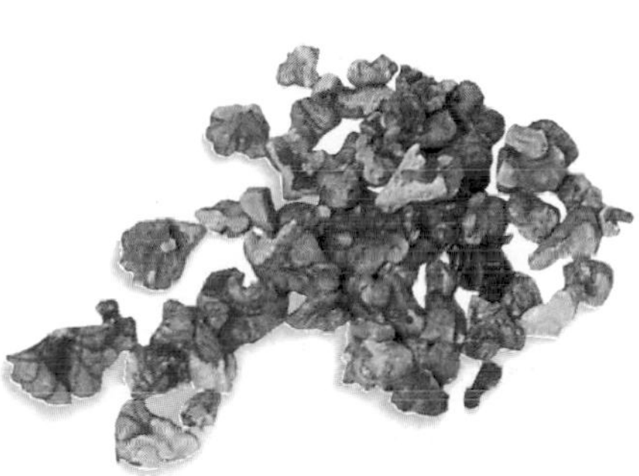

FATS

Fats are vital too, helping to form part of the cell structure and maintaining our inner organs and nerves. They also act to provide insulation and temperature regulation. It is, however, well-recognized that in the developed world much of our diet is too rich in fats, especially animal fats, and this is a major factor in heart disease, obesity and even some cancers, especially when we have such sedentary lives. Growing children, however, especially active ones, do need fats more than adults, and we should not reduce their intake so much.

Advice on fat-containing foods tends to be what to reduce rather than what to increase. Meat and dairy products can contain concentrated sources – a nice, juicy steak may have 30 per cent fat, for example. There are some differences between the effects of saturated fats (from animal products) and unsaturated fats such as are found in oily fish like salmon or plant oils like sunflower products. In general terms, move the emphasis towards the latter, using oils such as olive, sunflower, corn or safflower with salads or in cooking, but most people need to reduce all kinds of fats; they are the most concentrated sources of energy and anything over small amounts easily leads to obesity. There are plenty of reduced-fat items, particularly dairy products, which are now available and which can help in controlling fat intake.

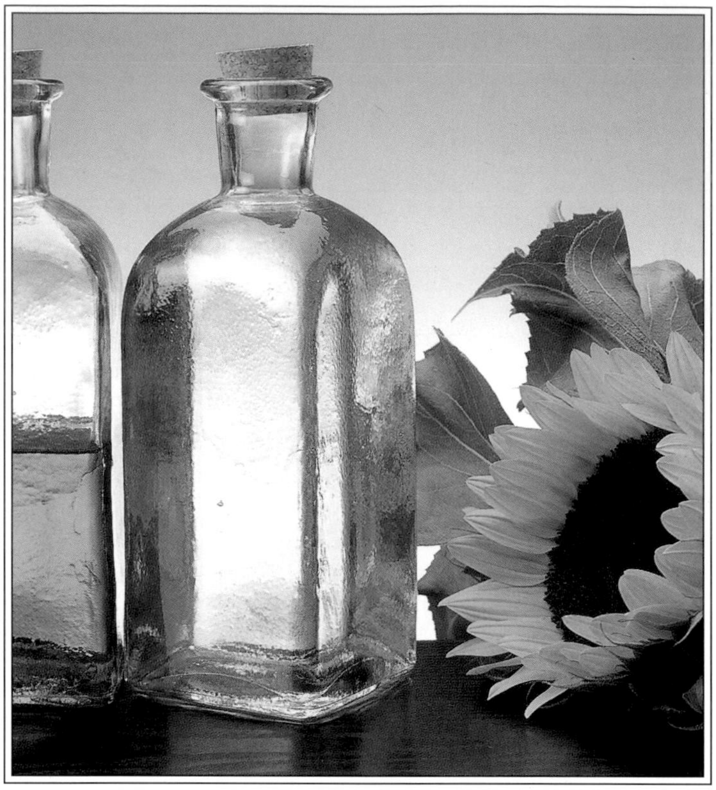

ABOVE: Oil made from the seeds of sunflowers is an unsaturated fat which should be used instead of animal fats in cooking. Avoid frying foods, however, and grill or steam instead.

EASY WAYS TO CUT DOWN FAT AND SATURATED FAT

EAT LESS	INSTEAD
Butter and hard fats.	Spread butter more thinly, or replace it with a low fat spread or polyunsaturated margarine.
Fatty meats and high fat products such as pies and sausages.	Buy the leanest cuts of meat you can afford and choose low fat meats like skinless chicken or turkey. Look for reduced-fat sausages and meat products. Eat fish more often, especially oily fish.
Full-fat dairy products like cream, butter, hard margarine, milk and hard cheeses.	Choose skimmed or semi-skimmed milk and milk products and try low-fat yogurt, low-fat fromage frais and lower fat cheeses such as skimmed milk soft cheese, reduced-fat Cheddar, mozzarella or Brie.
Hard cooking fats such as lard or hard margarine.	Choose mono-unsaturated or polyunsaturated oils for cooking, such as olive, sunflower, corn or soya oil.
Rich salad dressings like mayonnaise or salad cream.	Make salad dressings with low-fat yogurt or fromage frais, or use a healthy oil such as olive oil.
Fried foods.	Grill, microwave, steam or bake when possible. Roast meats on a rack. Fill up on starchy foods like pasta, rice and couscous. Choose jacket or boiled potatoes, not chips.
Added fat in cooking.	Use heavy-based or non-stick pans so you can cook with little or no added fat.
High-fat snacks such as crisps, chocolate, cakes, pastries and biscuits.	Choose fresh or dried fruit, breadsticks or vegetable sticks. Make your own low-fat cakes and bakes.

VITAMINS AND MINERALS

Vitamins and minerals are needed for proper growth and development and body maintenance. They control the absorption of other nutrients and without them a series of complaints can develop, from headaches to sterility. There are 13 major vitamins which, apart from K and D, must be obtained from the food we eat. The fresher the food the higher its vitamin content. Food loses its vitamins through cooking, exposure to light or cold and storage, so buy small quantities of fresh food and eat it as soon as possible.

RIGHT: Supplements are an important source of vitamins but do not rely on them for all your requirements.

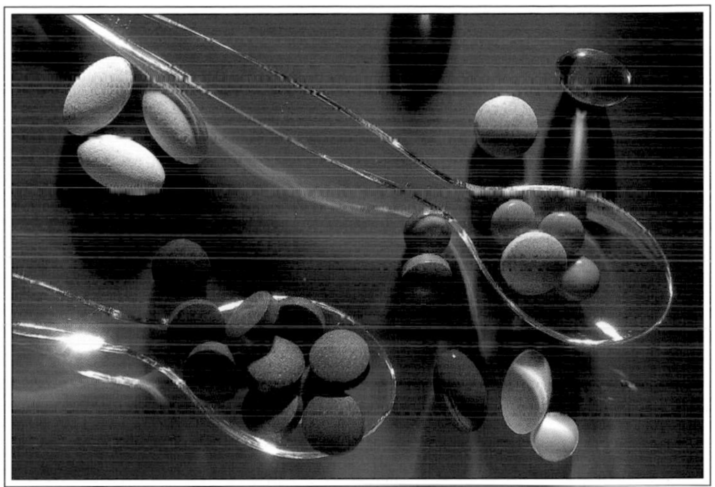

Mineral and Vitamin Values

Vitamin	Sources Include	Benefits
Vitamin A	Liver (especially fish livers), egg yolk, fortified margarine, oily fish, oranges, apricots, carrots, tomatoes, melons, dark green leafy vegetables.	Eyesight; skin; may protect against cancer.
Vitamin B1	Most foods – including wheatgerm and pulses, wholegrains, brewer's yeast, nuts, fortified breakfast cereals.	Helps break down carbohydrates; nervous system;
Vitamin B2	Brewer's yeast, liver, kidney, dairy produce, wheat bran, wheatgerm, eggs.	repairs body tissues.
Vitamin B3	Wheatgerm, wholegrain cereals, meat, fish	Essential for tissue chemical reactions.
Vitamin B6	Avocados, liver, wholegrains, egg yolk, lean meat, bananas, fish, potatoes.	Nervous system; skin; red blood cells.
Vitamin B12	Liver, kidney, some fish (including shellfish), eggs, milk.	Healthy blood and nerves.
Vitamin C	Citrus fruits, potatoes, tomatoes, leafy greens.	Helps heal wounds, may fight colds, flu and infections; protects gums, keeps joints and ligaments in good working order.
Vitamin D	Fish liver oils, fatty fish, eggs, fortified margarine, also synthesized by ultraviolet light.	Calcium deposits in bones.
Vitamin E	Vegetable oils, some vegetables, wheatgerm.	Cell growth; antioxidant.
Vitamin K	Most vegetables – especially leafy green ones, liver.	Essential in production of some proteins.
Mineral	**Sources Include**	**Essential for**
Calcium	Cheese, milk, yogurt, eggs, bread, nuts, pulses, fish with soft bones such as whitebait and tinned sardines, leafy green vegetables.	Healthy bones, teeth and nails; muscle and nerve function; blood clotting; milk production in nursing mothers.
Iron	Liver, red meat, oily fish, wholegrain cereals, leafy green vegetables.	Makes haemoglobin, the pigment in red bloods cells that helps transport oxygen around the body.

MOVE TO KEEP ALIVE

As far as exercise is concerned, the best phrase to sum up the importance of movement to your body and health is, "Use it or lose it". Inactivity, a sedentary lifestyle, means that our bodies steadily deteriorate and various health problems start to develop. Equally importantly, exercise helps to reduce the effects of stress and worry, and makes us feel better. The value of exercise is high at all times of life, for children growing up and developing strong bones and muscles, for adults to keep fit, active and healthy, and for older people to reduce problems like osteoporosis and simply to keep mobile and independent.

This is another area where official encouragement has occurred in recent years, with suggestions of a minimum of 20 minutes of brisk exercise three times a week as one example. Having activity goals can be very useful, but they should not act as a deterrent to getting started; any amount of exercise is better than none. It must be said, of course, that sudden, unaccustomed or inappropriate exercise can cause musculoskeletal problems, and people with certain conditions may need to seek medical advice before undertaking exercise. Nevertheless, steadily increasing exercise is likely to benefit the great majority of us, improving the efficiency of our heart, lungs and muscles, improving our posture and making us feel fitter and look healthier.

BELOW: Exercise in the fresh air as much as you can with walks and cycle rides in the country.

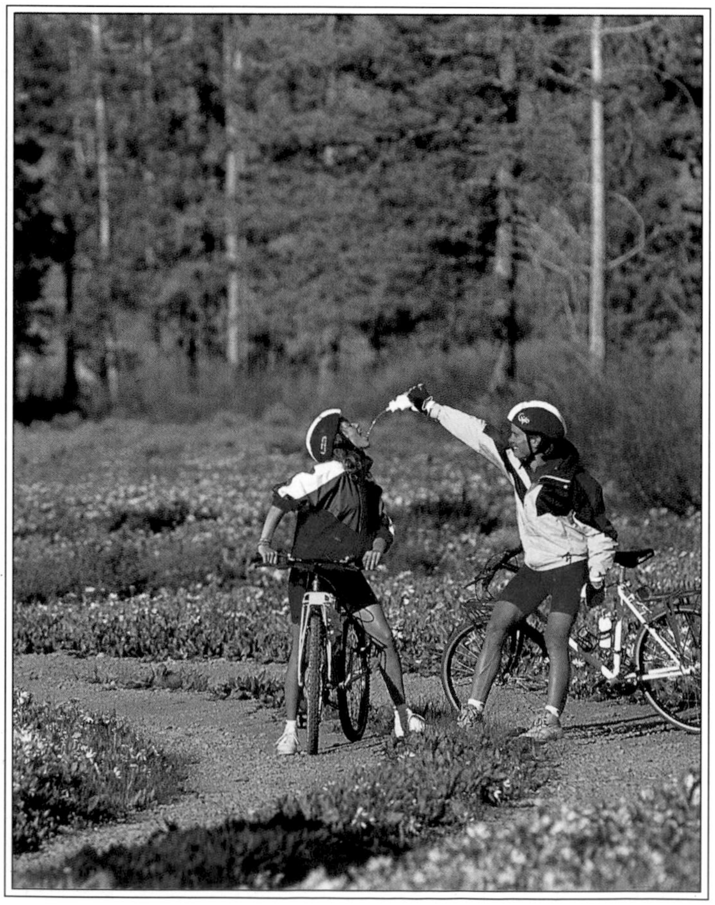

RIGHT: Take small amounts of regular exercise.

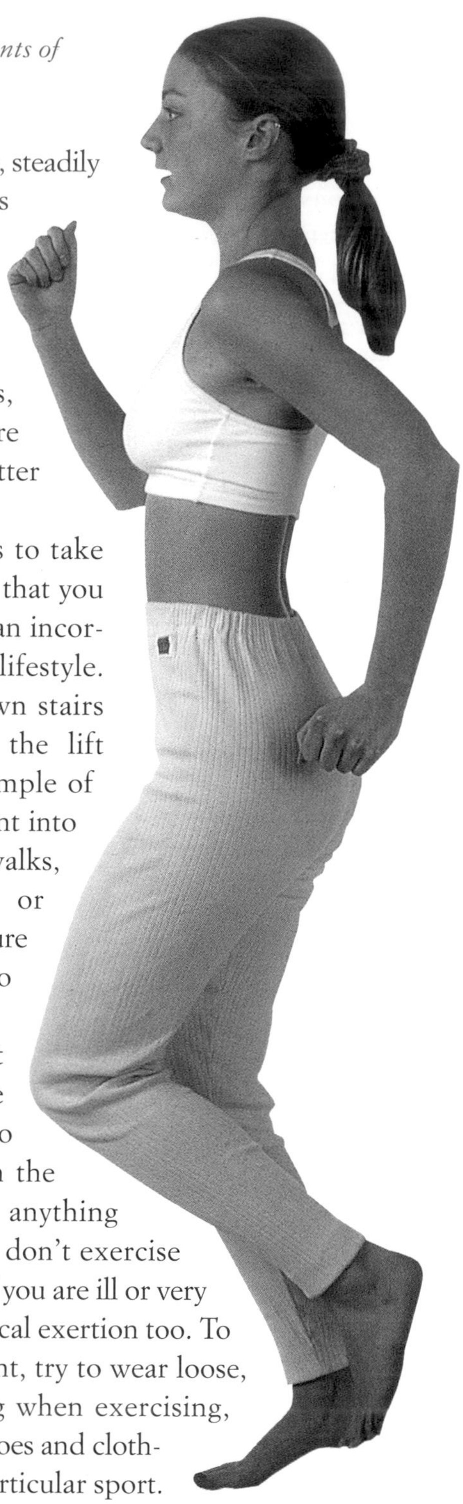

The first advice is to take the kinds of exercise that you enjoy and that you can incorporate into your lifestyle. Walking up and down stairs rather than taking the lift can be a simple example of fitting more movement into your life. Weekend walks, gardening, cycling or dancing are some leisure activities that can also help you to get fitter.

If you have not done much exercise for some time, do try to warm up and loosen the body before doing anything more strenuous, and don't exercise straight after meals. If you are ill or very tired, then limit physical exertion too. To allow easier movement, try to wear loose, comfortable clothing when exercising, and use the correct shoes and clothing when playing a particular sport. A good idea may be to join a class; with exercise like aerobics, low-impact exercises or weight-training, a class is essential to make sure that you are doing the movements safely and correctly. Personal trainers can provide detailed exercise programmes for you, with advice on the training zone, or optimal heart-rate, that you should aim for. Serious exercisers have access nowadays to all kinds of scientific back-up on how to plan and carry out exercise, but for most people it is most important to get fun and enjoyment out of physical activity.

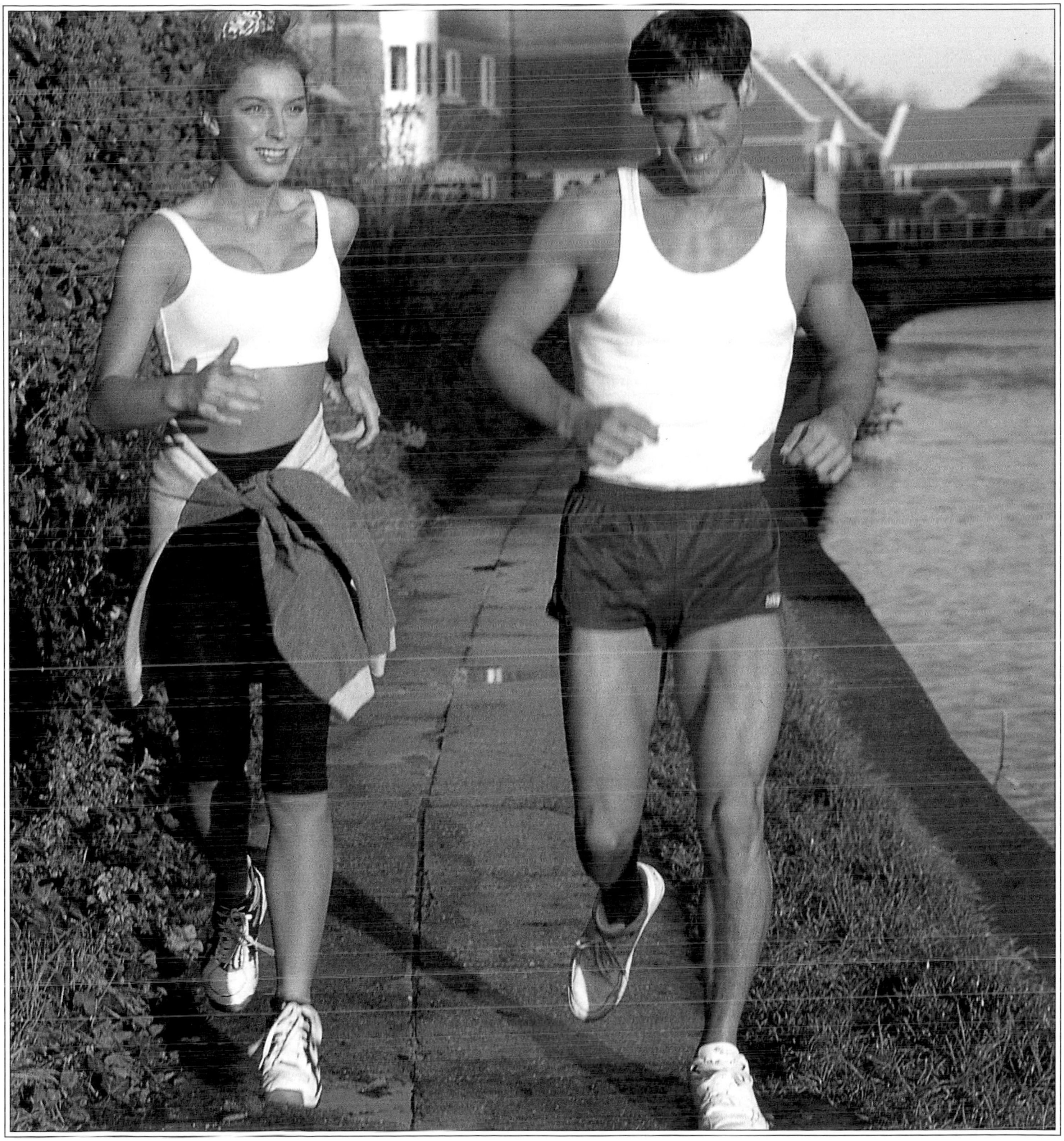

ABOVE: Exercising with friends adds encouragement and company.

Another important aspect of physical fitness is the effect it has on the way we feel about ourselves. Without becoming neurotic about your size and weight, try to take an interest in the state your body is in. An enjoyable and invigorating fitness regime, at a level you can sustain without undue stress, can enhance your mental and physical well-being. When you are unfit you tend to feel more lethargic and uninterested in the world and the people around you. A straight back, a spring in your walk and an alert, energetic expression will create a better impression than bad posture, slumped shoulders and uncoordinated movements. So improve your fitness and your self-esteem at the same time.

STRESS MANAGEMENT

It is probably fair to say that the greatest threat to our health today, at least in the developed countries, is having more stress than we are able to handle. The increasing pace of lifestyles, the complexity of many professions, not to mention changes and added strains in relationships due to greater mobility and thus distance from others, has placed considerable burdens on our stress-management systems.

Nearly all natural therapies place great importance on stress as a probable factor in ill-health, and yet people need a certain amount of stress in order to become motivated and develop; so what is the problem? Our internal stress-coping mechanisms originally developed to cope with potentially life-threatening situations, the so-called "fight or flight" adaptation. However, these biochemical changes are all too often brought into play by other factors nowadays, from meeting deadlines or work crises to receiving the latest bill. When the body is placed in an almost constant state of alert, the adrenal glands become tired eventually and people are depleted and panicky rather than stimulated and awake.

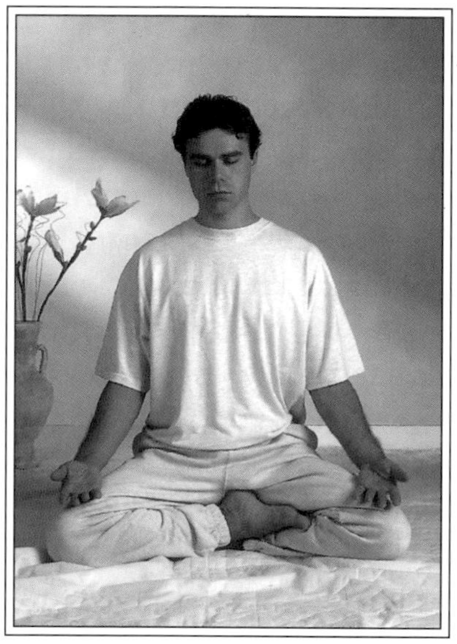

These problems have been recognized for a long time, and most natural therapies will offer some help with stress-related problems; in this section the focus is on some approaches which specialize in helping with stress-management directly.

ABOVE: Meditation is a well-known method for diffusing stress and tension.

OPPOSITE: Take time to relax and allow your body to rest during busy periods of life.

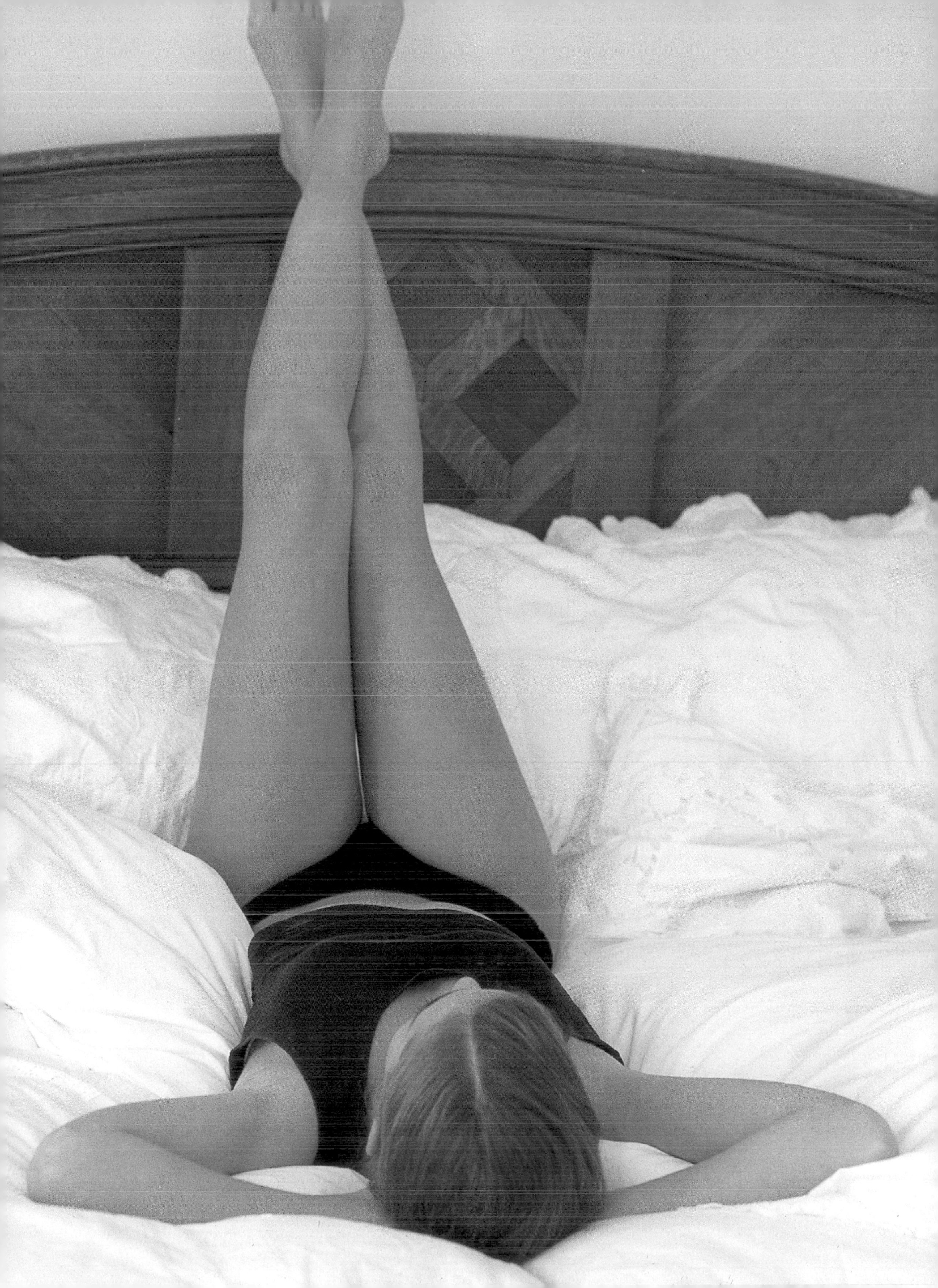

Hypnotherapy

A person in hypnosis is not "asleep"; indeed they are often more aware of what is taking place than normal. Anybody (with a very few exceptions) can enter this deeply relaxed state, and indeed will, naturally.

It is believed that the state of hypnosis was used in ancient Egypt, South East Asia, and the Pacific island cultures. The hypnotic state is described in Greek and Roman writings too. The advent of Christianity appears to have marked the decline in its use, as it was then classed as witchcraft. It was, strangely enough, a Roman Catholic priest, Father Gassner, who in the late 1700s renewed public interest by using hypnotic inductions as a means of "casting out devils". Around the same time Anton Mesmer began to theorize about "animal magnetism", and the use of this phenomenon for medical purposes. He believed that Gassner was magnetizing his clients with the metal crucifix which he held. Mesmer attracted a lot of attention in France, and was later investigated by the French government and denounced as a fraud. It was left to James Braid to investigate further in 1841, and he is responsible for renaming mesmerism as hypnosis, from the Greek word *hypnos* meaning sleep, later trying to rename it mono-idealism, as he recognized it was not sleep but a concentration of the mind upon one channel of communication. But the words hypnosis and hypnotism had caught on, and change was impossible. Many more people after Braid developed theories about hypnosis and used it in the medical world. Perhaps the best-known exponent is a surgeon called Esdaile, who performed many serious operations painlessly using only hypnosis as an anaesthetic; some three hundred of these are carefully recorded. This method might well have continued had it not been for the discovery of chloroform and ether as chemical alternatives. It is interesting to note that hypnosis as anaesthetic is returning to popularity, especially in the US.

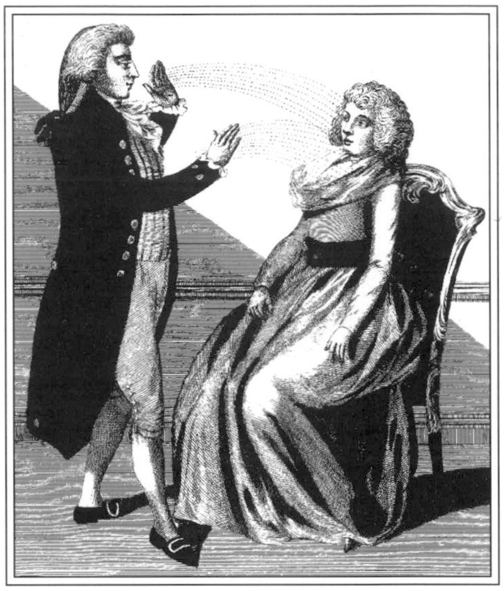

Above: Mesmerism: an operator and his patient from E. Sibly's A Key to Physic and the Occult Sciences, *London.*

What then is hypnosis? It is a state of deep relaxation, a state of heightened awareness, combined with a feeling of calm lethargy. It can be best described as similar to that state between sleep and wakefulness when you are aware of your surroundings but unwilling to move. Its characteristics are a heightened susceptibility to beneficial suggestion and a much improved memory with access to "forgotten" or repressed memories stored in the unconscious mind.

In itself, the hypnotic state is very pleasant, but nothing more than that. It is very similar to the mental states achieved during meditation and yoga. It is what the therapist and client do together within this state that makes it therapy.

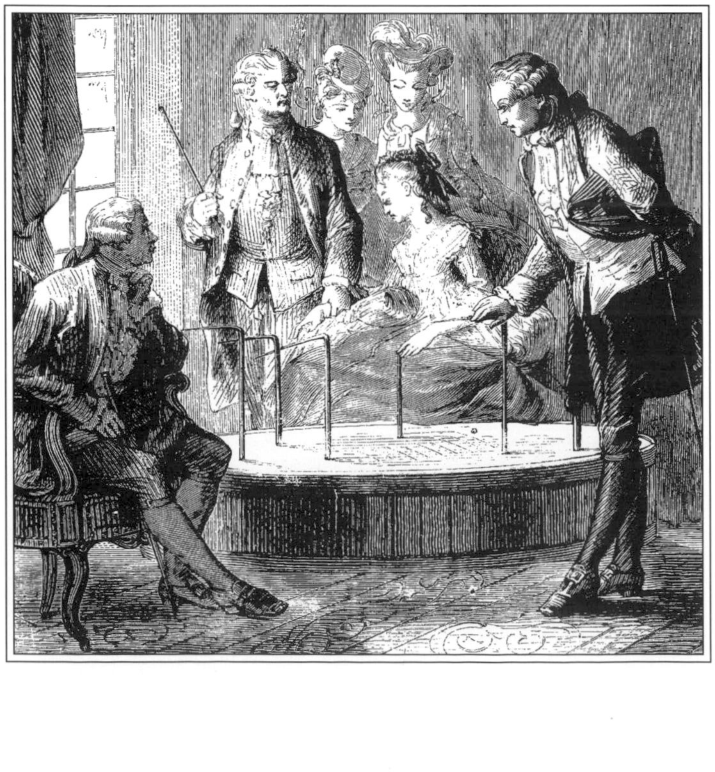

Left: Mesmer's tub at his consulting room in Paris which he opened soon after his treatise in 1779. The tub was a vat of dilute sulphuric acid and patients sat round it holding hands or holding on to one of the iron bars which projected from it.

SELF-HYPNOTIC INDUCTION

Self-hypnosis may not be suitable for anyone suffering from mental illness, or taking medication for a nervous condition. It is also potentially dangerous to use self-hypnosis to mask pain as this could lead to a serious illness going undetected. Ask your doctor's advice before using self-hypnosis in the above situations or if you have any doubts as to its suitability for you. It is also advisable to have one or more sessions with a properly qualified hypnotist to establish suitability and to receive instruction on how to use self-hypnosis.

Hypnosis as a natural state can be created in a number of ways, by audio, tactile or visual means. People can be shocked into hypnosis or coaxed or even bored into it. Self-hypnosis can be attained in many different ways too, but many therapists believe that by using the patterns outlined below, anyone can achieve a state of self-hypnosis. Initially, when learning these patterns, it may be useful to read them, slowly, on to a cassette tape, and then, preferably with headphones, use the tape to guide you into self-hypnosis. You may be reassured that should anything happen that requires your immediate attention, you will sit up straight away and deal with it as you would normally do: you are in control at all times. Non-intrusive music in the background can be helpful, too. Once you have learned to gain the state of hypnosis, you will be able to do so anywhere at any time that is useful to you.

STRESS MANAGEMENT

There follow three methods of self-hypnotic induction that can be highly beneficial to break a stressful day, to take five minutes to clear the mind before that important meeting, or just to unwind at the end of the day, so as to be clear thinking and able to enjoy the evening at leisure without carrying the worries of work into other areas of your life.

1 PHYSICAL RELAXATION

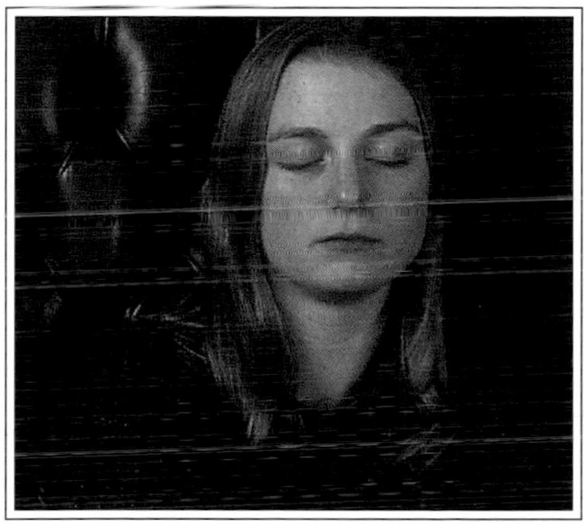

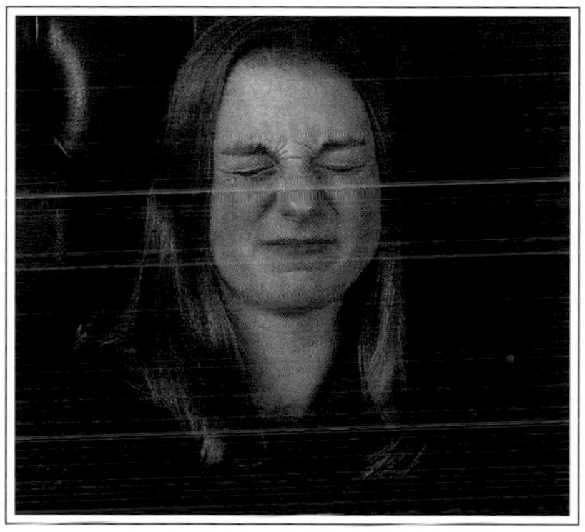

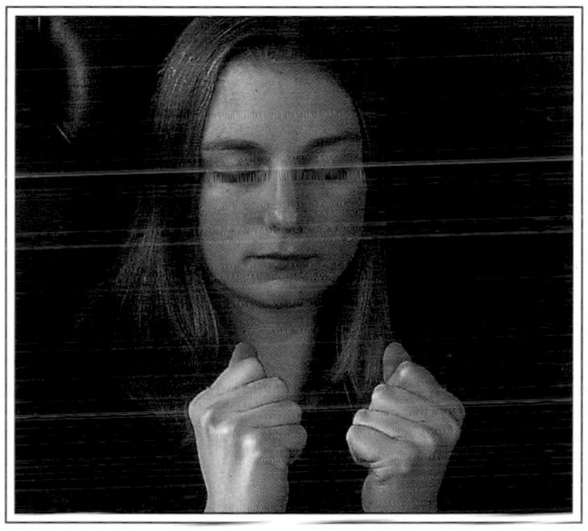

1 Settle back and relax in a chair or on a couch, or lie on your bed and just gaze upward, as if you were looking up through your eyebrows. Fix your gaze on a spot, either real or imaginary, and count down slowly from five to one. As you count down, imagine your eyelids becoming heavy, your eyes becoming tired, so that when you get to one, you can allow your eyes to close. Now begin to relax deeply. Think of the top of your head, your scalp, and concentrate on all the muscles, skin and nerve-endings there, deliberately relax them all and let go of all the tension.

2 Tense your facial muscles, scrunch them all up, around the eyes, the forehead, around the mouth, scowling and grimacing for a count of five seconds, and then release and let go, and feel that beautiful relaxation in all those muscle groups.

Thinking down through the neck and shoulder muscles and on into the tops of your arms, allow those muscles to sag down and become tension-free. Thinking over the muscles of the upper arms, tense those muscles for a count of five and let them go, let them relax down into the elbows and on to the forearms, just letting all those areas relax and let go.

3 Clench your fists, really tight, for a count of five, and release any tension, leaving the hands and arms heavy, easy and relaxed. With each breath you breathe out say to yourself, in your mind, the word "calm". Let any tension in the chest area drain away, as you think down into the stomach muscles, letting them relax too. Let all the muscles of your back relax. Thinking into your waist, your hips, and thigh muscles, let tensions drain away as you think down towards your knees … and on down into the shins and calves, allowing those muscles to relax, into the feet and toes, all muscles tension-free and feeling good.

What about ways of sitting? Generally, meditation seems to work best when the spine is straight, but relaxed and vertical. The reasons for this are several. First, sitting upright is a very good way of staying awake and alert while the eyes are closed and the attention drawn inwards. If the body is upright, the breath can begin to move in and out freely and without obstruction. Also the muscles of the torso and spine have a chance to unknot themselves of old tensions. This may not always be an entirely pain-free process. Until the body becomes used to sitting in a new more conscious way, it may fight to be allowed back to its habitual "comfortable" state. These conflicts will pass, perhaps aided by some exercises such as yoga, tai chi or chi gung.

Eventually, proper posture will prove to be the most genuinely comfortable way of sitting still for a period of time. Sitting upright sends a message to the unconscious that although your eyes are closed, you are not going to sleep, as you would when lying down. On a more subtle level the body's *qi* energy, or life force, is able to move more freely if the spine is straight. Energy cannot move through tense muscles, so as relaxed a way of sitting needs to be found.

There is not necessarily any inherent virtue in sitting on the floor to meditate. Some people are very comfortable doing so, but if this is difficult for you, sitting in a chair is perfectly acceptable. Given the basic requirement of an upright spine, the way of arranging the legs is a matter for personal preference and respecting the body's limits. If sitting cross-legged on the floor, you will probably find it helpful to have a firm cushion at least 5–7.5cm (2–3in) thick under your bottom. This lifts the spine so that it is easier to sit upright. You may choose to kneel, in which case a larger cushion or a meditation bench under your bottom would be advisable to prevent cutting off circulation to the legs. If you feel most comfortable sitting in a chair, choose one that is the right height for you, or use some books under your feet. A firm, straight-backed chair is better than an armchair and if you can sit up unsupported, all the better.

A major objective in this discussion of posture is to ensure the free flow of breath through an open posture. Why is the breath so important in meditation? On the physical level, if the body is taking in enough breath, the brain then has sufficient oxygen to function at its peak and thus remain alert and focused. Breathing in by allowing the lower abdomen to expand enables the lungs to expand to their full extent and also relaxes the muscles of the torso and the internal organs. Many people breathe in a very shallow way, using only their shoulders and the top part of the chest. This way of breathing can produce stress and anxiety as it provokes the "flight-or-fight" response, meaning that rather than being alert in a relaxed and open way, they are tense and watchful. Breathing deeply, with the muscles of the abdomen relaxed, enables you to let go of deep levels of stress and tension, continuing and deepening the process of relaxation that begins with an aligned posture.

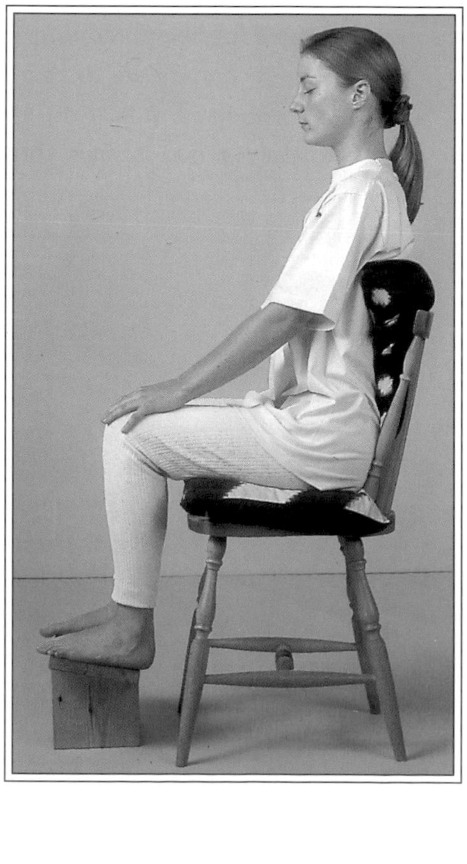

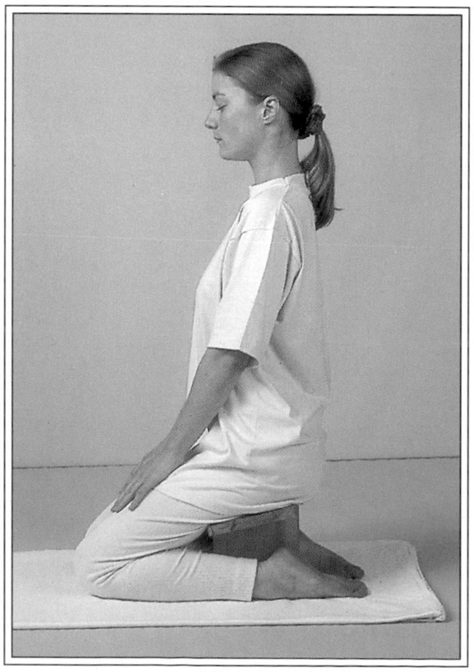

Above and left: Choose your posture, sitting on a chair or kneeling on the floor.

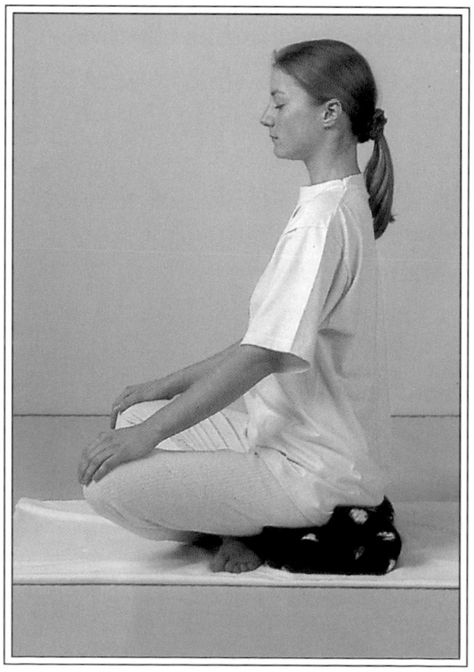

Above: The traditional meditation position is sitting on the floor, with legs crossed.

FOCUSING

Your breath also provides an ever present and easily accessible focus for concentration. One is always breathing! Many schools of meditation teach focus on the breath in various ways. This may involve imagining that the breath originates in one particular point in the body. The points most usually focused on are the *hara* or *tan tien* just below and behind the navel, or the heart – in the centre of the chest. The crown of the head, the base of the spine or the soles of the feet may all be included in the awareness. Focusing on the breath can also take the form of noticing the physical changes as the breath moves in and out, either at the nostrils or the abdomen. Meditation can be as simple as this, just breathing while sitting.

There are many ways of concentrating the mind in order to occupy that part of the mind that chatters incessantly, worrying and obsessing.

❦ Count the breaths from one to ten, then begin again.

❦ Notice the stillness at the changeover points at the end of the inhalation or the exhalation.

❦ Let an image arise that evokes a feeling of wholeness, joy and peace; perhaps a beautiful natural scene of mountains, the sea, a tree, the sun, a child or an inspirational figure and breathe this image into your heart.

FIVE MEDITATION STEPS

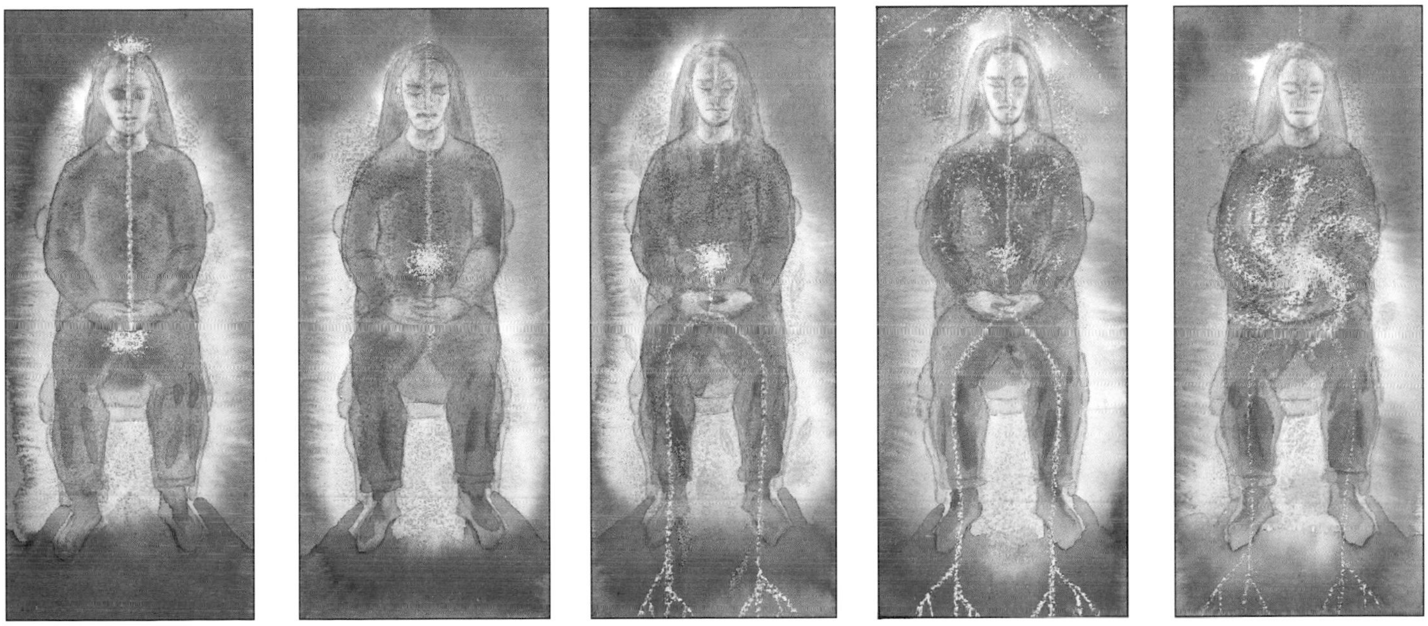

You can memorize these steps, have a friend read to you, or make a tape for yourself. Sitting comfortably but upright, feel your weight on the chair or cushion and relax into it. Imagine breathing in and out through your navel, taking a few deep breaths to settle in. Let your attention gather at a point at the base of your spine, imagine it as a point of energy. Notice what sensations you feel there.

1 Move your attention to the crown of the head, imagine a point of energy there. Notice what sensations you feel. Feel these two points align, connected by a line of light, inside the body near the spine. Allow energy to move freely between these two points.

2 Let your attention come to rest at a point of balance along this line, deep within you, at the centre of your being.

3 From this centre of your being, imagine the line of light extending downward through your legs and feet, relaxing the toes and sinking into the earth. Breathing out, let all tension and fatigue run down this line into the earth.

4 Breathing in, imagine drawing up, through the soles of your feet, fresh, transformed earth energy. Allow it to fill your whole body from the feet up to the crown of your head, bringing a feeling of being supported and cradled by the solidity of the earth. Return your attention and your breathing to the centre of your being. Imagine the line of light rising to the crown of your head and above, out into the clear blue sky, to the heavens. Breathe in fresh air.

5 Allow light and clearness from the heavens to radiate down the line of light to fill the whole body. Breathe into the centre of your being and feel the two energies, from the earth and the sky, mingling. From this centre let your attention be on your breath moving in and out (using one of the focuses suggested above).

BODYWORK

What is the special importance of bodywork? Simply, it provides the most immediate way to affect another person, to reassure and relax them, to help to reduce pain, influence our ability to build relationships, and even fight off disease. Touch is an absolutely primal, vital requirement that is sadly neglected in many of our societies. The continuing rise in the popularity of bodywork therapies shows how much this need is still there.

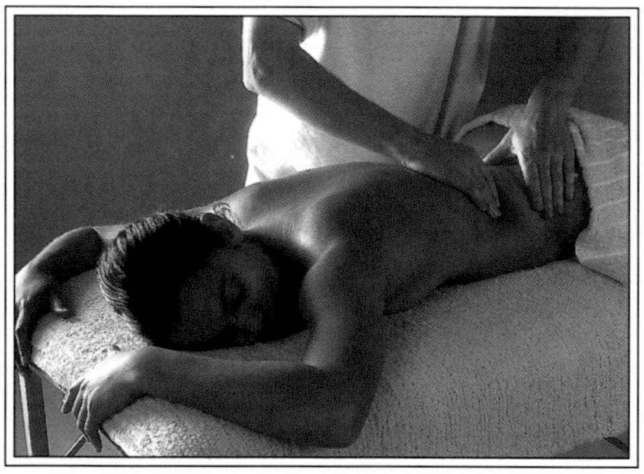

In the last 30 years researchers have started to look at the therapeutic effects of touch, and have shown that not only does regular physical contact lower anxiety levels and enhance the quality of life, but it affects physiological processes, too, ranging from lowered blood pressure, and even less arteriosclerosis, to reduced brain cell deterioration and memory loss with ageing. Musculoskeletal disorders are most often helped by manipulative or other physical treatments, and both pain levels and pain tolerance can often be aided with the help of bodywork therapies.

As if that were not enough, many therapies such as massage are also very enjoyable treatments to receive, and some techniques can be adapted for use at home, helping the giver too. A famous study in the 1960s looked at frequency of touch by couples in cafés around the world; in South America it was 180 times an hour, in the US twice an hour and in England never, so there is much room for improvement.

ABOVE: Professional massage is widely available at natural health centres.

OPPOSITE: Self-massage is often unconscious and with some practice can become part of our daily routine.

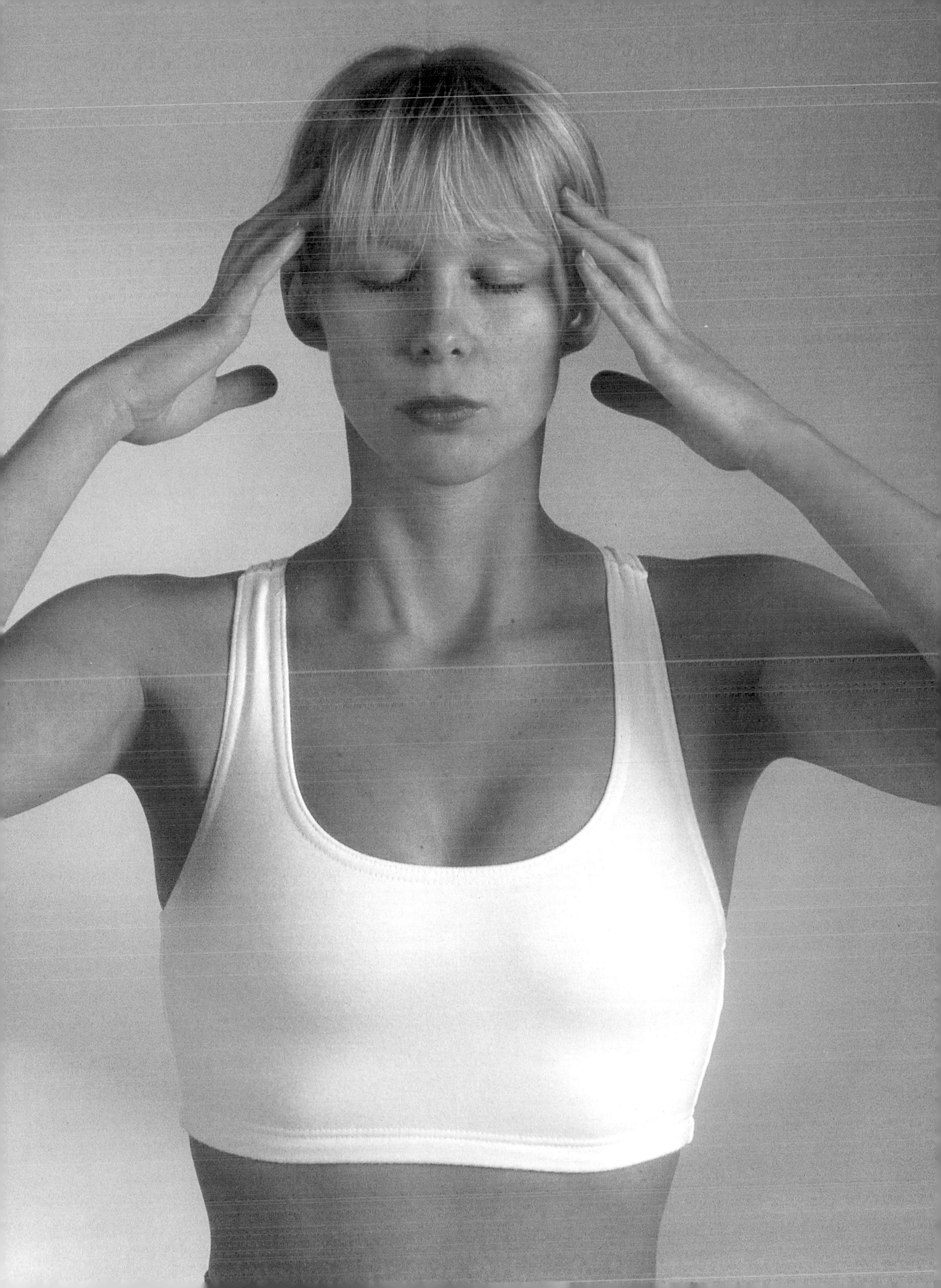

REVITALIZING ARM AND NECK MASSAGE

Even when we are not using our arms in a particularly physical way, tiredness induces aching limbs so that we feel physically drained. Use this quick self-massage routine to renew your energy levels during a busy day and prevent any build up of aches and pains.

1 Do a kneading action on the arms, working rapidly from the wrist to the shoulder and back with a firm, squeezing movement. Do this more quickly and briskly than usual in massage, to invigorate each arm and shoulder in turn, rather than soothe and relax the muscles.

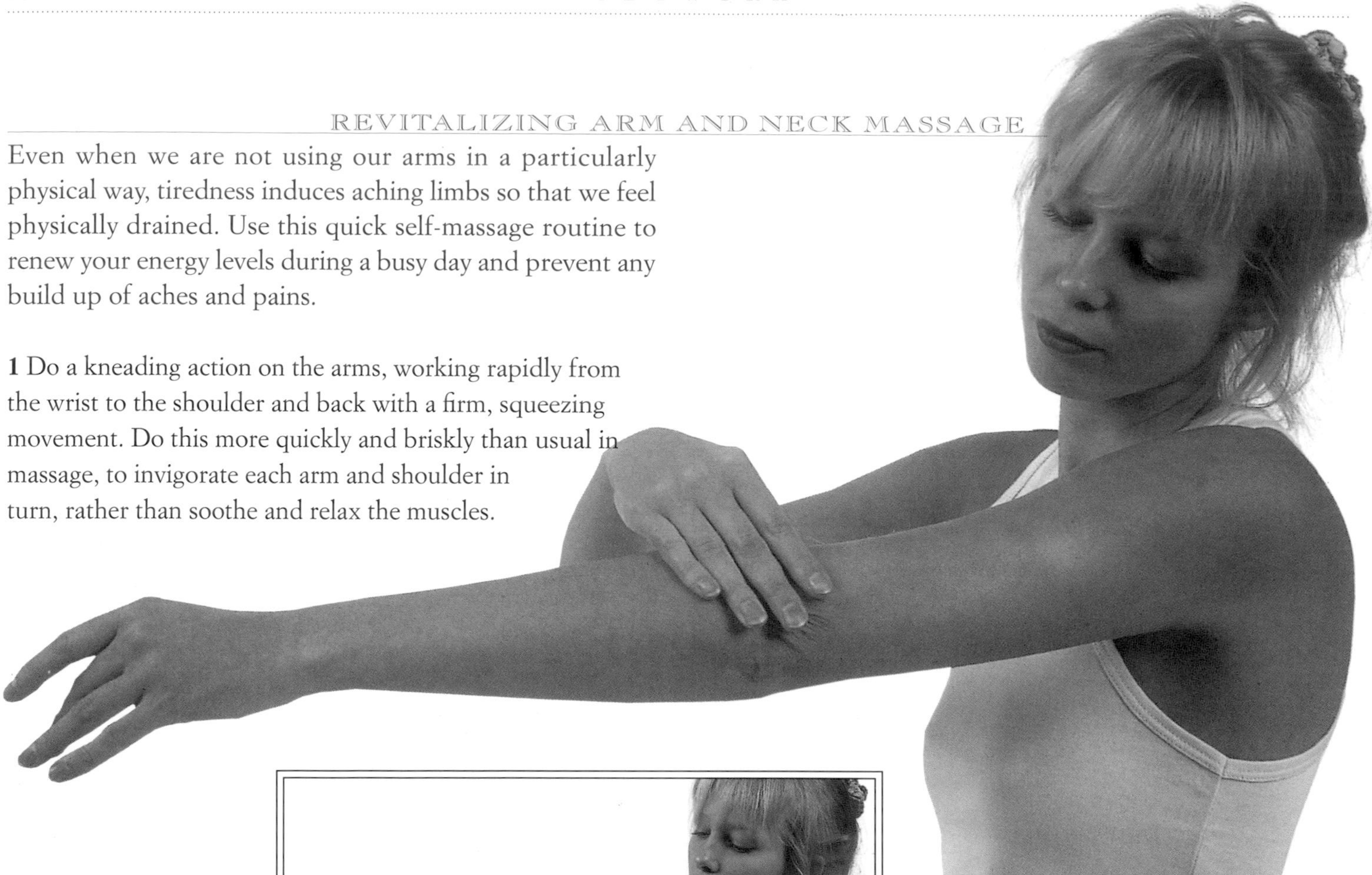

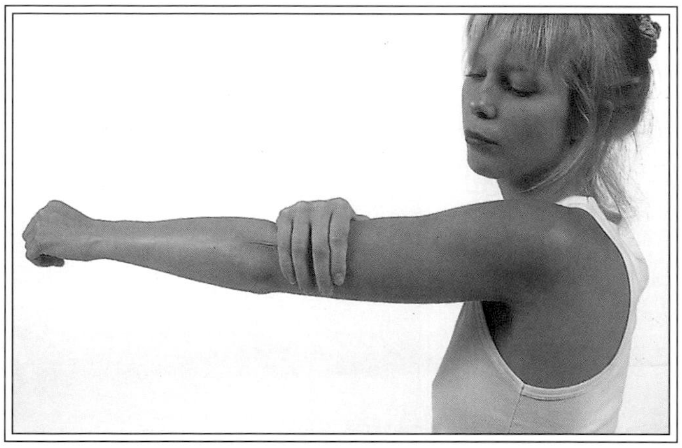

2 Swiftly rub up the outside of each arm using small movements to really stimulate the circulation. Repeat in an upwards direction each time.

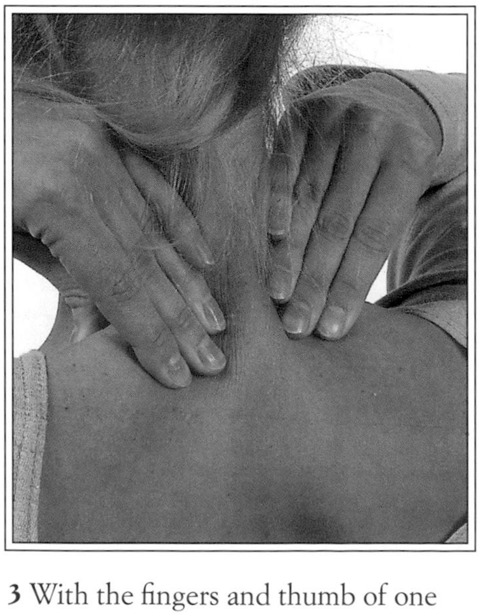

3 With the fingers and thumb of one hand, firmly squeeze the neck muscles with a circular motion.

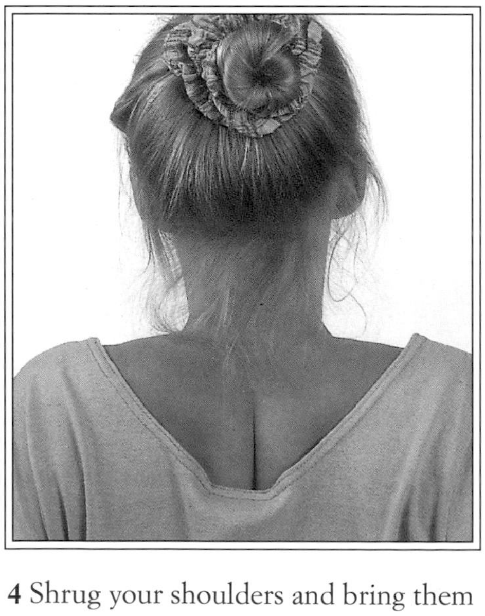

4 Shrug your shoulders and bring them up close to your ears, hold the position for a few seconds.

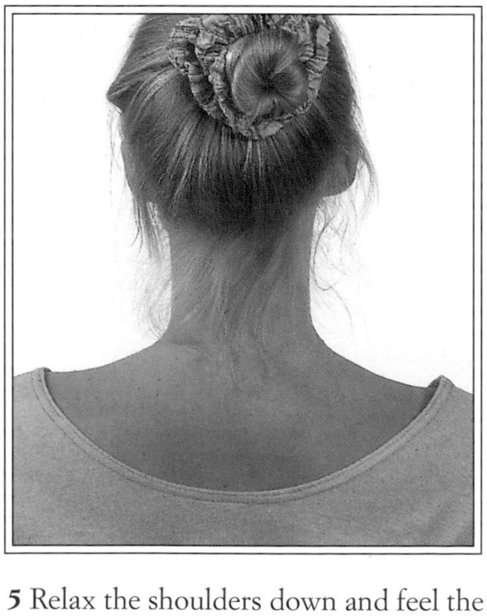

5 Relax the shoulders down and feel the tension ebb away. Repeat the exercise two more times.

LEG MASSAGE

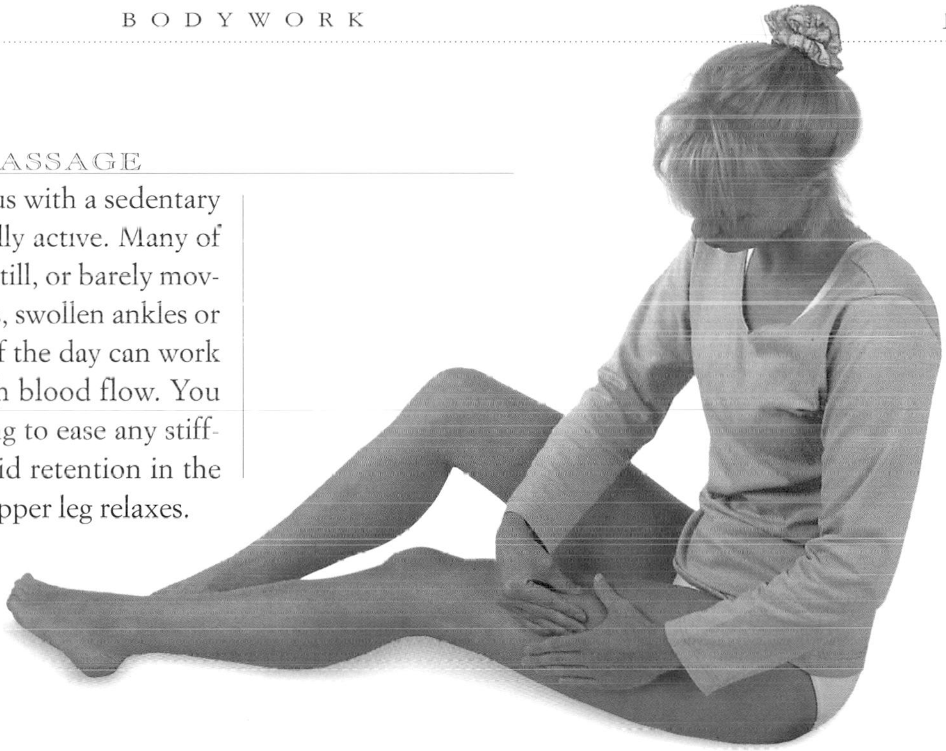

This massage is as beneficial to those of us with a sedentary average day as it is for the more physically active. Many of us spend far too long each day standing still, or barely moving around, leading to tired, aching limbs, swollen ankles or cramp. A quick leg massage at the end of the day can work wonders in reducing aches and sluggish blood flow. You could also use this routine in the morning to ease any stiffness. Start on the thighs, so that any fluid retention in the calves will have somewhere to go as the upper leg relaxes.

1 Using both hands, knead one thigh at a time, by squeezing between the fingers and thumb; squeeze with each hand alternately for the best effect. Repeat on the other thigh.

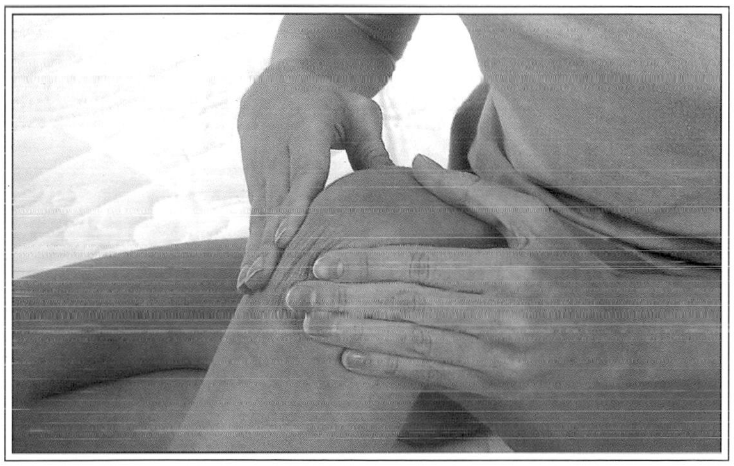

2 Do a similar action around both the knees, but using just the fingers for a lighter effect and working in smaller circles, again squeeze with each hand alternately.

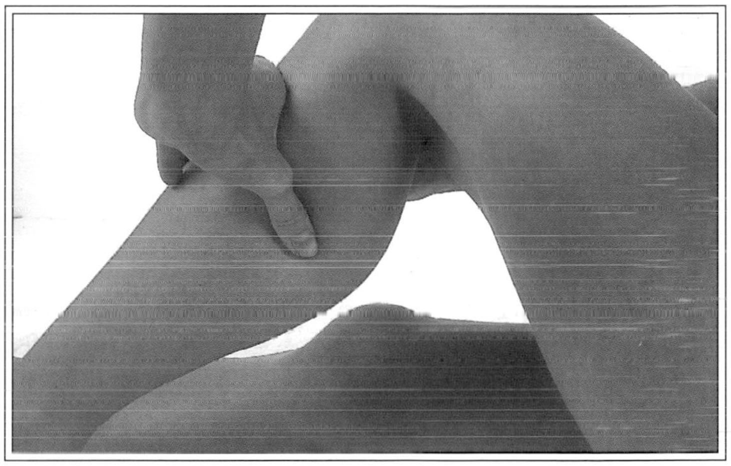

3 Bend the leg and with your thumbs, work up the back of the calf with a circular kneading action. Repeat a few times, each time working from the ankle up the leg.

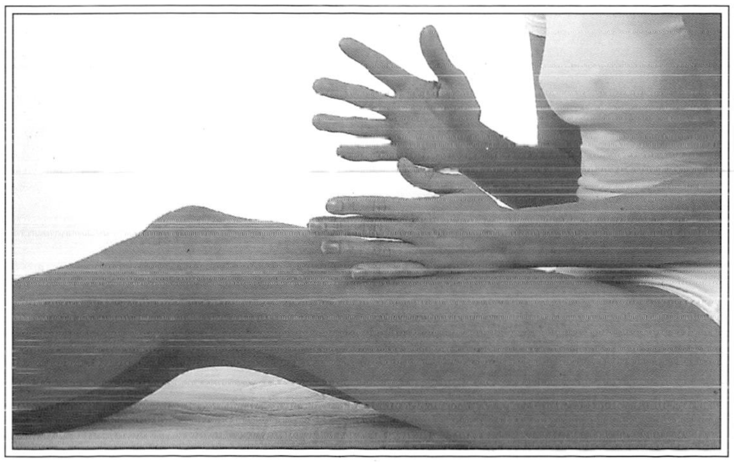

4 With the outside of the hands, lightly hack on the front of each thigh, using a very rapid, almost flicking motion. Keep this action gentle.

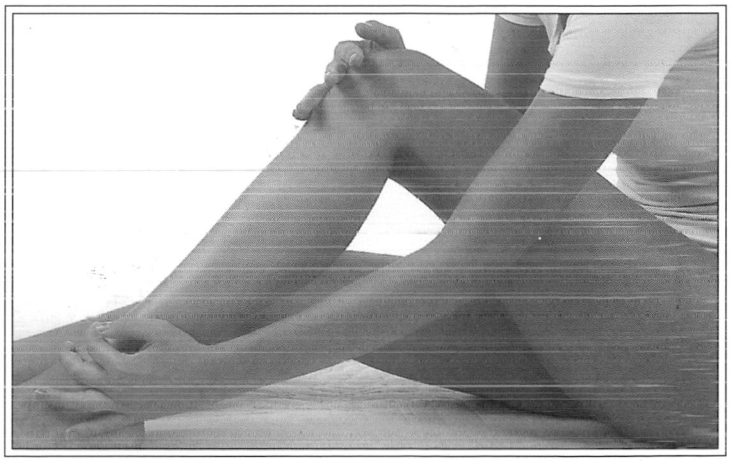

5 Stroke the length of your leg with the fingertips of both hands, from the ankle to the thigh to help blood flow back towards the heart.

Eastern Approaches

The traditional Oriental view of health is quite different from the reductionist standpoint of modern, technological medicine in the West. In Eastern philosophy, illness is placed in the context of a holistic approach to life, and in particular the concept of an energy-based system. From the idea of a universal energy, or the highest level of spirituality, down to the lowest forms of life, much of Eastern ideology is an energetic one, with all parts of the human body interconnected and infused with a vital energy, and all life-forms similarly interdependent on an exchange of energies.

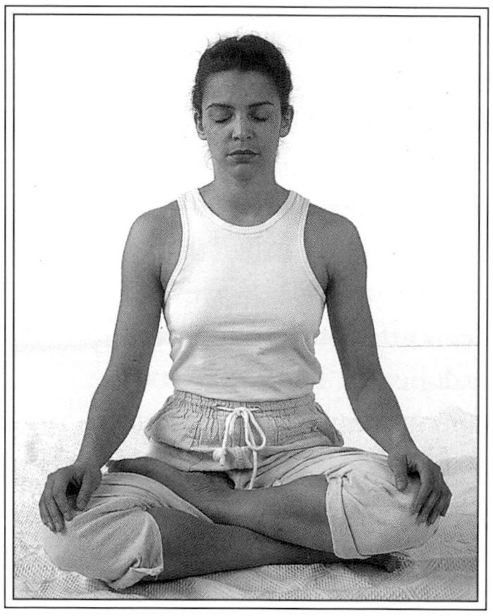

These concepts have led to the development of traditional therapeutic systems, such as acupuncture in China, shiatsu or acupressure in Japan, and yoga in India. Some of these are more suited to professional treatment of ailments, or imbalances in energy flow as they would be described, while practices such as yoga are very suitable for everyday life, in order to *prevent* illness as well as to promote self-development.

Modern medicine in many Far Eastern countries is now often an amalgam of conventional Western medicines alongside traditional approaches; they are quite happy to utilize the best of both worlds, and this is perhaps a useful pointer to the rest of us. Acute, severe illness may be treated with hi-tech medicine, but a more holistic approach can remedy most health problems.

Above: Yoga is one of the most ancient ways of releasing the mind.

Opposite: Acupuncture, once practised only in the East, is now available throughout the world.

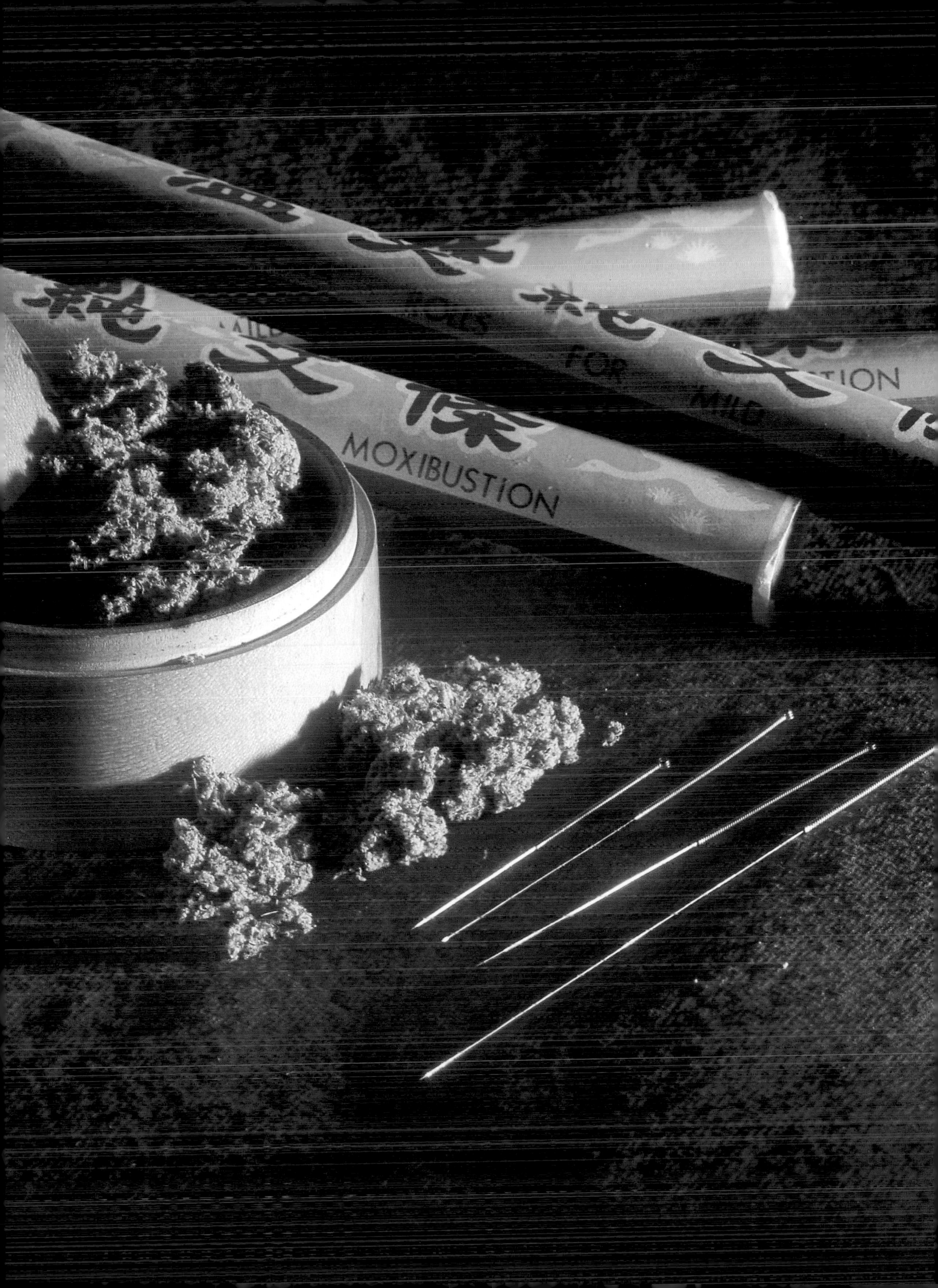
MOXIBUSTION
FOR

Shiatsu

Shiatsu is a contemporary therapy with its roots in Oriental traditional medicine. It is sometimes described as Japanese physiotherapy since it is primarily a physically based "bodywork" system of treatment. The actual treatment approach and philosophy is similar to acupuncture in its usage of the meridians (energy channels) and *tsubo* (pressure points) as well as diagnostic methods, but without the use of needles. Unlike most other forms of bodywork, in shiatsu the receiver remains clothed for the treatment and this is often a consideration for patients.

The word "shiatsu" is Japanese and literally means "finger pressure". The application of pressure is the underlying principle of shiatsu. This pressure can be applied using not only your fingers, but also the palms of your hands, thumbs, elbows or knees, depending on the amount of stimulation required and which body area is treated. Stretching exercises and other corrective techniques will also be included in the treatment with the intention of creating flexibility and balance in the body, both physically and energetically.

Shiatsu works on the flow of energy or *qi* that circulates through our bodies in specific energy channels or meridians. Essentially, we all have a "life force" or "life energy" which created our physical structure and regulates physical, emotional, mental and spiritual stability. This life force, called *qi* in Chinese and *ki* in Japanese, maintains a homeostatic balance in your body.

The flow of *qi* can be disturbed either through external trauma, such as an injury, or internal trauma such as depression or stress. This is when symptoms like aches and pain start to occur and we start to experience a state of "dis-ease". In shiatsu the physical touch is used to assess the distribution of *qi* throughout the body and to try to correct any imbalances accordingly.

Touch is the essence of shiatsu and a wonderful means of communicating our love and compassion for others in a very direct way. Touch can be of very different quality, ranging from aggressive, abusive and mechanical to more nurturing, caring and intuitive. We all need to be touched in some way and shiatsu helps to fulfil this need. The caring touch used in shiatsu will help to trigger the self-healing process within.

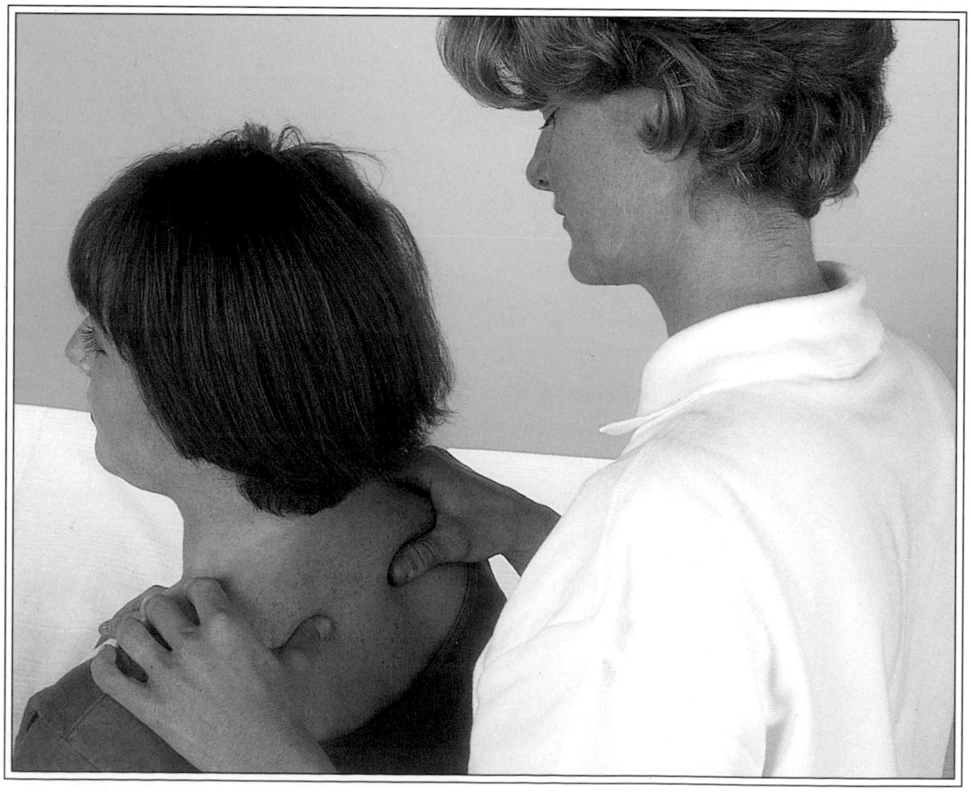

Left: The essence of shiatsu is touch. The practitioner will build up a relationship of trust and care with the patient.

Shiatsu at Home

The exercises in this chapter give two routines, one which you can do on yourself and one with a partner. You may find that during or at the end of these routines you feel slight mood changes. Other reactions experienced after a professional treatment include cold or mild flu symptoms which disappear after a day or so. Do not attempt any shiatsu techniques other than the following exercises without consulting a trained practitioner.

THE HISTORY AND PHILOSOPHY

Oriental medicine developed out of a need to maintain good health and prevent illness. Therapies such as acupuncture, herbalism, moxibustion (the burning of the mugwort herb on the skin) and *amma* (Chinese massage) developed in different geographical areas according to lifestyle and cultural considerations. In the earliest recorded writing on Chinese medicine, *The Yellow Emperor's Canon of Internal Medicine*, written over 2,000 years ago, the Yellow Emperor asked the master of Oriental medicine why there were so many methods to treat one illness and why each method was effective. The master replied that environment was the main reason for using different approaches. In the east where the people lived close to the sea, tended to eat more fish and protein and suffered skin diseases, acupuncture developed as an effective treatment. In the west, where there are mountains and deserts, the people tended to be fat and eat too much animal protein. This caused problems with their internal organs which were best remedied by herbal medicine. In the cold northern mountainous regions, moxibustion was most effective in driving out respiratory disorders associated with the climate, such as coughing and mucus. In the flat central regions, the people developed symptoms of general weakness which was most effectively treated with *amma* and corrective exercises.

Amma (*anma* in Japanese) has been used for centuries to deal with many common ailments, aches and pains as well as treating more serious "dis-eases". New influences from traditional Eastern medicine and Western science have gradually shaped it into what is today called shiatsu. There are several main styles of shiatsu found in the West: barefoot shiatsu, macrobiotic shiatsu, Namikoshi style, Ohashiatsu, Shiatsu-Do and Zen shiatsu. These are all valid and effective therapies using the basic shiatsu principles but with differing emphasis placed on techniques or philosophy. In Japan there are more than 87,000 registered shiatsu practitioners. This fact alone goes some way towards demonstrating its effectiveness in the prevention and treatment of disease.

QI – YOUR LIFE FORCE

Shiatsu acts on the subtle anatomy of the body described as *qi* in Chinese or *ki* in Japanese. The concept of *qi* might be a bit difficult to grasp at first as it is so little recognized in Western society, but everyone can learn how to perceive *qi* and appreciate its effects. *Qi* is a fundamental idea to Oriental medical thinking and is considered as our "life essence" which maintains and nurtures our physical body

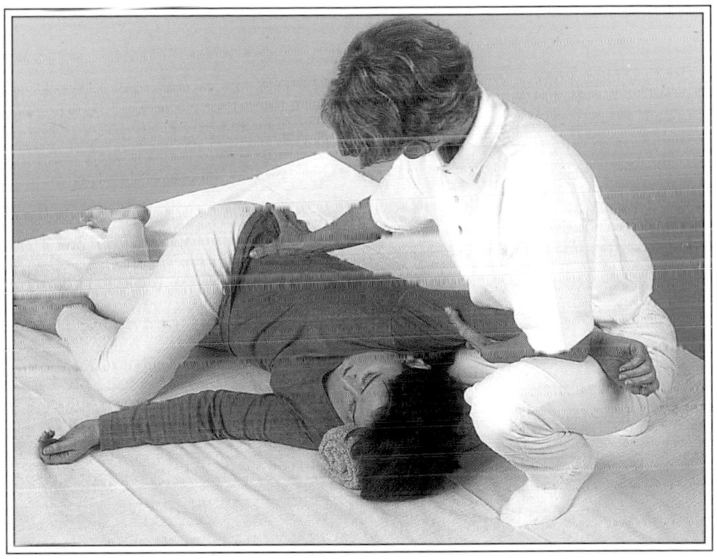

ABOVE: *Here the practitioner stretches the gall bladder meridian and opens the rib cage.*

and therefore also affects our mind and spirit. *Qi* is everywhere. It moves and changes quickly from moment to moment and can easily be replenished on a day-to-day basis. The human body is a field of continually moving energy, circulating through cells, tissues, muscles and internal organs.

The concept of *qi* was introduced to the West through acupuncture and the Chinese martial art of T'ai Chi Chuan. The Chinese word *qi* translates as "breaths". A Japanese dictionary defines *qi* as mind, spirit, or heart and lists hundreds of expressions which use the word *qi*, most of them ordinary ways of talking about human moods, attitudes, or character. For example, *genki* means "source of *qi*" or health.

It is much easier to demonstrate *qi* than to try to measure or contain it and there are a variety of exercises you can do to get in touch with *qi* and feel its affect on your body. *Qi* is a real force, made up of electric, magnetic, infrasonic and infra-red vibrations, which can be intuitively perceived and mentally directed. Like air that we breathe and depend on for our life and water that we take into our bodies, *qi* is the very source of our vitality. It is the force within us which gives us initiative, which drives and inspires us to move forward in life. When the *qi* leaves us, we die. According to the ancient philosophers, life and death is nothing but an aggravation and dispersal of *qi*:

"*Qi* produces the human body just as water becomes ice. As water freezes into ice, so *qi* coagulates to form the human body. When ice melts, it becomes water. When a person dies, he or she becomes spirit *(shen)* again. It is called spirit, just as melted ice changes its name to water."

WANG CHONG, AD 27–97

SHIATSU WITH A PRACTITIONER

A shiatsu session usually lasts for about an hour with the actual treatment taking between 35 and 45 minutes.

In the first session the shiatsu practitioner will ask you many questions about your state of health, your lifestyle, any symptoms, likes and dislikes you may have, to build up your case history. An assessment based on Oriental diagnosis will be compiled. Apart from this oral diagnosis, your practitioner will use visual diagnosis, looking at posture, movement and facial diagnostic areas; and touch diagnosis, feeling the body and the different meridians for areas of excess and deficiency. As touch is the most essential aspect of shiatsu, this diagnosis continues throughout the whole treatment, your practitioner gaining new information about you as the sessions proceed.

You will usually remain clothed during treatment, but your practitioner may need to examine skin surfaces for discolorations and/or swelling at some stage. As the treatment will involve stretches and different movements for you to practise in between sessions, it is advisable to wear loose, comfortable clothing, preferably of cotton. Avoid receiving shiatsu after you have eaten. Digestion will draw energy to the abdomen and disturb your practitioner in reading the energetic movements in your meridian system. There should be as little outside disturbance as possible to maintain the balancing effects of the treatment. It is also suggested therefore that you refrain from consuming any alcohol on the day

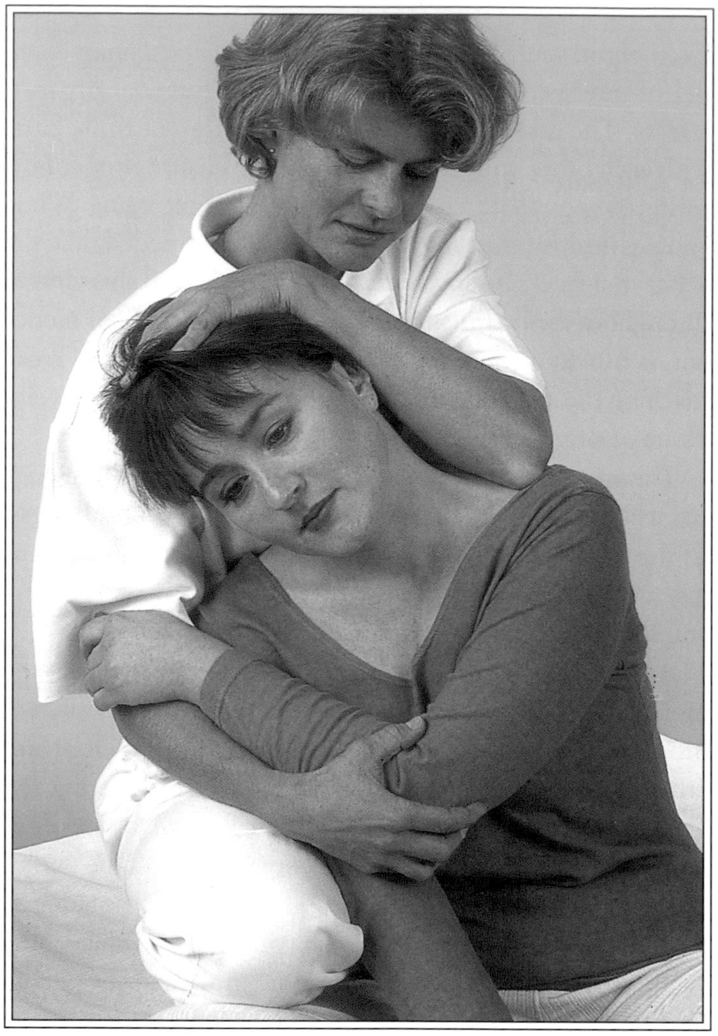

ABOVE: The sitting position is one of the different positions used in a shiatsu treatment. In a supportive way the practitioner is treating the trapezius muscle, affecting the large intestine and gall bladder meridian on top of the shoulder.

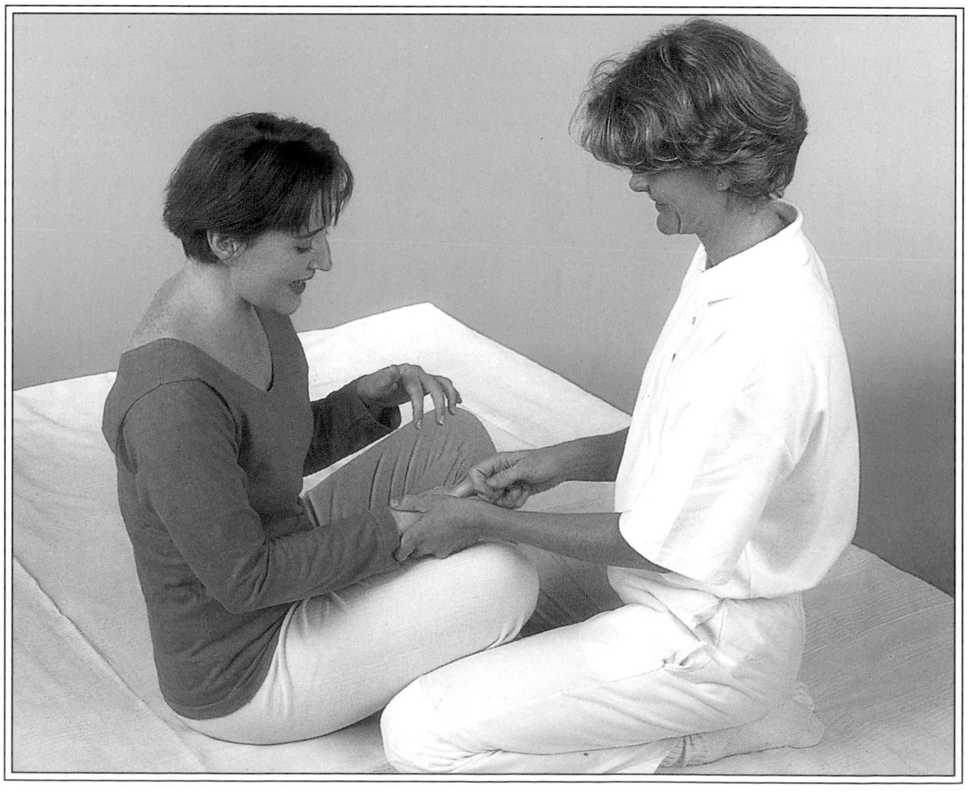

LEFT: All meridians – or energy channels – either start or end in the fingers and toes.

before your treatment as well as the actual day and avoid strenuous exercise following your shiatsu session.

HOW MANY SESSIONS?

A course of treatment usually involves four to eight sessions, preferably on a weekly basis. This depends on the nature of the problem. A long term imbalance might need more treatments, while a couple of sessions for an acute disturbance might be sufficient. Remember that shiatsu is also a preventive therapy, aiding the maintenance of good health, so you do not need to be unwell to receive treatments. This is why many clients continue their shiatsu sessions, after the initial course of treatments, every month or two for their general health and well-being.

BELOW: Here the practitioner is treating the bladder meridian in the back of the leg, using the knee.

EFFECTS AFTER YOUR SHIATSU TREATMENT

The immediate effect of treatments differs with each individual. Depending on your state of health, your symptoms and how accustomed you are to receiving bodywork, you will have different reactions after your shiatsu treatments. A sense of well-being is common.

Because of the deep relaxation that usually occurs and the stimulus to the major body systems, you may have some healing reactions. Some people feel cold or flu-like symptoms, aches and pains, or headaches after the first treatment. These symptoms will only last for a day or so and usually subside with each subsequent treatment. It is important to remember that any such effects you may experience are positive signs from your body telling you it is making an attempt to correct its own condition in a natural way. These are signs of elimination and the beginning of the healing process.

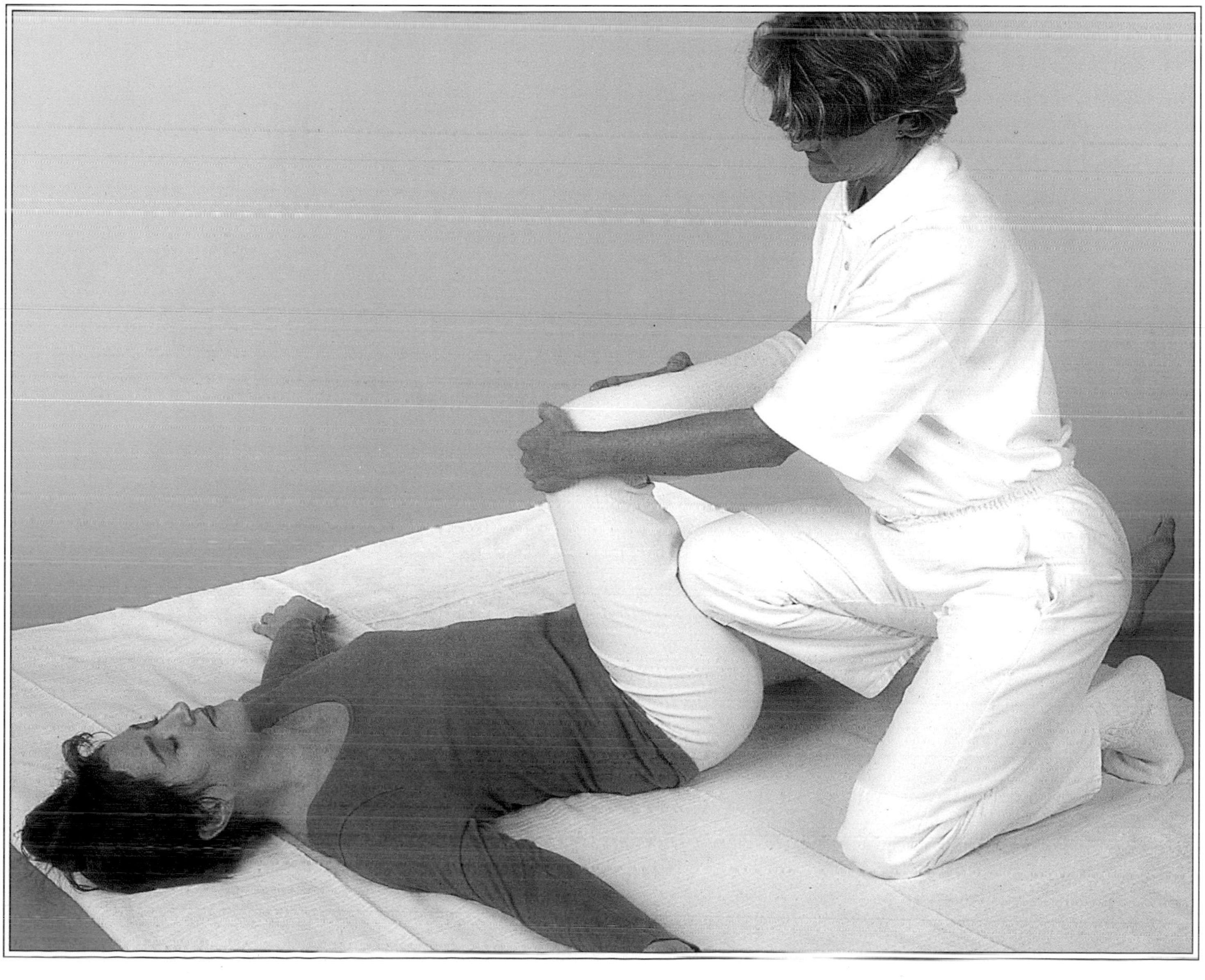

SHIATSU WITH A PARTNER

Here are some simple shiatsu techniques which you can perform on a partner. This is an ideal way to release tension without putting too much strain on the body. You may feel sleepy afterwards. Keep your touch gentle.

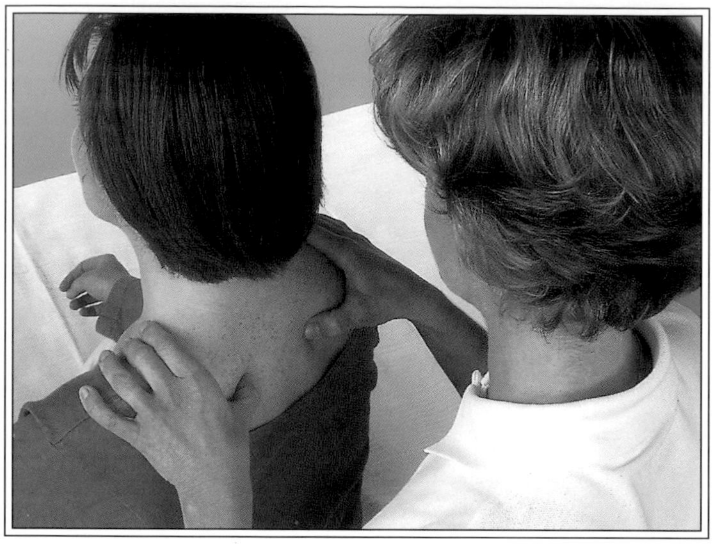

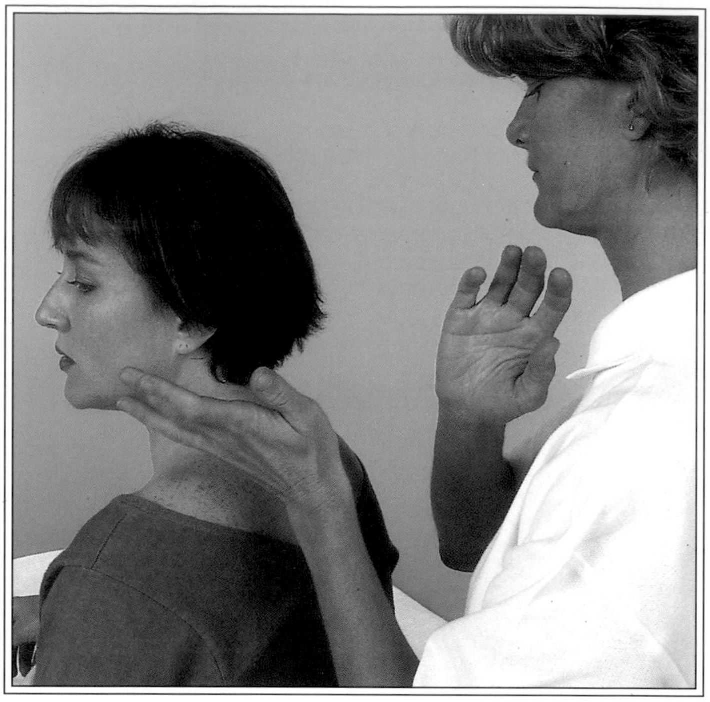

1 Gently place your hands on your partner's shoulders. Take a moment to tune into her energy. There may be tension in the area to begin with. Squeeze the trapezius muscle – the muscles of the shoulder and neck – using your thumbs and fingers in a rhythmic kneading action.

2 With the little finger side of your hand, gently hack across the shoulders and neck in a rhythmic motion. Gradually your partner's muscles will relax and you can increase the intensity and power of the hacking. Keep checking if this feels comfortable for your partner.

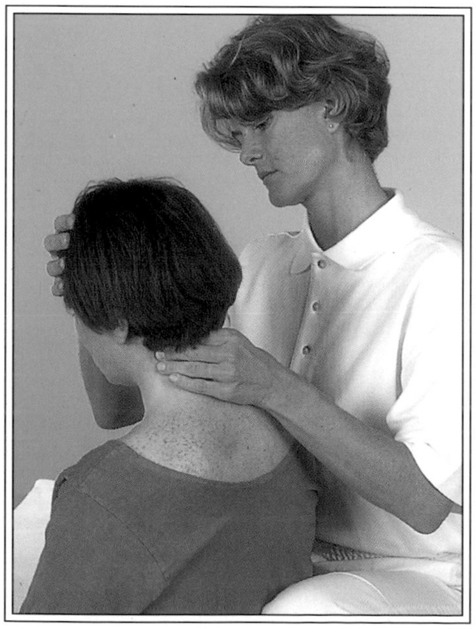

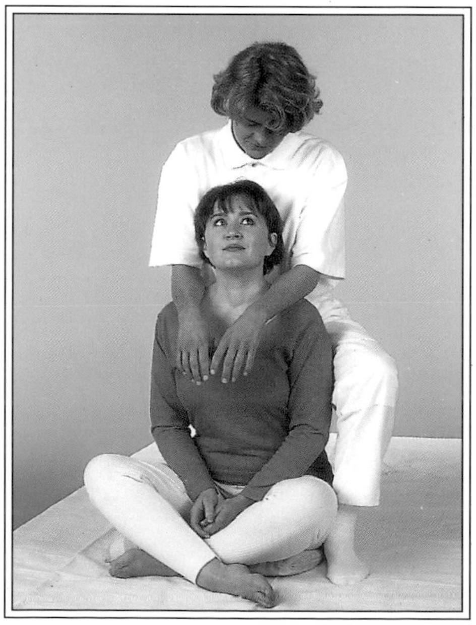

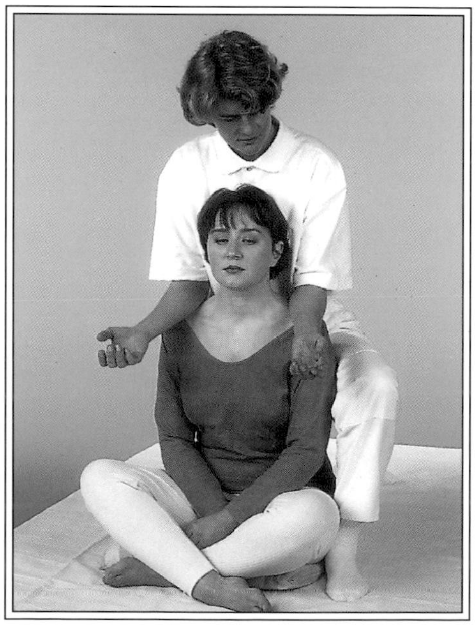

3 Kneel at your partner's side supporting the back with your leg. Place one hand on the forehead and encourage the partner to relax the head into your hand. With the fingers and thumb of the other hand, gently squeeze the neck muscles.

4 Kneel behind your partner and place your forearms on the shoulders with your palms facing to the floor. Lean into your forearms using your body to apply equal gentle pressure on to your partner's shoulders.

5 Ask your partner to breathe deeply. On the out breath, roll your arms across the shoulder, from the neck towards the shoulder joint, ending up with your palms facing up. Lift your arms up and repeat several times.

PRONE POSITION

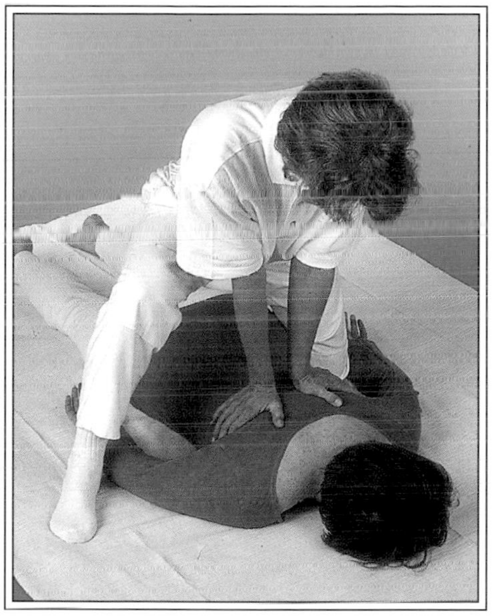

1 Using the palms of your hands, press down gently on your partner's back. Start at the top of the back in between the shoulders and gradually work downwards. Apply the pressure as your partner breathes out. Keep your elbows straight. Repeat three times.

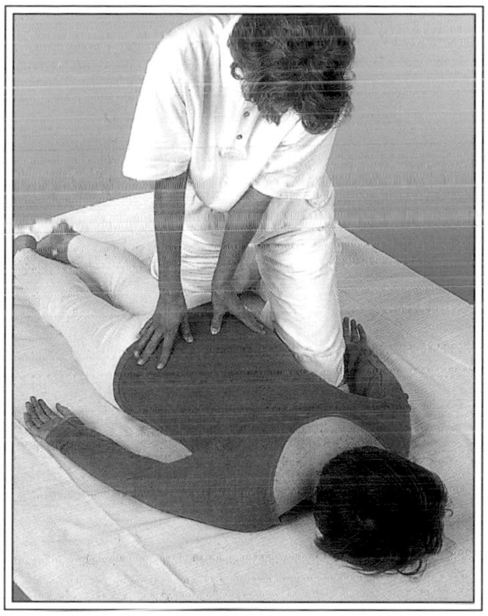

2 Measure two fingers' breadth from the centre of the spine to locate the bladder meridian. Use your thumbs and apply gentle pressure all the way down the back, working gradually from the top to the bottom.

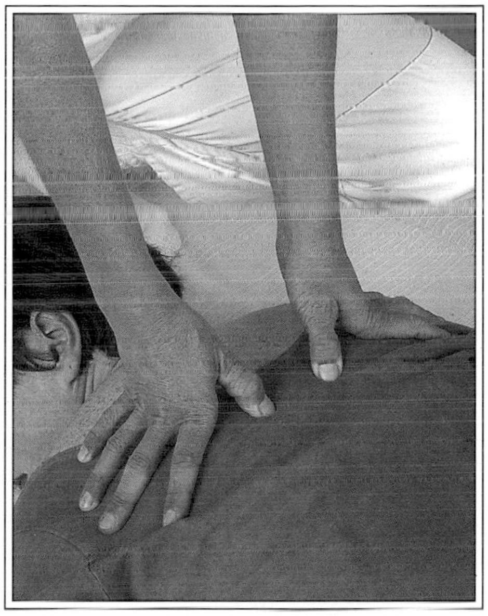

3 For the upper part of the back, kneel or crouch at your partner's head. Using your thumbs, apply pressure to the bladder meridian. Hold this gentle pressure for a few seconds.

COMPLETION

To complete the session, lie your partner down on the back. Rest your hand on the stomach. This is called the Hara in the Orient, and is thought of as the vital centre of ourselves. In this position "tune in" to your partner's breathing. Stay in this position for a few moments until you can sense that your partner is relaxed and peaceful, then slowly move your hand away and gently dissolve the contact.

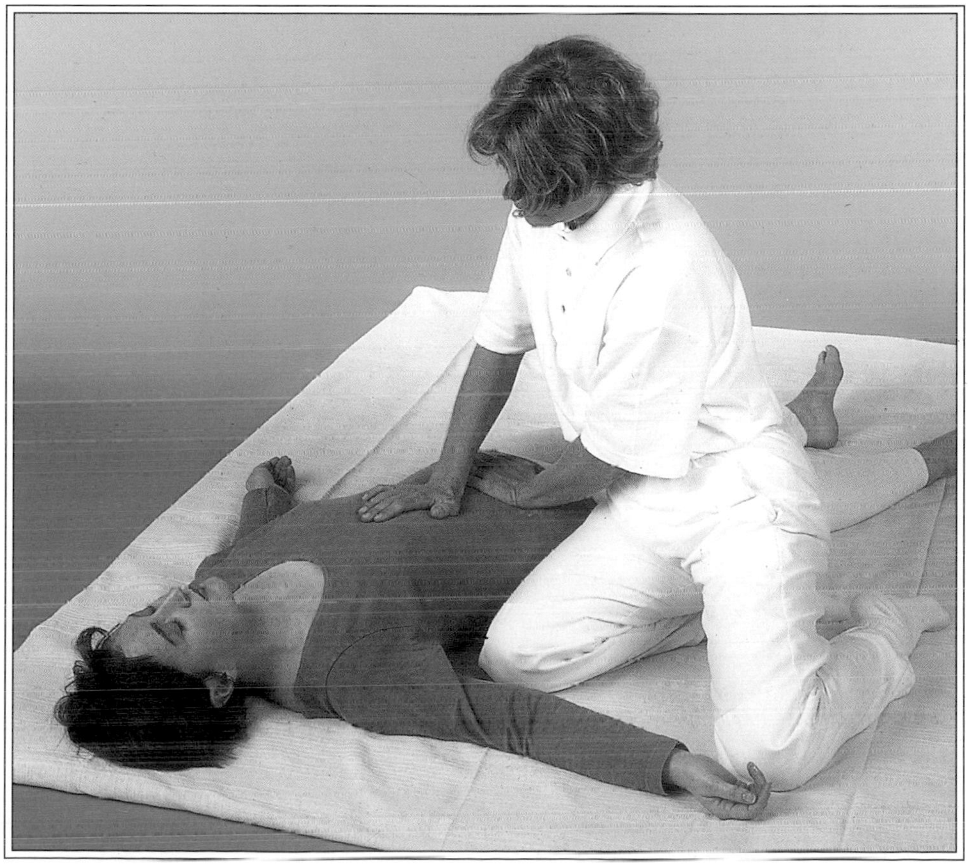

MERIDIAN STIMULATION

The following DoIn (a form of shiatsu) exercises are designed to improve, maintain and develop your general physical, mental and emotional health and well-being.

The exercises can be practised by anyone maintaining a normal daily life, at any time without any special effort. The DoIn exercises will open up the energy channels, release any blockages and facilitate the free flow of *qi* along the meridians, thus improving the circulation of energy throughout the whole body. You will feel invigorated and energized after performing the exercises, and it is recommended that you do them upon rising in the morning, or whenever you are feeling low and generally under par.

Although any part of the series of exercises can be practised independently, it is best to perform the whole sequence at one time to achieve the maximum benefit. Keep a natural posture and breathe normally throughout the exercises and try to maintain an empty mind, clear from any disturbing thoughts and feelings. Keep your focus on the exercise and feel the effect it has on your body. As you become accustomed to the routine, it will be easier to follow and you will find it takes even less time to complete.

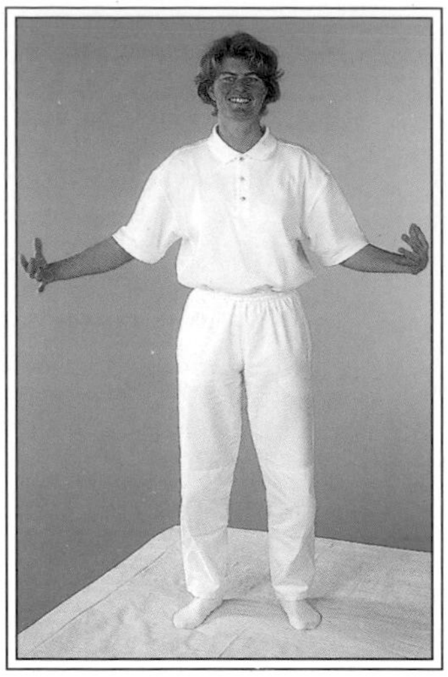

1 Prepare yourself by gently shaking your body. Shake your arms and hands. Lift your shoulders up to your ears as you breathe in; let them relax on exhaling. Repeat a few times.

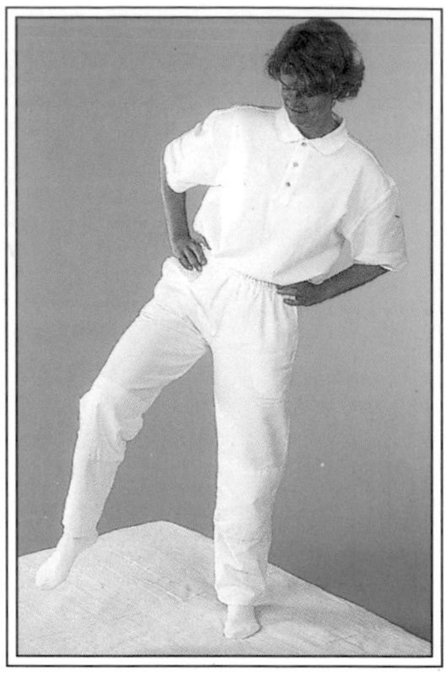

2 One at a time, gently shake each of your legs and feet. Then sit down in a chair or on a cushion on the floor, keeping your back straight. Keeping an upright posture allows a good energy flow.

HEAD

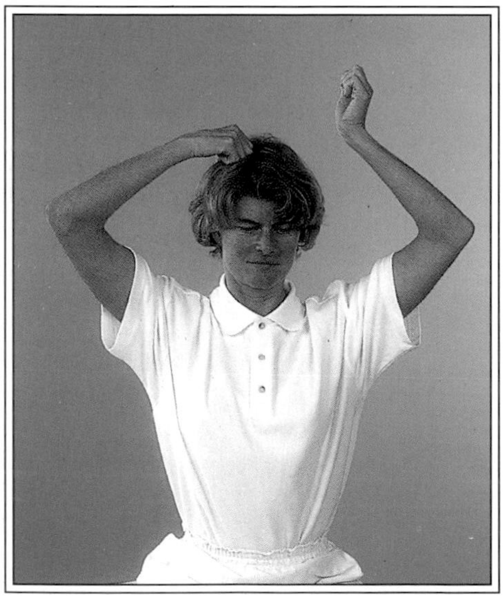

1 Clench both hands loosely and, with your wrists loose, start to tap the top of your head gently. Work your way slowly all around your head, covering the sides, front and back. Adjust the percussion pressure as needed. This exercise will wake up your brain and stimulate blood circulation which will be beneficial for your hair growth and hair quality.

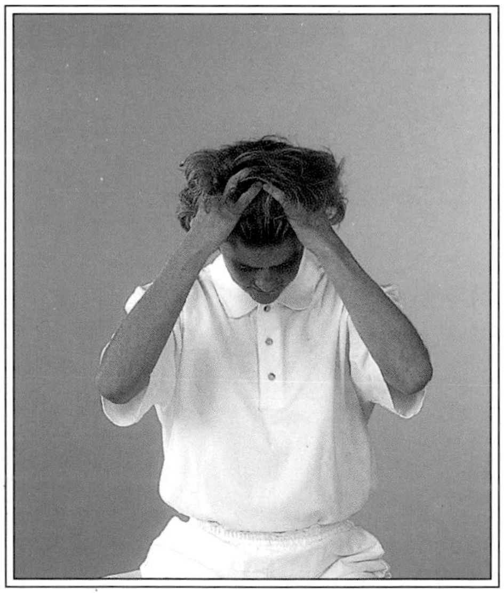

2 Pull your fingers through your hair, gently stimulating the meridians running across the top and side of your head (bladder and gall-bladder).

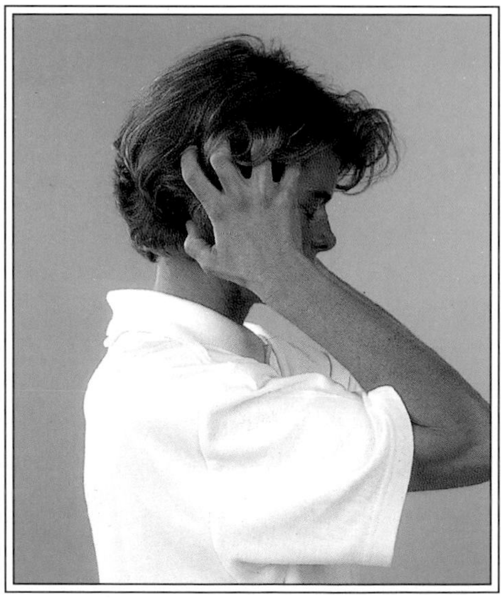

3 Place your fingers on either side of the mid-line of your skull and apply pressure with your fingertips to the bladder meridian, working from the forehead to the back of your neck. Then move your fingers down to just above the ears and apply pressure. Repeat this sequence three times.

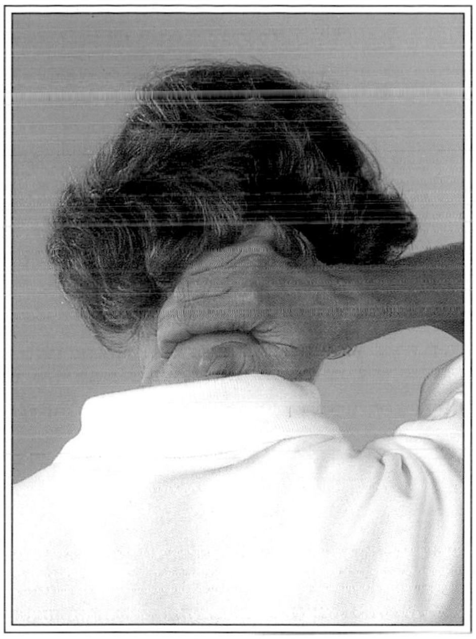

1 Now move your attention to the back of your neck. Bend your head down and using one hand, place your palm across the back of your neck and gently massage it using a squeezing motion.

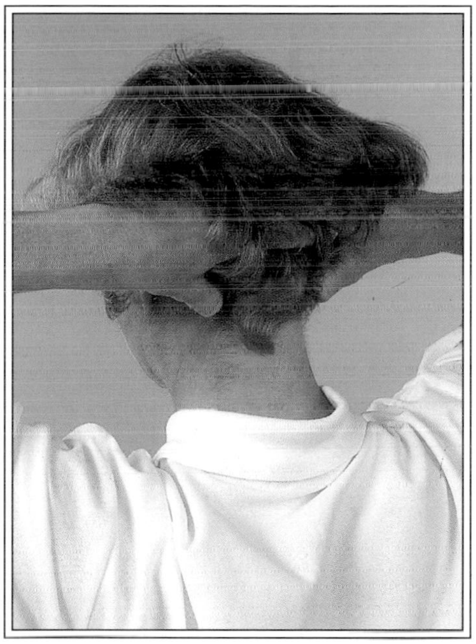

2 Lift your chin slightly and with your thumbs, press either side of the base of the skull, supporting your head with your fingers. The pressure should be directed up against the skull.

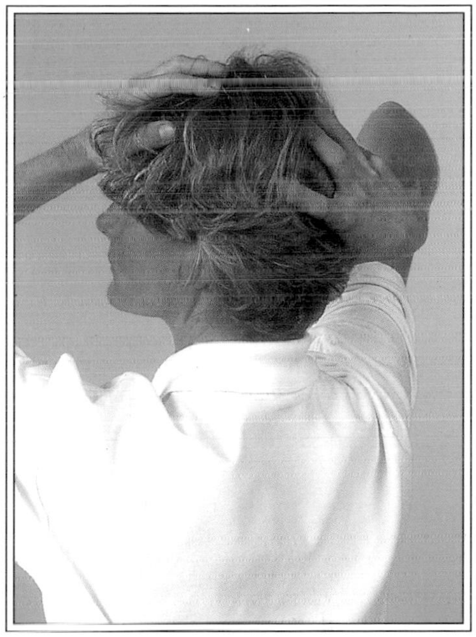

3 Use one thumb to stimulate the skull's mid-base, while the other hand supports your forehead, tipping the head slightly up and back. Vibrate your thumb gently as you apply pressure, then release. Repeat three to five times.

FACE

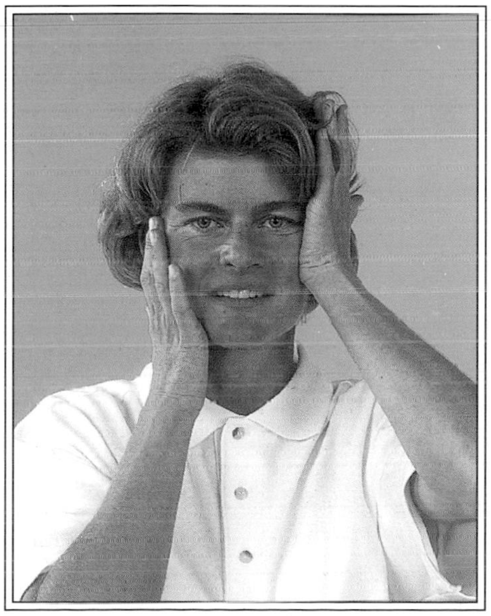

1 Apply both hands to your cheeks and using the palms gently rub your cheeks in an up-and-down motion until the skin becomes warm.

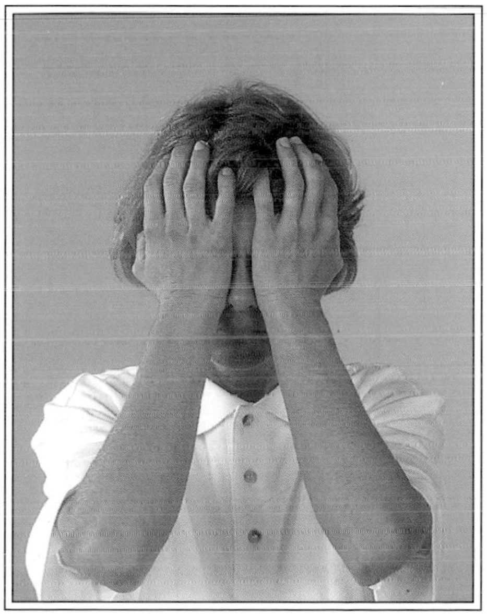

2 Bring your palms to your eyes, covering them and warming the area around the eyes. This stimulates blood circulation in the area and will be beneficial for tired eyes.

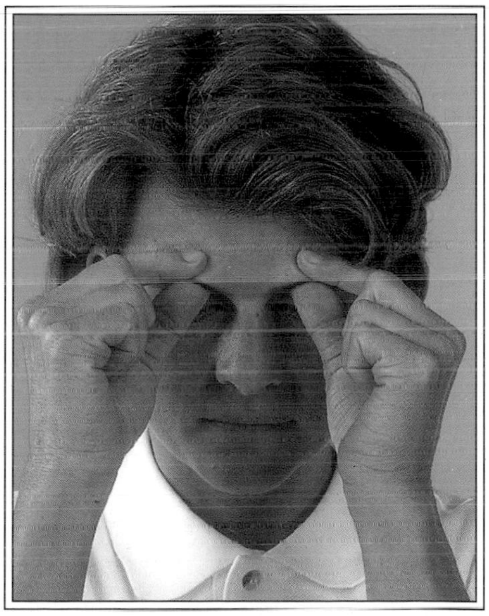

3 Using your index finger and thumb, squeeze your eyebrows starting from the centre line and moving laterally, three times.

►

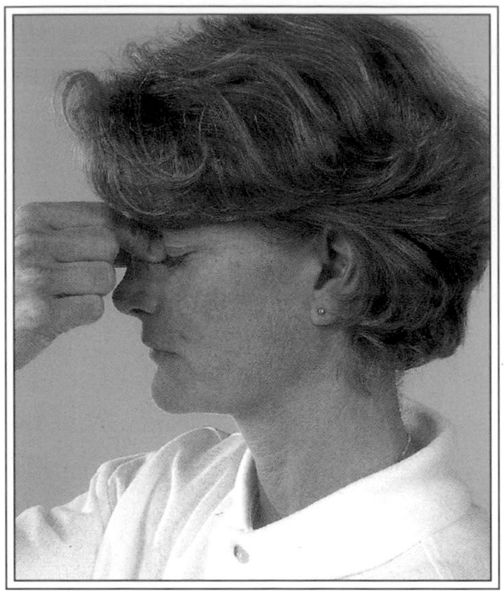

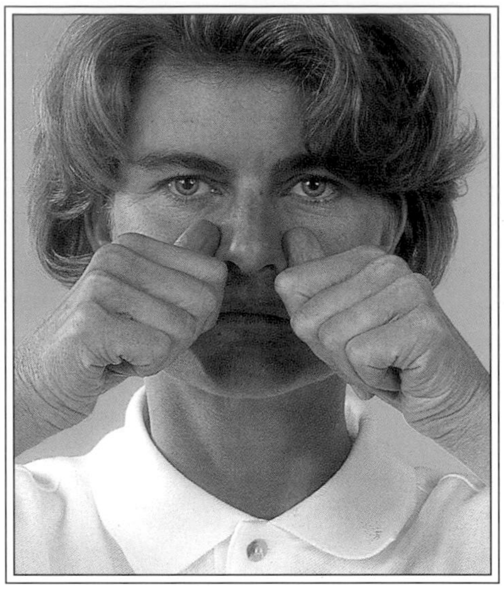

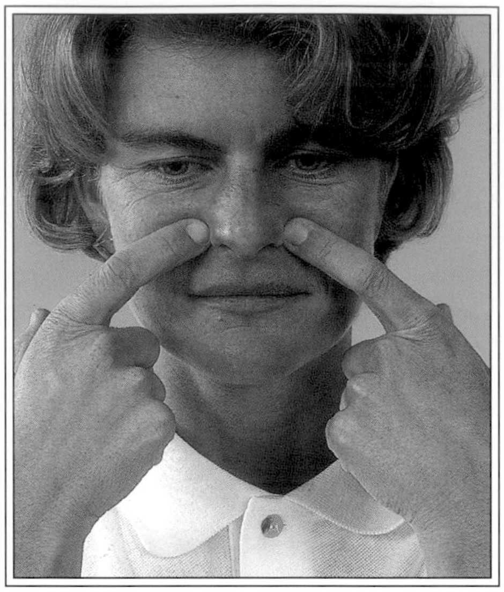

4 With an index finger and thumb, pinch the bridge of the nose and the corners of the eyes. This point is called "eye's clarity". It opens and brightens the eyes and clears vision and will be especially helpful if the eyes are tired.

5 Clench your fingers and apply your thumbs to the sides of your nose. Stroke down the side of your nose quickly at the same time as you breathe in. This will help to clear your sinuses and release any stagnation of mucus.

6 Use your index fingers to stimulate either side of the nose.

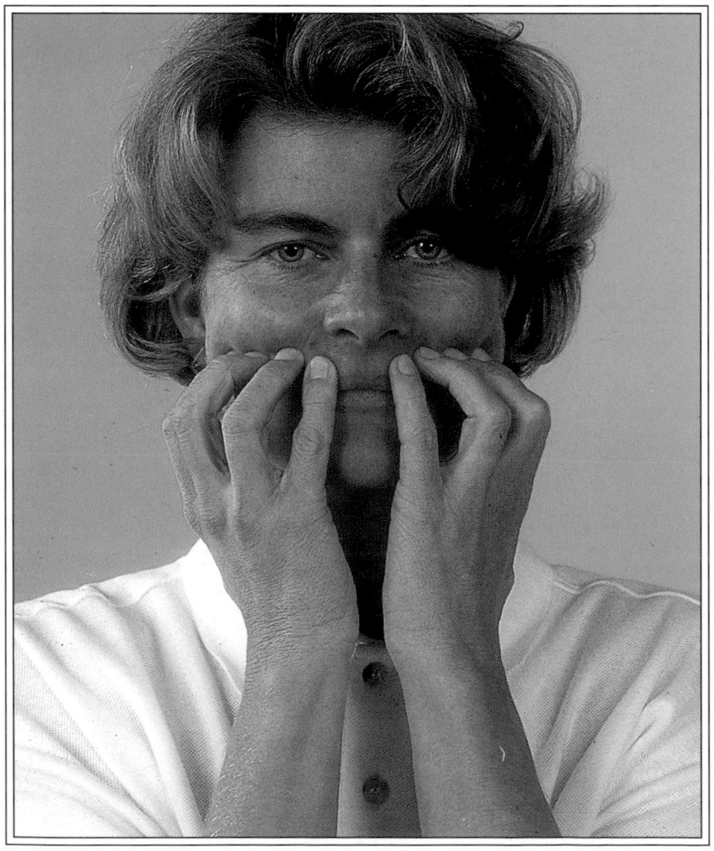

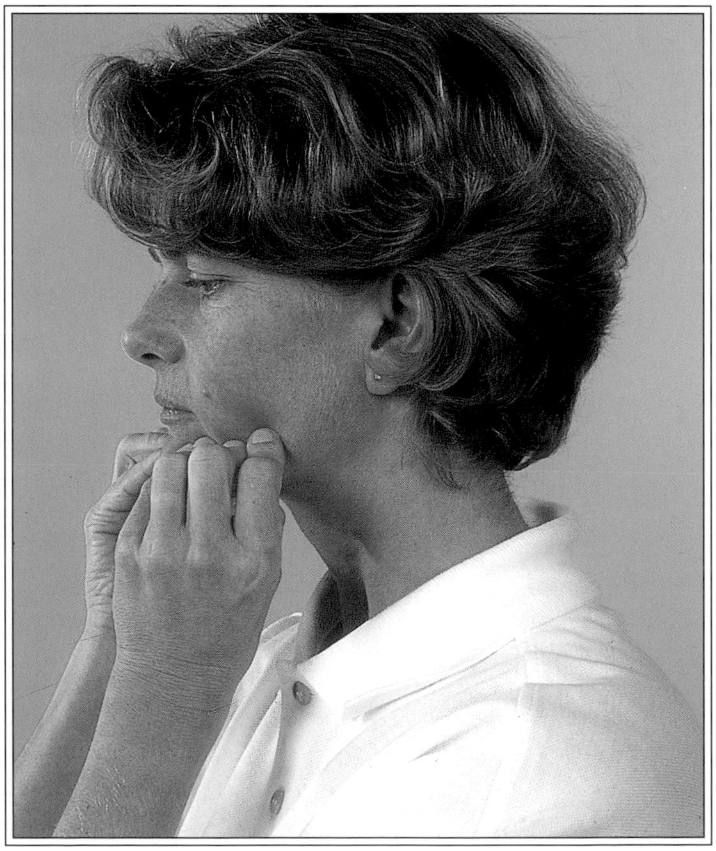

7 Using the four fingers of both hands, apply pressure around the mouth. This area of your face reflects the digestive system and these exercises will activate the production of saliva and strengthen the system.

8 Using your thumbs and index fingers, squeeze your lower jaw. Repeat three to five times. This will stimulate the glands which are directly related to the ears, saliva and lymph so that they function properly.

EARS

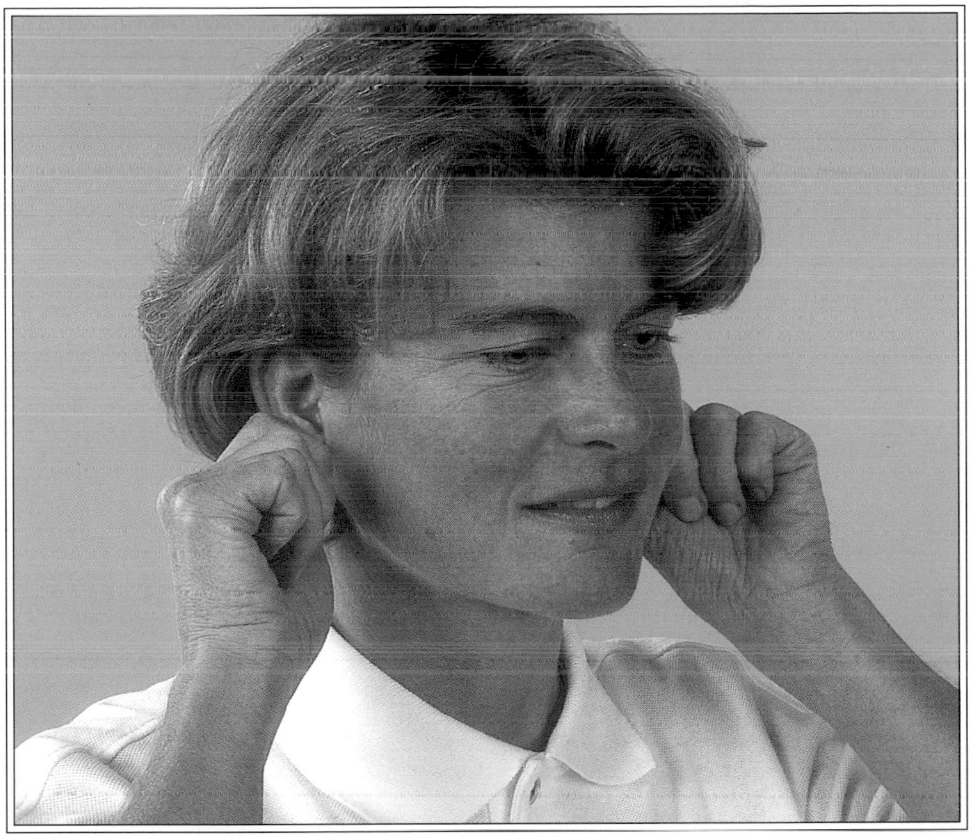

1 Move your hands to your ears and massage them gently, using your index fingers and thumbs. Your ears relate to your kidneys and these exercises will improve mental balance as well as kidney and excretory functions. First rub the peripheral ridge of the ear in order to activate circulation; then rub the middle ridge and finally move to the inner ridges and indentations.

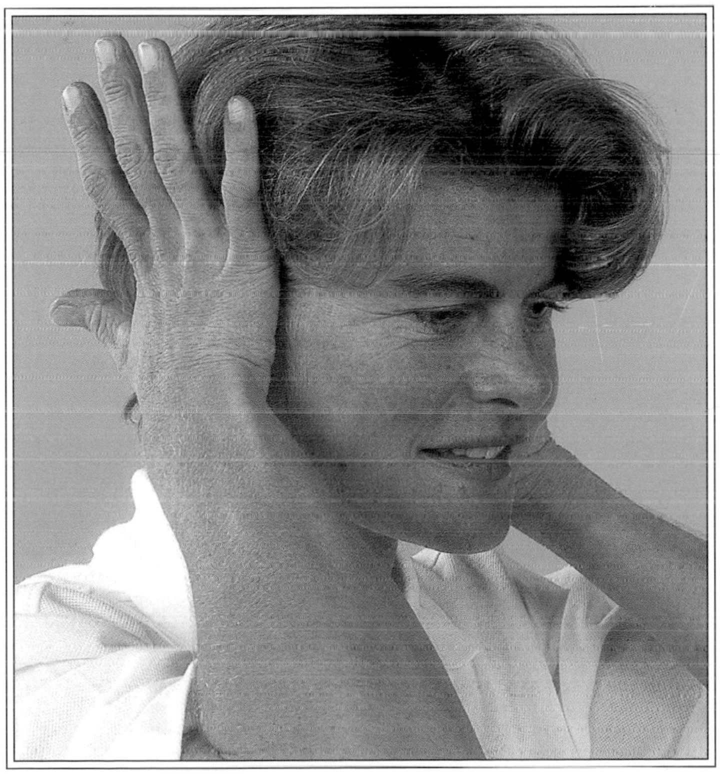

2 Squeeze your ear lobes and then, with the palms of your hands, vigorously rub the whole of both ears, up and down, until they become warm.

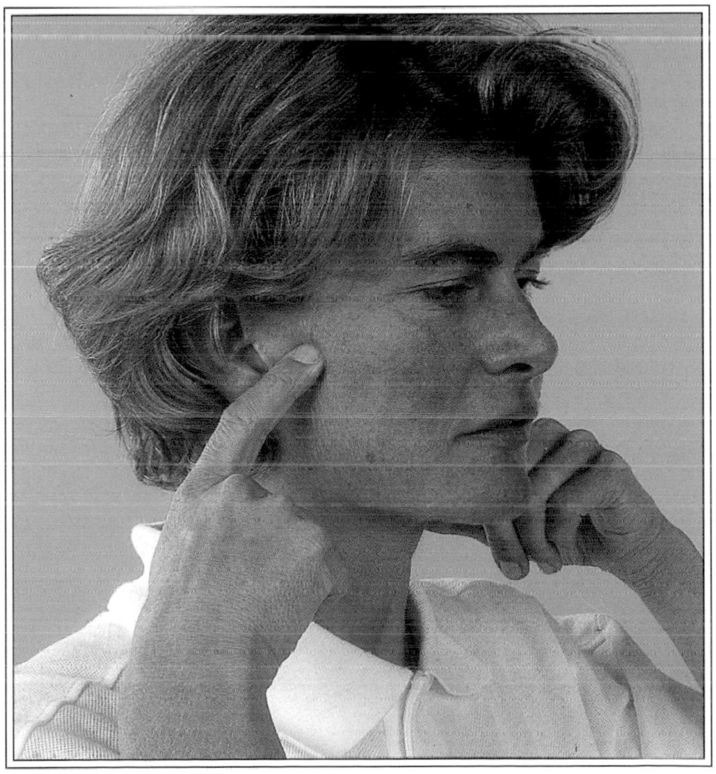

3 If you have a ringing in the ears, apply gentle pressure to the point in front of the middle of the ear.

SHOULDERS AND ARMS

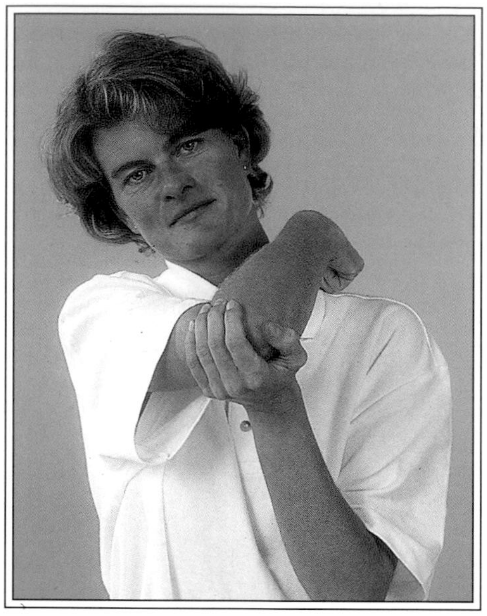

1 Using your left hand to support the right elbow, with a loose fist tap across the top of your left shoulder with your right hand and, as far as you can, reach over your shoulder-blade.

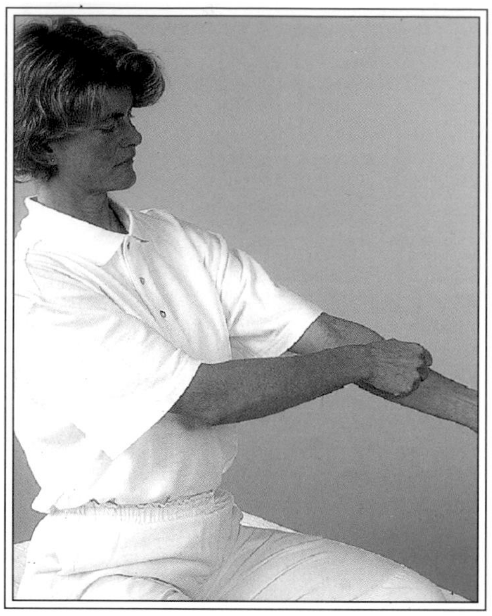

2 Release the elbow, straighten your left arm in front of you, open up your palm and tap down the inside of your arm from the shoulder to the open hand. This will stimulate the energy flow of the lung, heart governor and heart meridians.

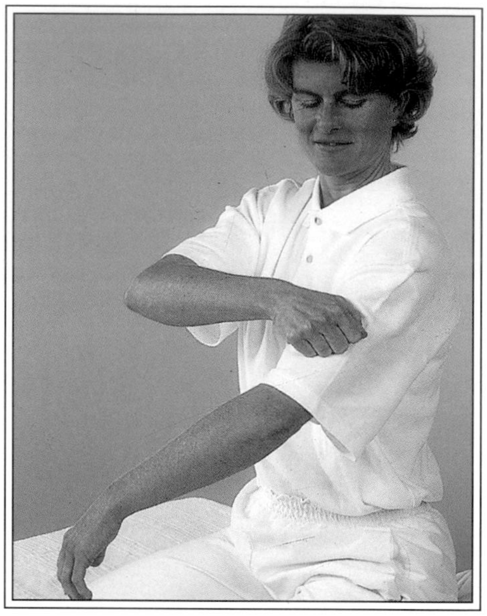

3 Turn your arm over and tap up the back of your arm, from the hand back to the shoulder again. This will stimulate the meridians on the back of your arm, namely the large intestine, triple burner and small intestine. Repeat three times.

HANDS

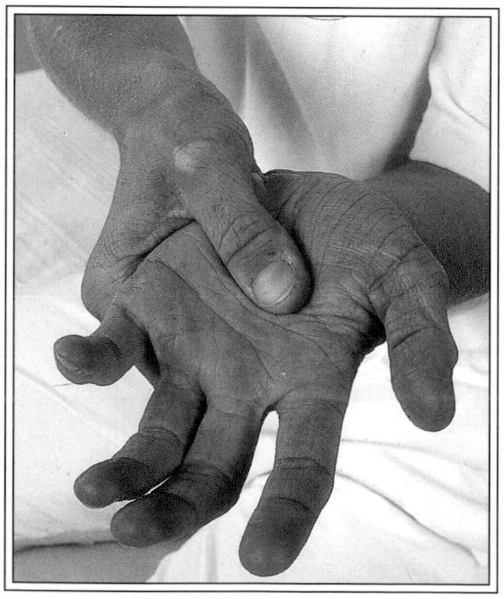

1 Use your right hand to work your left, massaging the centre of your palm gently with your right thumb. The point here is called "palace of anxiety", heart governor 8, and is good for relieving general tension.

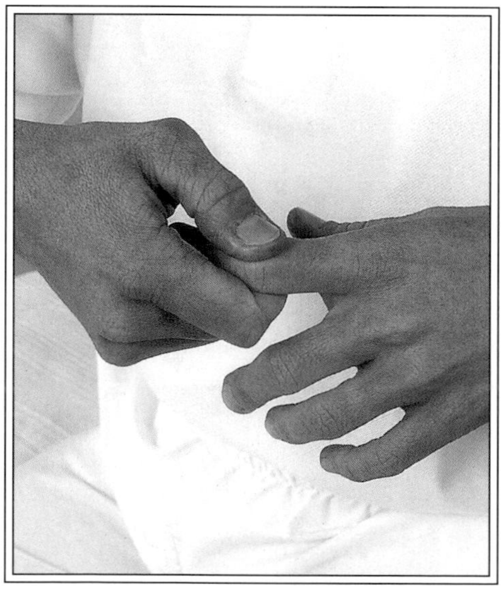

2 Rotate and massage the joints of each finger using your right index finger and thumb. This is a great way to release any tension in your hands and helps to prevent arthritis as well as improving flexibility in the joints.

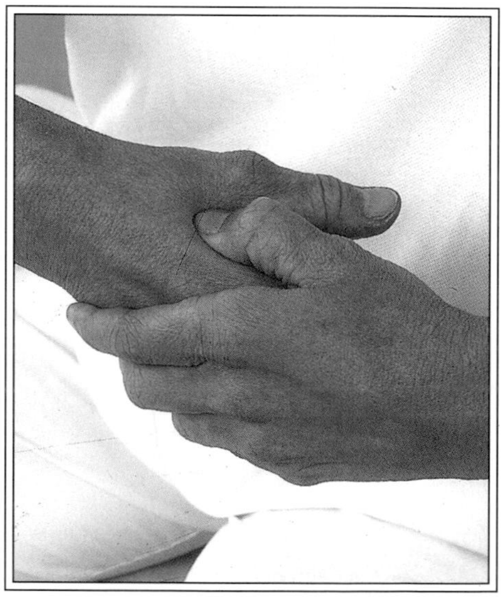

3 Apply pressure in between your thumb and finger. This point will help to relieve headaches, constipation or diarrhoea. It is a point sometimes used to expedite labour; therefore it should not be stimulated during pregnancy.

CHEST AND ABDOMEN

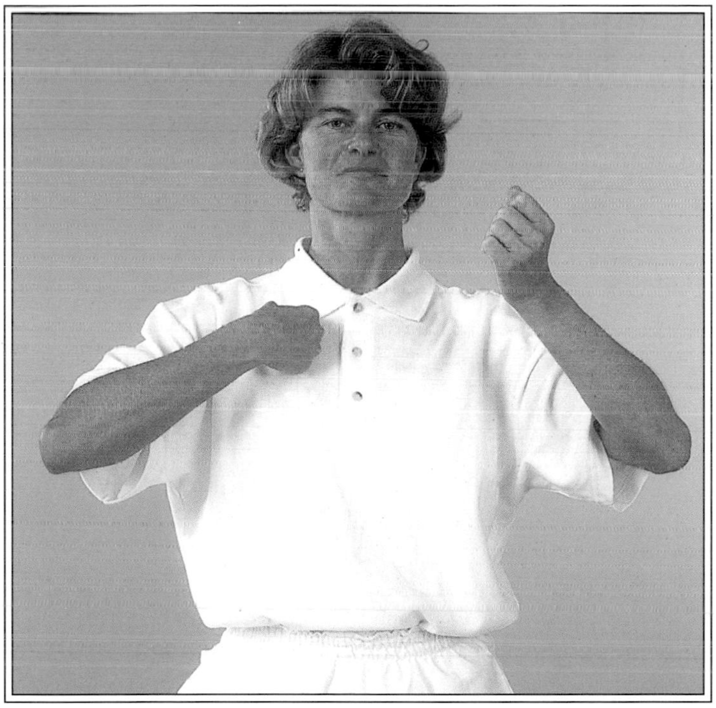

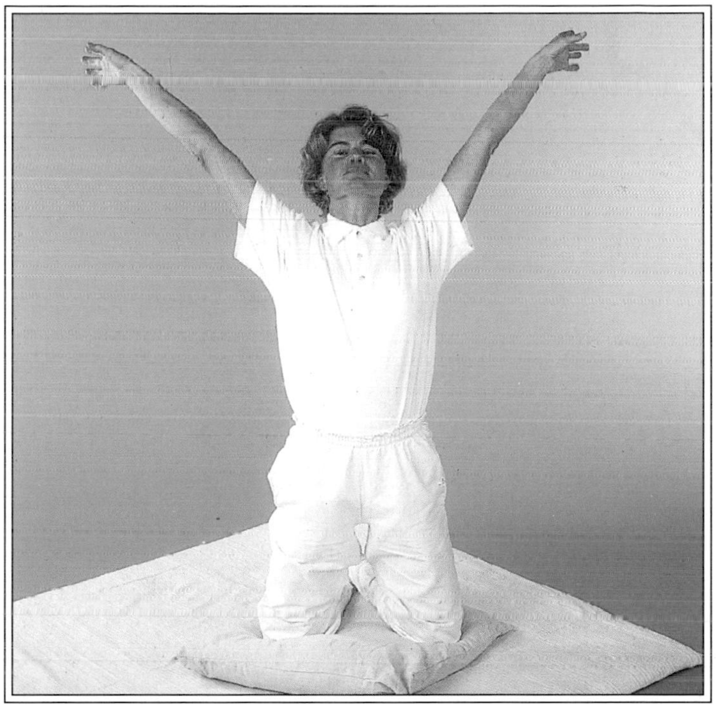

1 Open up your chest by tapping across it with loose fists, above and around your breasts and across the ribs. This will stimulate your lungs and enhance and strengthen your respiratory system.

2 Take a deep breath in as you throw your arms up over your head. Repeat the tapping. This is good for releasing tension in your chest and supporting you in expressing your thoughts and feelings.

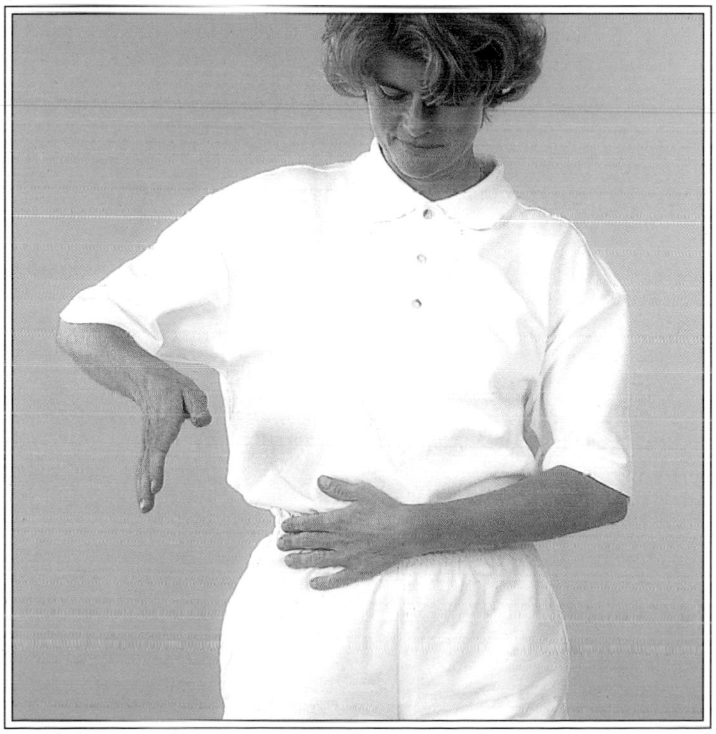

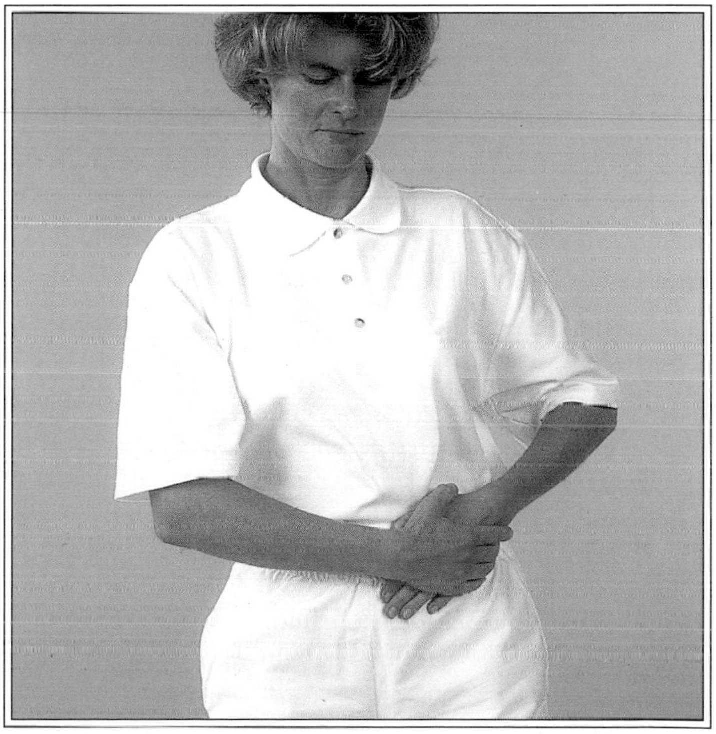

3 Proceed down towards your abdomen and with open hands tap around your abdomen gently in a clockwise direction, going down on the left and up on the right side. This follows the flow of circulation and digestion.

4 Place one hand on top of the other and make the same circular motion around your abdomen for a minute.

BACK

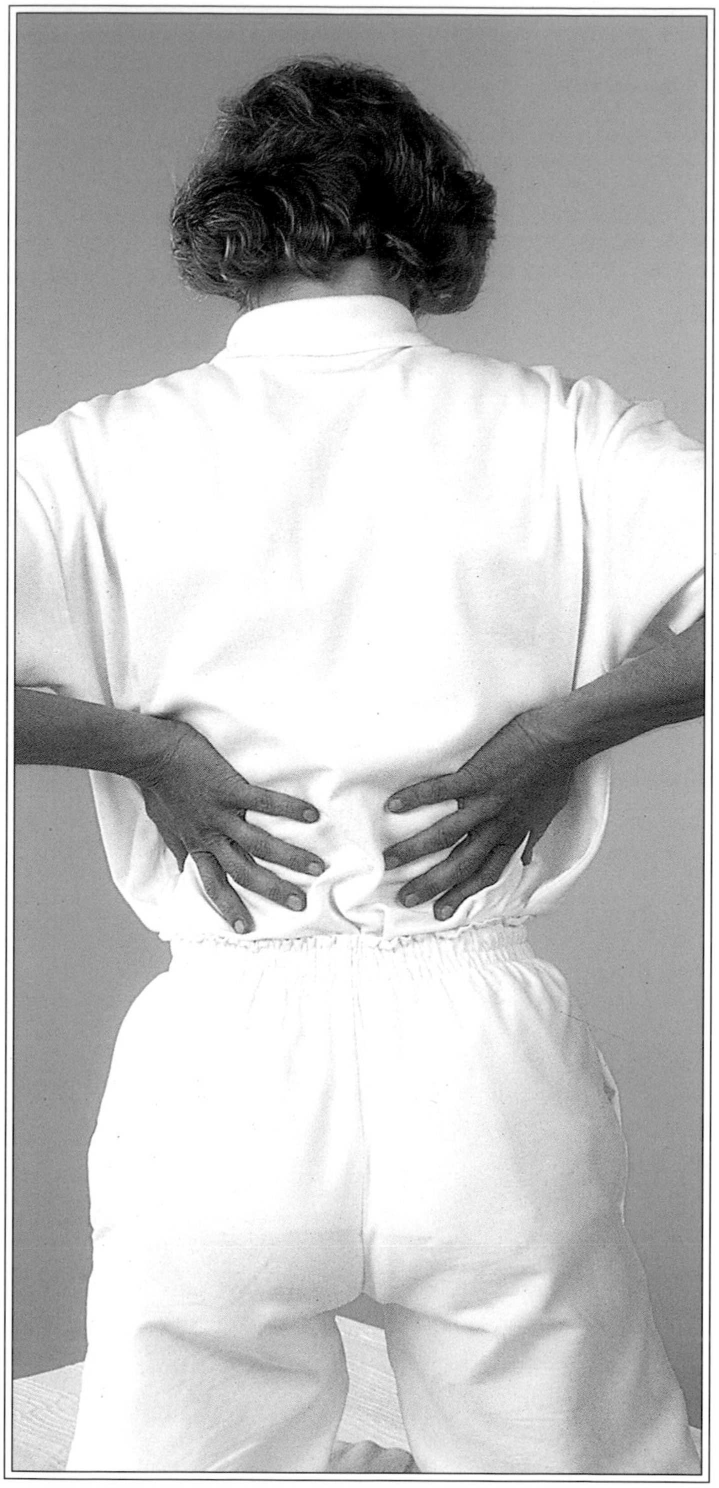

1 Place your hands on your back, just below the rib cage. This is the area of your kidneys. Start to rub the area slowly until you feel some warmth building up under your hands. This stimulates your kidney energy responsible for your vitality and also for warming your body.

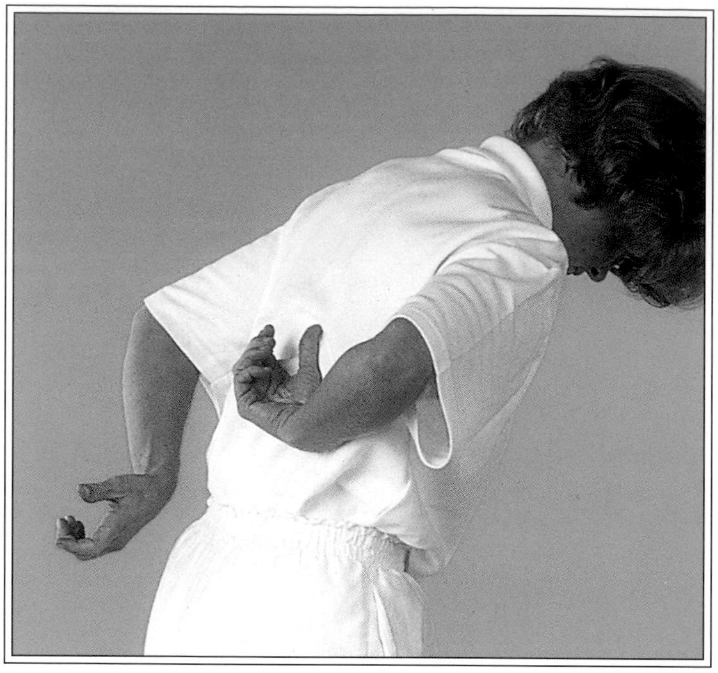

2 Stand up with your feet shoulder-width apart. Bend forward slightly and tap your lower back gently using your loose fists. Reach up as far as possible and move down to the lower part of your spine, your hips and the muscles of your buttocks. Releasing tension in this area will stimulate your digestive and elimination organs.

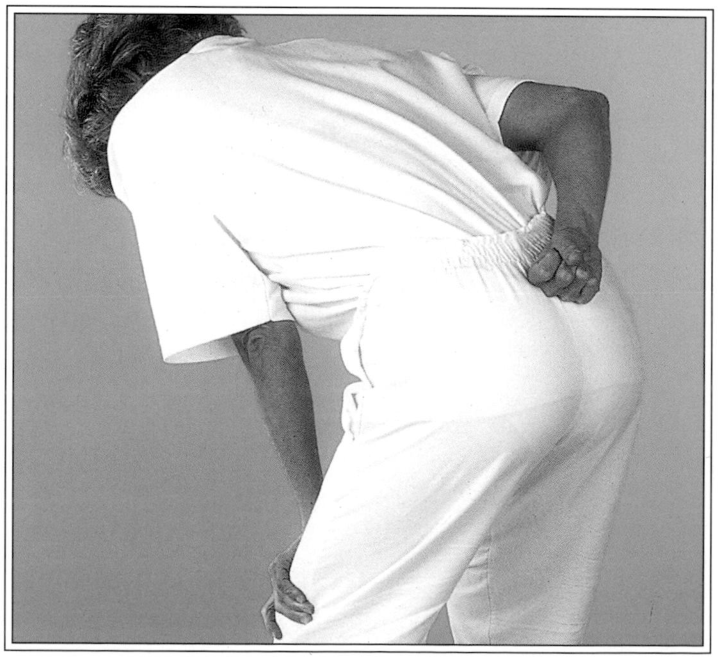

3 Using the back of your hand, tap across the sacrum bone at the base of your spine. This activates your nervous system and sends energy vibrations up the spine to your brain. Tapping the coccyx also decongests the sinuses, so breathe deeply through the nose when practising this exercise.

LEGS AND FEET

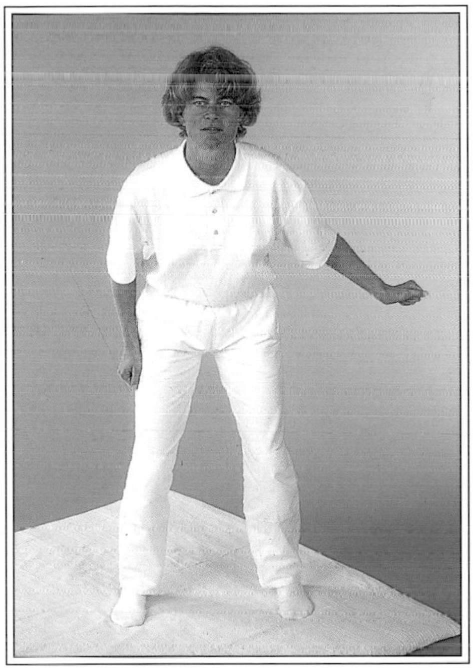

1 Stand with your feet wider apart. Keeping your knees slightly bent, start tapping with your fists down the outside of your legs from the hips to your ankles. This is where your gall-bladder meridian is located.

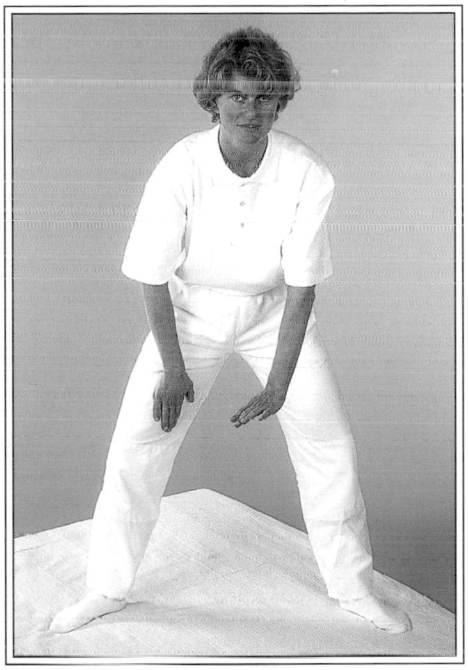

2 Now tap up the inside of your legs from the ankle to the groin area, stimulating your liver and spleen meridians. Use the palms of your hand rather than a fist if you prefer.

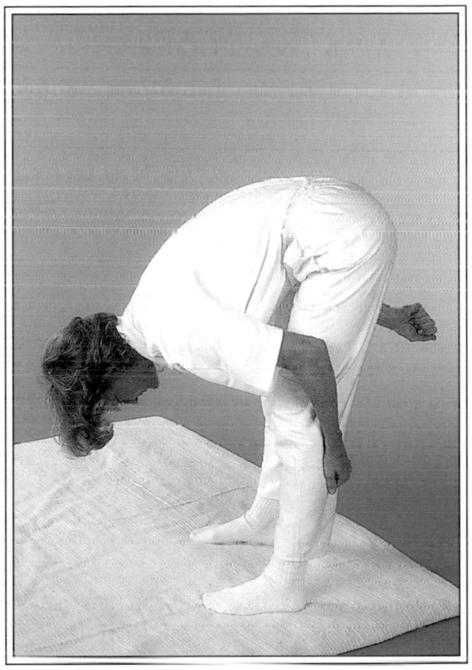

3 Then tap down the back of your legs following the flow of energy in your bladder meridian, from your buttocks to your heels. Come up the inside of your legs again.

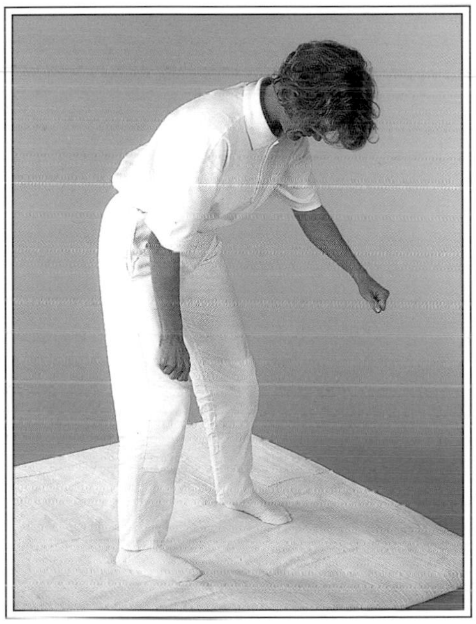

4 Tap down the front of your legs, slightly outside the big quadriceps muscle. Tap all the way down to the front of your ankles and then come up the inside of your legs. Repeat this whole sequence three times.

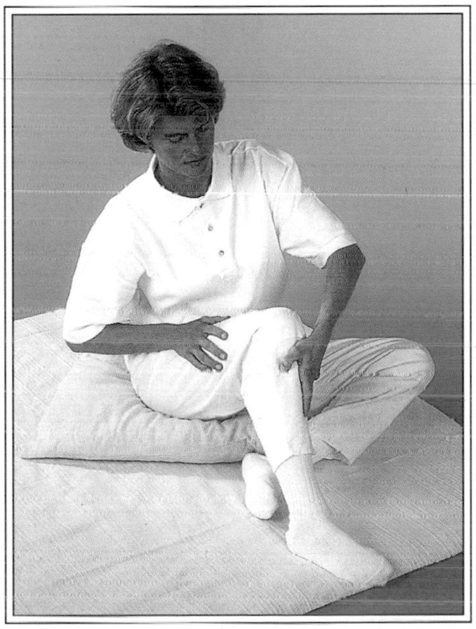

5 Along the stomach meridian there is a good point for general well-being, on the outside of your leg, below your knee. Apply gentle pressure for a few seconds.

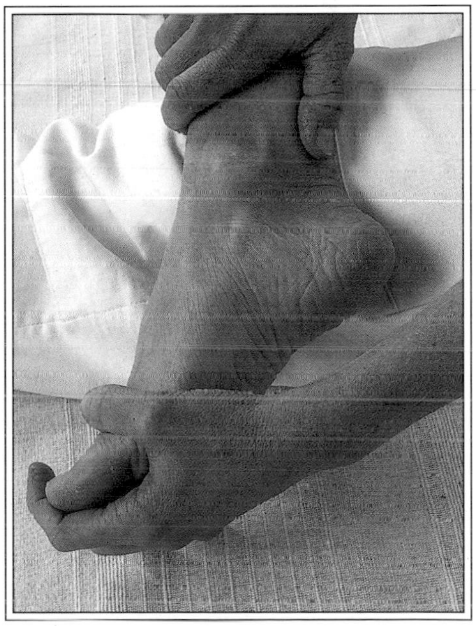

6 Remain seated on the floor, hold your foot and make a circular movement at the ankle to free up joint mobility.

▶

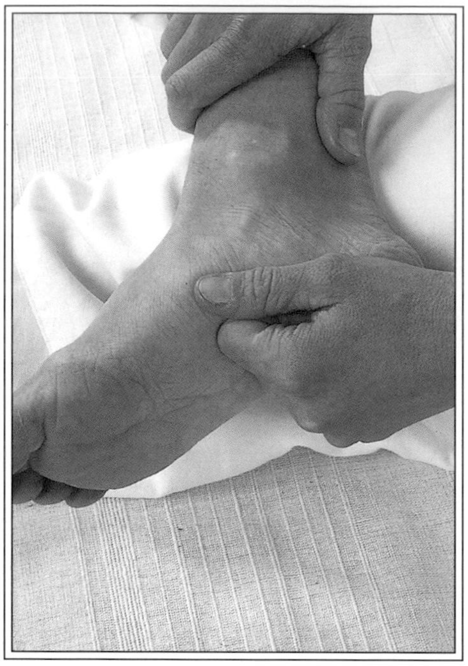

7 Tap the sole of the foot, with a loose fist, then massage the whole foot with both hands.

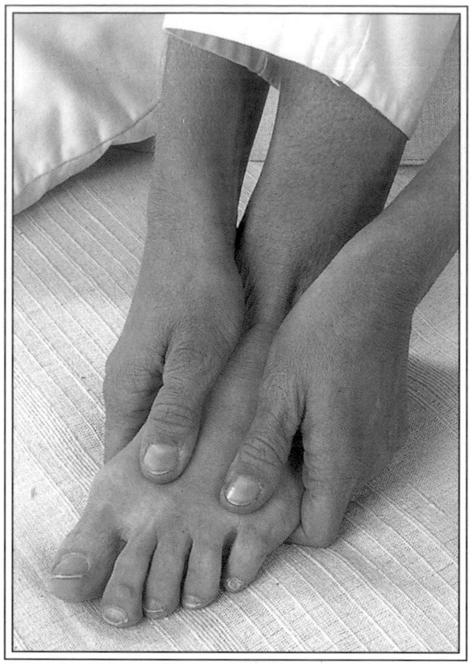

8 Hold your hands under the bottom of your foot and use your thumbs to rub downward along the top of your foot, in between each metatarsal bone to your toes.

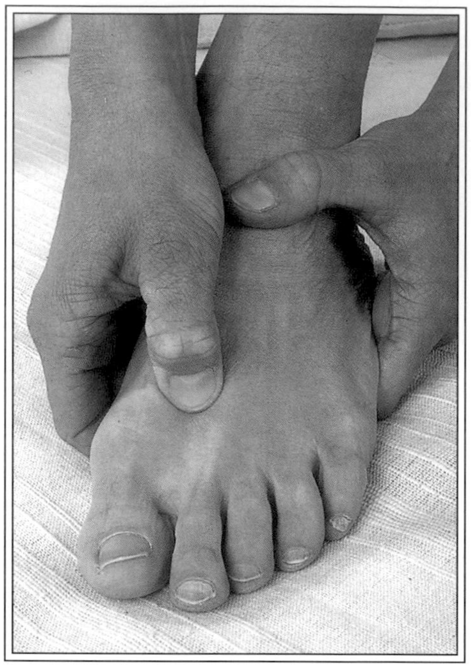

9 Massage the web between each toe and then massage the toe joints gently. The point between the big toe and the second toe is good for abdominal cramps: do not use during pregnancy.

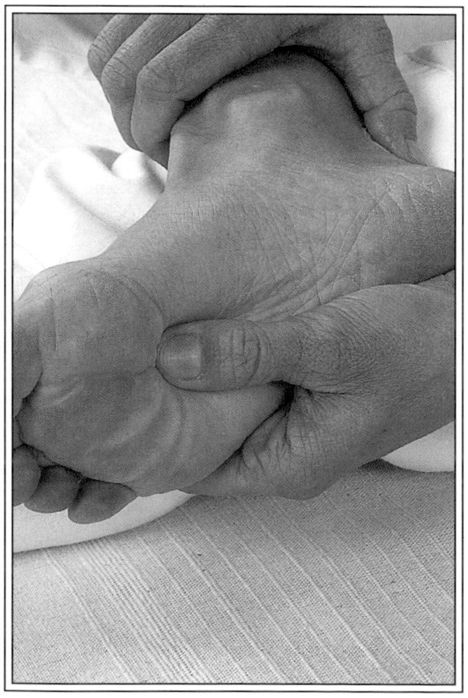

10 Come to the sole of your foot and apply pressure to this point with your thumb. This will have a revitalizing effect upon your body and stimulate energy flow.

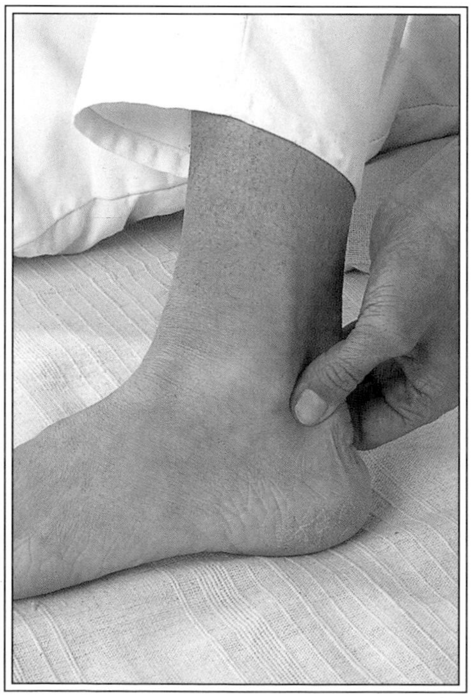

11 Use your thumbs to massage the area under the ankle bone. This area, spleen 6, located four fingers' width up from the inside ankle bone, is a great point to use for any menstrual disorders.

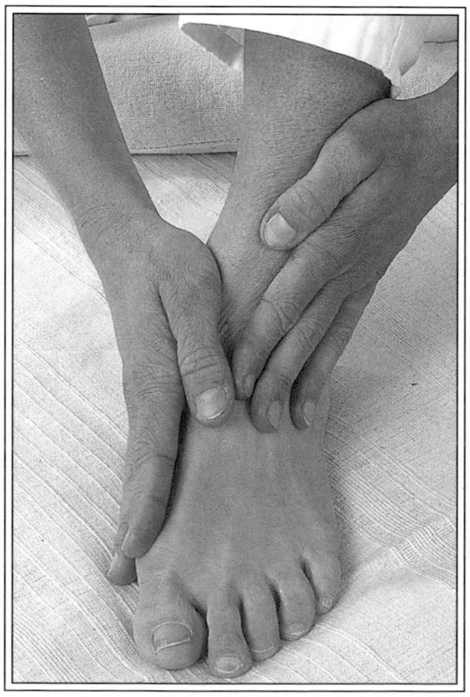

12 Give the whole foot a good rub. Then grab hold of your ankle with both hands and shake out your foot. Now repeat this whole sequence with your other foot.

COMPLETION

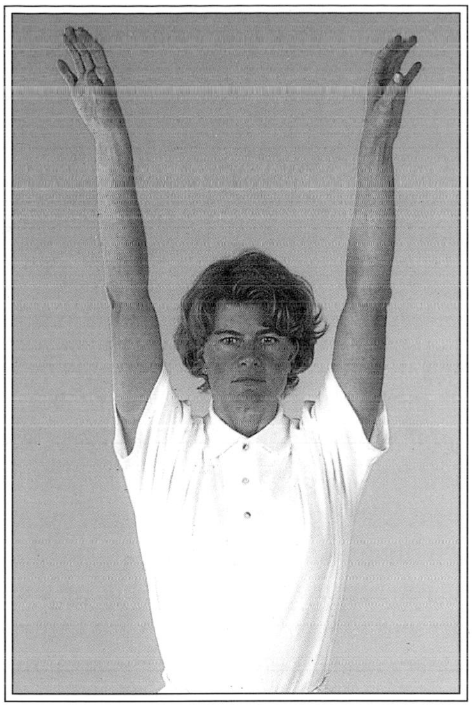

1 After having worked your body, stroke your meridians gently. First stand up with your feet apart. Take a deep breath in and lift your arms up.

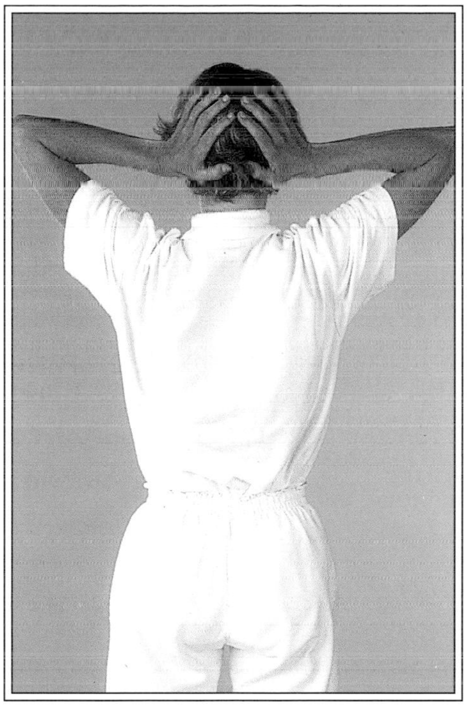

2 As you breathe out, bend your arms and place your hands on your head. Stroke down the back of your head to your neck.

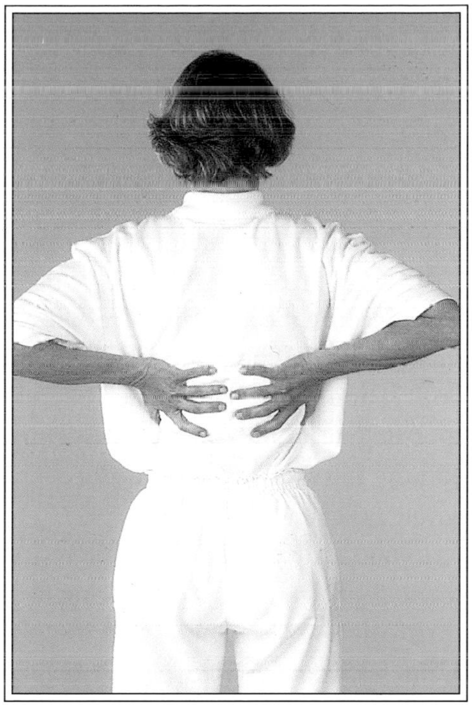

3 Bring your hands as high up as possible underneath the shoulder-blades and stroke down the whole of your back, buttocks and legs.

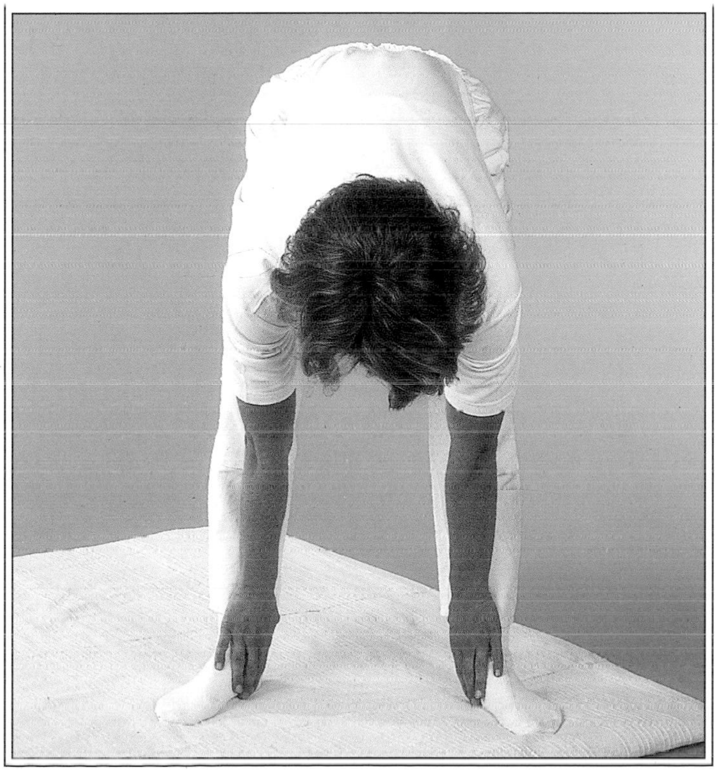

4 Open your legs and come up the inside of your legs to the groin area. Proceed up the front over your abdomen and up to your chest.

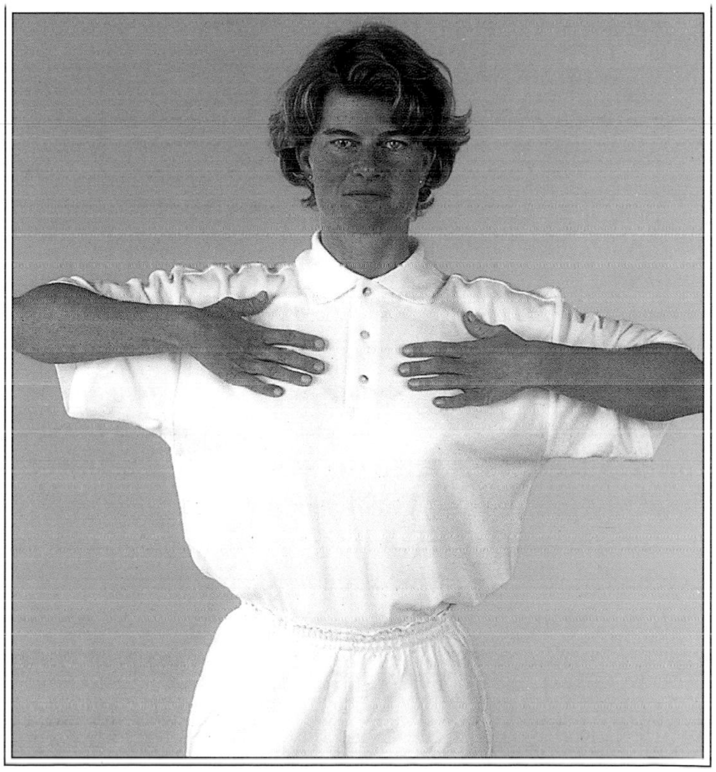

5 Stroke out to the sides and open up your chest. Open your arms to the sides and then repeat the whole completion sequence again, three to five times.

LUNGS AND LARGE INTESTINE

The lung and large intestine meridians are concerned with exchange of air and elimination of waste products. They represent the metal element which is connected with the air, breathing, boundaries and the emotion of grief. Be especially aware of the breath and the qualities of taking in and letting go in this exercise. Remember to keep observing your sensations and feelings. This exercise will help with breathing problems and regulate elimination.

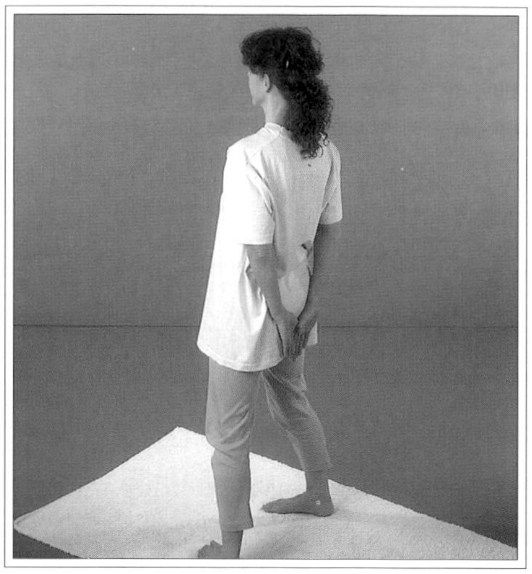

1 Stand with feet shoulder-width apart, toes turned slightly inwards, and feel your connection to the earth. Link your thumbs behind your back and check that your jaw is relaxed.

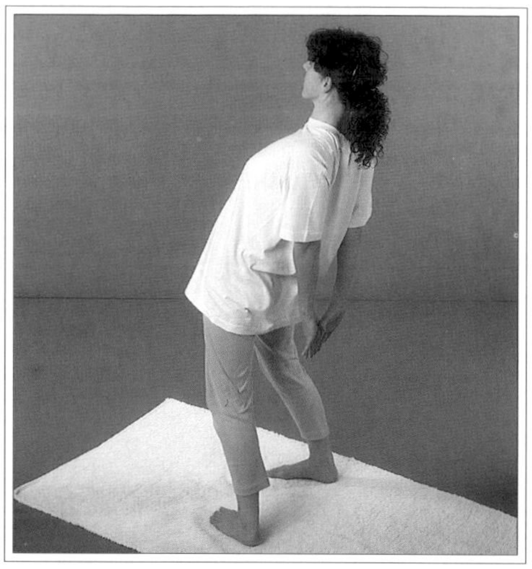

2 Breathe in, feeling the breath fill your body and lungs. Breathe out, straightening your arms, open the chest and lean slightly backwards.

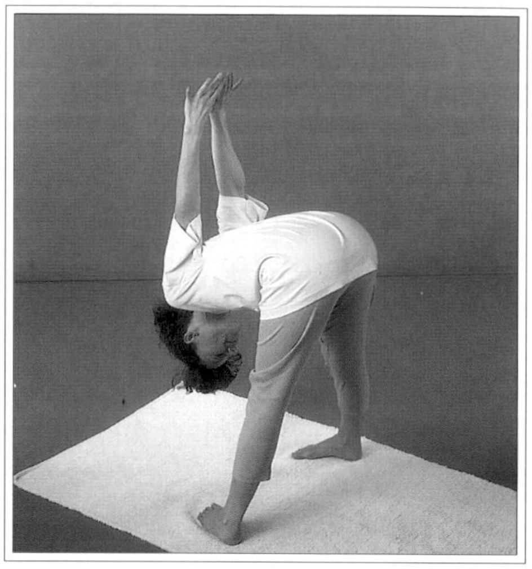

3 Breathe out, bending forward with your back, arms and legs straight. Keep this position for three breaths. On the third exhaled breath, return to your original position. Repeat twice more.

SPLEEN AND STOMACH

The spleen and stomach meridians represent the earth element which is concerned with digestion and nourishment. Be aware of your connection to the earth and the support it gives your body in this exercise.

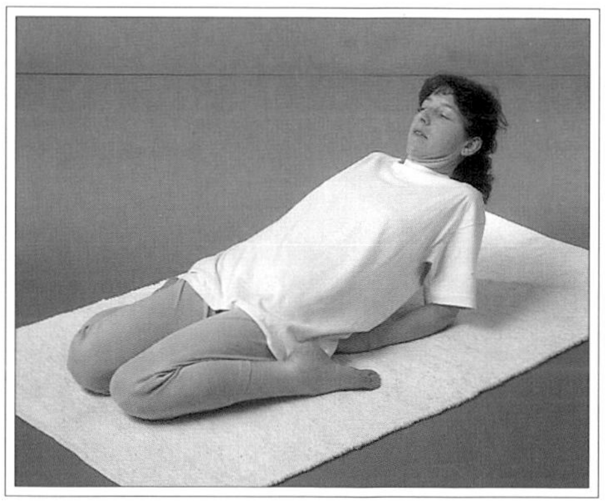

1 Kneel between your feet with your buttocks resting on the floor and your knees close together. If this is not possible, sit on a small cushion. On an exhaled breath gradually lean backwards, easing your body down by supporting yourself with your arms, and then elbows. Do **not** strain your knees or back, if you experience discomfort do not push. Use your breath to relax.

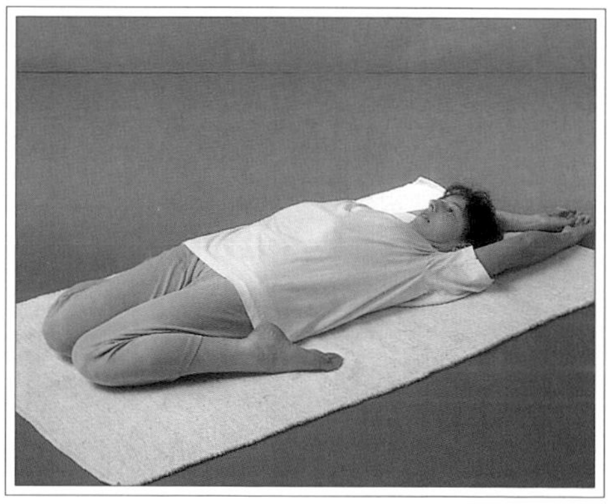

2 Ease down to the floor, without straining, keeping your knees close together on the floor. Stretch both arms over your head, interlock your fingers and stretch. Breathe deeply three times in this position, be aware of the movement of the belly as you breathe, your connection to the earth and the nourishment received through the breath.

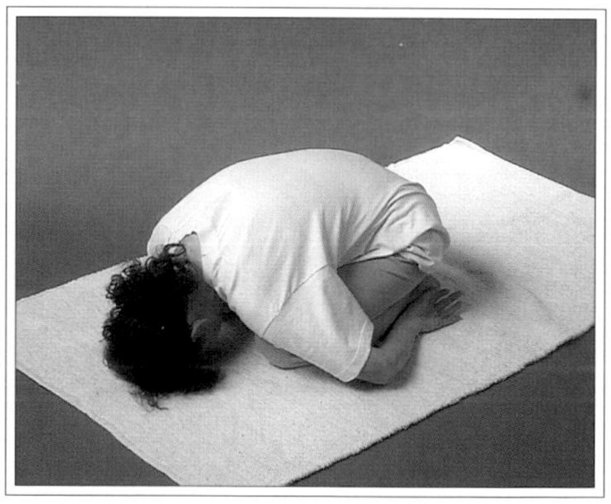

3 On the third exhaled breath ease out of the position and bend forward to ease out the lower back. Repeat twice more.

ALTERNATIVE SPLEEN/STOMACH EXERCISE

If you are unable to kneel you may try this alternative sequence. Stand with your feet together and feel your connection to the earth. Lift your left foot and clasp it behind you. Breathe out and draw the leg upwards behind you, keeping the knee close to the other leg. Hold and feel the stretch. On the third exhaled breath release the stretch and place your foot on the ground.

Repeat twice more, then carry out the sequence with the other leg.

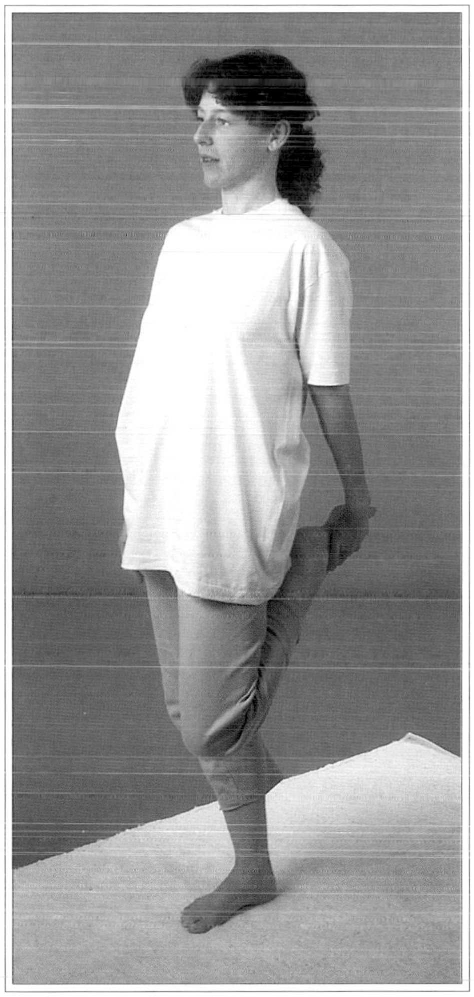

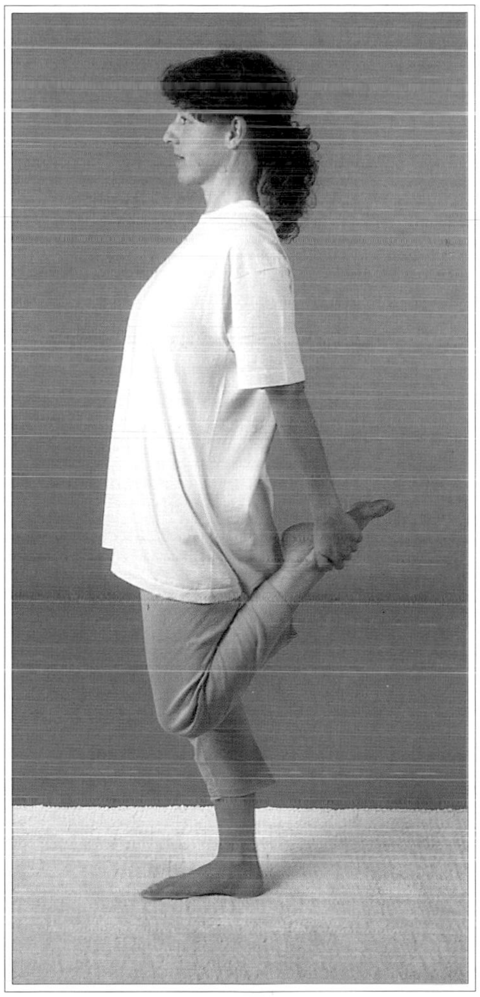

HEART AND SMALL INTESTINE

The heart and small intestine meridians represent the qualities of assimilation of food and integration of external stimuli and emotions in the body. Representing the fire element, they promote warm-heartedness and joy in our lives. Be aware of an alive warmth and increased circulation in this exercise.

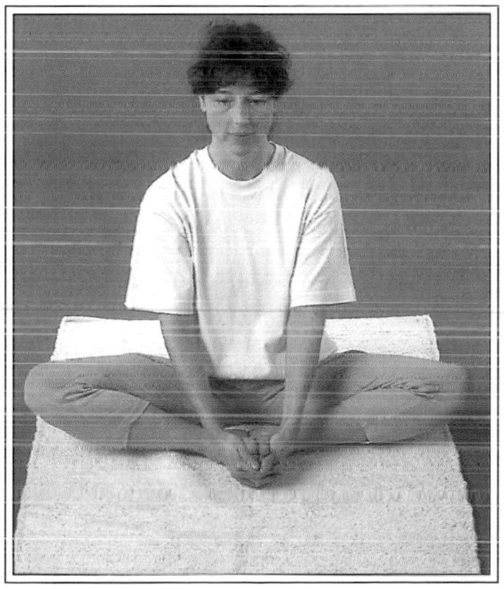

1 Sit on the floor, place the soles of your feet together, hold them and draw them close to your body. Breathe in, feeling a warm expansion in your body.

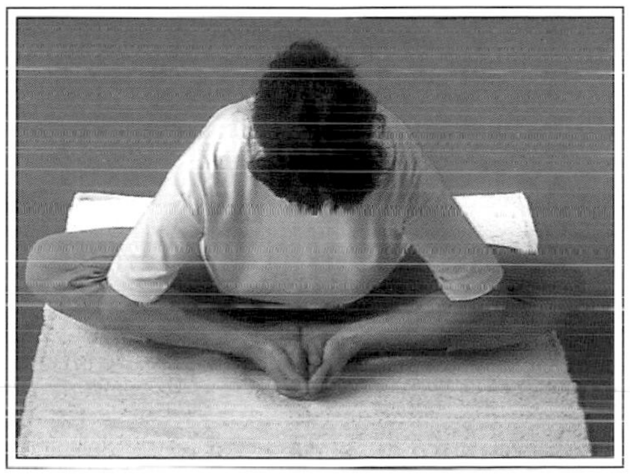

2 On the exhaled breath, draw your body down, bending your elbows and easing your knees towards the floor. Do not strain your hips. Keep your back straight. Breathe fully three times in position, feeling expansion in your back and observe how you feel. On the third exhaled breath, return to the original position. Repeat twice more.

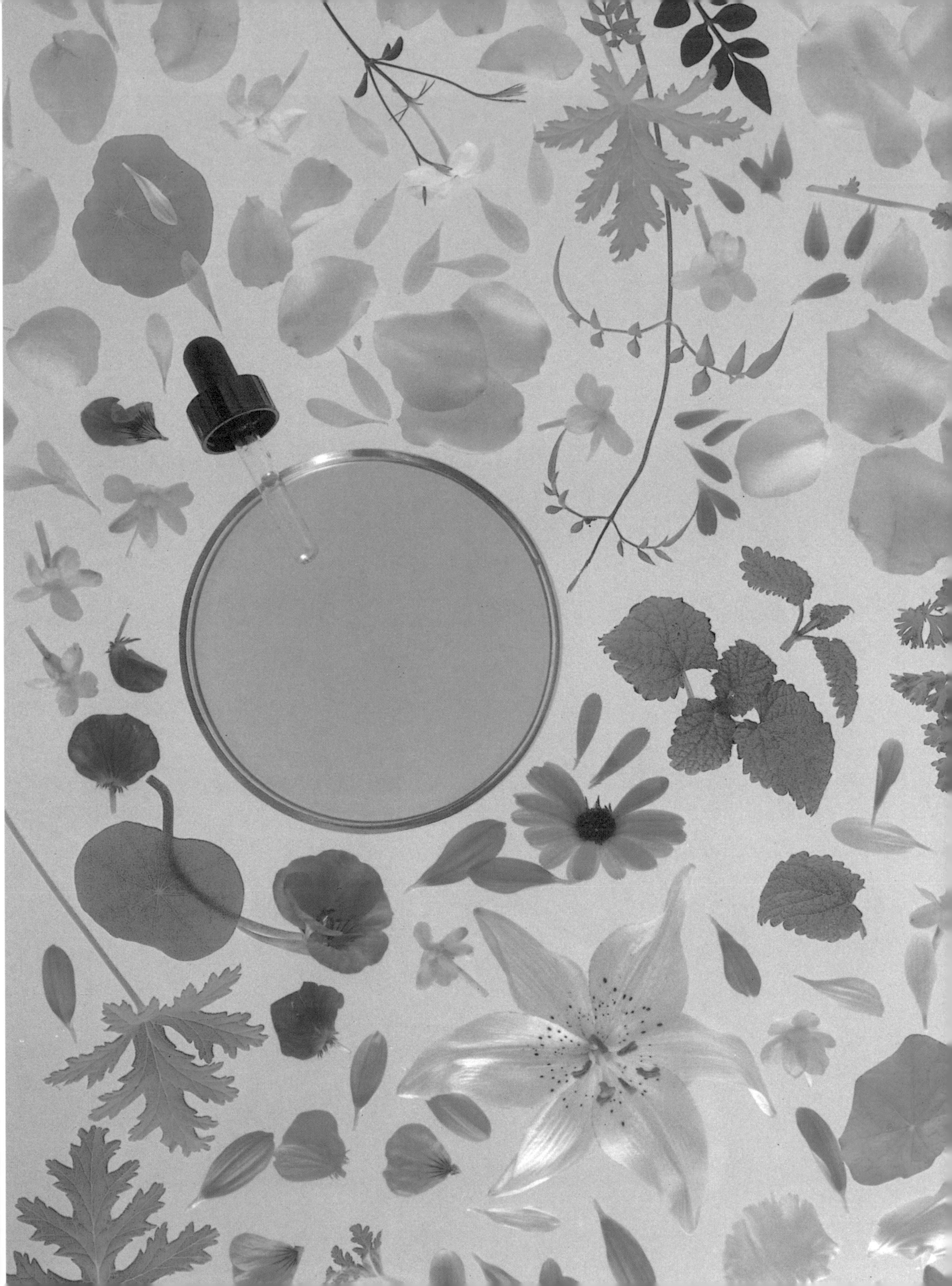

AROMATHERAPY

The pure essences of aromatic plants have been prized for thousands of years for their health-giving properties and heady scents. This section of the book takes an in-depth look at the ancient art of aromatherapy which has been refined through many centuries. Each individual essential oil is described in full detail; its origins and its therapeutic effects and uses are revealed. After a detailed look at the many qualities of essential oils, you can learn how to harness their therapeutic powers through massage, beauty treatments and perfuming your home, to enhance every aspect of your life. These potent, volatile essences are nature's gift to mind and body.

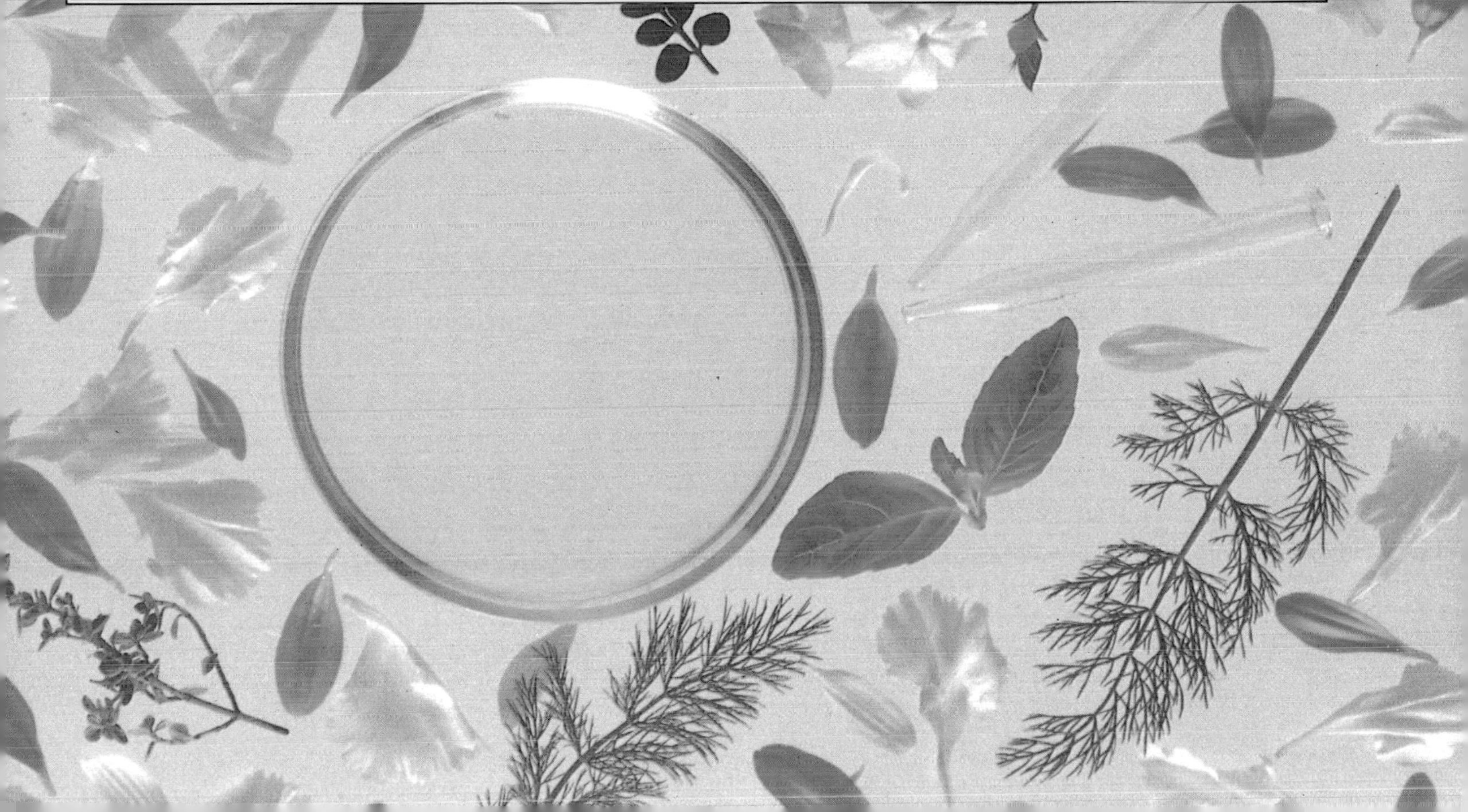

AN ANCIENT ART

The value of natural plant oils has been recognized for more than 6,000 years, for their healing, cleansing, preservative and mood-enhancing properties, as well as for the sheer pleasure of their fragrances. Today, these properties are being rediscovered as we look to the wisdom of past eras and civilizations to restore the balance that has been lost in modern-day life. Stress, pollution, unhealthy diet, hectic but sedentary lifestyles – all these factors have adverse effects on our bodies and spirits. The art of aromatherapy harnesses the potent pure essences of aromatic plants, flowers and resins, to work on the most powerful of senses – smell and touch – to restore the harmony of body and mind.

SECRETS OF THE OILS DISCOVERED

The origins of aromatherapy can be traced through the religious, medical and social practices of all the major civilizations. It is likely that the Chinese were the first to discover the remarkable medicinal powers of plants around 4500 BC. However, it is the Egyptians who must take the credit for recognizing and fully exploiting the physical and spiritual properties of aromatic essences. From hieroglyphs and paintings we know that aromatic preparations were used as offerings to the gods. Furthermore, the natural antiseptic and antibacterial properties of essential oils and resins, particularly cedarwood and frankincense, made them ideal for the purpose of preserving corpses in preparation for the next world. The discovery of remarkably well-preserved mummies up to 5,000 years after their preparation is a tribute to the embalmer's art.

By around 3000 BC priests who had been using the oils in religious ceremonies and embalming rites became aware of the usefulness of their properties for the living, too. Closely guarding their secrets, they became the healers of their time, mixing and prescribing "magic" medicinal potions. Use of essential oils gradually permeated all levels of society as cosmetics and perfumes became widespread.

From Hippocrates we know the Greeks had some awareness of the therapeutic properties of the oils and their value as sedatives and stimulants was certainly recognized. The Greeks and Romans used aromatics widely in rituals and ceremonies and the oils played an important role in the rise in popularity of baths and massage and body-culture generally. However, with the fall of the Roman Empire the use of essential oils died out in Europe.

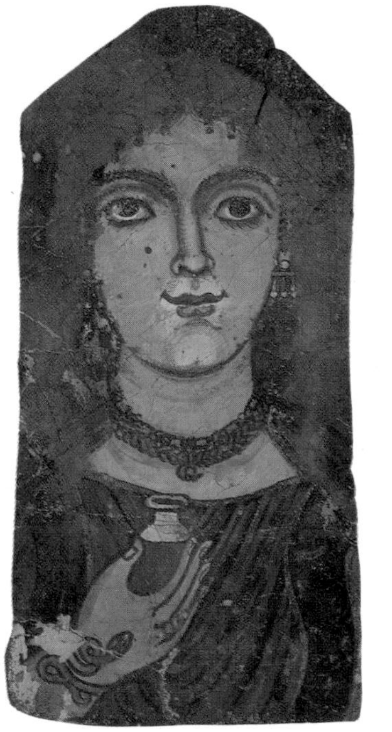

LEFT: The personal use of perfume was widespread in ancient Greece and Rome. The Roman girl in this portrait (from around AD 350) carries a small pot of aromatics.

RIGHT: From the tomb of the Noble Senedjem, ancient Egypt. The cones of unguent worn on the heads melted in the heat, waxing and scenting the hair and body.

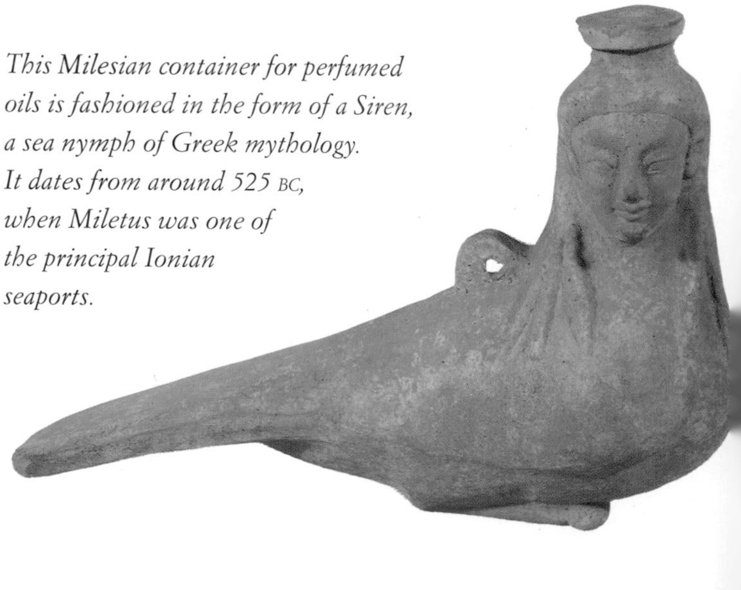

This Milesian container for perfumed oils is fashioned in the form of a Siren, a sea nymph of Greek mythology. It dates from around 525 BC, when Miletus was one of the principal Ionian seaports.

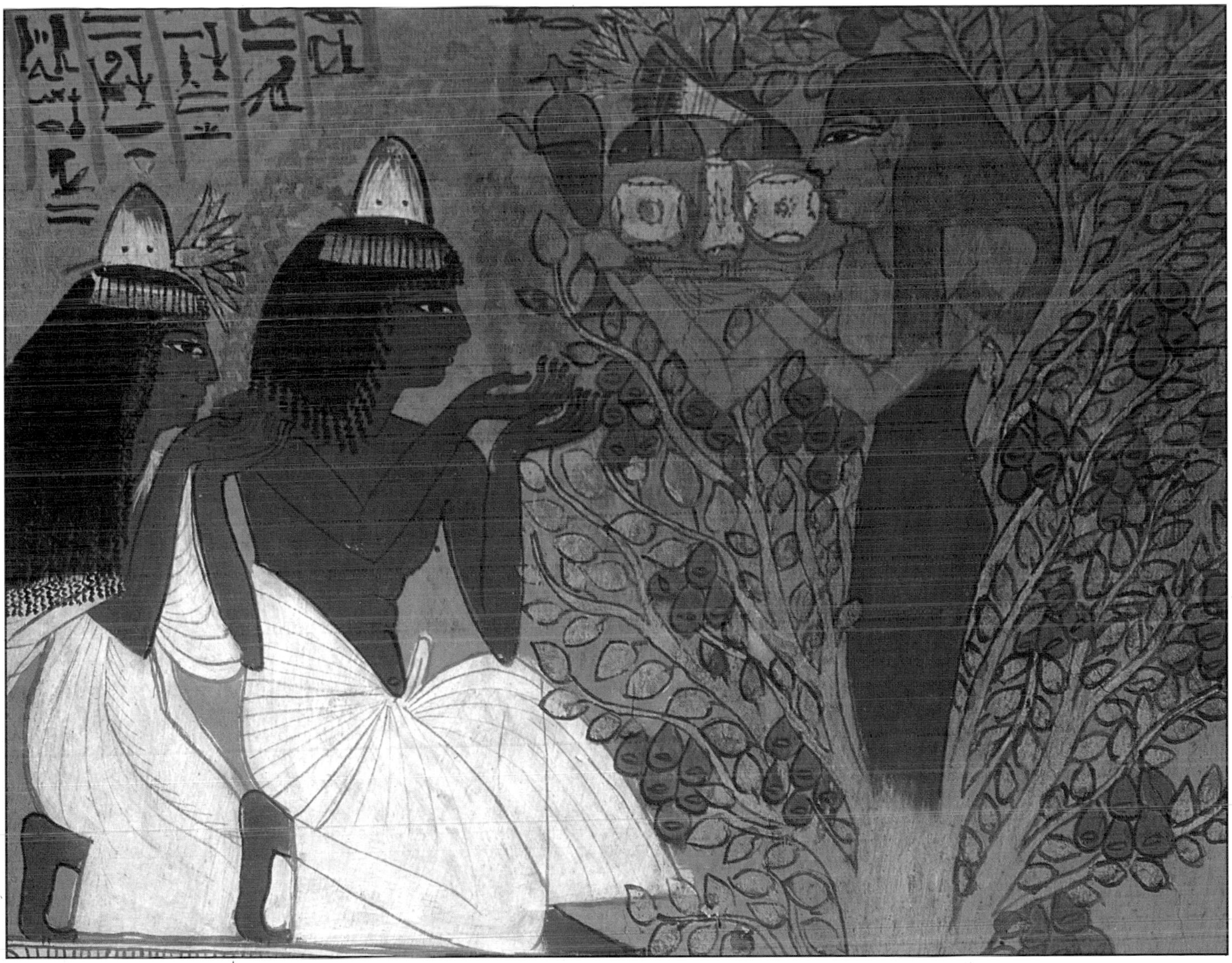

The art flourished elsewhere, though, particularly in Arabia, where Avicenna first distilled rose essence in around AD 1000. Arabia became the world's centre for production of perfume, importing raw materials from Egypt, India, Tibet and China, and trading their products internationally.

With the Crusaders the art of perfumery was reintroduced to Europe around the twelfth century. Records show that aromatics were used as protection against the plague and the lower incidence of death among perfumiers suggests they were to some degree effective. The fifteenth century saw the rise of the great European perfumiers, and their wares were widely used to disguise body smells and ward off sickness. By the seventeenth century the aphrodisiac properties were well recognized, and with the work of herbalists, such as Culpeper, the therapeutic properties also started to be recorded, laying the foundation for modern aromatherapy.

THE MODERN RENAISSANCE

The term "Aromathérapie" was first used in 1928 by a French chemist, René-Maurice Gattefossé, to describe the therapeutic action of aromatic plant essences. His work was taken up by Dr Jean Valnet who found the essences' remarkable regenerative and antiseptic properties effective for healing the wounds of World War II soldiers.

The application of aromatherapy to beauty therapy and health care was pioneered by Marguerite Maury in her influential book, *The Secret of Life and Youth*. She also developed the method of applying the oils through massage.

Today there is a world-wide revival in the art of aromatherapy and contemporary research is beginning to understand the scientific foundations of the oils' properties and applications, discovered by trial and error over thousands of years.

AROMATICS

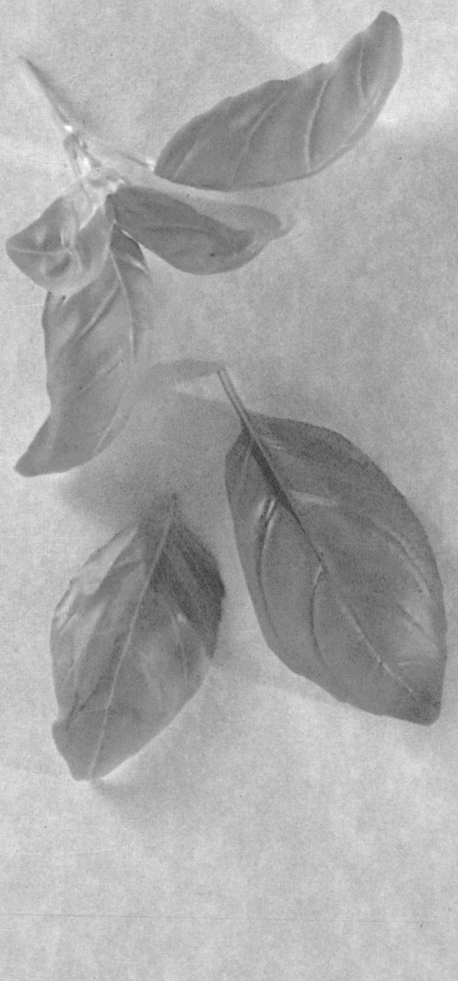

Aromatic oils extracted from flowers, fruits, leaves, barks, resins and roots have been used throughout the centuries for their healing properties and marvellous fragrances. Hundreds of essential oils are used today in such industries as food, cosmetics, pharmaceuticals and perfumery. Modern-day aromatherapy uses a much smaller selection, but the range of aromas and applications is nonetheless remarkable.

This section is a connoisseur's guide to thirty-five of the most popular, versatile and safe oils. Get to know their individual characters, their origins, their therapeutic values and discover your own favourites. Lavender, geranium and rosemary are excellent all-round oils and provide a good basis for any collection. Rose, though expensive, is also well worth the investment if you would like to explore the benefits and delights of aromatherapy.

BASIL

OCIMUM BASILICUM

Origins Basil was used in baths and body massage by ancient Greek nobles. The Egyptians used the aromatic fragrance in their offerings to the gods and also mixed it with essences of myrrh and incense to embalm bodies. In India it is believed to offer protection to the soul and is sacred to the Hindu gods Krishna and Vishnu.

Description Native of Africa and the Seychelles and now grown as a popular culinary herb in Europe, it can grow up to 90 cm (3 ft) in height and has small white flowers. The essence is distilled from the leaves and is a greenish-yellow with sweet green overtones.

Therapeutic effects Ideal as a nerve tonic, to lift fatigue, anxiety and depression. Also good for bronchitis, colds, fever, gout and indigestion, and reputed to soothe snake bites.

Uses Inhalation, baths and massage. It has both hot and cold qualities. When used in the bath or smoothed over the body it has an invigorating effect – great for sluggish skin and pepping up circulation. Combined with other oils such as thyme it also acts as a powerful antiseptic.

Cautionary note A powerful depressant if over-used. Also best to avoid during pregnancy.

Bay

Pimenta racemosa

Origins Roman emperors wore sprigs of bay, known as *Laurus nobilis* (Roman laurel), not only as a sign of wealth, but to ward off evil spirits. Greek priestesses chewed the leaves for their soporific effect, and after gastronomic banquets it was chewed as a breath freshener.

Description Popular as a culinary herb, bay is an attractive evergreen shrub whose shiny leathery leaves produce clusters of yellowish-green flowers in spring. The spicy-smelling oil is extracted from the leaves and is yellowish-brown in colour.

Therapeutic effects As a pulmonary antiseptic, it helps relieve bronchitis, colds and flu. Also used to aid digestion and sleep, to soothe rheumatic aches and pains, and as a general tonic.

Uses Inhalation, baths and massage. Widely used in perfume and exotic bath essences for its uplifting effects.

Benzoin

Styrax benzoin

Origins In the Far East the gum from the benzoin tree was one of the main ingredients used in incense to drive away evil spirits. The compound tincture is highly potent, pharmaceutically used in friar's balsam and as a fixative in perfume.

Description The benzoin tree is cultivated in Borneo, Java, Malaysia, Sumatra and Thailand. Like the rubber tree, its gum is taken from the bark by making a deep incision in the trunk. The gum is dark, with reddish-brown coloured streaks. These pigments contain the fatty oils which exude a delicious aroma similar to vanilla.

Therapeutic effects Valuable for treating urinary infections, it has a warming, relaxing, action suitable for respiratory conditions such as bronchitis, coughs and colds. Also effective for relieving skin conditions, and for gout.

Uses Inhalation, massage and in cough medicines. This is an energizing oil which can be used in one of two forms: simple tincture or compound – the former is not so toxic and is preferable for skin conditions.

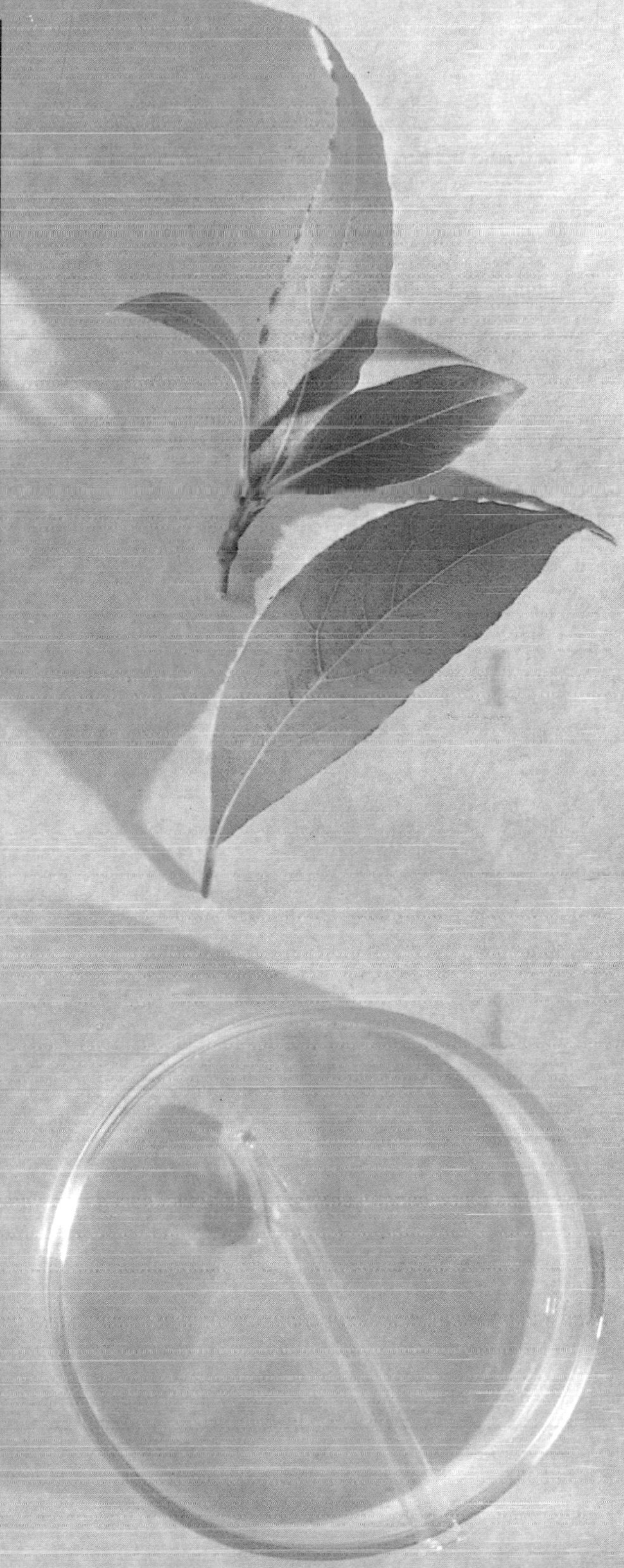

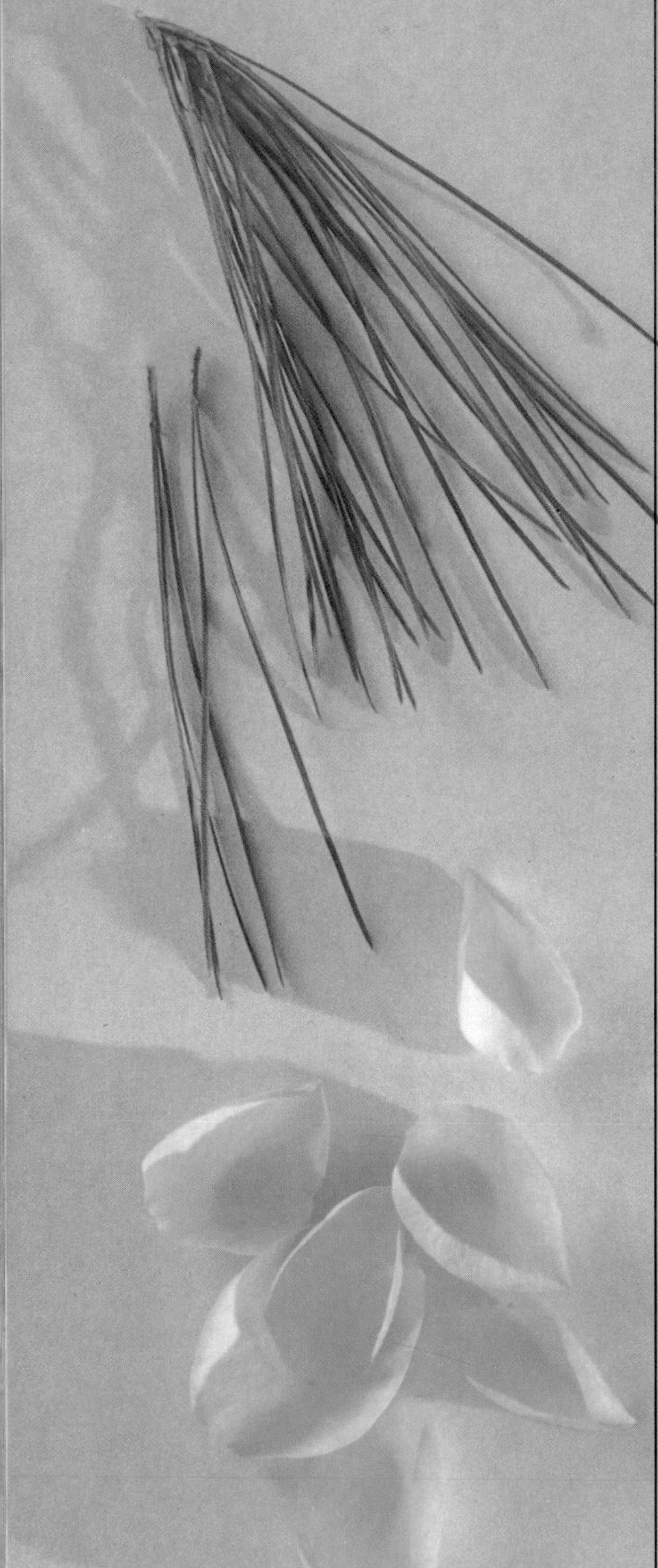

Pine

Pinus sylvestris

Origins The Scandinavians have traditionally used pine in the sauna or steam bath for its refreshing and antiseptic qualities.

Description This species of conifer grows wild all over Europe, North America and the former Soviet Union. General pine oil comes from the heart of the wood but the best essences are distilled from the pine needle. The oil has a fresh fragrance with a resinous woody undertone.

Therapeutic effects Acts as an antiseptic, and is particularly valuable for treating the respiratory tract, for bronchitis, catarrh, colds and sinusitis. Will also help relieve cystitis, arthritis and muscular aches and pains.

Uses Inhalation, baths and massage. Widely used to give coniferous fragrance in household products and in some masculine perfumes, this oil is popularly used throughout the cosmetics and pharmaceutical industries in balms, body rubs, soaps and bath oils. The oil can be used as an antiseptic deodorizer (add a few drops to freshen shoes) and in saunas or hot tubs for its invigorating steam.

Rose

Rosa centifolia, Rosa damascena

Origins The rose has been loved for its fragrance at least since Roman times, when it was used in garlands, scented baths and perfumes, often in ostentatious public displays. But the rose has its private uses too: Cleopatra reputedly carpeted her bedroom in rose petals to aid her seduction of Mark Antony.

Description The *Damascena* rose is cultivated in Bulgaria. The flowers are picked at dawn and the yellowy-brown oil is extracted within 24 hours. It takes approximately 5 tonnes (5 tons) of blossoms to produce just 1 kg (2 lb) of oil – not surprisingly one of the most expensive in the world. *Centifolia* roses, also yielding a richly fragrant oil, are cultivated in France, Algeria, Morocco and Egypt.

Therapeutic effects An aphrodisiac and mood enhancer, rose is a general tonic and fortifier, useful for circulatory problems, constipation, headaches and mental fatigue, menstrual and menopausal problems and skin disorders.

Uses Baths and massage. One of the least toxic of all essences, it is particularly good for older, drier, skins, and is useful for pot pourri or to perfume bed linens and underwear (add a few drops to the final rinse).

Rosemary

Rosmarinus officinalis

Origins First favoured by the Egyptians, rosemary was popular with the Greeks and Romans who believed it symbolized love and death. During the plague it was burned in public places and worn around the neck for its antiseptic qualities.

Description A small shrub, it grows to around 90 cm (3 ft) high, with grey-green leaves and pale blue-white flowers. The clear oil is steam-distilled from the flowers and leaves, and has a powerful, warm, woody aroma.

Therapeutic effects A good stimulant, especially for the circulation and memory. Also helps alopecia, bronchitis, burns, colds, dandruff, diarrhoea, flatulence, headaches and obesity.

Uses Inhalation, baths and massage. Inhale from a handkerchief to clear headaches and fatigue. In massage it stimulates the lymphatic system.

Cautionary note Use in low concentration, as excessive doses may bring about epileptic fits or convulsions. Do not use in early pregnancy or if you have high blood pressure.

Sage

Salvia officinalis, Salvia sclarea (Clary sage)

Origins A sacred herb, its properties were used by the Egyptians to help cure infertility in women. The Chinese have used it medicinally for centuries.

Description The many varieties of common sage are all shrub-like herbs with rough, wrinkled leaves. The oil is distilled from the dried leaves and has a powerful, spicy fragrance with a hint of camphor.

Therapeutic effects A tonic, particularly renowned for regulating menstruation, it can also help relieve arthritis, bacterial infections, throat infections and water retention.

Clary sage (*Salvia sclarea*) is also used for its sedative and euphoric effects, and in treating insomnia, anxiety and depression, as well as menstrual and menopausal problems. It has a spicy fragrance, rather more floral than common sage.

Uses Bathing and massage. A sage bath helps muscular aches and the effects of prolonged stress or mental strain.

Cautionary note In high doses, sage can overstimulate and should be avoided by anyone who suffers from epilepsy. Both sage and clary sage should be avoided in early pregnancy.

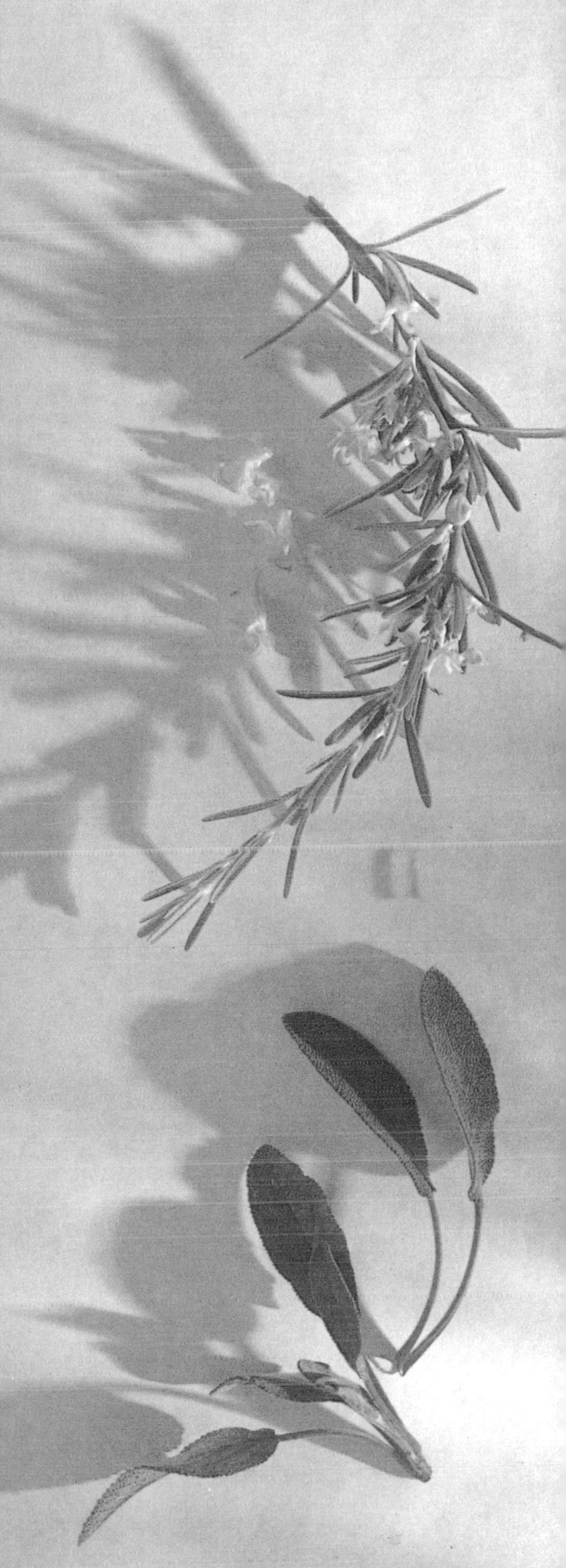

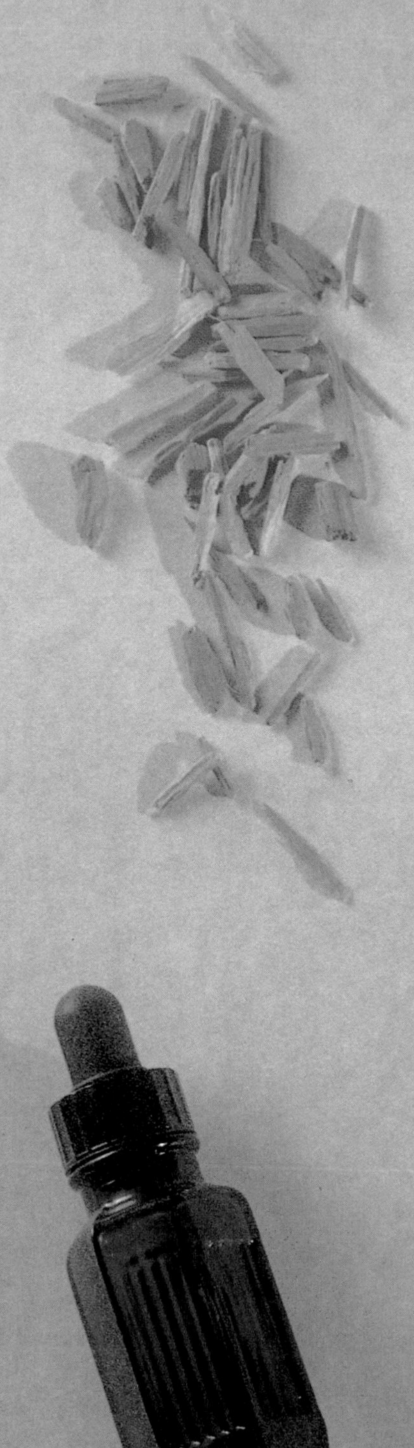

SANDALWOOD

SANTALUM ALBUM

Origins In China, India and Egypt sandalwood was used in perfumes and cosmetics. It has also been prized by furniture makers, and in India many of the temples were built with this lovely wood. Worshippers also covered their bodies with its essence, along with rose, jasmine and narcissus.

Description The evergreen sandalwood tree grows to a height of up to 8 m (30 ft) in Indonesia, South East Asia and in particular East India. The syrupy, balsamic oil is extracted from the roughly chipped and powdered wood by steam distillation. It has a rich, warm, woody odour. It is used as a fixative in perfumes and gives the lingering classic base notes in many expensive fragrances.

Therapeutic effects Sandalwood's sedative properties are good for treating depression and tension. It is also an expectorant and antispasmodic; useful for bronchitis, coughs, nausea, cystitis and skin complaints. Regarded as an aphrodisiac.

Uses Inhalation and massage. Apply in a warm compress to revitalize dehydrated skin. Blends well with neroli and rose. Massage enhances its soothing effects.

TEA TREE

MELALEUCA ALTERNIFOLIA

Origins The antiseptic properties of the tea tree were discovered centuries ago by the Aborigines of Australia who used it medicinally for treating sunburn and many bacterial/fungal infections, from ringworm to athlete's foot. It was known as an antidote for venomous snake bites.

Description A native of Australia and Tasmania, it is often referred to as the swamp tree. It produces white hanging flowers on a long spike, but the pale green oil is extracted from the twigs and leaves, which have a strong aromatic odour. The oil itself has a camphorous smell, reminiscent of eucalyptus.

Therapeutic effects A strong disinfectant and antiseptic, it is ideal for skin complaints, including athlete's foot, burns, cold sores, mouth ulcers, verrucas, thrush and warts. Also effective for many respiratory complaints.

Uses Inhalation and baths. Tea tree can be used to kill fleas on pets but is more commonly used as a deodorizing/antiseptic foot bath. Dab on cold sores. Inhale to alleviate laryngitis and bronchitis. Diluted in water, it can be used as a mouthwash (not swallowed) to soothe ulcers.

Thyme
Thymus vulgaris

Origins The ancient Egyptians incorporated the essential oil of thyme into their embalming fluids. The Greeks drank a herbal infusion of the leaves after banquets to aid digestion. Culpeper considered it a great lung strengthener and a remedy for shortness of breath.

Description This common low-growing wild herb has dark green leaves, woody stalks and small pink flowers. It is cultivated throughout the Mediterranean, Algeria, former Yugoslavia and in Egypt for culinary and pharmaceutical uses. The oil is extracted from the whole flowering herb by steam-distillation and has a pungent, sweet herbaceous smell. It is an important component in colognes and herbal perfumes.

Therapeutic effects Helps fatigue and anxiety, but best known as a natural antiseptic for treating coughs and infections of the respiratory tract. Good too for rheumatic aches and for skin problems such as sores and swellings.

Uses Massage and baths. When added to a bath, its invigorating effects help revive tired muscles.

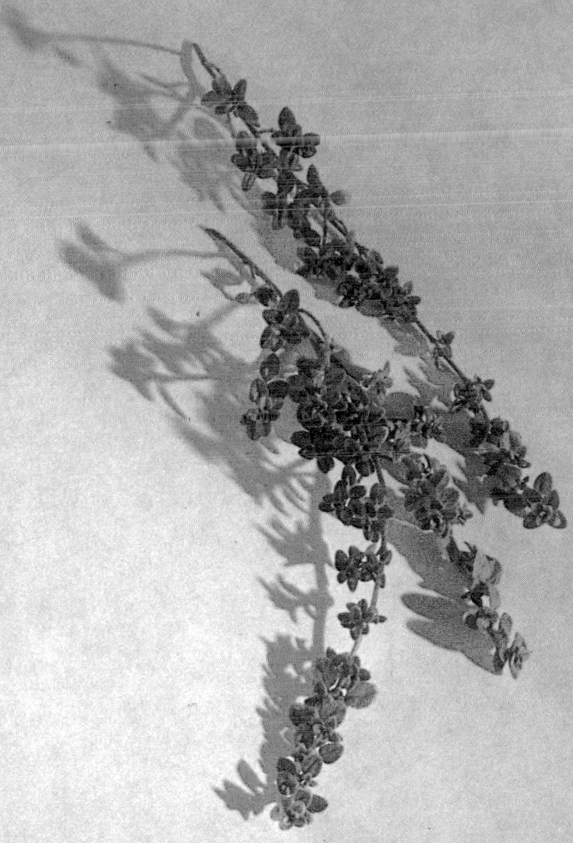

Ylang-Ylang
Cananga odorata

Origins A tropical tree, its first medicinal uses were to treat malaria, soothe insect bites and generally fight infections. Its antiseptic qualities were appreciated but it was also recognized as an aphrodisiac and a tonic to the nervous system. In the past, the flowers were mixed with coconut oil to perfume and condition the body and hair.

Description A native of Indonesia and the Philippines, the ylang-ylang tree reaches a height of 20 m (60 ft). The yellow flowers are freshly picked in the early morning and the oil extracted by steam-distillation. It has a narcotic, floral-sweet, jasmine-like aroma which adds warmth to perfumes.

Therapeutic effects A great relaxer (if used sparingly) and highly recommended for anxiety, depression, insomnia and frigidity. It also has benefits in treating high blood pressure and skin conditions.

Uses Baths and massage. This oil can soothe away all forms of stress when used as a bath oil or massaged onto the body. Its lasting fragrance is often used in facial and skin preparations, pot pourri and pomanders. It blends well with bergamot, melissa, sandalwood and jasmine.

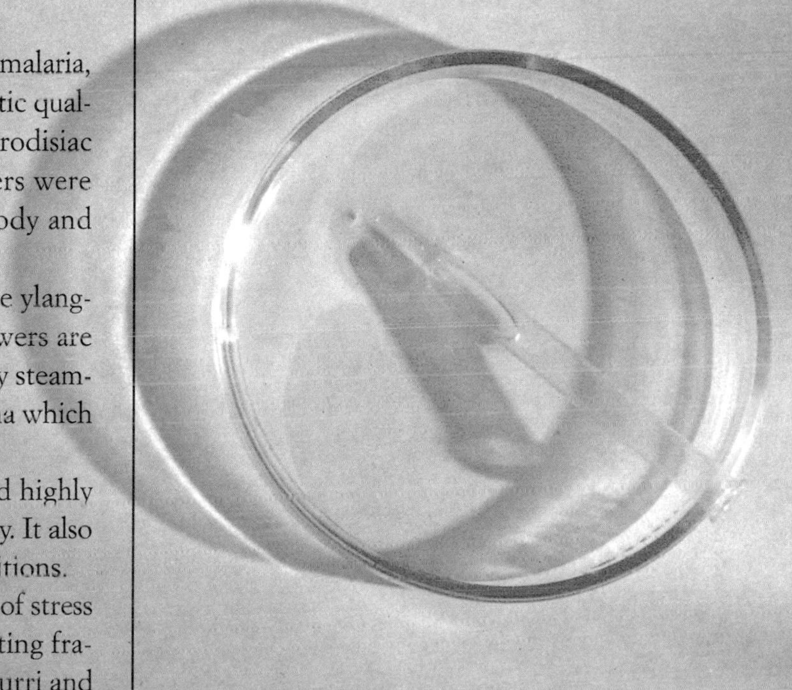

Oils for Common Problems

KEY

R	*Relaxing oil*
S	*Stimulating oil*
U	*Uplifting oil*

Some oils have more than one of these properties, tending to balance or normalize the emotions and bodily systems.

Caution

This chart is a general guide only. For the treatment of persistent problems, seek the advice of a qualified aromatherapist. Chronic conditions should be referred to a medical practitioner.

Never mix more than three oils in any one treatment as the synergistic effects are less predictable. Do not exceed the proportions of essential oil to carrier oil suggested in this book.

The following oils should not be used during pregnancy:
Basil • Bay • Clary Sage • Comfrey
Fennel • Hyssop • Juniper
Marjoram • Melissa • Myrrh
Rosemary • Sage • Thyme

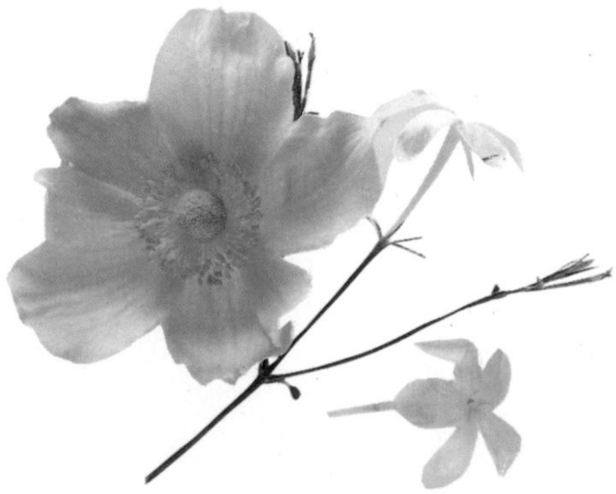

		Acne	Anxiety	Arthritis	Athlete's Foot	Blood pressure: High	Low	Body odour	Bronchitis	Cellulite
Basil	R, U		❀						❀	
Bay	R			❀				❀	❀	
Benzoin	S			❀				❀	❀	
Bergamot	R, U	❀	❀							
Cedarwood	R	❀							❀	
Chamomile	R	❀	❀	❀						
Cinnamon	R						❀			
Comfrey	R				❀					
Cypress	R		❀					❀		❀
Eucalyptus	S	❀		❀					❀	
Fennel	S									
Frankincense	R									
Geranium	R, U		❀							
Hyssop	R, S					❀	❀		❀	
Jasmine	R		❀							
Juniper	R, U	❀	❀							❀
Lavender	R, U	❀	❀	❀	❀	❀		❀	❀	
Lemon	S	❀				❀				
Lemongrass	S	❀			❀			❀		
Marjoram	R		❀	❀		❀			❀	
Melissa	R, U		❀			❀				
Myrrh	S								❀	
Neroli	R		❀					❀		
Orange	U		❀			❀				
Parsley	S									
Patchouli	R	❀	❀		❀					❀
Peppermint	S						❀	❀	❀	
Pine	S			❀				❀	❀	
Rose	R		❀	❀						
Rosemary	S						❀			❀
Sage	S		❀	❀			❀		❀	
Clary Sage	R, S		❀			❀				
Sandalwood	R	❀	❀						❀	
Tea Tree	S				❀				❀	
Thyme	S		❀						❀	
Ylang-Ylang	R		❀			❀				

Water retention									❀				❀			❀	❀								❀			❀		❀	❀					
Warts																	❀	❀									❀							❀		
Varicose veins									❀							❀		❀	❀								❀			❀						
Travel sickness																	❀																			
Throat infections				❀						❀		❀	❀				❀	❀	❀			❀									❀	❀	❀	❀		
Stress						❀							❀				❀			❀	❀						❀						❀			
Sinusitus										❀							❀						❀					❀								
Sexual problems					❀		❀						❀		❀											❀			❀			❀	❀			❀
Rheumatism		❀				❀			❀	❀						❀	❀	❀		❀			❀					❀		❀					❀	
Pre-menstrual syndrome	❀					❀			❀				❀			❀	❀				❀		❀						❀	❀	❀	❀	❀		❀	
Obesity									❀		❀															❀				❀	❀				❀	
Nausea	❀										❀						❀				❀						❀		❀				❀			
Muscular aches							❀	❀	❀	❀							❀			❀								❀		❀	❀					
Mental fatigue	❀															❀					❀							❀		❀	❀	❀			❀	
Painful periods						❀		❀	❀						❀	❀				❀	❀								❀			❀				
Irregular periods						❀										❀	❀				❀								❀	❀	❀	❀				
Menstrual problems (general)	❀					❀								❀		❀	❀				❀								❀	❀		❀			❀	
Menopausal problems						❀		❀	❀		❀		❀				❀	❀			❀		❀	❀					❀		❀	❀				
Insomnia					❀	❀			❀			❀		❀			❀			❀			❀						❀			❀	❀			
Influenza	❀						❀		❀	❀				❀														❀						❀		
Indigestion	❀					❀										❀	❀	❀	❀	❀	❀	❀		❀			❀			❀						
Hormonal regulation						❀							❀								❀			❀												
Headache	❀					❀				❀							❀		❀	❀	❀						❀			❀						
Hayfever						❀				❀											❀								❀							
Haemorrhoids									❀													❀					❀						❀			
Flatulence				❀		❀					❀			❀		❀	❀	❀									❀			❀		❀			❀	
Fainting	❀					❀											❀										❀			❀						
Eczema					❀	❀		❀	❀				❀	❀	❀	❀						❀				❀							❀			
Diarrhoea						❀	❀		❀	❀			❀			❀	❀	❀			❀	❀					❀									
Depression	❀			❀		❀			❀				❀		❀		❀		❀				❀	❀		❀			❀	❀	❀	❀	❀			❀
Dandruff					❀								❀			❀	❀	❀								❀				❀			❀	❀		
Cystitis			❀	❀					❀	❀						❀									❀			❀			❀		❀			

THE ESSENTIAL MASSAGE

An aromatherapy massage using essential oils is a therapeutic treatment for both mind and body which works mainly on the nervous system. Aromatherapy is both holistic and practical in that it helps to protect the body's life-saving immune system and energize or stabilize emotions. It is often called the "sensual science" because it combines the powers of touch with the sense of smell. More effectively than any other massage, aromatherapy can either relax or stimulate the body and mind. The highly potent essential oils penetrate the body via the skin and are also inhaled as the massage progresses.

SETTING UP

Any massage is relaxing but you can enhance the experience by following a few simple steps to help create the right mood.

An aromatherapist uses a massage bench, but at home you can work comfortably on a cushioned floor or a futon (Japanese mattress). An ordinary bed is not really firm enough. Prepare the floor or surface with a large cotton sheet covered with a bath towel. You should also have to hand a pillow, a large wrap-around towel for the body, and a warm blanket or even a hot-water bottle by the feet.

RELAXING YOUR PARTNER

Additional touches help to establish a calming atmosphere. You could fragrance the room with a burner, using a relaxing oil, and switch on some background music: play instrumental tracks, voices can be distracting.

The room temperature should be warm. Once the oils are gently massaged in, the whole body responds by slowing down and, although the skin may feel warm to touch, the body feels colder. It is important to keep your partner comfortable, so offer to cover parts that are not being worked on if you think your partner may be getting cold. Being at ease with one another is an important part of any treatment.

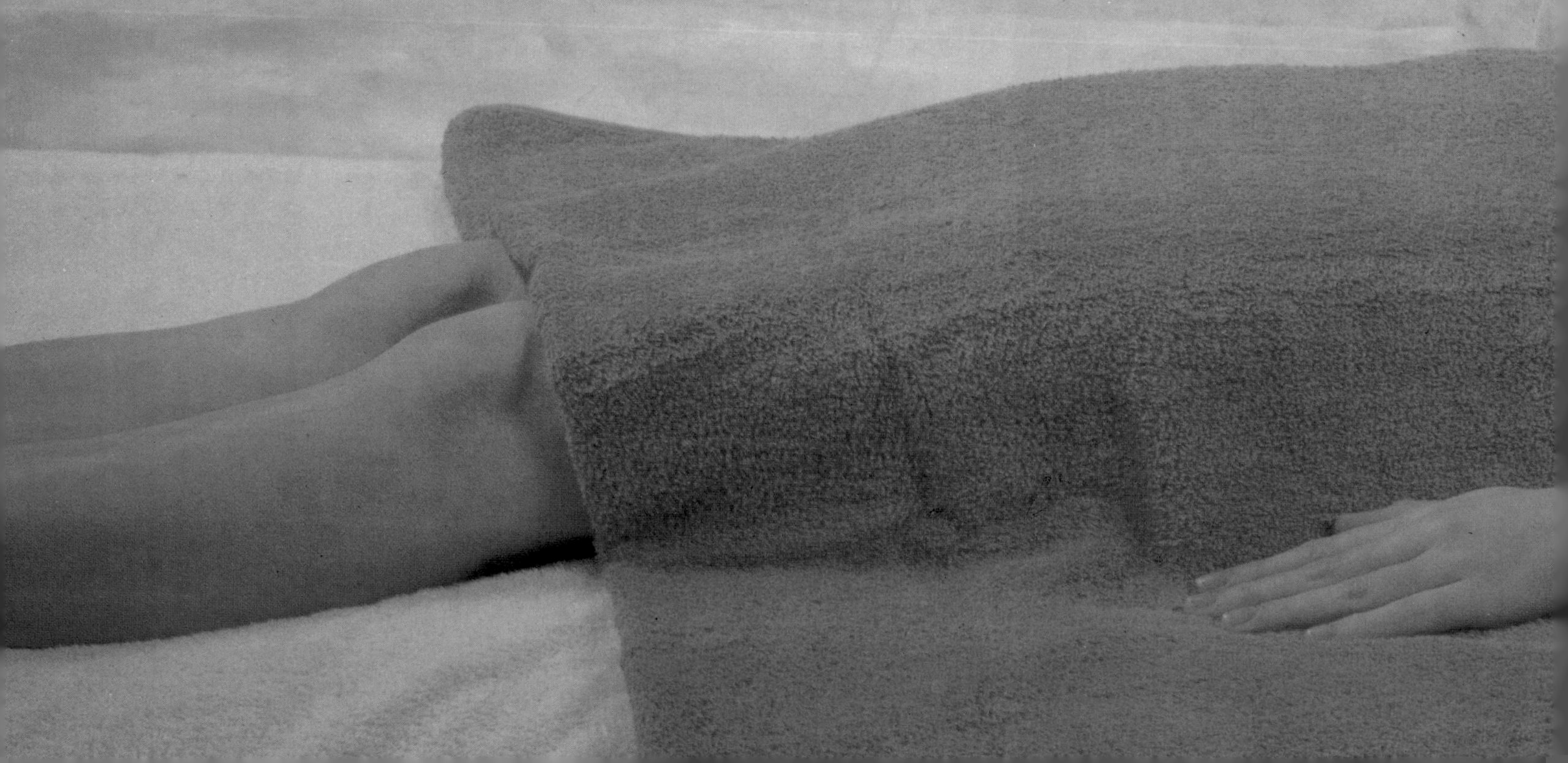

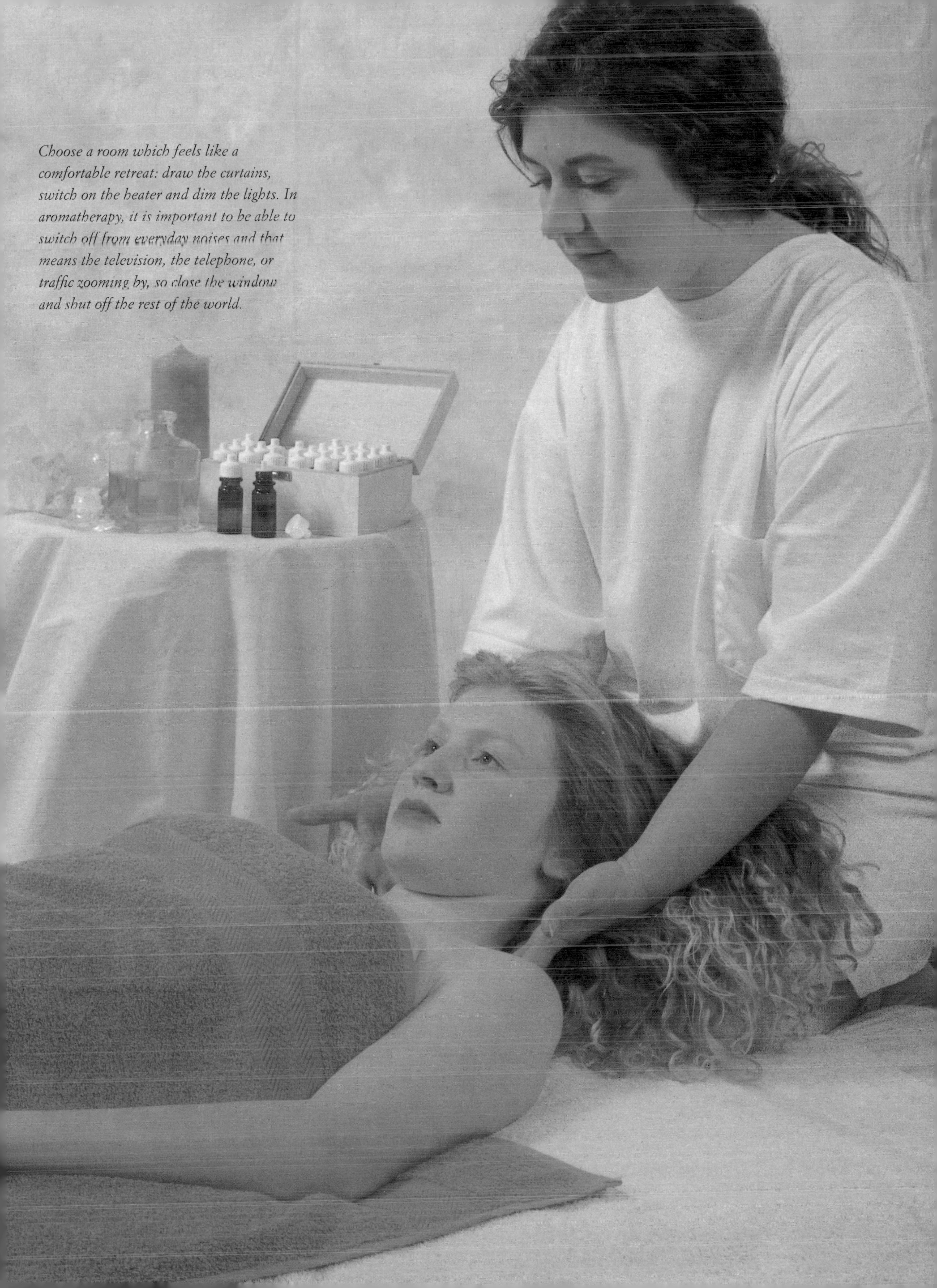

Choose a room which feels like a comfortable retreat: draw the curtains, switch on the heater and dim the lights. In aromatherapy, it is important to be able to switch off from everyday noises and that means the television, the telephone, or traffic zooming by, so close the window and shut off the rest of the world.

ABOUT THE TREATMENT

A complete aromatherapy massage takes just under an hour from top to toe. It is important to find out before massage about physical aches and pains, in particular back injuries, recent operations or whether the person you are massaging is in an "emotional" state of mind at the time.

GIVING THE MASSAGE

❦ Make sure you have read through the step-by-step instructions several times to familiarize yourself with the sequence. You do not want to keep stopping to refer to the book.

❦ Try the movements on your own body to get a sense of how the strokes should feel and how much pressure to use.

❦ Massage movements should be slow to help relaxation and eliminate tension which tightens the muscles.

❦ Remember that the movements should flow into each other. If you find you have missed out a step or gone on to the wrong part of the body, do not panic. Finish the part you are working on before going back to it, or leave it out altogether, rather than interrupting the flow of the massage.

❦ When you give the massage, make sure *you* are relaxed and comfortable, as well as the person being massaged, or you will transmit your own tensions to your partner and it will not be an effective massage.

❦ Try to maintain contact with your partner's body as much as possible; even as you move into a different position try to keep a hand on the body.

❦ When massaging different parts of the body keep the areas not being worked on covered with a large towel or blanket. The heat helps the body to absorb the oils and make the massage more therapeutic.

Choosing the Essential Oil

Aromatherapists never start a massage immediately. In order to provide the most effective treatment, the therapist has to ascertain the state of mind and body of the individual, and establish whether there are any specific problems to attend to. Is the problem physical? Is it mental? Is it a combination of both? To help them to treat a wide variety of complaints, aromatherapists have many oils at their disposal, but they never mix or use them until they have worked out a prescription for the receiver's individual needs.

Mixing the oils is a trained art, yet there are simple recipes you can use at home to deal with specific problems from muscular aches and pains to headaches and stress. With potent essential oils it is far better to use less, rather than more, so if in doubt, start the massage technique with a base oil like sweet almond and add 2 or 3 drops of just 1 essential oil. Lavender, rosemary and geranium are good all-purpose oils, or use chamomile for particularly sensitive skin.

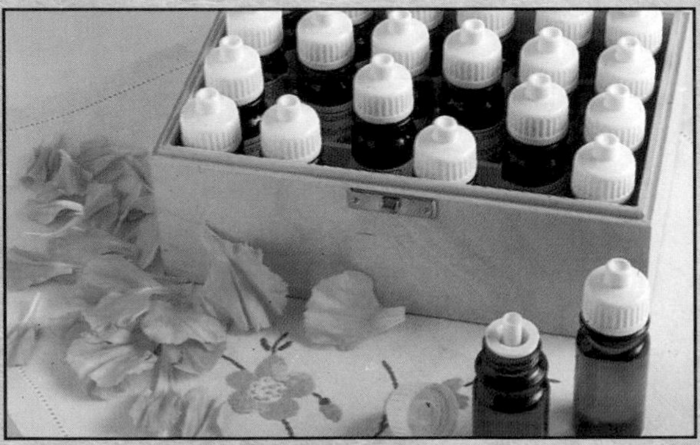

Applying the Oils

❦ Keep the oil in an easy dispenser or bowl so you do not have to worry about lids during the massage. But keep the oil covered in some way as essential oils will quickly evaporate.
❦ Always warm your hands before applying oils.
❦ Some therapists recommend warming the oil in your hands before applying it to the body as a courtesy to the recipient. Others advise against this on the grounds that it hastens evaporation of the essential oil and that the oil takes on your own energy rather than your partner's.
❦ If the part of the body you are working on is particularly hairy or the skin is very dry you will need to apply more oil.
❦ Keep your touch light and sensitive. Remember that your hands are the main channel of communication.
❦ If you become tired while masssaging, sit back for a minute but don't let your hands leave your partner's body as it is essential to maintain the continuity.

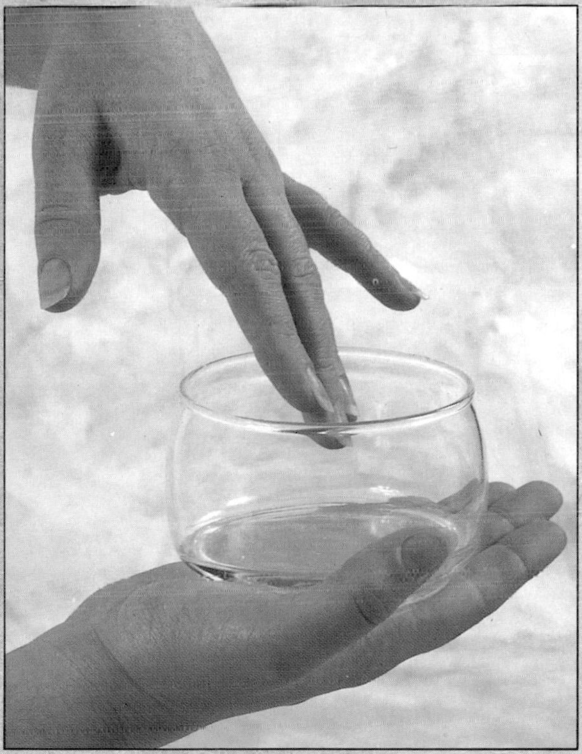

❦ If the recipient's back is stressed in any way, place a pillow under the knees when lying on the back, and under the pelvis when lying on the stomach.
❦ Wear loose, comfortable clothing to give the massage, so your movements are not hampered.
❦ If oil is accidentally spilt on clothing, dab off quickly with a tissue. It will soon evaporate, but it may leave a stain so rinse out clothing in warm soapy water.
❦ For complete relaxation avoid chatting during the massage: play music if you do not like silence. But do encourage feedback from your partner – you must be told if something does not feel good.
❦ Ensure that the person you are going to work on is given the following set of guidelines.

Receiving the Massage

Before the Massage
❦ Have a cool shower or wash before a massage. Do not soak in a hot bath, or the oils will immediately seep into the skin.
❦ Do not use an underarm deodorant or body spray before the treatment, as this will block the effect of the oils.
❦ Do not have a large meal just before an aromatherapy massage as the body's systems will have to work too hard at digesting to be thoroughly relaxed.
❦ Do not drink alcohol before a treatment.
❦ Do not have a massage if you have flu or a fever or any serious condition (see Caution, page 278). Wait until you are over the worst and then let an aromatherapy treatment help restore your system's balance.

After the Massage
❦ Drink a glass of still water immediately after a treatment.
❦ Lie still for at least five minutes before getting up.
❦ Do not bathe or shower for at least 12 hours after a treatment to allow the oils to be absorbed by the skin and begin the all-important work of detoxifying the body.
❦ Drink plenty of water for the rest of the day as the kidneys will be active in eliminating the toxins.
❦ Avoid alcohol for at least 12 hours after the treatment to give the body a chance to detoxify thoroughly.

THE MASSAGE STEP-BY-STEP

Following your assessment, select the oils you are going to use and blend 10–15 drops of your chosen oils with 4 tablespoons of base oil. The massage starts with your partner lying face down, with the back uncovered and the rest of the body covered with a towel or light blanket.

ESTABLISHING CONTACT

Take a few moments to create a bond of communication with your partner and to prepare yourself for the massage. Focus or "centre" yourself by becoming aware of your whole body and its role in giving the massage, and letting go of outside concerns to concentrate on the task in hand.

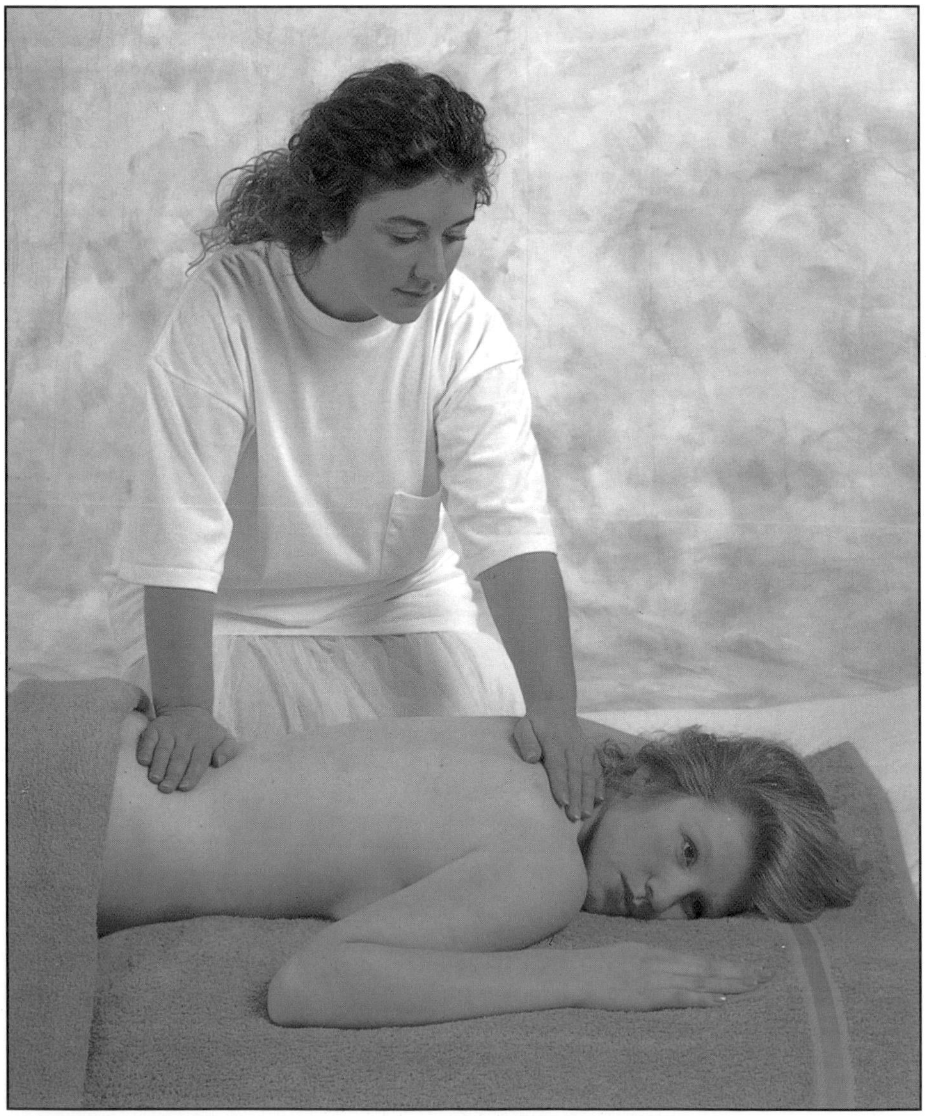

CAUTION

Aromatherapy is an holistic therapy in that it works on the person as a whole. Though it is an excellent way of treating minor ailments, stress and negative emotional states, it is not a substitute for conventional medical treatment. If symptoms persist, always consult a medical doctor.

Never attempt to treat the following conditions:

- cancer
- progressive neural disorders
- heart conditions
- advanced asthmatic conditions
- post-operative states
- severe varicose veins
- very high blood pressure
- epilepsy

For oils to avoid during pregnancy see Pregnancy Treatments on page 297.

LEFT: With your partner face down, rest one hand lightly at the base of the neck (the occipital bone) and place your other hand on the lower back (the sacral area). Hold the position for a count of 20, while you focus on your breathing and clear your mind. This is carried out with dry hands.

THE LEG

EFFLEURAGE (SMOOTHING STROKE)

This is a smooth, sliding movement which soothes the skin and distributes the oil. Always worked in the direction of the heart, *effleurage* improves circulation, lymph flow and the function of the muscles. It is used between movements throughout the massage to provide continuity and to prepare a new area with oil.

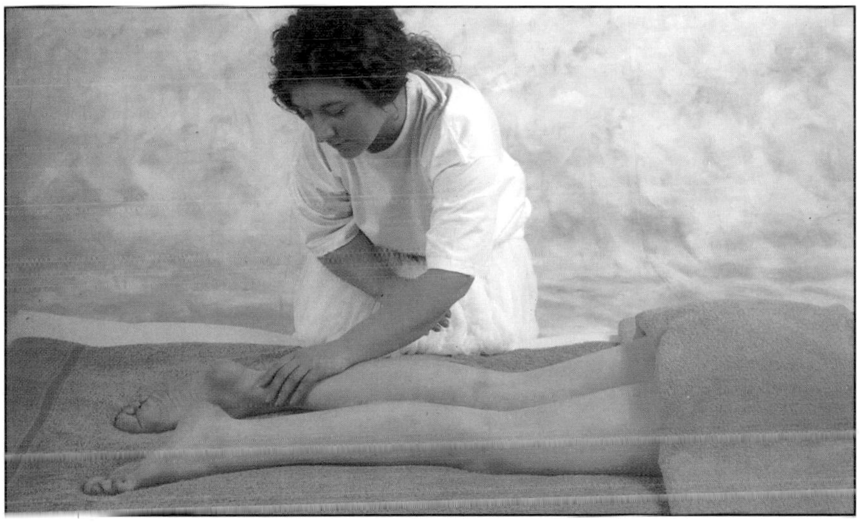

1 Seated to the side of your partner, begin with one hand at the heel, brushing in an upward, sweeping movement to the buttock ridge and sliding round to the thigh.

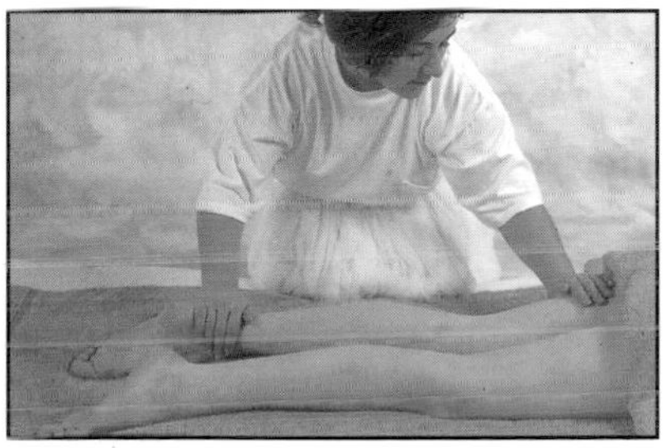

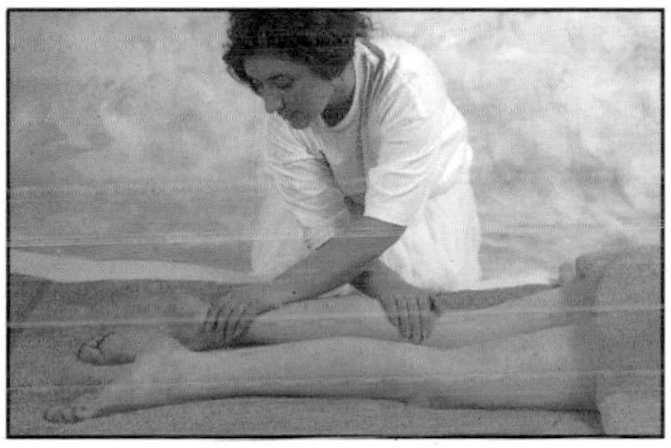

2 As the first hand comes round the thigh, place the other hand at the heel and brush with an upward sweep, ending at the back of the knee.

3 As the second hand comes off, cross the first hand over and begin the movement again from the heel up to the thigh.

Repeat the sequence about six or seven times, keeping the movements continuous and flowing, and then repeat on the other leg.

ANKLE THUMBING

The ankles are an important centre of energy, and this movement helps to relieve congestion.

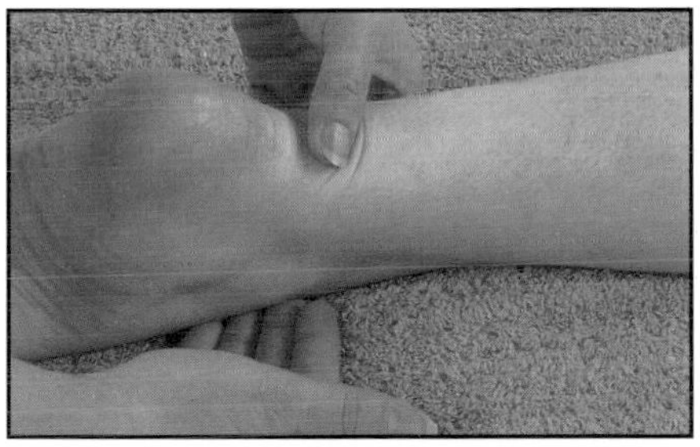

1 Sitting at your partner's feet, cradle one ankle gently with your hands, allowing the thumbs to sit naturally above the heel.

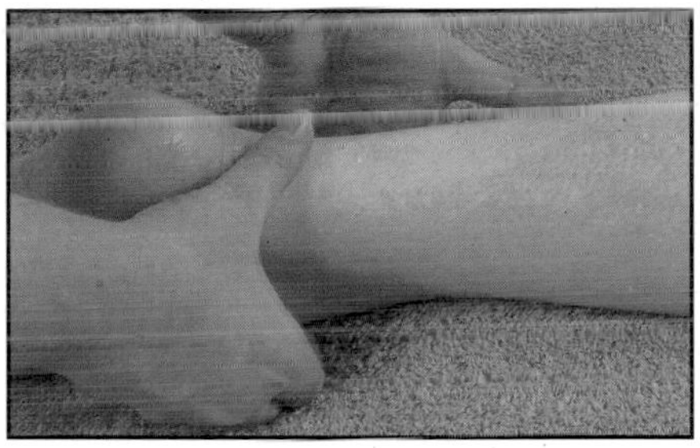

2 Keeping the rest of the hand still, apply a light pressure with the thumb as it brushes in an upward and outward movement.

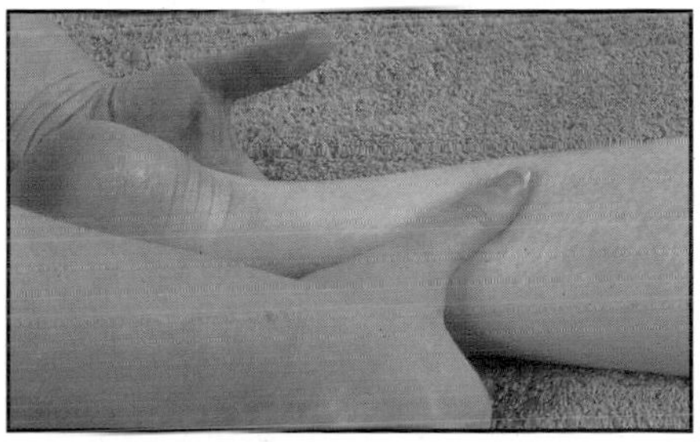

3 Repeat with alternate thumbs, continuing in a rhythmic sequence for about 30 seconds.

FLUSHING

Flushing drains the lymph channels and stimulates the circulation. This movement should not be used on anyone with severe varicose veins.

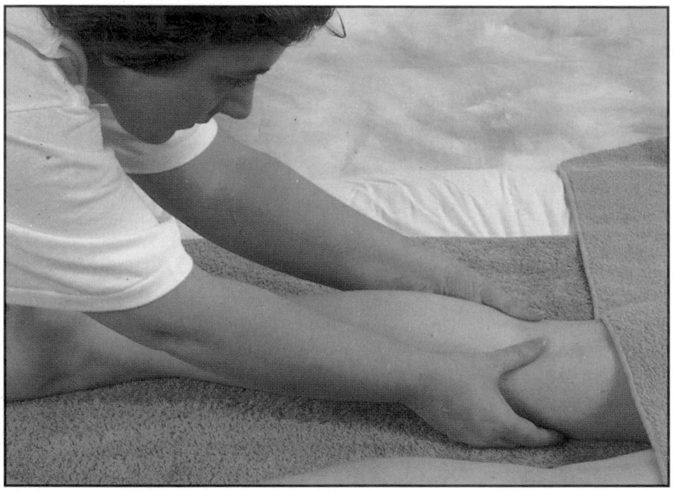

1 Sitting at your partner's feet, gently slide the thumbs up the middle of the leg, ending at the back of the knee.

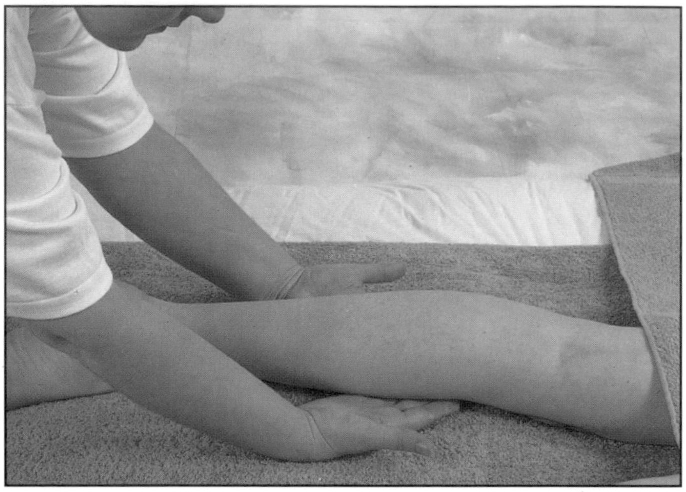

2 Slowly bring the hands back down to the ankles by brushing down the sides of the calf muscle, taking care not to drag.

Repeat the movement five or six times.

KNEADING

Move back round to the side of the leg for this movement. It is particularly effective for relieving tension at the back of the legs.

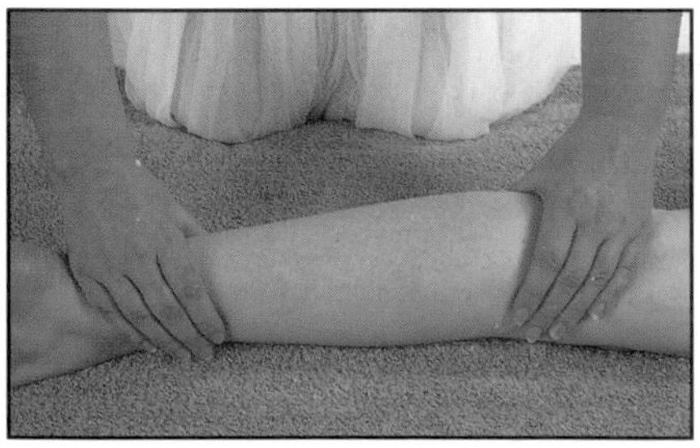

1 Place the hands gently on the calf, one at the top and one just above the ankle.

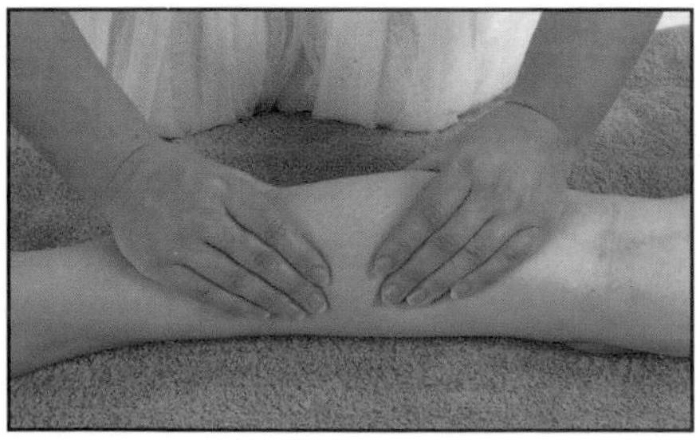

2 Grasp the calf muscle firmly with both hands and slide them toward the centre of the calf, lifting the muscle.

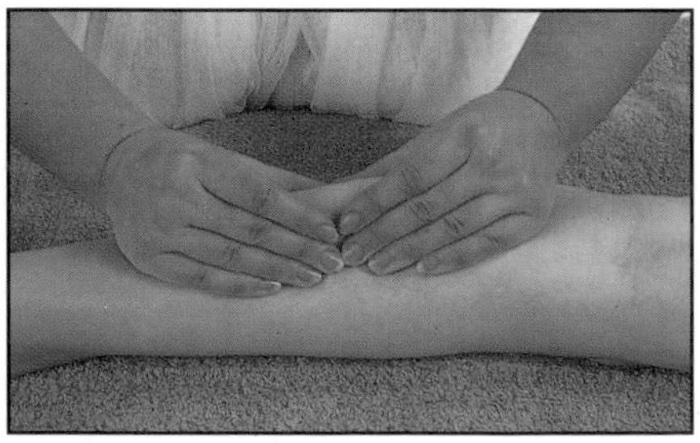

3 Using gentle pressure, knead the area by bringing the fingers and thumbs together and raising the muscle further.

Continue kneading for about 30 seconds.

WRINGING

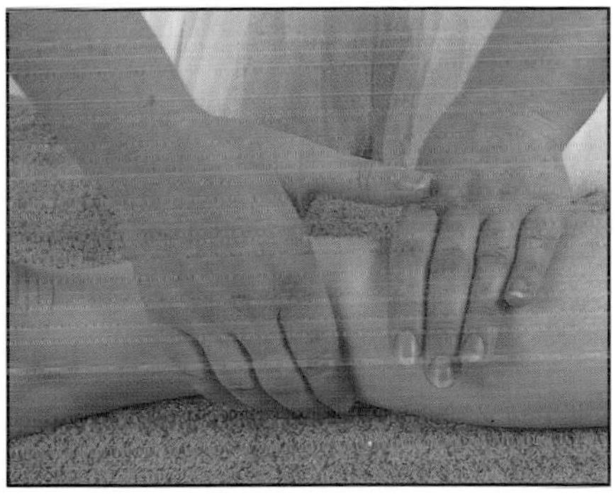

1 Place the hands on opposite sides of the calf, just above the ankle. Gently glide the hands past each other so the heel of one hand is pushing away from you while the other hand is pulling.

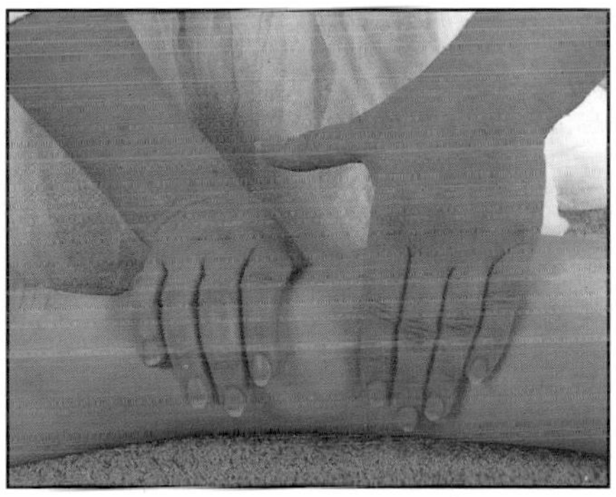

2 Keep the thumb of the pulling hand raised so the thumbs do not collide as they pass each other each time.

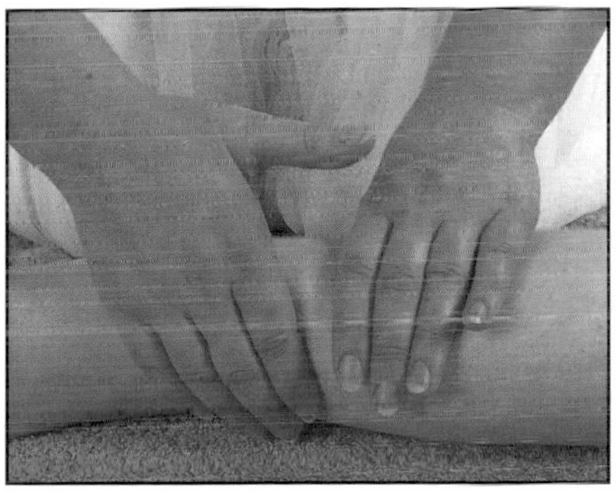

3 The hands alternate the pushing and pulling as you work all the way up the calf and down again. The pressure should be firm but gentle.

Clear these movements by flushing through again from ankle to back of knee.

THUMBING THE KNEE

This is the same action as the thumbing performed at the ankle base. It is helpful for people who suffer from cold feet as it stimulates the circulation.

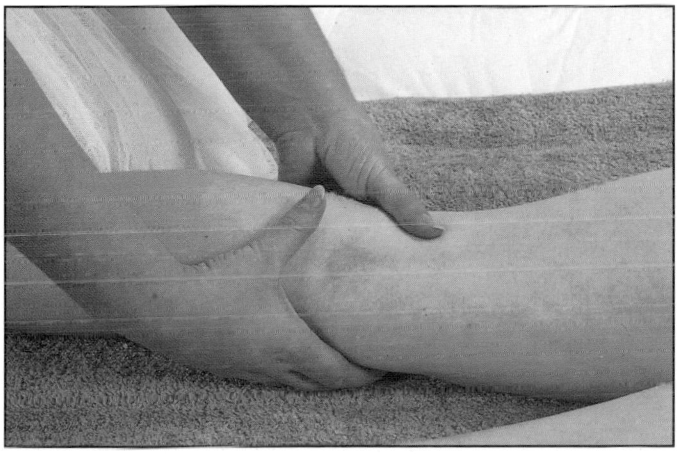

1 Cup the hands gently around the knee, allowing the thumbs to sit naturally on the fleshy part at the back of the knee.

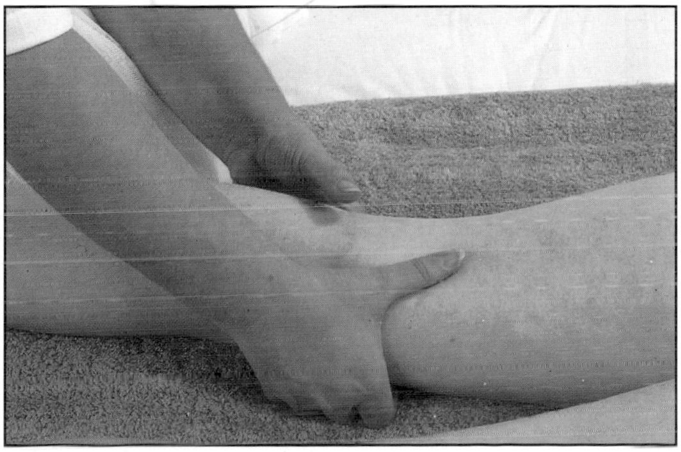

2 With the same thumbing movement used on the ankles, brush one thumb upward and outward, covering the full width of the knee, and follow immediately with the opposite thumb.

FLUSHING

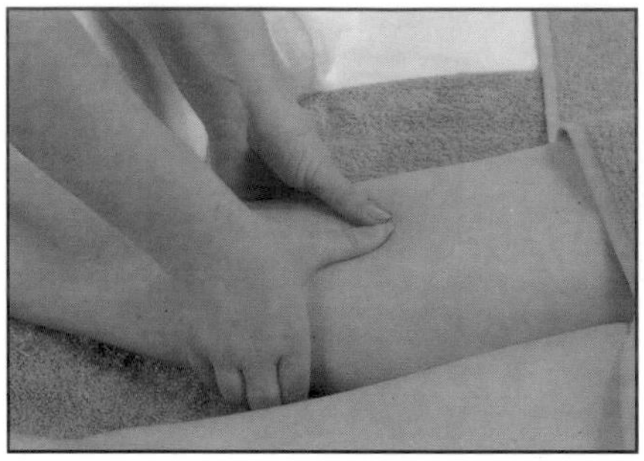

Flush through with the thumbs together from the back of the knee to the top of the thigh.

WRINGING

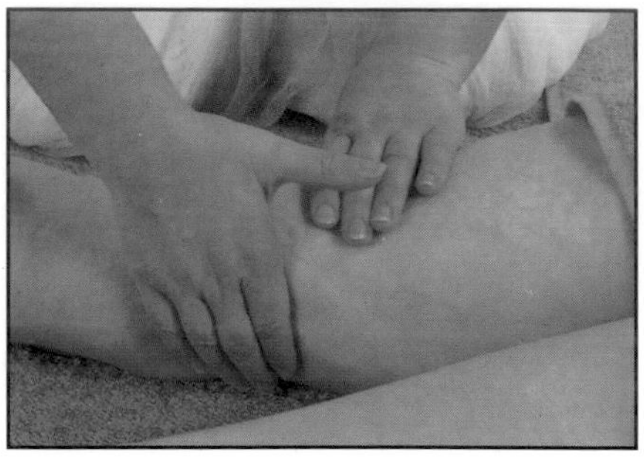

Wring the leg from the knee to the top of the thigh with the same action as used on the lower leg.

THIGH PUSH

This knuckling movement is very effective for breaking down cellulite, helping to disperse the fatty tissue and improve the circulation.

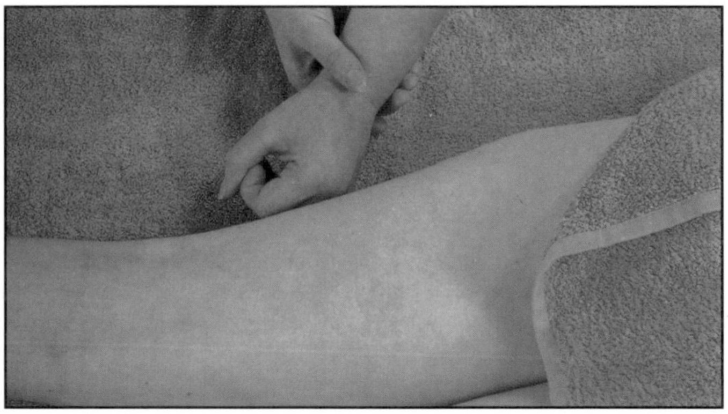

1 With the supporting hand wrapped around the wrist of the working hand for stability, place the clenched fist on the side of the thigh, just above the knee.

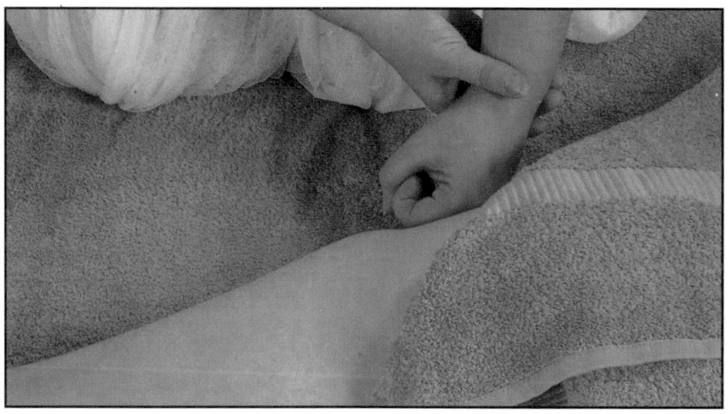

2 Drag the fist slowly up the side of the thigh toward the hip bone. This is not a heavy action – all you need is a little gentle pressure.

Repeat five or six times, working slightly different parts of the thigh each time.

Finish the leg massage by repeating the opening *effleurage* movement and then repeat all the steps on the other leg.

Cover the legs with towels before proceeding to the next stage. An extra blanket or hot-water bottle at the feet might also be appreciated.

BACK MASSAGE

The back carries a lot of strain and these relaxing movements are often the most appreciated part of the massage. Do not be tempted to use too much pressure: it is better to keep the strokes broad and flowing.

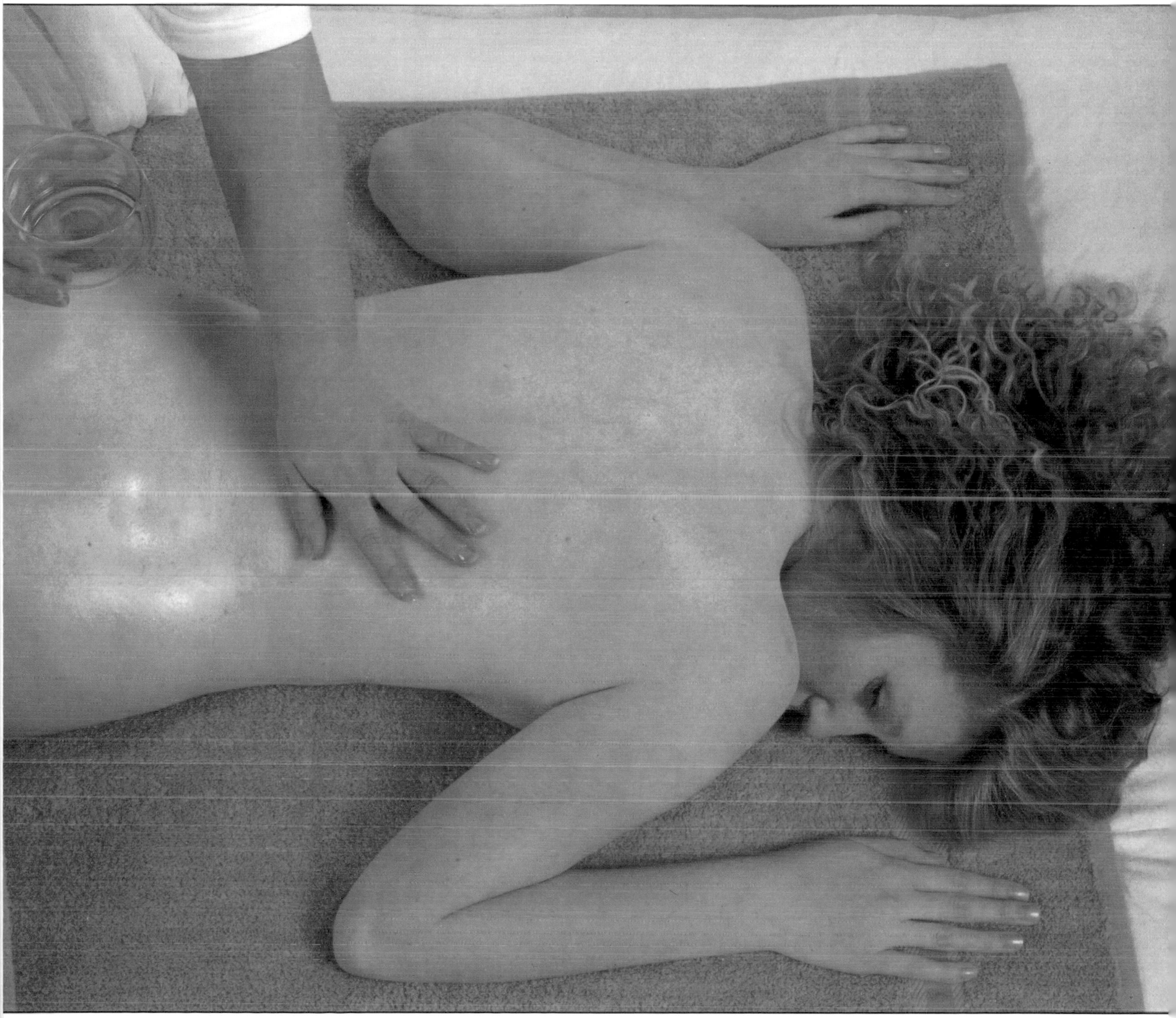

Seated to the side of your partner, apply oil evenly over the back with smooth upward strokes, following the direction of the lymph flow.

CHIN MASSAGE

This not only tones the jawline, but also stimulates the energy points that govern the stomach and small intestine.

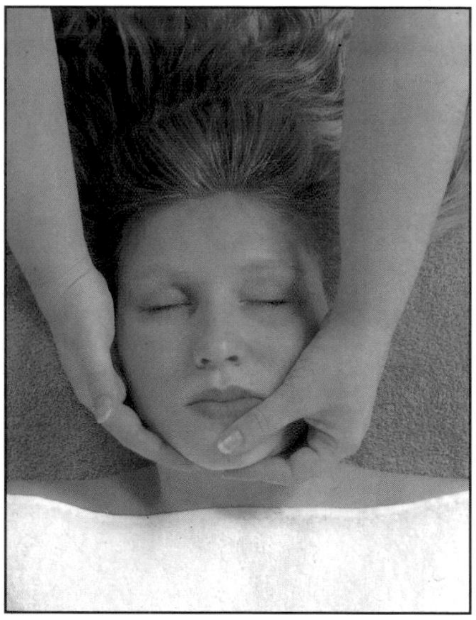

1 Place the thumbs on the chin, allowing the rest of the fingers to cradle the jaw.

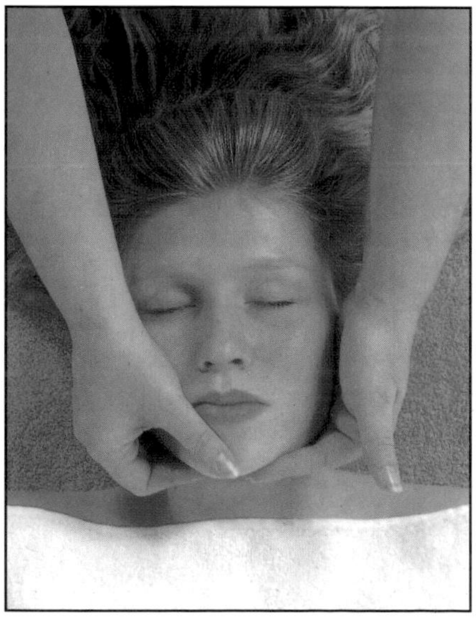

2 Brush alternate thumbs down and outward, with a light stroke. Repeat the movement six or seven times with each thumb.

NECK SWEEP

This is an extremely soothing stroke which improves the tone of the muscles as well as flushing the neck.

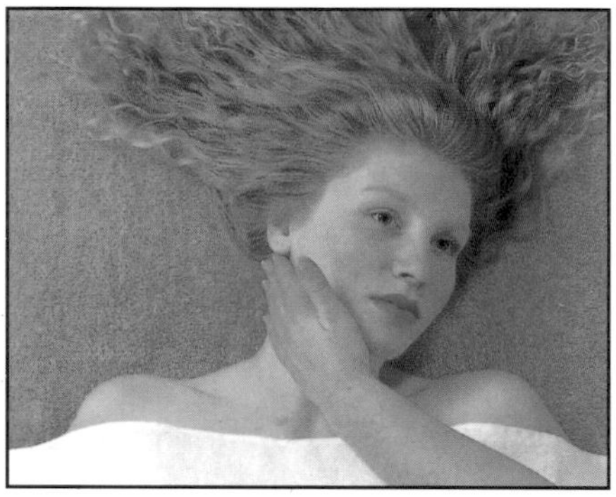

1, 2 Above and right: Apply a little facial oil to the neck, upper chest and shoulder areas using the flat of the hand. Gently brush down with the hand from the side of the ear out to the shoulder, using a broad sweeping stroke to cover the area.

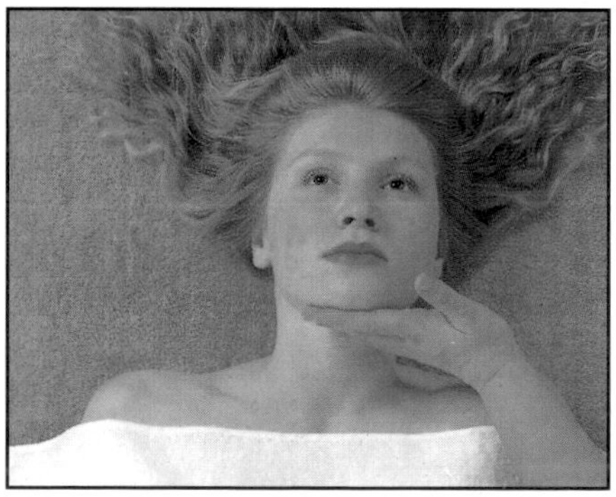

3 Repeat the movement working around the front of the neck, down from the chin to the top of the chest, and then sweep from the other ear to the shoulder.

The sequence of sweeps around the whole neck should be repeated three times.

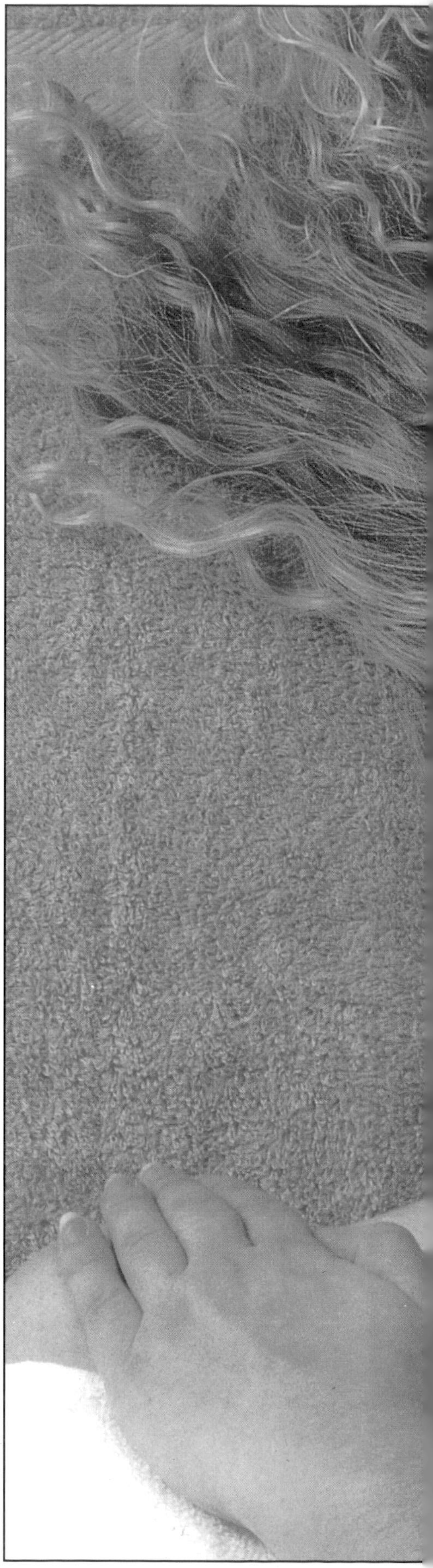

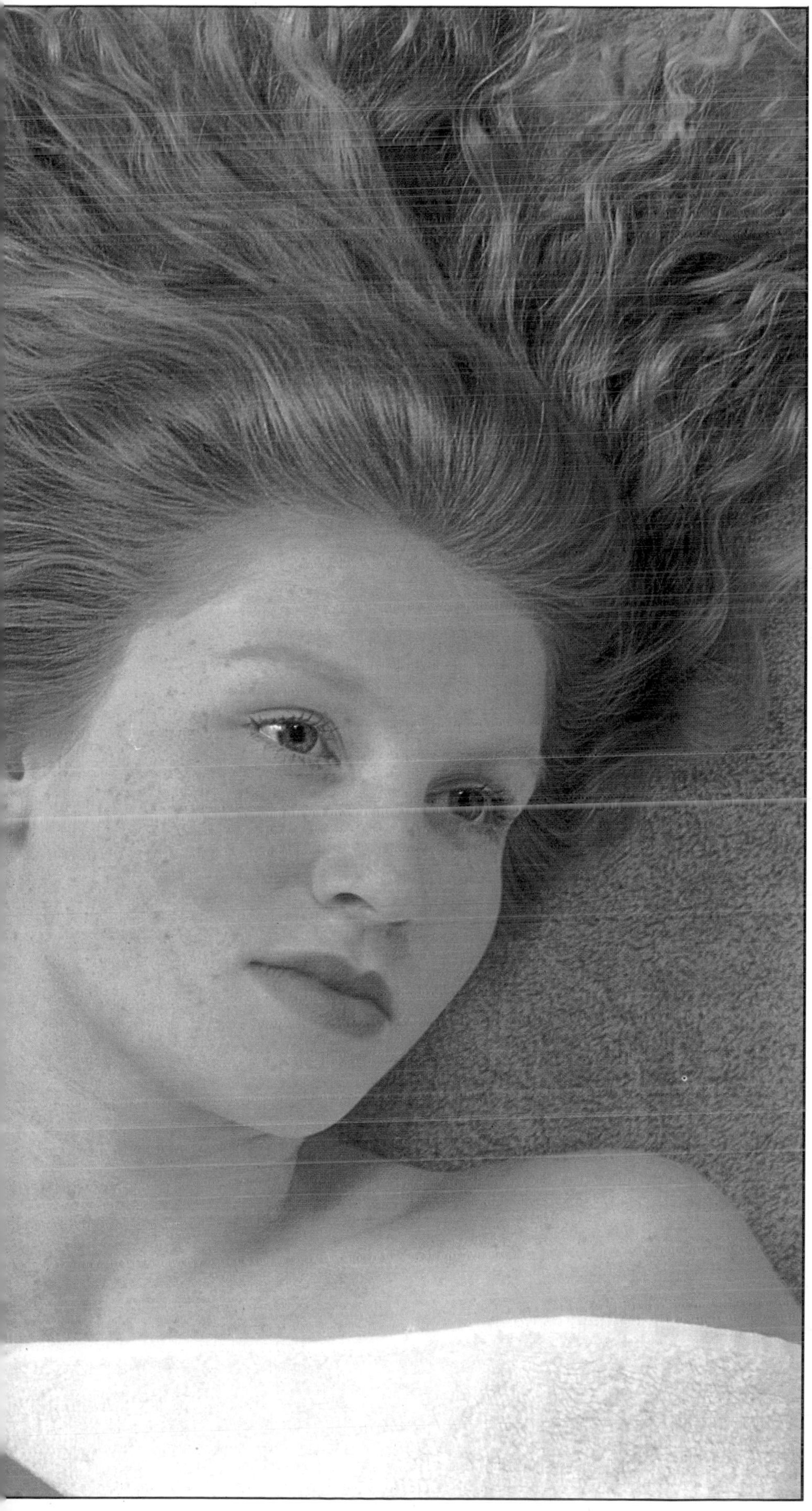

FANNING THE SHOULDERS

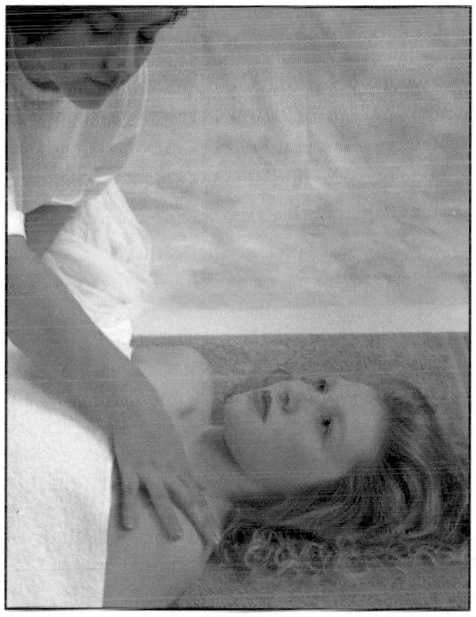

1 With fingers spread, brush with the flat of the hand across from the breastbone and out over the shoulders.

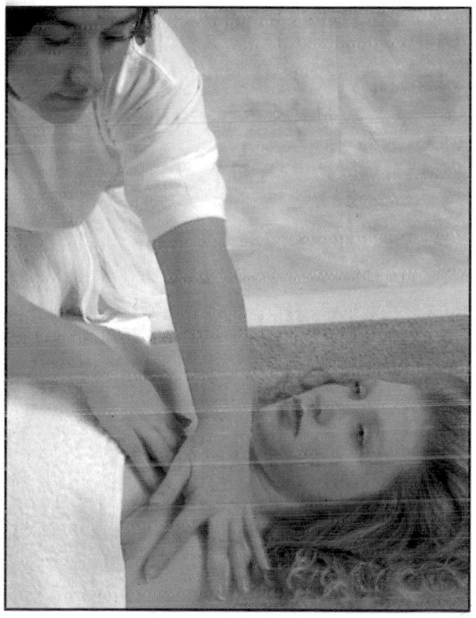

2 The second hand follows closely behind the first, so they are draining simultaneously toward the armpit.

Repeat twice before moving onto the other shoulder.

STOMACH AREA

ABDOMEN

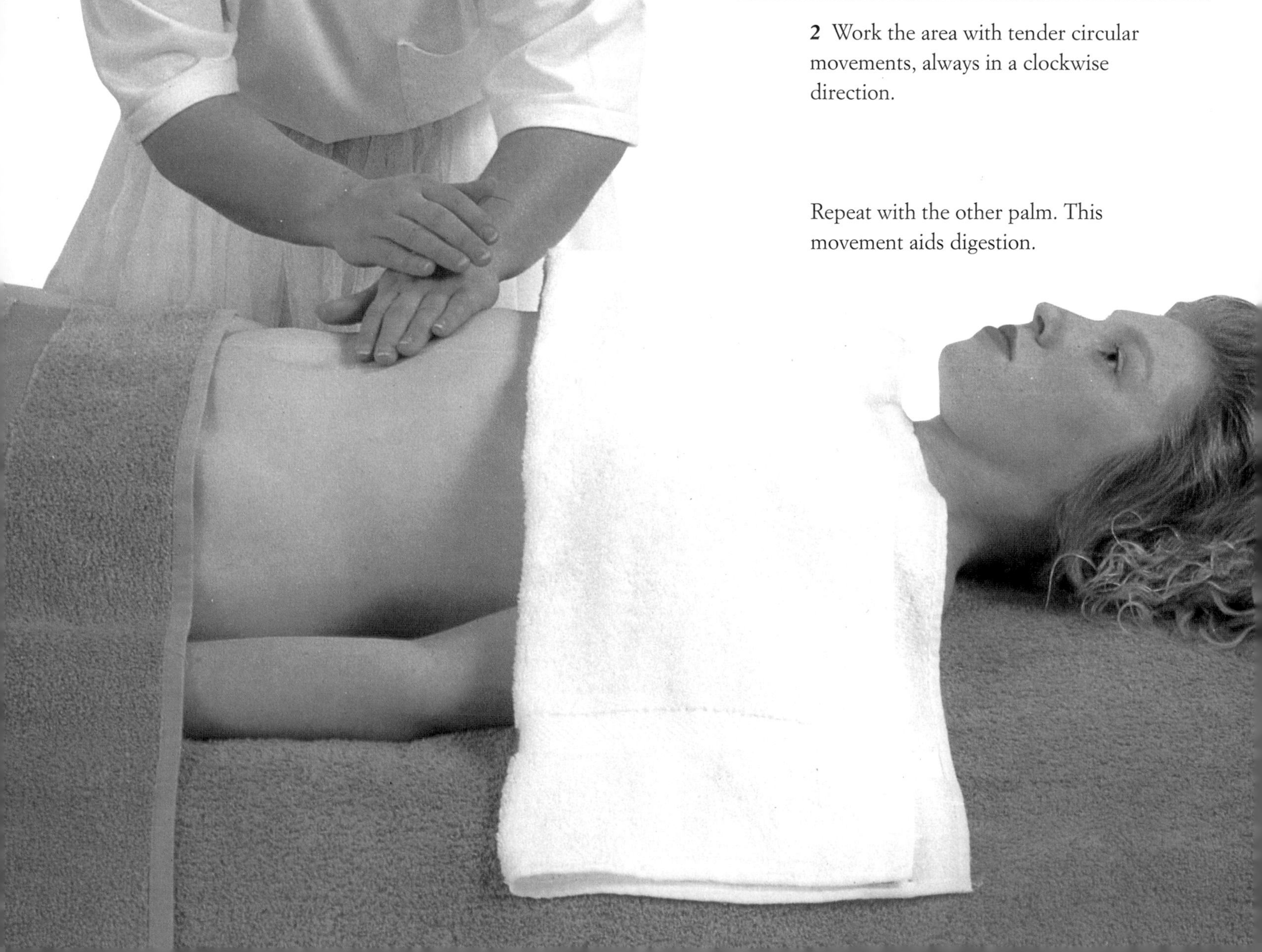

1 LEFT: Apply a little oil evenly over the stomach. Place the palm of a hand on the centre of the abdomen.

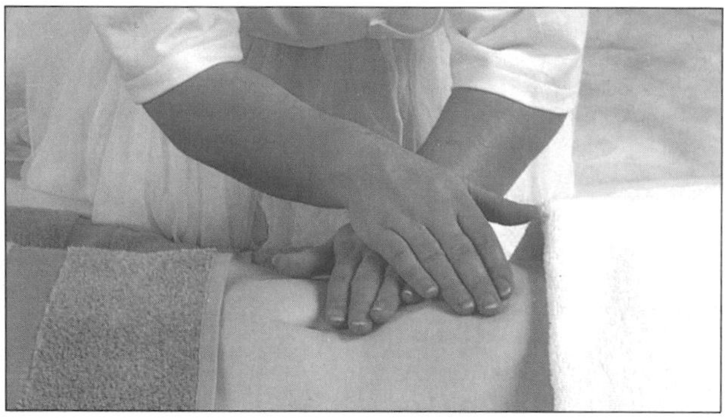

2 Work the area with tender circular movements, always in a clockwise direction.

Repeat with the other palm. This movement aids digestion.

RIB CAGE SWEEP

This movement helps to cleanse the stomach and spleen by pushing the lymph away from these areas.

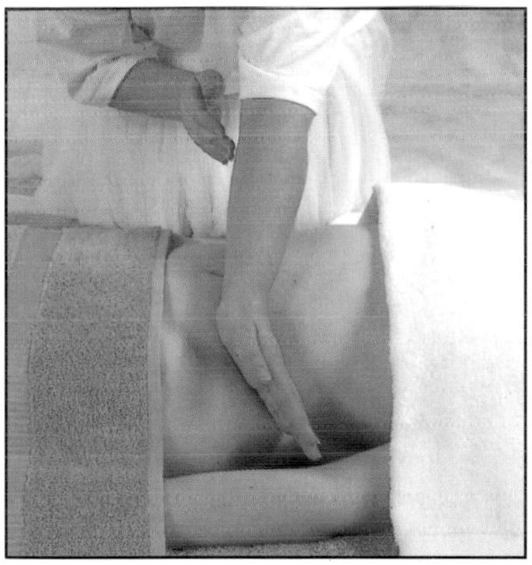

1 Starting with the outer edge of the hand placed at the centre of the rib cage, sweep away from you, following the line of the ribs with a long sweeping movement out to the waist.

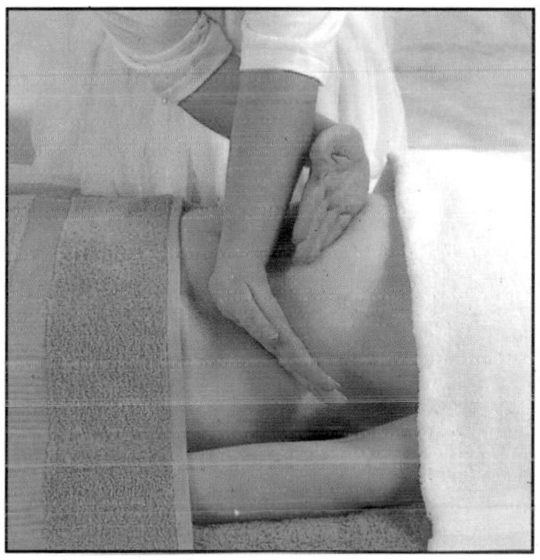

2 As the first hand finishes the movement, the other hand follows on the same side.

Repeat the movement with both hands six or seven times and then move around the body to work the other side of the rib cage.

WAIST PULLS

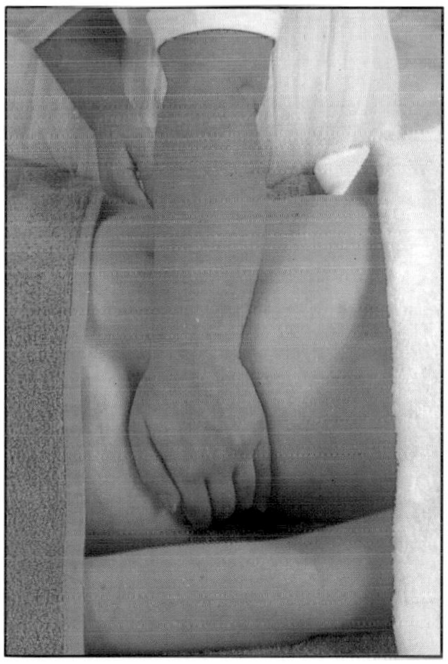

1 Reach across your partner, placing a firm grip around the waist with one hand. Reinforce your grip by placing your other hand on top of the first hand.

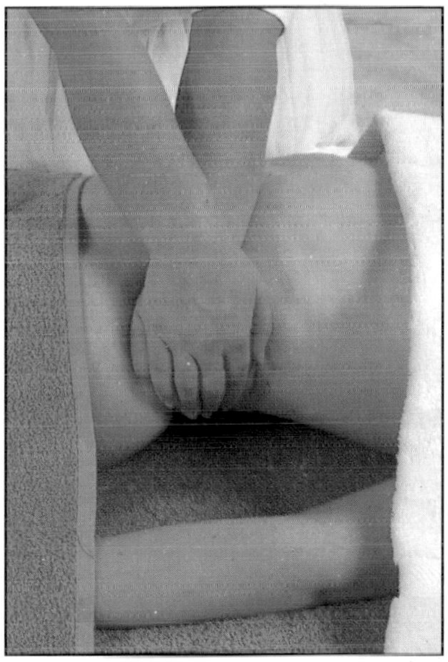

2 Lift the waist by pulling your partner's body-weight toward you, then gently release while sliding the hands around the hipbone. This cleanses the liver and gall bladder.

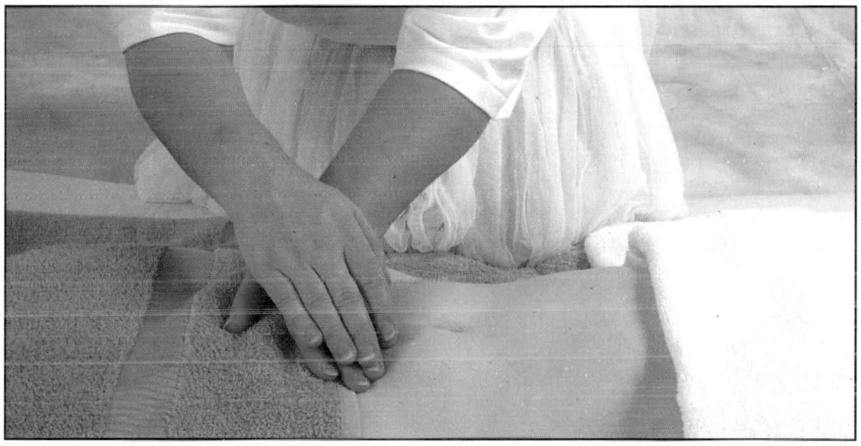

3 Complete the movement by sliding the hands across and around the pelvis, draining toward the major glands in the groin. Be careful not to dig with the fingers as this is an extremely tender area. Keep the pressure light and even over the whole hand. This is particularly beneficial for women who suffer from menstrual problems.

Repeat five or six times before moving around to the other side of the body.

FRONT OF LEGS

EFFLEURAGE

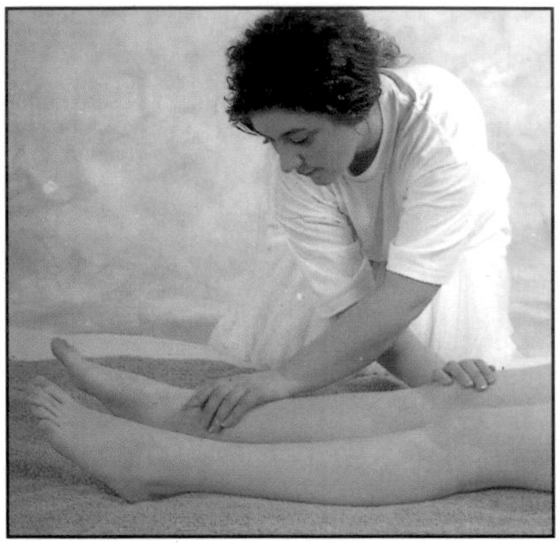

Apply oil to both legs using an *effleurage* movement working up from the ankles, as used on the back of the legs.

Repeat the *effleurage* strokes sequence several times to ensure an even distribution of oil.

LEG STRETCH

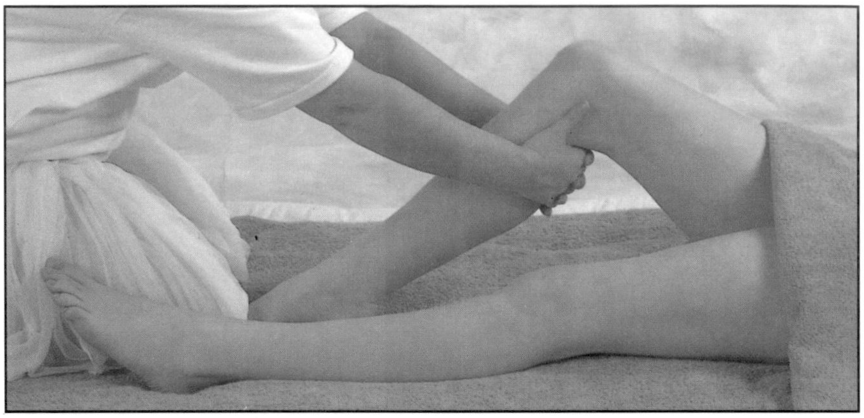

Supporting the leg at the ankle and behind the knee, bend the leg up and place it in line with the shoulder.

Clasp the hands around the back of the knee. Ask your partner to inhale deeply, then pull the calf muscle toward you.

Hold for a slow count of 3. As your partner breathes out, release the pull on the calf.

Repeat the whole movement three times, then gently lay the leg down and repeat the stretch on the other leg.

ARMS AND HANDS

EFFLEURAGE

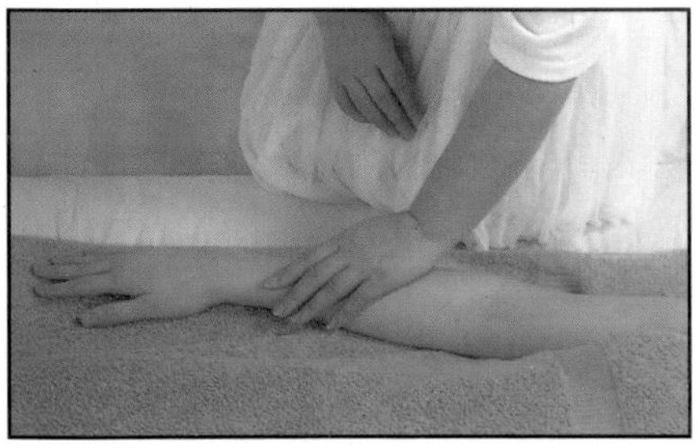

1 Seated to the side of your partner, move the arm slightly away from the body. Apply the oil by sweeping from just above the wrist, up to the shoulder and round.

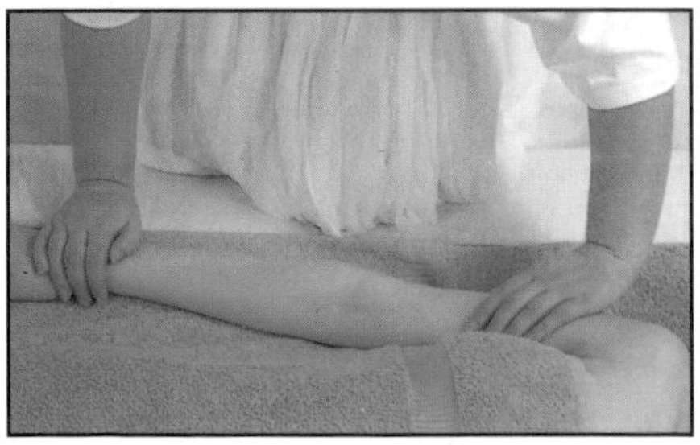

2 As the first hand comes off the arm, the other hand starts at the wrist and sweeps upward to the gland sited in the elbow joint.

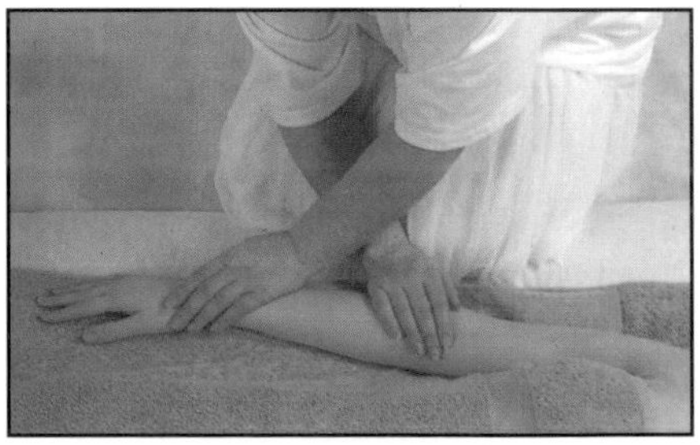

3 The first arm crosses the second as it reaches the elbow and again sweeps from wrist to shoulder.

Repeat six or seven times.

You can follow the *effleurage* with flushing to the inside of the arm, using the same movements performed on the leg, working from the wrist to the elbow. Before going on to the second arm, massage the hand of the first arm.

HAND MASSAGE

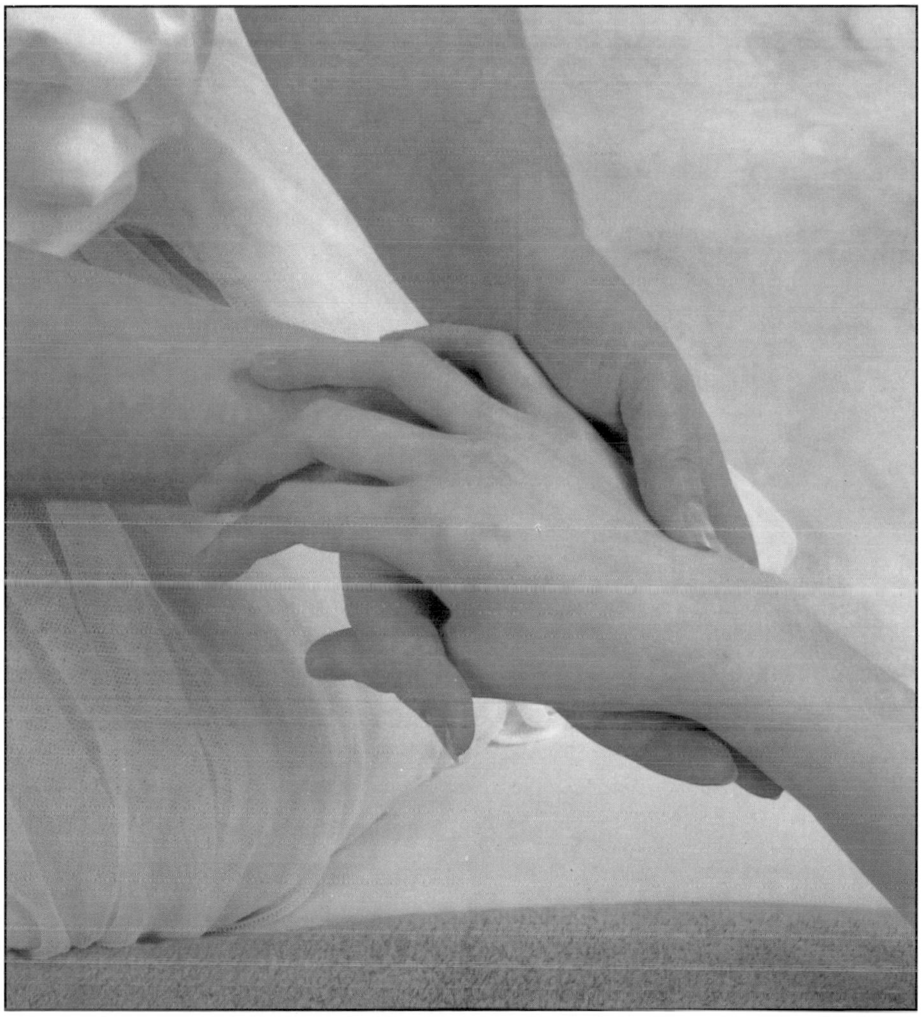

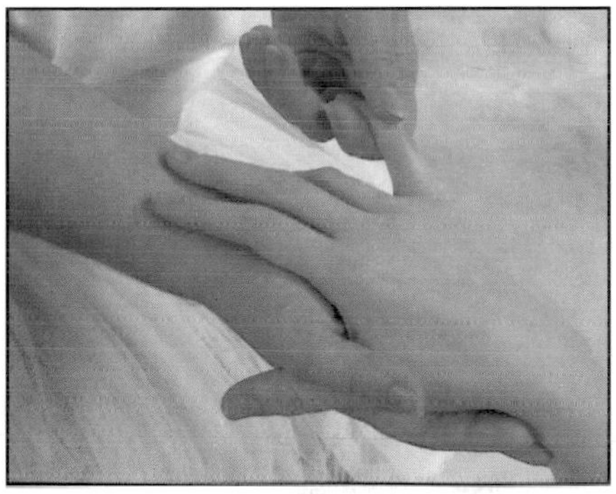

2 Pull back to the fingers, gently massaging the joints between your thumb and forefinger as you draw toward the tips. Finish with a slight pull to the finger to stretch it out.

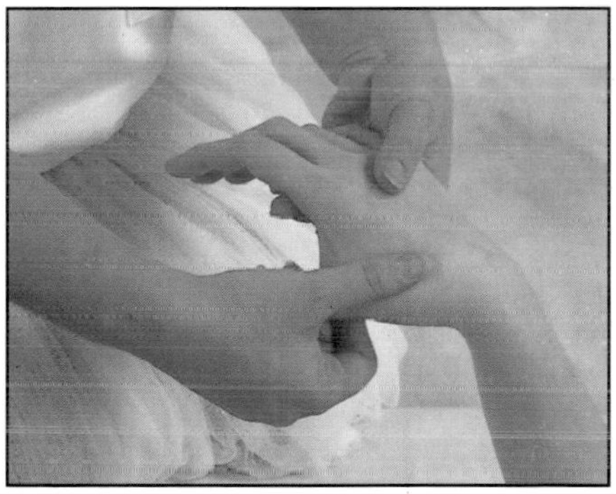

1 Resting your partner's hand palm down over your own palm, use small brushing movements with your thumbs to work upward between the joints of the fingers toward the wrist.

3 Repeat with each finger, finishing with the thumb.

Now repeat the movements on the other arm and hand.

To finish the massage, cover your partner to the neck, check he or she is warm and comfortable, and leave to rest for a minimum of 5 minutes (up to 15 minutes is preferable). Upon returning, help your partner to sit up carefully and offer a glass of water.

PREGNANCY TREATMENTS

Pregnancy can be one of the most exciting and fulfilling times of a woman's life. The joy of bringing another human being into the world creates a tremendous feeling of contentment and anticipation, but it is also a time of great physical and emotional upheaval. Together with the ever-important trio of exercise, good diet and rest, essential oils can play an important role in helping a woman cope with the stresses of nine months of pregnancy, the pain of labour and post-natal recovery.

COMMON AILMENTS

Surging hormone levels and changes in your swelling body can bring a host of discomforts, many of which can be alleviated by aromatherapy treatments and other simple steps.

Backache

The lower back region takes a lot of strain during pregnancy, and will benefit from a firm massage with 4 drops each of lavender and sandalwood in 30 ml (2 tbsp) base oil. 6 drops of lavender in the bath will help to soothe away the aches.

Morning Sickness

Eat little and often during the day, avoiding junk food and heavy meals late at night. Choose fresh foods which are free from preservatives or chemicals. Try herbal tea infusions such as chamomile, peppermint or orange blossom, which are good for the digestion.

Heartburn

Avoid heavy meals and particularly rich, spicy foods. Peppermint tea infusions help, and you can rub the solar plexus with a blend of 2 drops each of lemon and peppermint essential oils in 15 ml (1 tbsp) of base oil.

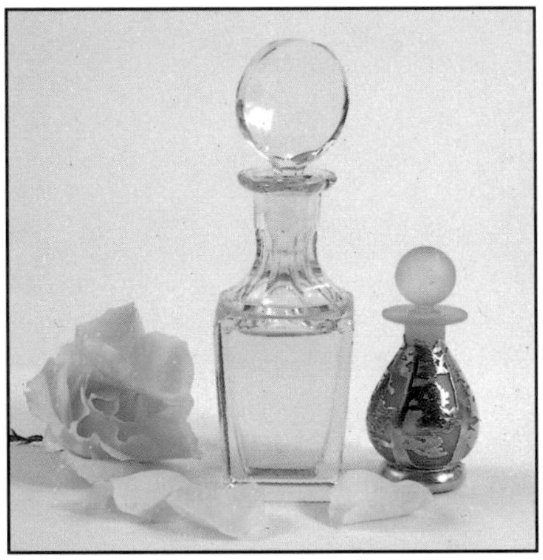

Spoil yourself with the luxurious and relaxing scent of rose for body and facial oils, to keep your spirits up during pregnancy.

Sore Breasts

These need extra care and attention during pregnancy as they expand. Use a gentle massage oil with rose and orange, 3 drops of each in 15 ml (1 tbsp) sweet almond oil; or if breasts are swollen, make a cool compress using rose water and place over the breasts while having an afternoon rest. Sweet almond oil on its own is excellent for sore, cracked nipples during breast-feeding. Never use pure essential oils on the breasts during this period as they can easily be transferred to the baby while feeding.

Constipation

Make sure your diet contains plenty of fresh and high fibre foods and drink plenty of still water. Tension can also be a contributory factor, so try a relaxing bath with 3 drops of lavender and 4 drops of rose. Massage your abdomen and the small of the back with a blend of 4 drops of chamomile or orange in 15 ml (1 tbsp) base oil.

Sleep Problems

In the last few months of pregnancy, because of various discomforts it is often difficult to get a good night's sleep. A relaxing bath with neroli and rose is soothing, and you can add ylang-ylang for its calming, sedative effect – a maximum of 8 drops in total. Sprinkle 2 drops of rose or lavender on the edge of the pillowcase to help induce sleep.

Stretch Marks

When the stretched skin returns to the body's normal shape it can leave tiny jagged scars. A daily massage around the hips and expanding tummy, using 5 drops of lavender in 15 ml (1 tbsp) jojoba, wheatgerm or evening primrose oil, will help keep skin smooth and supple. Start around the fifth month of pregnancy and continue after the birth until you return to your normal weight.

Swollen Ankles

These can be reduced with a cool to warm footbath of benzoin, rose and orange. Add 2 drops of each directly to the bowl or mix with 15 ml (1 tbsp) base carrier oil such as sesame seed. Rest with feet raised on cushions or pillows.

Varicose Veins

During pregnancy the blood flow to the legs is often slowed down, causing the veins to dilate. Mix 2 drops each of cypress, lemongrass and lavender with 30 ml (2 tbsp) apricot kernel base oil, and smooth gently over the legs for relief. If veins are prominent then one of the best oils for the circulation is geranium, though this should always be very dilute for use in pregnancy. Add 4 drops to the bath or to 15 ml (1 tbsp) carrier oil to massage the leg with upward movements. Do not work directly on the veins or apply too much pressure to the leg.

LABOUR

To create a relaxing atmosphere in the labour room, use a few drops of lavender in a fragrancer, or try rose, neroli or ylang-ylang to fortify you as the labour progresses. Any of these oils can be used in a massage blend for the lower back to help with contractions. If labour is progressing slowly, try marjoram as a massage oil or compress across the abdomen to stimulate contractions.

AFTER THE BIRTH

The "baby blues" often occur around the third or fourth day after childbirth, though some women can suffer a more severe form of post-natal depression for up to a year. A bath of jasmine and ylang-ylang will help you feel better, or use a body oil of chamomile, geranium and orange (5 drops to 30 ml (2 tbsp) sweet almond oil), which is a good mix for hormonal imbalance.

To ease any perineal pains, a bath with lavender is soothing. Tea tree can also be added, since this is a powerful antiseptic and helps heal internal wounds and stitches.

CAUTION

The following oils should be avoided during pregnancy (particularly the first five months) because of their strong diuretic properties or tendency to induce menstruation:

Basil • Bay • Clary Sage • Comfrey Fennel • Hyssop • Juniper Marjoram • Melissa • Myrrh Rosemary • Thyme • Sage

Use all essential oils in half the usual quantity during pregnancy and take extra care in handling them. Ensure that the oils you are using are pure essential oils, as adulterated blends or synthetic oils can sometimes have less predictable effects.

If you have a history of miscarriage you could also avoid chamomile and lavender for the first few months, although in general these are excellent oils for pregnancy.

Because of their potentially toxic nature and strong abortive qualities the following oils should never be used except by a qualified aromatherapist, and must be avoided during pregnancy;

Oreganum • Pennyroyal • St John's Wort • Tansy • Wormwood

Recommended Oils for Pregnancy

Chamomile • Geranium (in low doses) *Lavender • Lemon • Neroli Orange • Rose • Sandalwood*

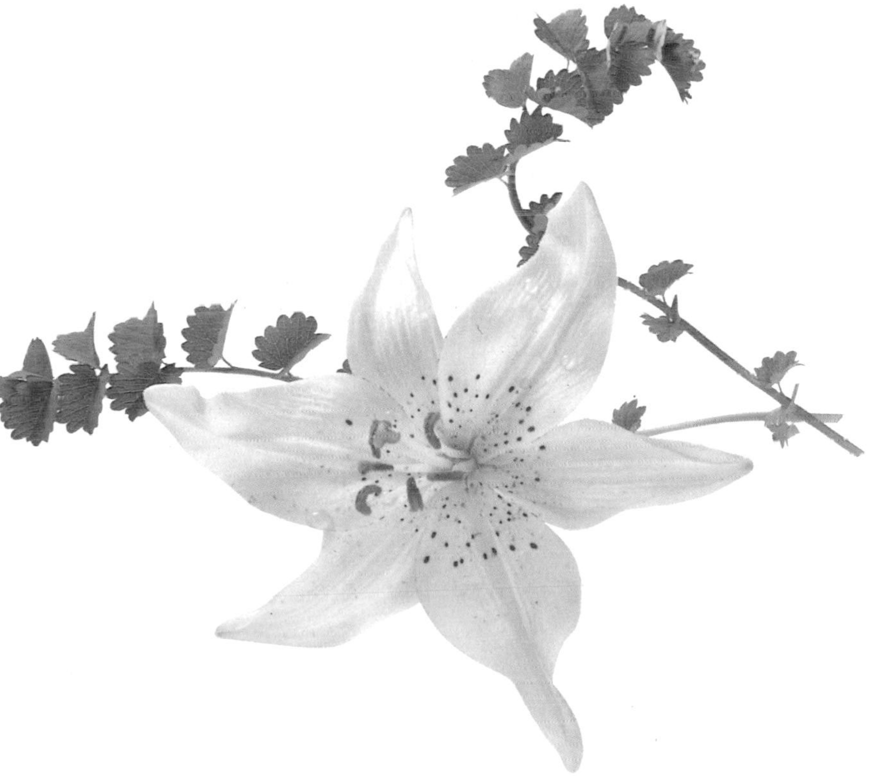

THE ABDOMEN

For a pregnant woman, the weight of the uterus can constrict important blood vessels if she lies down flat on her back, so provide plenty of pillows, cushions, bolsters or rolled towels to support your partner behind the back, under the neck and knees and anywhere else she needs to feel comfortable.

1 BELOW: It may seem alarming to massage the abdomen during pregnancy but, providing the strokes are light and careful, it is safe and relaxing for mother and baby. Gentle massage all over the abdominal area can be very soothing and is beneficial for relieving the stretched feeling often experienced during pregnancy. Apply oil evenly over the area to help feed the tissues and lessen the possibility of stretch marks.

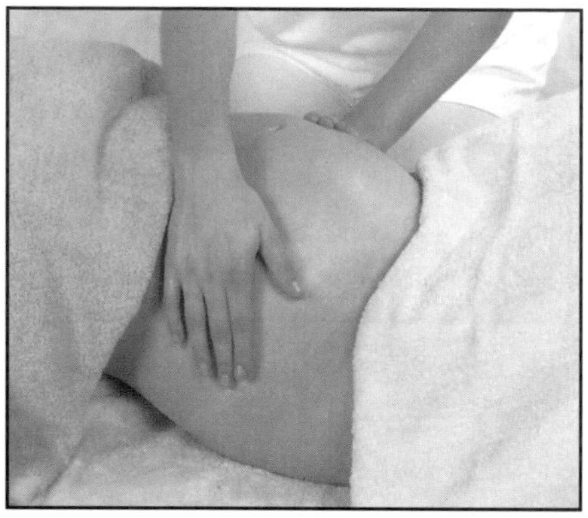

2 Using the flat of your hands, carefully glide them up from either side of the waist, lifting your hands off as they reach the navel, and then start again. Continue to stroke the area with a light, soft touch, working over the whole of the abdomen to soothe and calm.

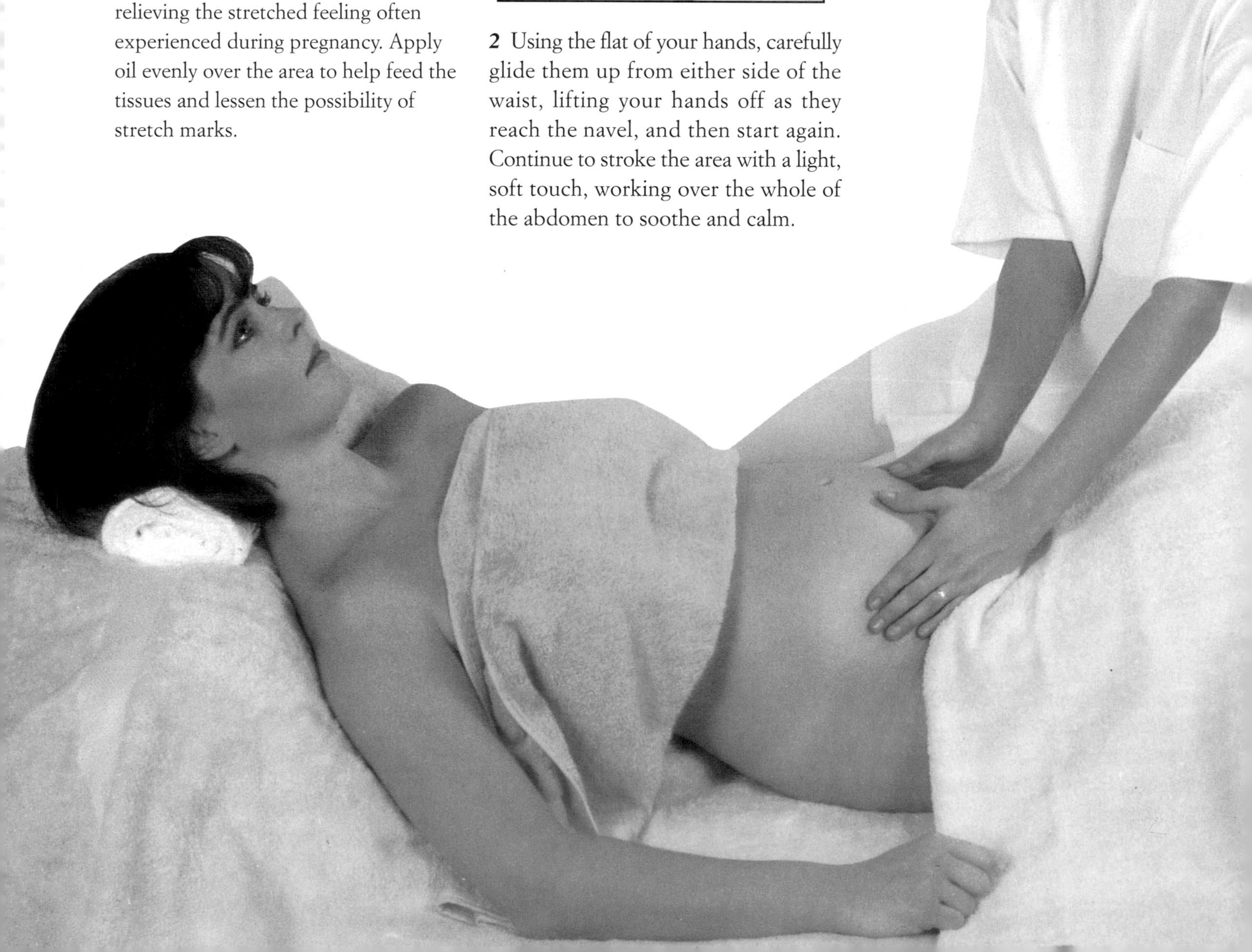

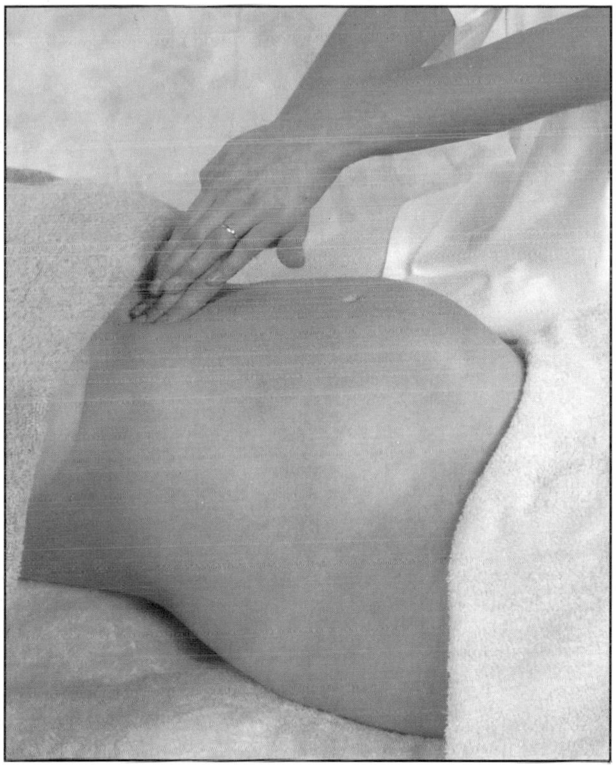

3 After a minute of gentle circular movements, place the fingertips of your left hand on the higher section of the solar plexus region and cover with your right hand. Rest both hands for a moment and then release to help alleviate stress.

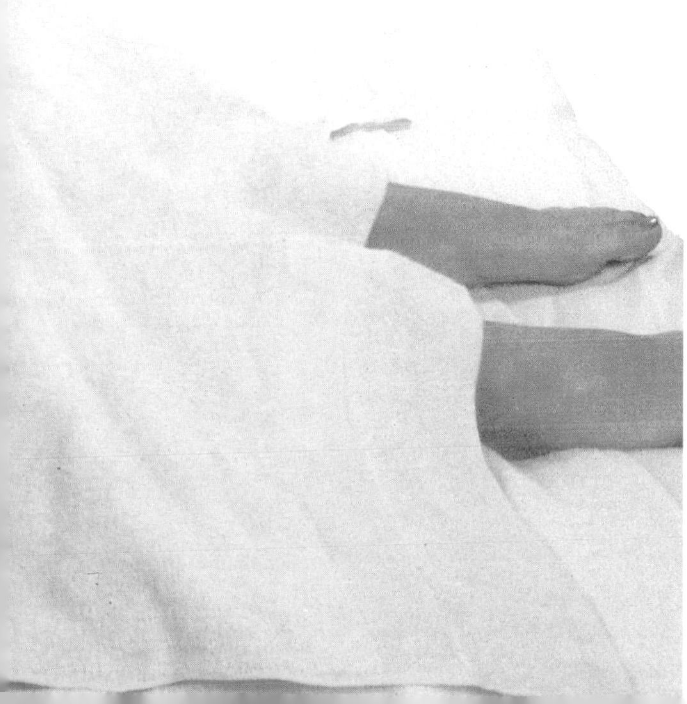

LEGS

Make sure your partner is comfortable, with the knees supported by cushions.

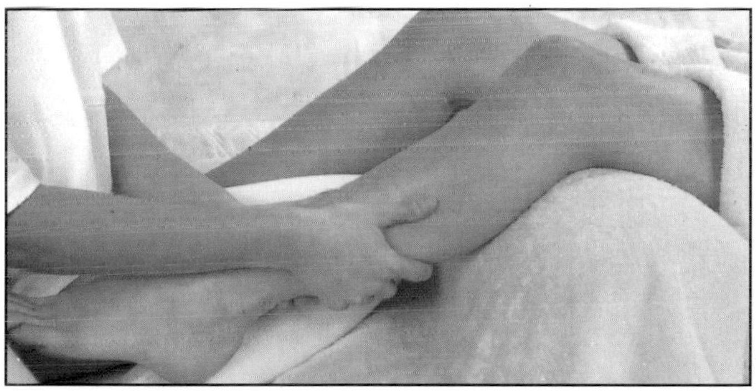

Begin gently stroking the leg with an *effleurage* from the ankle to the knee, smoothing up the shin and then glide around the calf.

It can help to relieve the swelling, varicose veins or cramp which afflict many pregnant women. Do not use any heavy movements to the legs and avoid any reflexology movements to the feet, though gentle stroking around the ankles may well be appreciated.

TO FINISH

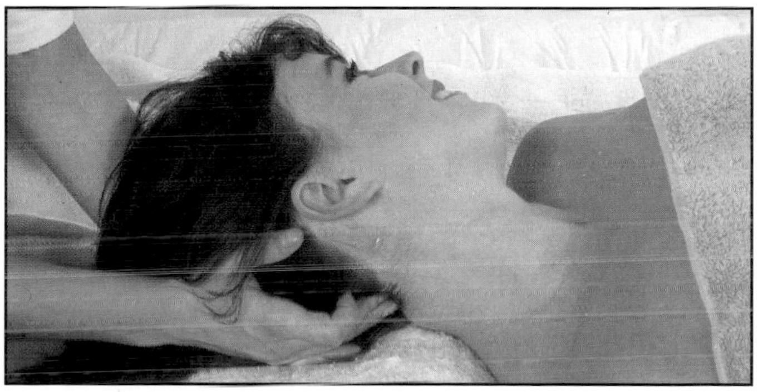

With both hands positioned at the back of the neck, apply light circular pressures to the cranium (skull) with your fingertips working in an upward direction to help release tension.

End the massage by smoothing the hair away from the neck and forehead, releasing all the negative energy. Allow your partner to rest for 15 minutes and then help her to get up very gently.

Beauty Basics

Looking good starts with great skin, and aromatherapy can help you achieve this in various ways: the remarkable penetrative properties of essential oils make them excellent moisturizers, and the wide range of their properties means there is always the right oil for the right condition. For instance, rosemary stimulates the circulation and thyme helps the cells to regenerate. As well as being stimulating to the lymphatic system, which helps cleanse the tissue that causes sluggish skin, essential oils can be used as part of your daily skin-care routine and to treat specific problems such as acne.

FEED YOUR SKIN

Skin needs to be fed and nourished – inside and out. Healthy diets can keep the body in shape but to keep skin in peak condition it needs to have a ready supply of valuable vitamins and minerals. Many factors can drain the body of this valuable resource – canned and over-processed foods, caffeine, alcohol, nicotine, sunlight, central heating, carbon monoxide and habitual drug taking. The effects of these can build up and attack the skin so from time to time you need to give it a break.

A one-day fruit and vegetable diet is an excellent regime to adopt once a month to cleanse your body and give a boost to your system.

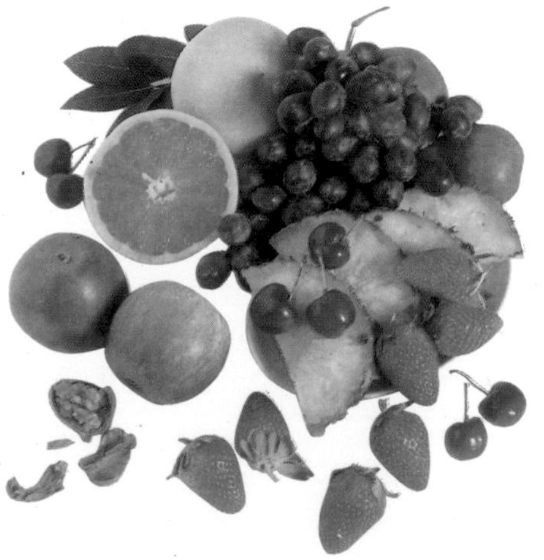

SKIN TYPES

Choose the right oils for your skin type and use them to blend your own cleansers, toners, masks and moisturizing facial oils. Remember that skin types can vary: skin may be drier in winter or more prone to oiliness around the time of your period, and it can change several times between puberty and menopause. So review the oils you use to suit your skin now and vary them to meet your changing complexion.

Few people are blessed with normal skin and even those who are may tend towards dryness or oiliness at times. Letters in parentheses indicate what other skin types an oil is suitable for. *D* = dry, *S* = sensitive, *O* = oily, *A* = all skin types.

Oils for Normal Skin

Chamomile (D, S) • Fennel (O)
Geranium (A) • Lavender (A)
Lemon (O) • Patchouli (D)
Rose (D, S) • Sandalwood (D, S)

Oils for Dry Skin

Chamomile • Geranium • Hyssop
Lavender • Patchouli • Rose
Sandalwood • Ylang-Ylang

Oils for Sensitive Skin

Chamomile • Lavender • Neroli
Rose • Sandalwood

Oils for Oily Skin

Bergamot • Cedarwood • Cypress
Frankincense • Geranium • Juniper
Lavender • Lemon • Sage

Combination skin has an oily T-zone panel from the forehead down to the nose and chin area, and may be normal or dry elsewhere. Double up on the treatments, using oils for oily skin on the greasy patches and oils for normal skin on the rest of the face area.

CLEANSERS

Choose the correct essential oils for your skin type and blend them in with an ordinary unperfumed brand of cleanser, liquid soap, or tissue-off lotion/cream, and they will do nature's work of rebalancing the skin.

FACIAL STEAM

Add 5 drops of chamomile for a soothing steam or try lavender, peppermint, thyme or rosemary to stimulate; or use comfrey or fennel for their healing properties.

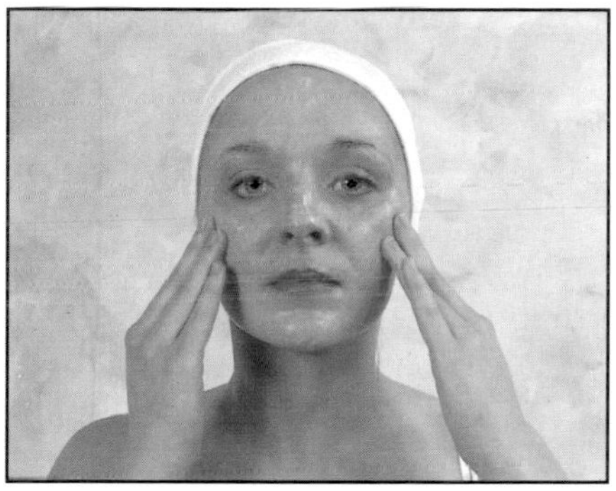

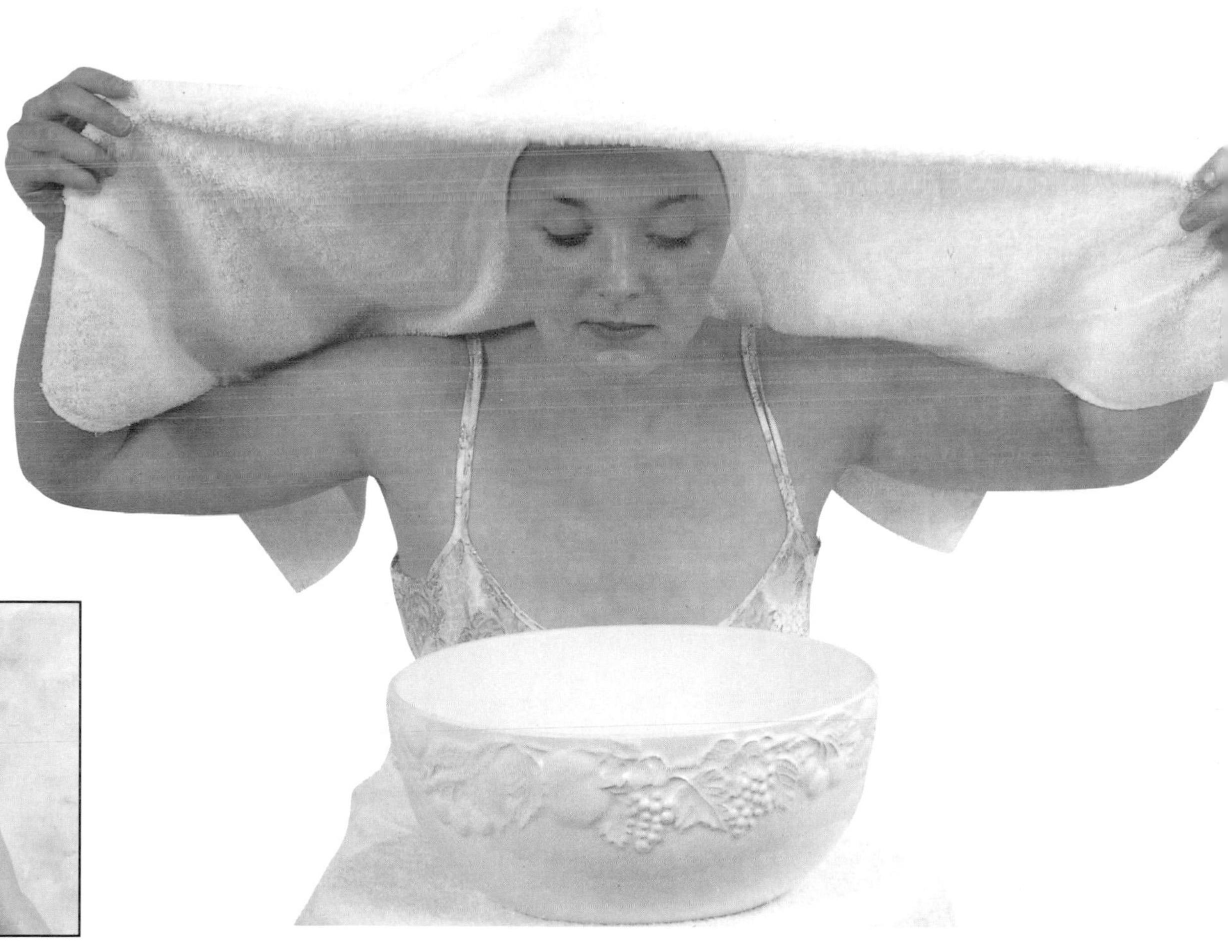

ABOVE: Cleanse the face, paying particular attention to the oilier areas.

ABOVE RIGHT: For a facial steam, boil the water, cool slightly and add the oils. Steam for 5 minutes.

TONERS

Essential oils are the gentlest way of toning up. Rose water for normal or dry/sensitive skin or witchhazel for oilier skins are ideal bases for fresheners. These can be applied with cotton wool or for a more refreshing tone, sprayed on to the face.

Herbal tea infusions are also ideal toners. Boil a cup of water and infuse chamomile, marigold, rosehip or nettle teas (you can use herbal tea bags if you cannot get hold of the herbs), add 2 drops of orange or lavender oil and leave to cool. Oily skin benefits from juniper or lemongrass whereas drier skins would appreciate rose or sandalwood.

FACIAL OILS

Well-moisturized skin is soft and supple, reflects a healthy glow and ages less quickly. Younger skin only needs light conditioning whereas older skin needs specific nourishing treatments. Most moisturizers soothe and sit on the surface of the skin, but essential oils, with their fine molecular structure, work their way through from the surface to the inner dermis (the skin's deeper regenerating layer). Mixed with the correct amount of base oil, these pure essentials do not clog up pores on lubrication: they are light enough to be absorbed spontaneously by skin.

Use 30 ml (2 tbsp) of base oil and add 6 drops of essential oil (maximum of 3 different oils) to suit individual needs.

MASKS

Both clay and oatmeal are ideal ingredients for any face mask. A natural powdered clay is fuller's earth, which can be mixed into a paste with hot water. Cool and then add yogurt for a smoother consistency. Similarly, finely ground oatmeal can be mixed into a paste and left to cool. Add 15 drops of essential oils to suit your skin type per cupful of paste. Smooth on to your face, leave to dry slightly and then sponge off. For particularly dry/sensitive skins add 15 ml (1 tbsp) evening primrose base oil to give a more moisturizing mask. When applying, avoid the eye area.

HEALTHY HAIR

Hair can define your image and style but it is also a mirror of your health. Emotional or physical problems can soon result in a lack of bounce or shine. Keeping hair in peak condition is a combination of caring for it on the surface and nurturing it from inside with a well-balanced diet.

SCALP MASSAGE OILS

Dry hair is rough to touch, thick in texture and dries out at the first sign of heated rollers or tongs. Avoid chemical colourants and perms and opt for shampoos and conditioners with jojoba and almond oils. Hot oil treatments allow essential oils to soak in easily and condition the hair. After massaging warm oil into the scalp, wrap the head in a warm towel and leave on for half an hour.

OILS FOR DRY HAIR

Geranium • *Lavender*
Rose • *Sandalwood* • *Ylang-ylang*

Greasy hair tends to look dull, lank, lacks body and will not hold a style. Central heating and environmental elements aggravate the condition but it can stem from a hormonal imbalance. Check your diet and avoid harsh degreasing shampoos. Clean brushes and combs weekly. Plastic brushes are better for brushing through as bristle continually stimulates the scalp. Choose light conditioning rinses to detangle but try a scalp massage to regulate the oil-producing sebaceous glands.

OILS FOR GREASY HAIR

Basil • *Cedarwood* • *Chamomile*
Cypress • *Eucalyptus* • *Lemongrass*
Rosemary • *Sage*

Normal hair is glossy with plenty of natural body and bounce. An occasional

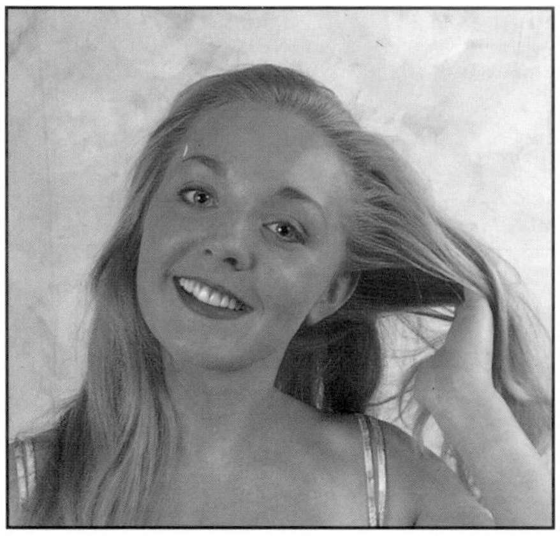

hot-oil scalp treatment will keep it looking good and growing healthily.

OILS FOR NORMAL HAIR

Geranium • *Lavender*
Lemongrass • *Rosemary*

Combination hair has ends that are dry or normal and the roots are greasy. Avoid using hot appliances near the scalp and keep the ends regularly trimmed and conditioned. Use a scalp treatment with oils for greasy hair but do not comb through to the ends.

HOW TO MIX

Base oils Choose from sweet almond, apricot kernel, avocado, jojoba, evening primrose or sunflower.

Essential oils For one scalp treatment, choose up to 3 oils and use 5 drops of each for 30 ml (2 tbsp) base oil (for very long hair you may need more oil). Warm the blended oils by placing the container in a bowl of boiling water, and then massage into the scalp. Wrap with a hot towel, leave for 15 minutes and then shampoo.

HAIR PROBLEMS

DANDRUFF

There are two types: dry and the more common oily. It is not catching! It can be caused by factors such as chemical body changes, stress, poor eating habits or wrong application of hair products. Both flaky and dry scalps can be treated with essential oils. Use special dandruff shampoos and conditioning rinses and treat the scalp by gently massaging with oils to suit. Use a base oil formula with patchouli and tea tree. For a dry, itchy scalp try cedarwood and lavender.

GREY HAIR

Grey hair is more porous and needs extra conditioning, particularly if it is chemically treated or coloured. Use a scalp formula for dry hair adding essential oil enhancers like chamomile to lighten or sage to darken any discoloration.

HAIR LOSS

Hair coming out in handfuls is often due to a hormonal imbalance, stress or anxiety, so first, learn to relax. Any unusual thinning patch should be looked at by a trichologist but, as a general remedy, use a scalp massage with lavender and rosemary oils.

SCALP MASSAGE

This is a wonderful way to condition hair, stimulate the scalp and relieve tension. You can use these steps to treat your own hair but it is even more relaxing if you can persuade a friend to help, especially if you have long hair.

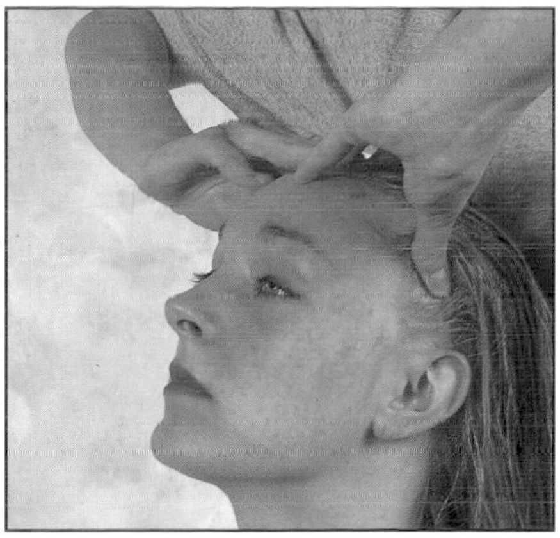

1 Shampoo the hair and towel dry to absorb excess water. Comb through with a wide-tooth comb. Tilt your head back and pour some oil on to the hairline, massaging in with thumbs on the temple and fingers spread apart over the centre of the head.

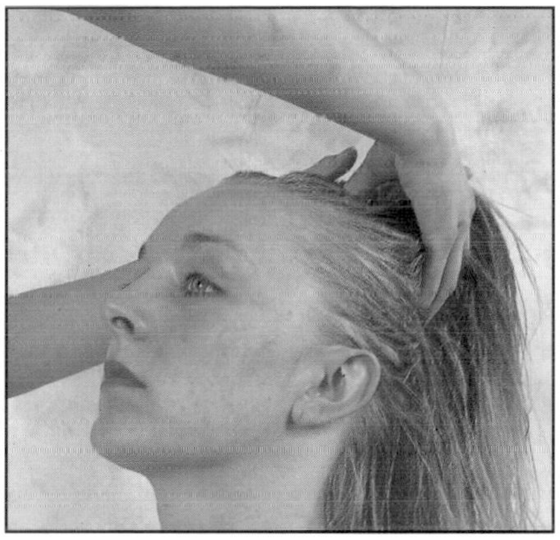

2 Loosely run fingers and oil over the top of the scalp from front to back, lifting hair at the crown. Keep dipping your fingertips in the treatment oil to spread through the hair while massaging.

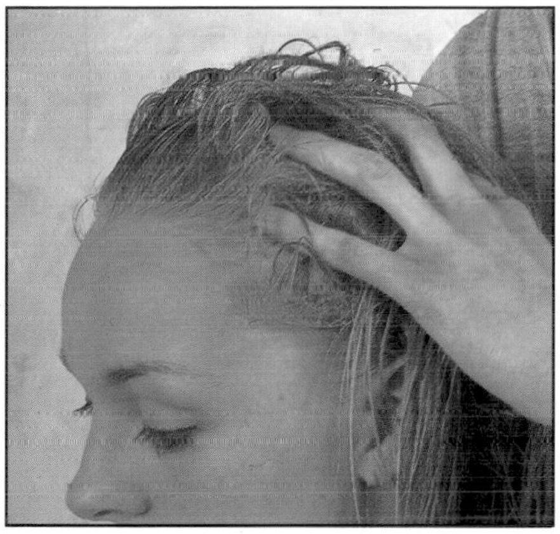

3 Massage the head by kneading. Grip and push (with fingerpads, rather than fingernails) against the scalp. The scalp should gently rotate against the skull. Concentrate on one area at a time, with the hands positioned on either side of the scalp.

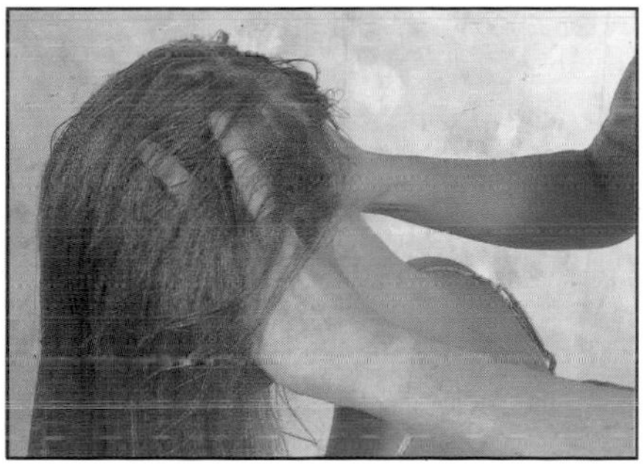

4 Scalp massage works from front to back, from the forehead, frontal hairline, temples and sides, over the crown of the head to the base of the neck, following the natural flow of blood. If the scalp feels particularly tight then concentrate on areas where the scalp does not want to move. At the base of the skull, press firmly and push the whole scalp up toward the crown to release tension.

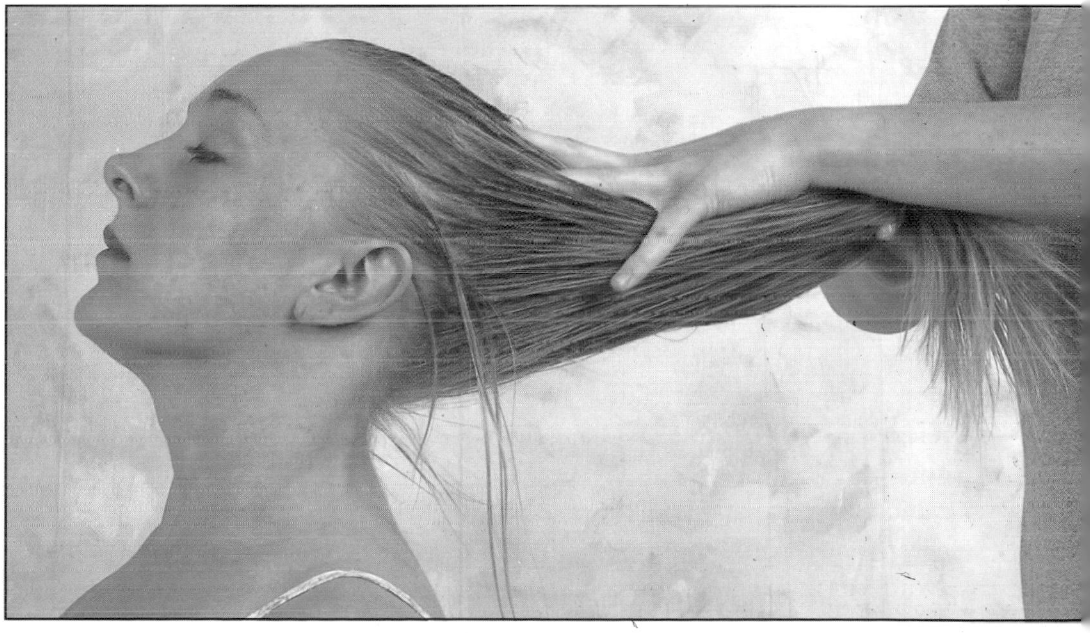

5 Pull any extra oil through the hair, working out from the roots to the tips. Make sure all the hair is well oiled, and then leave towel-wrapped for at least 15 minutes before shampooing.

Ambient Aromas

A lingering smell, whether pleasant or foul, is usually the first thing we notice when we enter a room, and it can strongly affect the way we feel. Fragrancing the home to cover unpleasant smells and delight the senses is an old tradition. For centuries the Chinese have suspended balls of jasmine flowers over the bed to clear the air and promote pleasant dreams, while posies of jasmine were handed to guests to refresh them on leaving banquets or dances. Lavender sachets placed in drawers and bowls of pot pourri to scent a room were particular favourites of the Victorians.

Studies and Offices

Work-places are often stuffy and full of unpleasant smells, but if you work in an open-plan space fragrancing the whole area may not be a viable option. Inhaling a few drops of oil from a handkerchief is the most personal way of using a fragrance, or you can spray your immediate environment with a room spray, or add a couple of drops of oil to a cup of hot water on your desk. Useful oils for the work-place are basil, rosemary, bergamot, lemon and melissa. Bergamot and lemon are particularly antiseptic, and lemon has the added advantage of helping efficiency. Basil stimulates a tired brain and rosemary is a great aid to concentration. Rosemary is also helpful in relieving headaches. If you are feeling overwrought, try clary sage or juniper, but watch the dosage as too much will cause sleepiness.

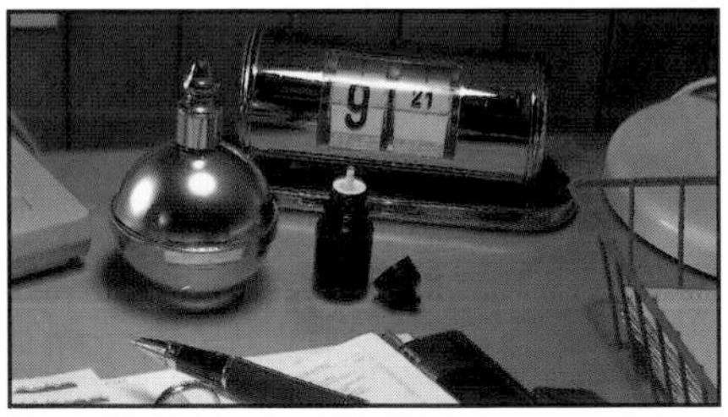

Living Rooms

The methods for fragrancing a room are many and diverse. Those that involve evaporating the oils, such as fragrancers/diffusers, water bowls, light-bulb rings and room sprays, are best for preventing ill-health, balancing the emotions and disguising unpleasant smells such as cigarette smoke or cooking odours. All these methods disperse the fragrance through a large space extremely quickly and effectively. For more lingering and subtle scents, blend your own pot pourri or, alternatively, use pomanders.

Rose, geranium, orange and lavender are pleasing and uplifting scents for a room, used individually or blended together. For an exotic, intimate atmosphere use sandalwood or patchouli, or to unwind in the evening try geranium, lavender, sandalwood or ylang-ylang.

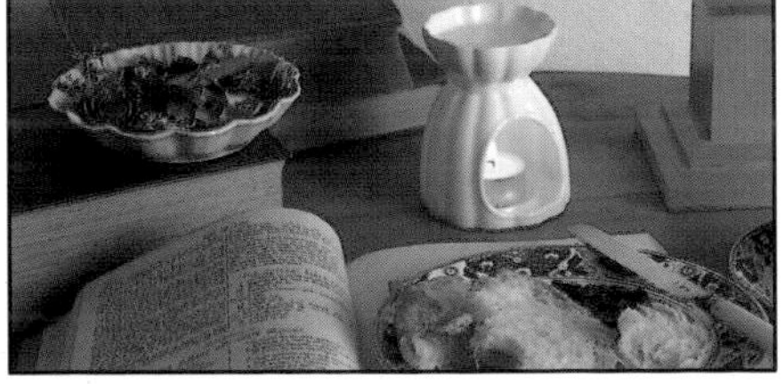

Perfumes for Parties

Clary sage or jasmine will create a heady, "feel-good" atmosphere for a party, or use orange, lemongrass or neroli for a lighter, fresher touch.

For a festive blend choose from the spicier oils such as frankincense, cedarwood, sandalwood, cinnamon and orange.

Bedrooms

Whether to ensure a restful night's sleep or to turn your bedroom into a place of passion, fragrancing the bedroom just before retiring will create an appropriate atmosphere. Rose, neroli and lavender are delightful all-purpose oils for the bedroom. Use lavender to freshen a musty spare room to make it welcoming for guests.

Insect Repellent

Use tea tree, eucalyptus, melissa, lemon grass or the closely related citronella in a diffuser to keep insects at bay.

Disinfecting

Vaporized molecules of any essential oil will neutralize airborne bacteria, but some – such as tea tree, bergamot, lemon, pine and lavender – are particularly antiseptic. Use these in a fragrancer or room spray. Pine, lemon and tea tree can be used on a damp cloth to disinfect surfaces in the kitchen or bathroom. Clear the atmosphere of a sickroom with bergamot, eucalyptus and juniper.

POT POURRI

To make your own pot pourri assemble fully-dried flowers, petals, herbs, leaves and other plant materials. There are no hard and fast rules about quantities and proportions, but an allowance of 30–40g (2–3 tbsp) ground spices, 30g (2 tbsp) orris-root powder, 10g (2 tsp) dried lemon, orange or lime peel, and 6 drops of essential oil to every 4 cups of dried plant material makes a pleasant, balanced mixture.

If your pot pourri loses a little of its aroma over a period of time, it can be revived. Simply stir in another 2 or 3 drops of essential oil. And if the mixture loses its colour sharpness just stir in a few dried flowers such as miniature rosebuds, santolina flowers or tansy clusters.

Cottage Garden Mix

1 cup dried lavender flowers
1 cup dried rose petals
1 cup dried pinks (*Dianthus*)
1 cup dried scented geranium leaves
15g (1 tbsp) ground cinnamon
10g (2 tsp) ground allspice
5g (1 tsp) dried grated lemon peel
30g (2 tbsp) orris-root powder
3 drops rose oil
3 drops geranium oil
Mix ingredients together in a covered container, and set aside for 6 weeks. Stir daily to distribute the fragrances.

Woodland Mix

1 cup lime seedpods, or "keys"
1 cup cedar bark shavings
1 cup sandalwood shavings
1 cup small cones
15g (1 tbsp) whole cloves
15g (1 tbsp) star anise
1 stick cinnamon, crushed
30g (2 tbsp) orris-root powder
4 drops sandalwood oil
2 drops cinnamon oil
Mix ingredients together in a covered container and set aside for 6 weeks. Stir daily.

Ingredients which can be used to make pot pourri. From the left: dried rosemary, lavender, and bay leaves, dried ground orris-root powder, dried rosemary leaves, a selection of essential oils, ground cinnamon, dried chillies and cinnamon sticks, whole cloves, a blend of dried flowers, limes and lemons. The dried peel of citrus fruit is finely grated or chopped for use in the spice mixture.

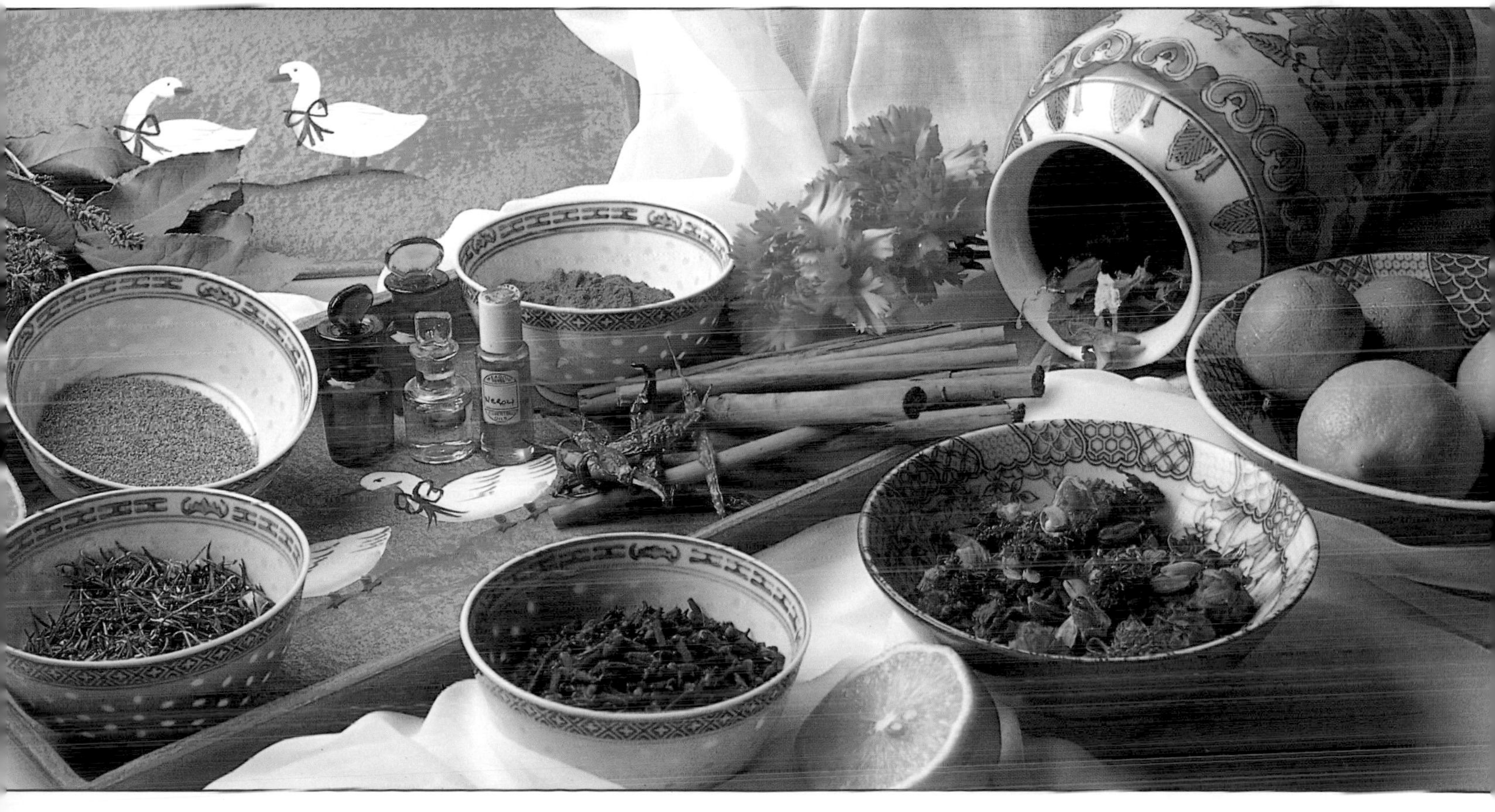

THE STRESS FACTOR

Pressure can be stimulating, challenging and motivating, but if it builds up we may be left feeling unable to cope. Our response is often to deny the pressure and ignore the physical signs of stress such as fatigue, self-doubt, sleeplessness and headaches. If the symptoms and causes of stress are left untreated they will affect your general health and well-being, and can even lead to serious illness, such as ulcers, heart attacks and clinical depression, so it is important to start tackling problems at an early stage, before they erupt. De-stressing requires a positive tactical plan for learning how to cope and retain a balanced outlook on life. Aromatherapy is a marvellous antidote to many of the problems associated with stress.

ANXIETY

Whether it is a temporary bout of nerves, caused by something like an impending examination or interview, or an ongoing response to a persistent problem, anxiety can be a debilitating response to stress. It prevents you from dealing effectively with a problem and makes you feel tense. Essential oils, when inhaled, stimulate the lymbic portion of the brain which is responsible for all our feelings of well-being and discontent. They can balance the senses before deep depression sets into a more serious state. Temporary anxiety can also trigger skin eruptions so watch your diet and boost levels of Vitamin C and E and B-complex.

Anxiety can be alleviated with a combination of uplifting and calming oils.

Basil (uplifting) • *Bergamot (uplifting)* • *Geranium (relaxing)* • *Lavender (soothing)* • *Neroli (sedative)* *Sandalwood (calming)*

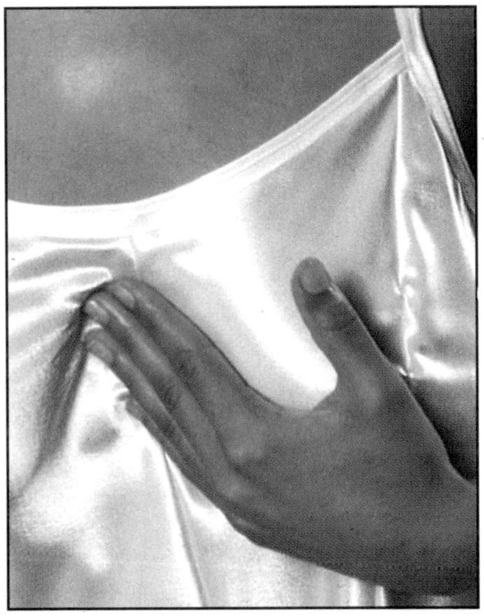

SOLAR PLEXUS STROKE

A marvellous way of unlocking tension by calming the main nerves that run through this area. Use your left hand (for calming) to stroke the solar plexus (located just below the breast bone) in anti-clockwise circles. Close your eyes as you do this and try to empty your mind. It can help soothe you even if you are clothed, but the effect is enhanced if you use a relaxing oil such as lavender or geranium. Try it while your bath is running, or when lying in bed before you go to sleep.

You can use the oils individually or mix them, using two relaxing oils to one uplifting oil. A good combination is basil, neroli and lavender. Stick to the same blend and proportions for bath and body, mixing 5 drops of each of the three oils in 15 ml (1 tbsp) of base oil for the bath and 30 ml (2 tbsp) for the body. All of the oils can be used individually in light-ring burners or fragrancers.

MILD SHOCK

This is a temporary form of stress, but the impact on the system can nonetheless be very strong, so a fast-acting remedy is needed.

Chamomile (calming) • *Melissa (anti-depressant)* • *Neroli (relieves anxiety)* *Peppermint (invigorating pain-reliever)* *Rosemary (stimulating)*

Use only two essential oils: both camphor and melissa work well individually with neroli, and peppermint has an affinity with melissa. Use a total of 6 drops in 20 ml (1½ tbsp) of base oils, with smaller quantities of rosemary (for example, 4 drops of rosemary to 6 drops of melissa). For fast relief add 4 drops to a handkerchief and inhale.

HEADACHES

Often one of the first signs of stress and a regular affliction for many people. Cold compresses of lavender or geranium across the forehead provide pleasant relief. Add 5 drops of one oil to a small bowl of cool or warm water, soak a cloth in the water, wring out and lay it across the forehead. To help a headache caused by tension in the neck, try a sandalwood compress across the neck. Scalp massage is soothing, or try the shiatsu headache relief steps (see page 318).

DEPRESSION

The blues can hit us all from time to time, as financial, emotional or work problems hang over like a dark cloud. In the long term, if problems are not resolved, depression lowers the immune system, leaving you prone to a spiral of worsening mental and physical health. Essential oils can work wonders in lifting the spirits to prevent this.

Uplifting Oils

Bergamot • *Cypress* • *Lemongrass*
Rosemary • *Sage*

Soothing Oils

Chamomile • *Geranium* • *Jasmine*
Lavender • *Marjoram* • *Neroli*
Patchouli • *Rose* • *Sandalwood*
Ylang-Ylang

Start off with three soothing oils, and then drop one of these in favour of an uplifting oil to give an element of stimulation, and eventually introduce two stimulating elements. Geranium, lavender and bergamot can make up a good combination. Use your formula for bath and body treatments.

Depression can be difficult to lift and if it persists you should consult a doctor or mental-health professional.

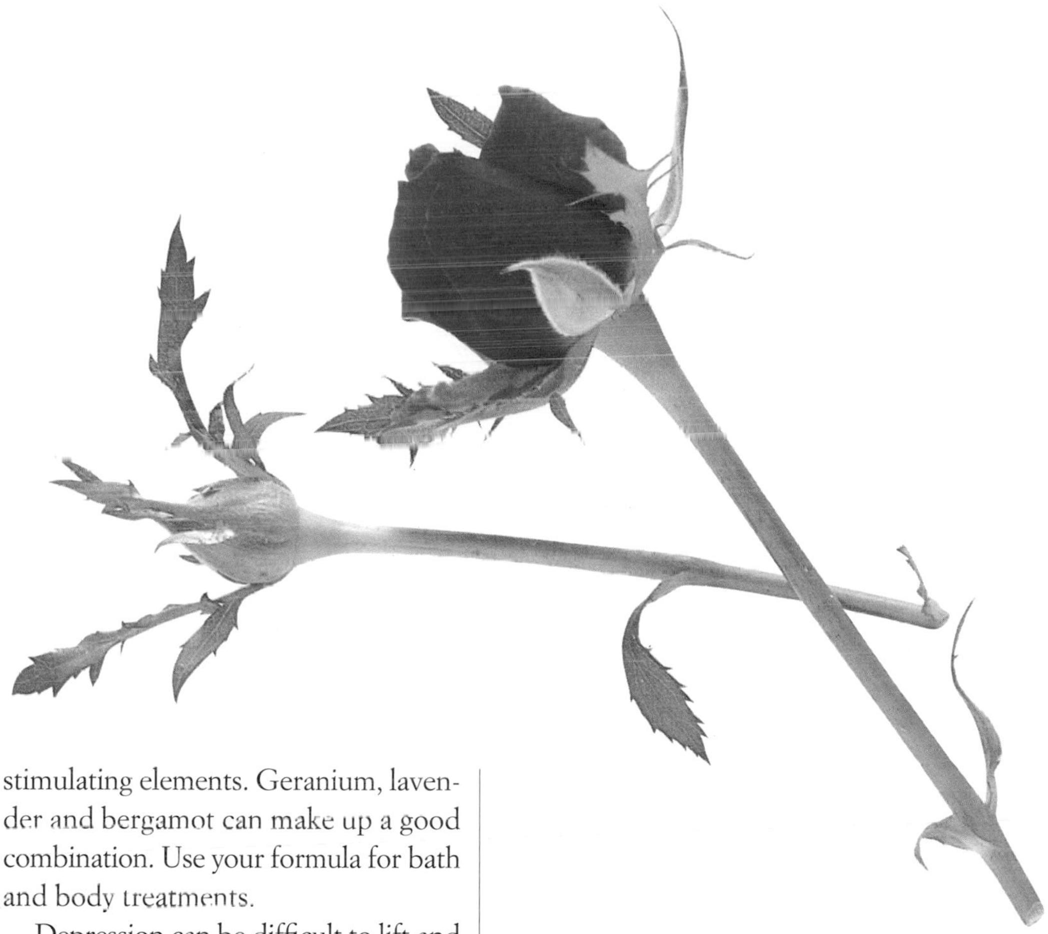

MENTAL FATIGUE

When you feel near to exhaustion or cannot concentrate on one thing at a time because problems seem to be crowding in on you, listen to your body's warning signals. Take time to unwind (try a bath with any of the soothing oils listed for depression), clear your head with a walk or deep-breathing exercises, and then revive yourself with oils such as eucalyptus and peppermint. Rosemary is helpful in concentrating the mind and stimulating the body so that you can continue to work if you feel you really cannot afford to take a break.

INSOMNIA

Sleeplessness is a common response to stress, as your mind and body refuse to let go enough to give you the rest that you need. Learning to relax has to be built into a daily pattern with a healthy diet, regular exercise, and a calming routine to wind down before bedtime. Try a milky drink or herbal tea last thing at night. Have a relaxing bath and massage, drawing on the sedative powers of up to three of the following oils:

Cedarwood • *Chamomile*
Frankincense • *Hyssop* • *Lavender*
Marjoram • *Melissa* • *Neroli*
Orange • *Patchouli* • *Rose* • *Sage*
Sandalwood • *Ylang-Ylang*

Breathing aromatic vapours in the bedroom helps to induce sleep:

❦ *Frankincense* is warming and relaxing, and encourages tranquillity. Use in a fragrancer.

❦ *Lavender*'s relaxing quality can be harnessed by dabbing 2 drops on the edge of your pillow.

❦ *Marjoram* has excellent soporific properties. Release in a light-bulb ring or fragrancer.

❦ *Neroli*'s wonderful floral fragrance is also sedative. Disperse unpleasant thoughts with 2 drops on the pillow or in a fragrancer.

HEADACHE RELIEF

Headaches and migraines are common symptoms of stress. Follow these simple shiatsu steps to sweep away the tension, relieve pain and clear the head. The sequence is quick and easy to administer; it can be used anywhere and friends and colleagues will be grateful for the relief of their pain. You can perform some of the steps on yourself, though the healing touch of another's hands is more effective.

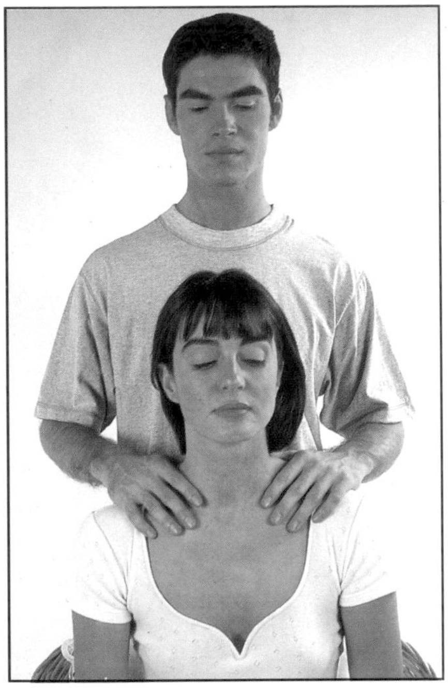

1 Establish communication with your partner by placing both hands loosely on either side of the neck. Gently massage the shoulders; this helps to relax the breathing and creates a feeling of well-being.

2 RIGHT: Tilt the head to the side and support with the palm of the hand so that the neck muscles can relax. Place the forearm across the shoulder and apply gentle downward pressure; hold for 5–10 seconds and then repeat with the other side. This movement is particularly good for opening the meridians running along the shoulders and neck.

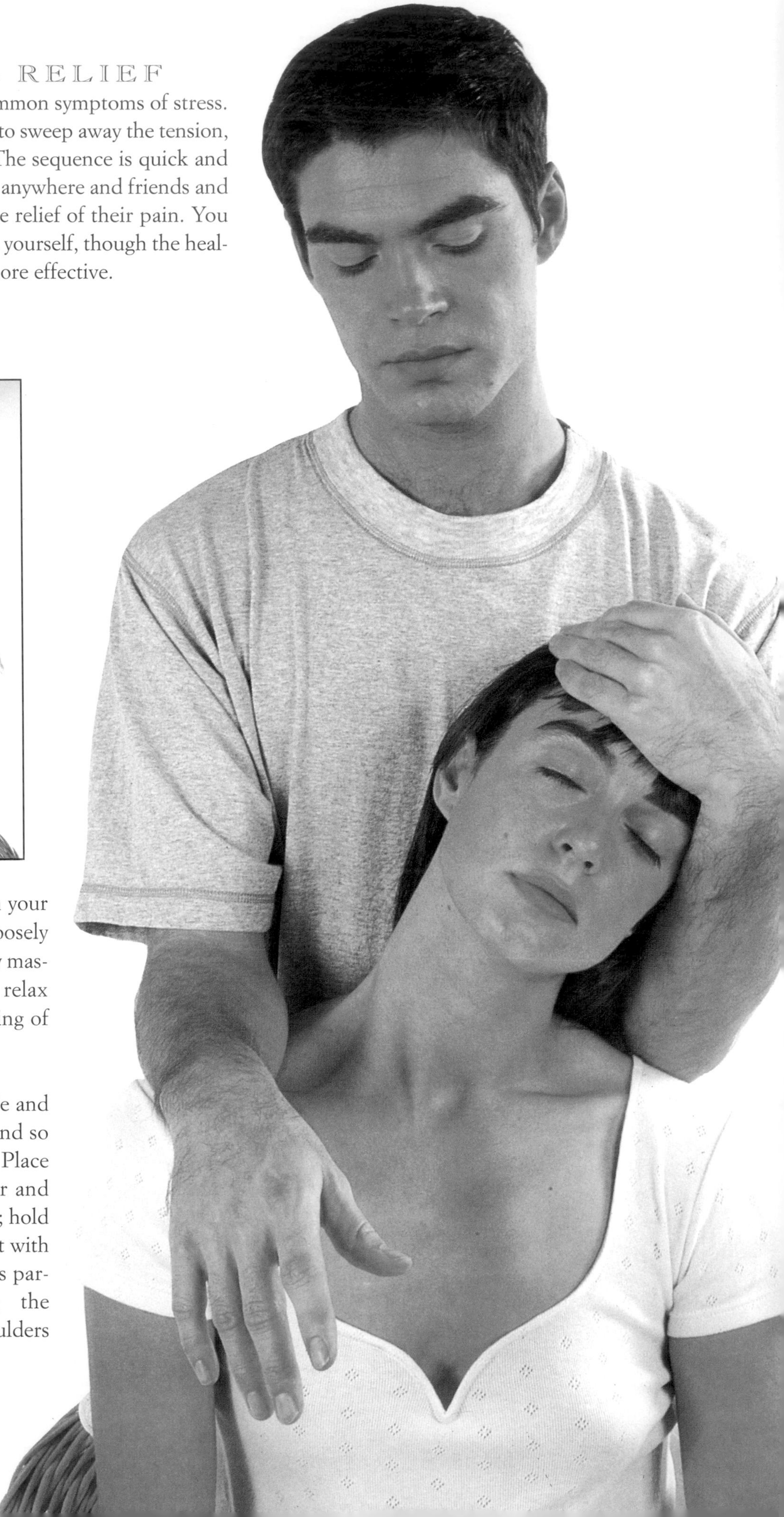

3 Supporting the head with the left hand, work with thumb and forefinger applying gentle pressure from the base of the neck to the nape. Hold at the nape of the neck for 5 seconds and then release the built up tension.

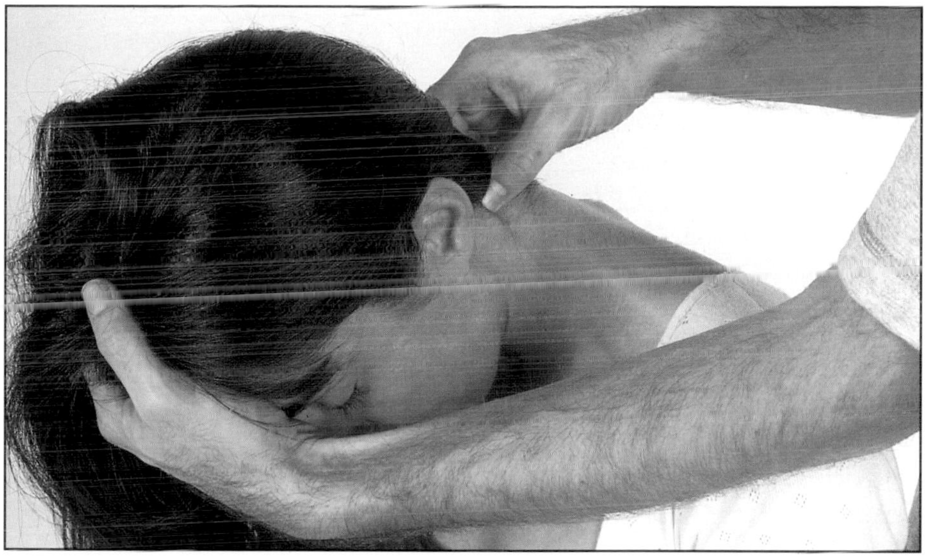

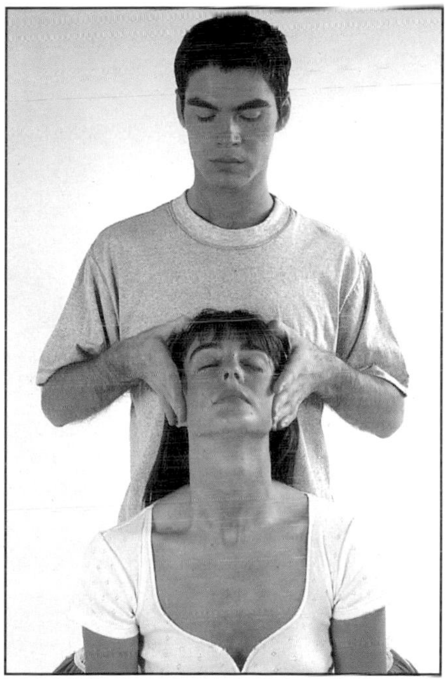

4 Tilt the head back slightly, supporting it on your chest. Place your thumbs on the temples with the fingers loosely resting on either side of the face. Gently rotate the thumbs in small forward movements.

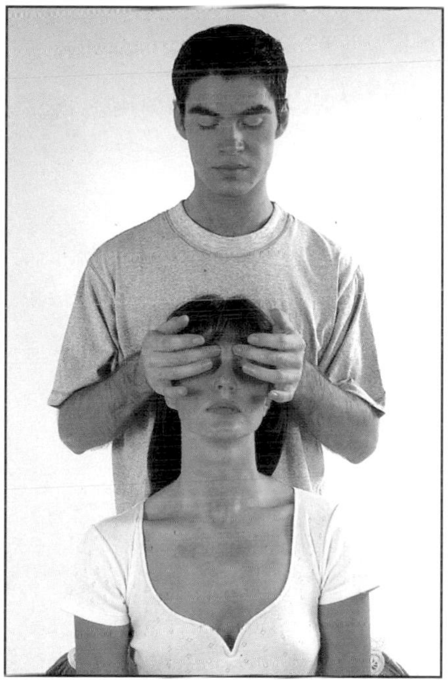

5 Find the pressure points just above the inner corner of each eye. Apply gentle pressure with the middle fingers to help disperse the pain. Hold the pressure points for 5 seconds.

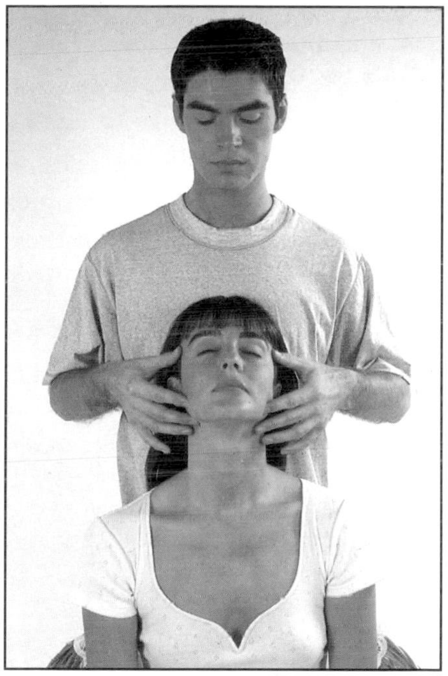

6 Position your thumbs on either side of the head just above the hairline – approximately 5 cm (2 in) apart – with palms pressed flat along the sides of the face. Press the thumbs evenly back along the top of the head.

A shiatsu treatment is usually very effective for relieving stress and headaches but if your headache persists, consult a doctor. Avoid the treatment during pregnancy.

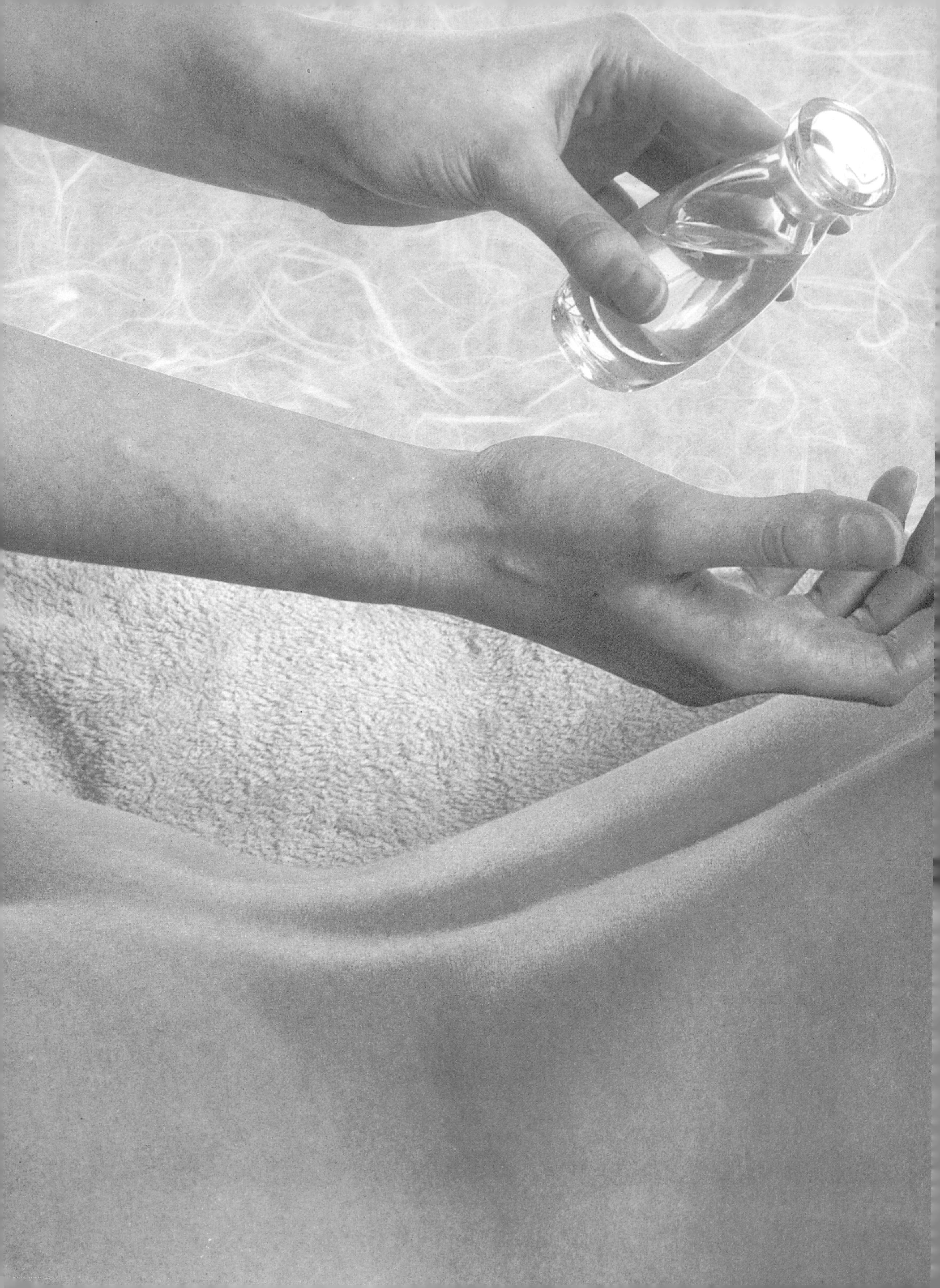

MASSAGE

Massage techniques are described in other parts of the book but this section presents the system developed by the Swede, Per Henrik Ling, who was inspired by the massage tradition of the Chinese. Using a few simple techniques and strokes, you can learn how to do a whole-body massage, designed especially to be practised at home. Ideas are given for massaging babies, elderly people, even yourself! Learn, too, how massage can be a highly pleasurable and sensual experience.

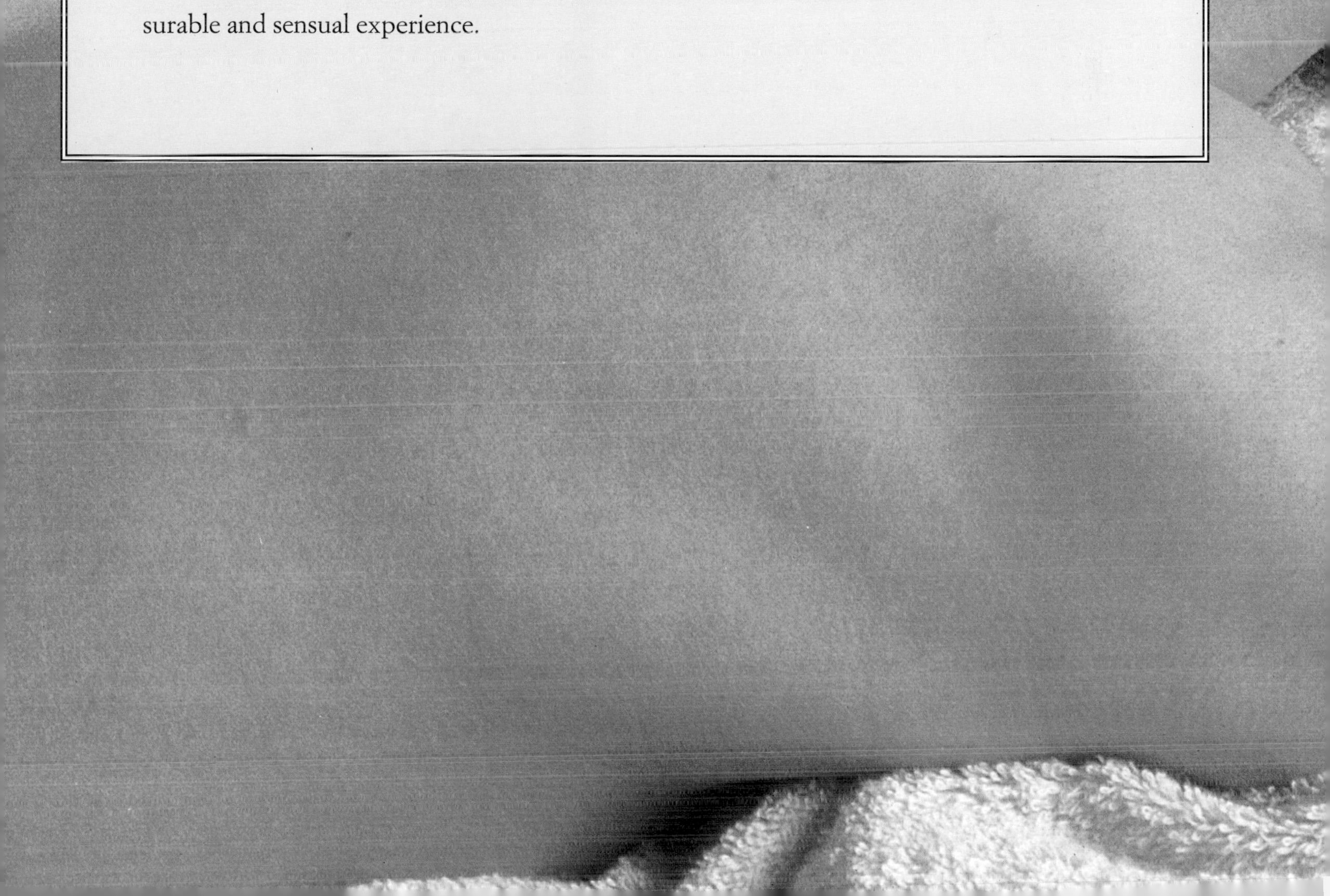

THE HUMAN TOUCH

The sense of touch is a powerful and highly sensitive form of communication. It is a natural reaction to reach out and touch, whether to feel the shape or texture of something, or to respond to another person, perhaps by comforting them. A mother cuddles her baby, family pets are stroked, sexual partners caress, and if we accidentally knock a limb we instinctively "rub it better".

Fortunately, we are now rediscovering the healing power of massage and other touch therapies which have been understood in other cultures for thousands of years.

THE DEVELOPMENT OF MASSAGE

History shows that although the early Egyptians made references to the benefits of massage, the Chinese were among the first to recognize its healing value at around 3000 BC. Roman and Greek philosophers and physicians prescribed it both for its restorative powers after battle and for general preservation of the body and mind. Although the Romans believed in its curative powers, the art of massage also became part of a daily ritual for relaxation. After bathing, oils would be used to anoint the body from head to toe, followed by a luxurious massage.

Herbalists throughout history have used massage to heal body and soul, both by applying balms and by laying their own hands on the afflicted to expel evil spirits and clear the mind. It was not until the eighteenth and nineteenth centuries, though, that massage became popular throughout Europe, thanks to the work of Per Henrik Ling (1776–1839). Ling was a Swede who travelled to China and returned with a detailed insight into their massage techniques. From these he developed his own system of massage based on a variety of movements, involving pressure, friction, vibration and rotation.

This wealth of practical knowledge soon spread, and medical and non-medical professions worldwide began exploring the benefits of massage. This eventually established the basis of massage today, which in many ways remains much the same now as those early Swedish techniques.

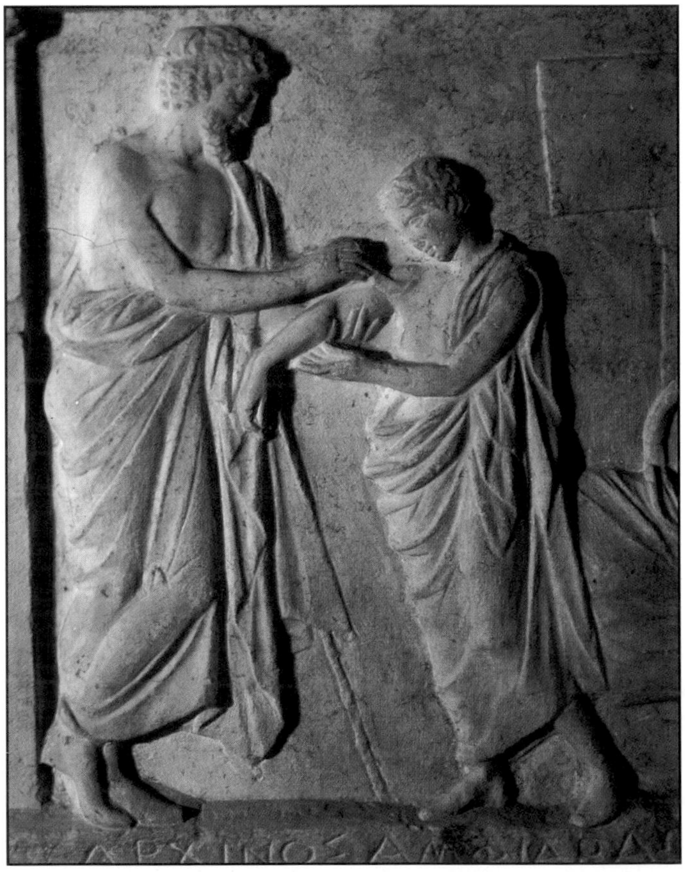

Along with basic massage we are now experiencing a revival of interest in many of the ancient arts which place such great importance on touch. These include aromatherapy, reflexology and shiatsu – all distinctive natural therapies which have a specific role to play in "alternative" health-care and are described in this book.

BELOW LEFT: *This Greek stone relief from the fourth century BC shows the physician Aesculapius treating a patient by "rubbing", as recommended by Hippocrates.*

RIGHT: *As Europe emerged from the Middle Ages, massage once again became part of the bathing ritual, as shown in this sixteenth-century German woodcut of a public bath house.*

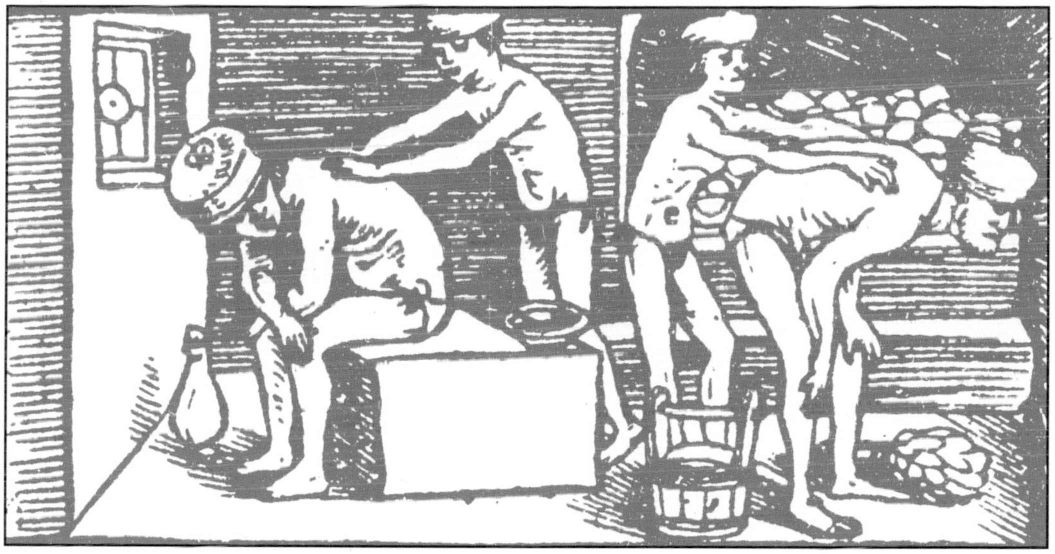

EFFECTS OF MASSAGE

Massage can stimulate and relax the body and the mind. The skin, blood and lymphatic systems are stimulated, which boosts circulation, aids cellular renewal and removes toxic wastes. As tense muscles relax, stiff joints loosen and nerves are soothed, an all-over feeling of relaxation and well-being comes about.

THE NERVOUS SYSTEM

The nervous system is a highly complex network which relays messages from the brain to the rest of the body. The part of the nervous system which regulates many physiological functions leaves the brain at the base of the skull and runs down the spinal cord, protected by the spine's bony vertebrae. Millions of nerve endings run throughout the body, controlling much of the way it functions. Depending on the depth of the massage movements used, the nerve endings can be stimulated or soothed.

THE SKIN

With massage comes an increase in blood circulation. This helps the exfoliation of superficial dead skin cells, tones the skin and encourages its renewal process. Massage helps maintain the collagen fibres, which give skin its elasticity and strength, and keep wrinkles at bay. The activity of the sweat and sebaceous glands, which lubricate and moisturize the skin, is regulated.

MUSCLES

With the increase in blood flow, the blood's vital nutrients circulate more efficiently. Massage is popular with sportsmen and women because it can improve muscle tone, restore mobility, and ensure the elimination of waste products after exercise. With regular massage, strains and sprains heal more rapidly, while calf cramps and stiff muscles can become a thing of the past. Massage before an exercise session will help loosen and warm up the muscles, or afterwards it will ease sore, aching limbs.

CIRCULATION AND LYMPHATIC SYSTEMS

By dilating the blood vessels, massage increases the blood circulation. A good circulatory system means that an efficient supply of the blood's constituents, including oxygen and nutrients, reaches the billions of individual cells. This is vital for the healthy functioning of the whole body, from the muscles to internal organs such as the kidneys and liver.

At the same time the increase in blood circulation helps accelerate the lymphatic system, which absorbs and eliminates waste substances. Unlike the blood circulation, which has the heart to pump it around, the lymphatic system has no pump of its own and is dependent on muscular action for its efficiency. Massage is an important means of speeding up the flow of the lymph, encouraging a more effective filtering and elimination of waste throughout the body. An efficient lymphatic system provides the body with a strong immune system to fight against infections and disease.

DIGESTION

Massage mobilizes the digestive system so that the processes of assimilation and elimination are improved, helping problems like constipation and flatulence. The digestive system is quick to respond to stress, and the reduction in anxiety and tension which comes with regular massage has a regulating effect on the digestion.

THE BASIC TECHNIQUES

When many people think of massage they picture the vigorous pummelling and slapping often associated with puritanical health spas. In truth, firm massage can be highly beneficial without causing discomfort. You can alternate firm and gentle flowing strokes to create a combination that will alleviate tension and muscular aches and pains whilst energizing and invigorating the body.

In Swedish massage there are four basic types of movement. Familiarize yourself with these different techniques before beginning the step-by-step, whole-body massage.

EFFLEURAGE

Effleurage describes long, soothing, stroking movements using the flat of the hand (or fingers if working on small areas). These are often used to apply oil evenly to the body. You can use one hand on its own or with the other providing support on top of it, both hands simultaneously, or one hand alternating with the other.

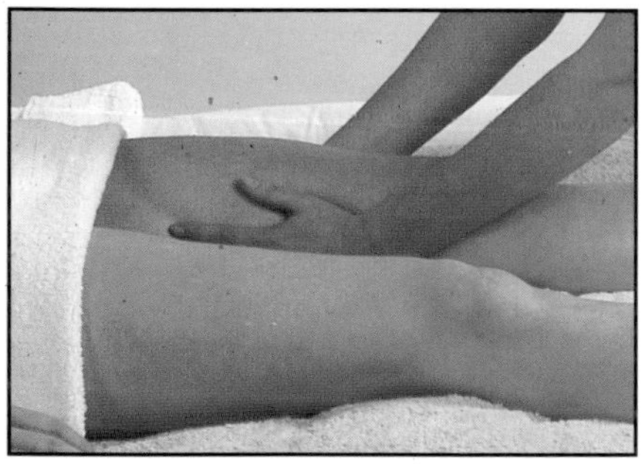

Relax the hands and mould them to the contours of the body. Apply slightly more pressure when you take the stroke in the direction of the heart to improve circulation and lymph flow. If you are working away from the heart, keep the pressure firmer on the return stroke. The movements should be fairly slow and continuous.

Effleurage is used to start off a massage, soothing the nerve endings and helping your partner get used to your touch. It is used again at the end of a massage for a relaxing finish. In between, *effleurage* movements provide an important link between other more stimulating strokes and are used to make first contact with a new area of the body. If you feel hesitant about what to do next, you can always insert some *effleurage*, so the continuity is not lost.

You repeat *effleurage* strokes several times. Each time try to start the first complete stroke with fairly light pressure, then apply slightly more pressure with the next complete stroke. Where there are larger muscle areas, such as the thighs and back, you can apply the most pressure for a more stimulating effect.

PETRISSAGE

Petrissage describes a number of movements which involve various ways of kneading, rolling and picking up the skin and muscles. These firm and strengthen the structures by stimulating the deep layers of tissue, and increasing the supply of blood to the area. They also improve the flow of lymph. Generally a single group of muscles, or an individual muscle, is worked on at one time.

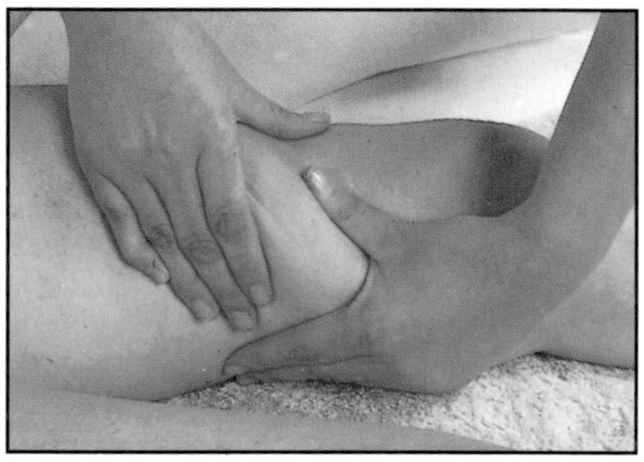

For petrissage, *start with your fingers pointing away from you, press down with the palm, grasp the flesh between fingers and thumb and push it toward the other hand. As you release the first hand your second hand grasps the flesh and pushes it back toward the first hand. It is a continuous action, alternating the hands to squeeze and release.*

With light kneading you are tackling the top muscle layers, whilst firmer kneading works on the deeper muscles, easing taut muscles and breaking down congested tissues to help the elimination of waste products.

FRICTION

Friction, or "connective tissue massage", is a penetrating circular movement which applies deep direct pressure to one particular site of muscular tension, using the thumb, fingertips or knuckles. It is a valuable technique for concentrating on specific areas of tightness and muscle spasm in the back.

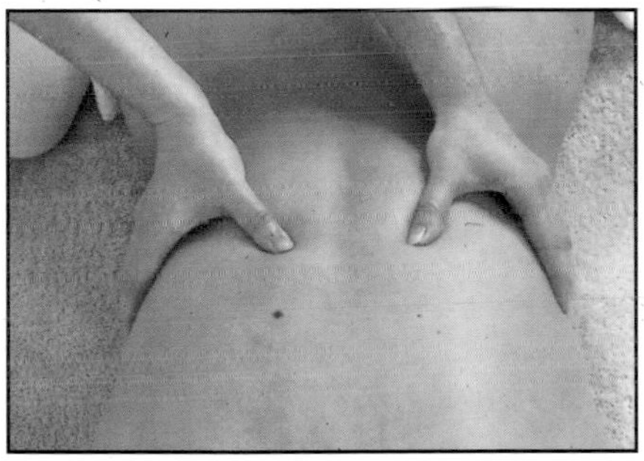

As you make the circular rotations you should actually feel the underlying tissues moving; you are not simply sliding over the skin's surface.

A variation on circular friction pressures is static pressure, where you lean gradually into the muscle, slowly deepening the pressure without the rotation action. Press for a few seconds, then gradually release.

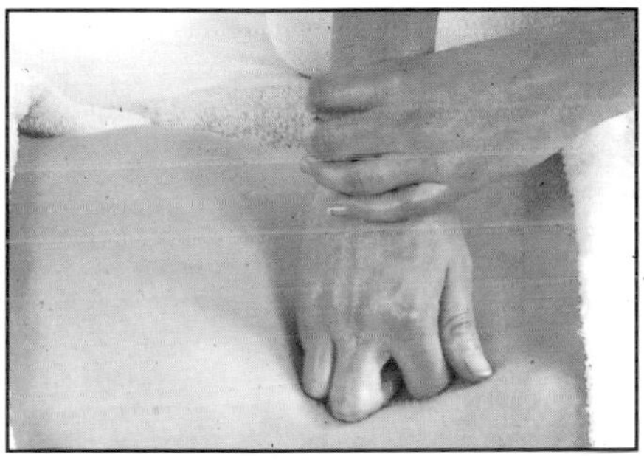

Another friction movement is knuckling: use the knuckles in a loosely clenched fist to produce rippling, circular motions. This is used to release tension up the sides of the spine and in other areas. Remember not to work right on top of the spine bone.

TAPOTEMENT

Tapotement, or percussion movements, are fast and stimulating. They include cupping, hacking, pounding (also called pummelling), which all sound like painful practices but when carried out properly should certainly not cause bruising or pain. (Do not use *tapotement* on particularly bony areas or on broken or varicose veins.) For all the movements, remember to keep the hands and wrists relaxed. All the percussion techniques are fast, precision actions, bringing one hand quickly after the other into contact with your partner. It is particularly important at the beginning to ask your partner whether you are applying the right degree of pressure.

These sequences stimulate the blood circulation, tone and help strengthen sagging skin and muscles. In particular, *tapotement* can tighten up soft tissue areas, such as thighs and buttocks, which are prone to cellulite.

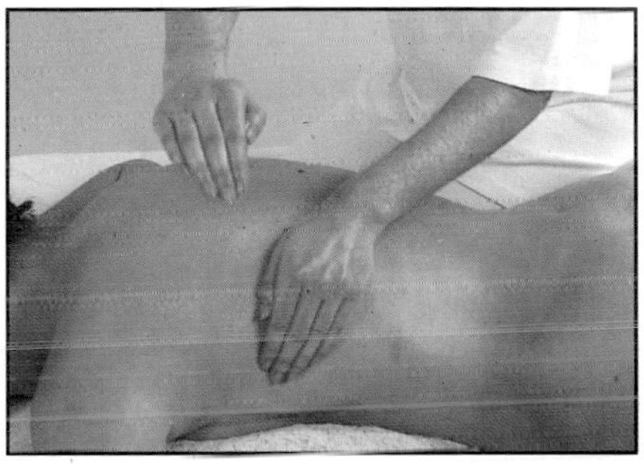

For cupping, gently curve the hands to make a loose cupped shape, bending at the knuckles while keeping the fingers straight and firm. Do not bend the fingers too far over. Using the cupped palm, make a bouncy, brisk, cupping action against a fleshy area, alternating the hands quickly. The fast, cupping action creates a suction against the skin. Try this movement on the back, buttocks and thighs.

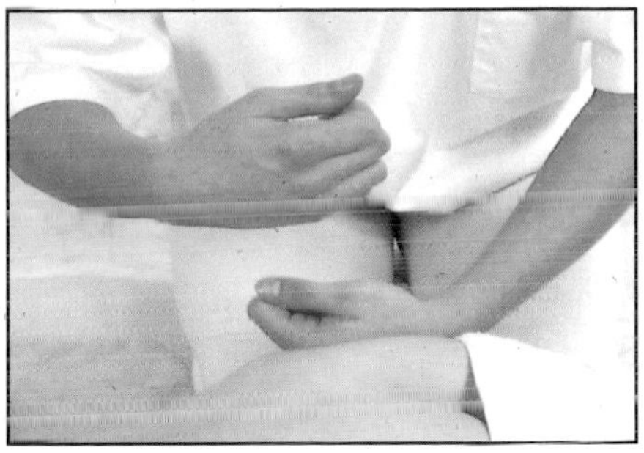

For pounding (or pummelling), loosely clench your fists, but keep the wrists relaxed. You can use the wrists in two ways: either striking your partner with the outer edges of the loose fist or with the front of the knuckles. Either way, the speed and rhythm of the movement is similar: brisk and firm, alternating the hands, without thumping your partner too enthusiastically. Once again, keep to the fleshier parts of the body, particularly cellulite zones such as hips, buttocks and thighs.

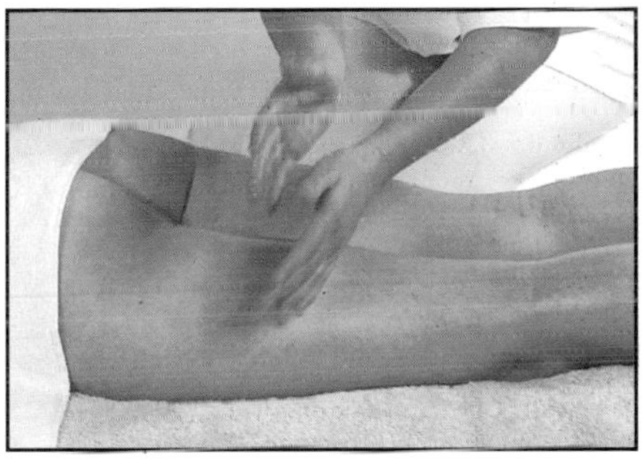

In hacking, the outer edge of the hand is used to stimulate the area by striking it quickly with alternate hands. You need to practise a brisk, bouncing movement, working rhythmically and rapidly over a fleshy area of the body. You need to have very relaxed wrists and fingers, and use the sides of the palm rather than the fingers. Used over the buttocks and thighs, hacking tones up muscles and disperses fluid.

Intersperse these brisk movements with the gentler, *effleurage* strokes, then go back to the pounding or pummelling for as long as you both feel comfortable.

WHOLE-BODY MASSAGE

Our whole-body massage is a comprehensive, top-to-toe sequence based on Swedish massage techniques, specially adapted for home practice. At first, you may find the full sequence too tiring. Until your hands and wrists build up their strength and you get used to positioning your own body comfortably to perform the massage, it is best to work on just a few parts of the body or to perform fewer movements on each part of the body. Always include *effleurage* strokes to begin and end a sequence, and never leave the body unbalanced – if you work on one leg or arm, you should repeat the same movements on the other side of the body.

COMFORT AND CLOTHING

If you are going to massage on the floor, put down a thick layer of blankets or towels, or a futon, to provide your partner with a firm, comfortable cushion. There is nothing more likely to reverse the relaxation process than a hard surface, a cold room and noise. Choose a quiet time, when you will not be disturbed. Your partner may need the room quite a lot warmer than you might expect. Being massaged on the floor might be extremely comfortable for your partner, but it can put a strain on the masseur's back and knees so, if you prefer, set up the same cushioning surface on a large table. It is not a good idea to massage on a bed – the give of a soft mattress can counteract much of your effort.

Have ready several towels, so that you can cover areas of the body which are not being worked on. Often a sense of modesty is crucial to relaxation, and the towels will also keep your partner warm. Move the towels around to cover most of the body, and especially an area you have just finished working on. You will need a cushion or towel to support the head, and it can be helpful to put a roll of towel under the knees when your partner is lying on their back. This relaxes the lower back. When your partner turns over on to the front, a towel under the chest can improve comfort.

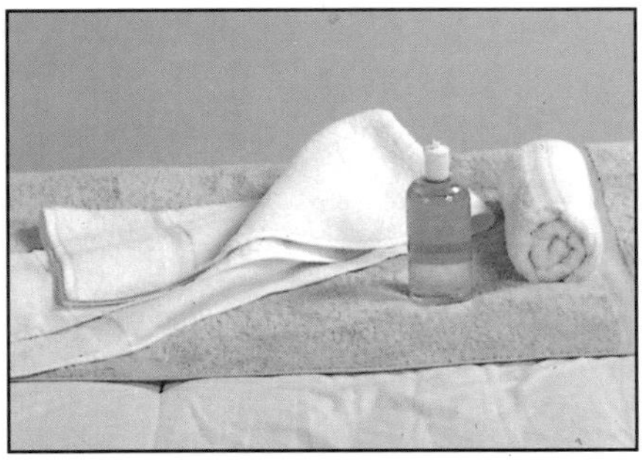

Massage in loose-fitting clothes, with soft-soled, flat shoes, or work in bare feet. Take off rings and jewellery, so there is nothing to distract your partner, and make sure your nails are short! The more relaxed you are, as the masseur, the better. If you feel keyed up, try some deep, regular breathing exercises before you start. Take a few stretches, shake your hands to loosen any tension, and you are ready to start.

OILS

There are several oils which are appropriate for body massage. Stick to vegetable oils, rather than mineral oils such as baby oil. Grapeseed, sunflower or almond oil are good, basic vegetable oils, which are light and therefore not too sticky. Jojoba is a good oil for the face, especially if your partner has oily skin. Avoid oils with strong smells, such as olive oil. Also try experimenting by adding a little avocado, apricot or peach kernel oil if you wish, or buy ready-mixed massage oil.

Measure 45–60 ml (3–4 tbsp) oil into a saucer or small container before starting your massage. You will quickly get used to how much oil to apply. The amount varies with the dryness of the skin, and how readily it absorbs the oil, but in general you need enough to facilitate the strokes without applying so much that your hands simply slide over the skin. If you need to apply more oil during a sequence, simply smooth a little oil into the palms of your hands and do some extra *effleurage* strokes.

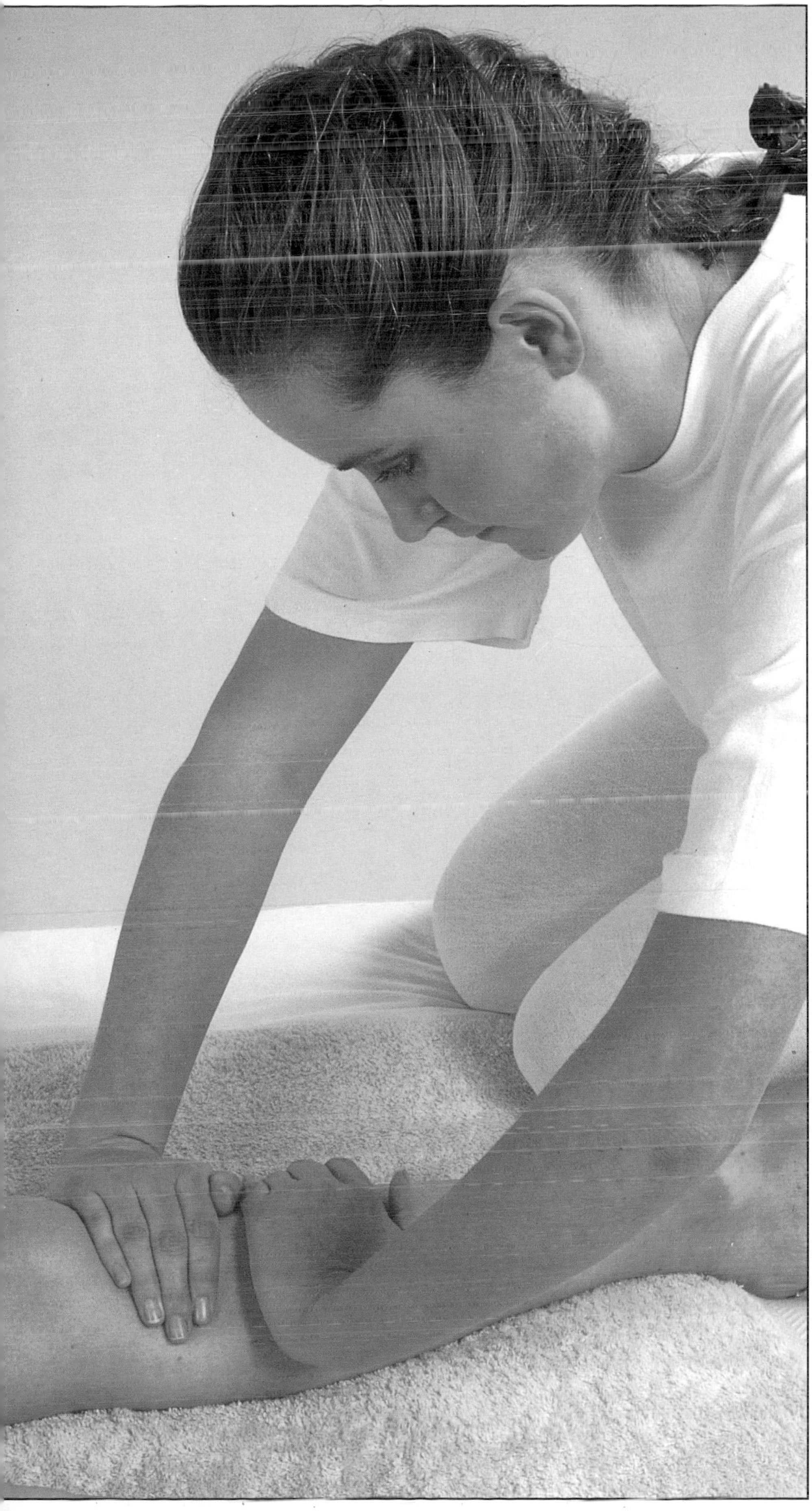

CAUTION

Exchanging a regular basic massage is a luxury for both giver and receiver. However, specific problems should be tackled by a trained practitioner. Never massage right on top of the spine. Working down each side of the bony spinal column is fine, and produces many benefits, but you should avoid working directly on top of the spine.

There are occasions when it is not appropriate to massage. Avoid if there are any of the following conditions:

- heart condition
- high blood pressure
- bacterial or viral infection
- nausea or abdominal pain
- severe back pain which may be caused by the spine, especially if there are shooting pains in other limbs
- temperature or fever
- open wound or skin infection
- cancer
- post-operative recovery

If you are in any doubt, it is always best to check with your doctor first.

THE FULL MASSAGE SEQUENCE

Front of Body

1 Legs 2 Feet and ankles
3 Arms and hands • 4 Chest, shoulders and neck • 5 Face
6 Abdomen and waist

Back of Body

7 Legs and buttocks
8 Back and shoulders

FRONT OF BODY

The full massage begins with the front of the body, so your partner should lie face up with cushions or rolled towels wherever needed for support.

LEGS

Since legs carry the full body weight, the bones and muscles in the legs are the largest and strongest we have. A good leg massage can not only help to relieve strain and tension in the legs, but can benefit the well-being of the whole body. It is not unknown for backache to be traced to problems in the legs, and for a good leg massage to help alleviate the pain.

Leg massage stimulates both the blood circulation and the lymphatic system, and done regularly it helps to prevent varicose veins. Any congestion in the lower legs will be lessened with *effleurage* movements taken up toward the lymph nodes at the back of the knee and in the groin. If legs feel puffy or swollen to the touch, make sure you use the gentlest of pressure. Firm massage on the larger muscles, such as those around the thighs, can dispel tiredness and stimulate a sluggish lymphatic system. Work more lightly over bony areas such as the shins and knees.

VARICOSE VEINS

You need to take certain precautions if your partner has varicose veins. Never knead or put any pressure on varicose veins, and only massage the part of the leg which is higher than the area with veins (that is, only massage closer to the heart); never on or below the vein.

EFFLEURAGE

1 BELOW: Kneel beside your partner's left ankle. With a little oil in the palm of your hands, start with your hands crossed over the ankle, in readiness to begin several long *effleurage* strokes. You will need more oil if the legs are particularly hairy or dry, but do not add too much in the first instance.

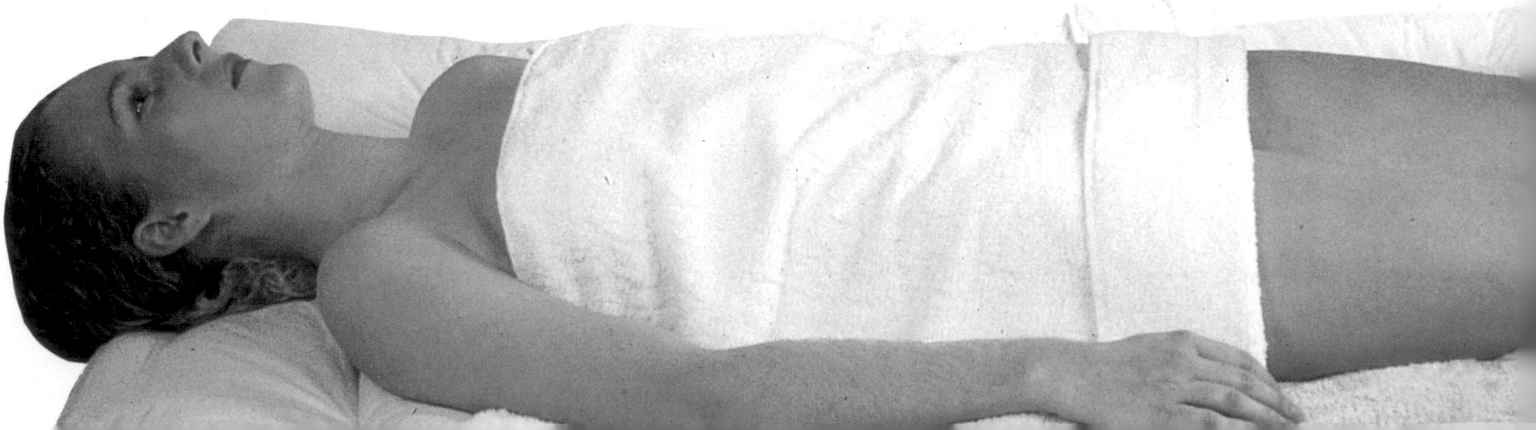

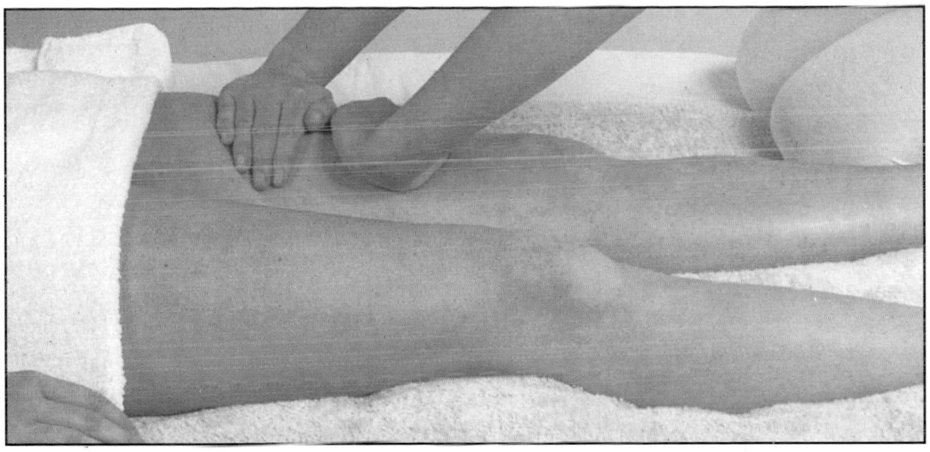

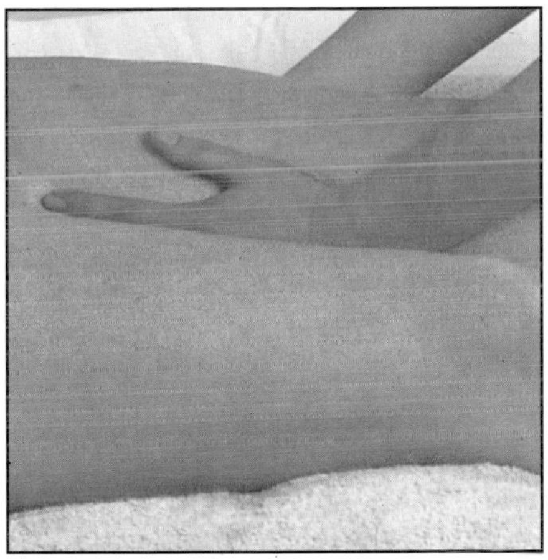

2 Keeping your hands crossed over the leg, slide the palms up the front of the leg, over the knee and up to the thigh, in one continuous, sweeping movement to oil the front of the leg evenly.

3 Turn the hands outward around the hip, separate them and bring the hands back down each side of the thigh.

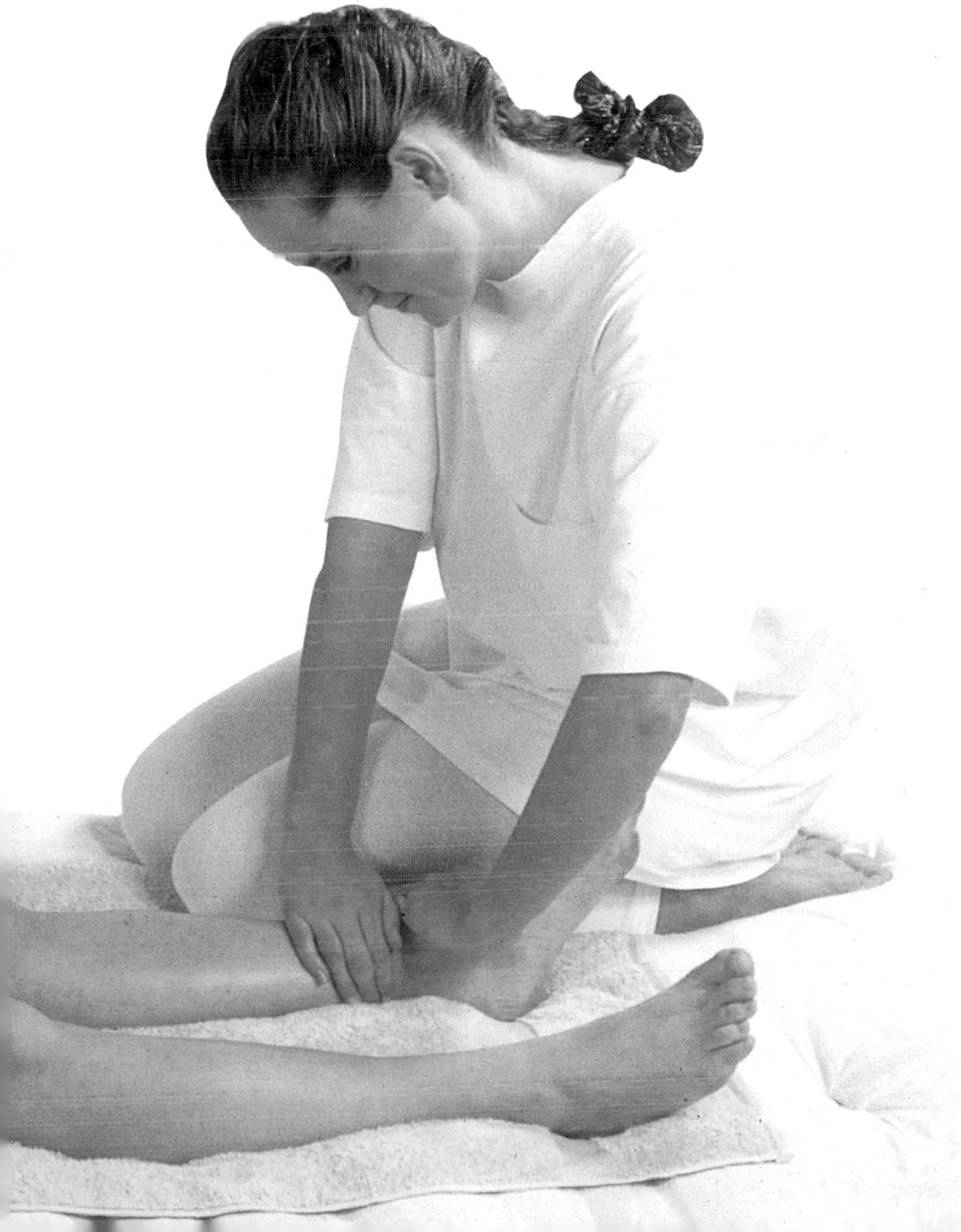

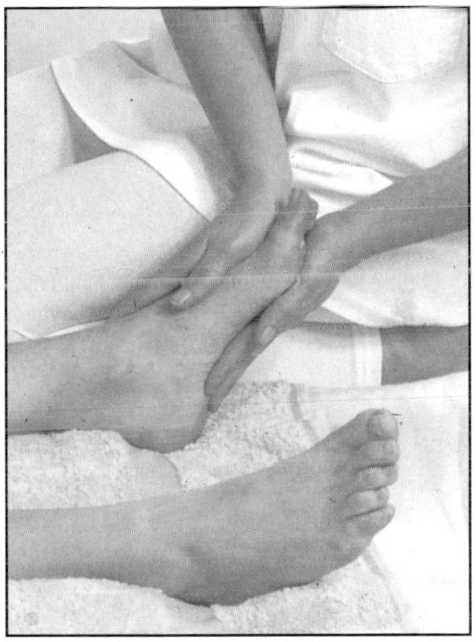

4 Continue to sweep the hands back to the ankle, and then over the foot to the toes. Then place your hands crossed over the ankle again, ready to repeat the entire movement.

Use some more oil if necessary, and this time use slightly firmer pressure on the upward stroke, then lighter again for the return. The stroke is smooth and continuous throughout.

Repeat the sequence over the whole leg once again.

THIGHS

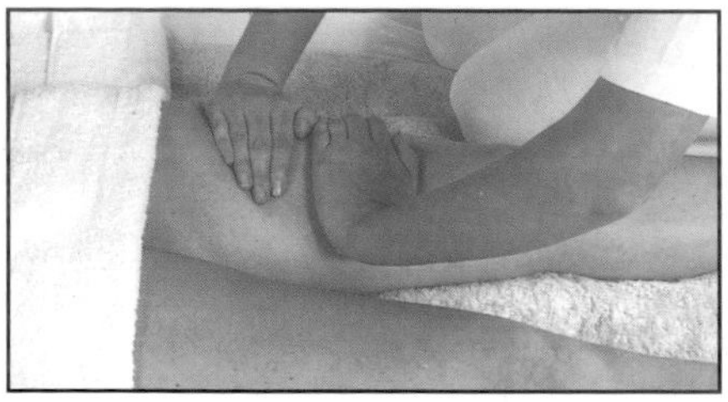

1 Bring both hands up to just above the knee and move them up together, pressing the muscles firmly toward the upper thigh. You should apply enough pressure to see movement in the muscles.

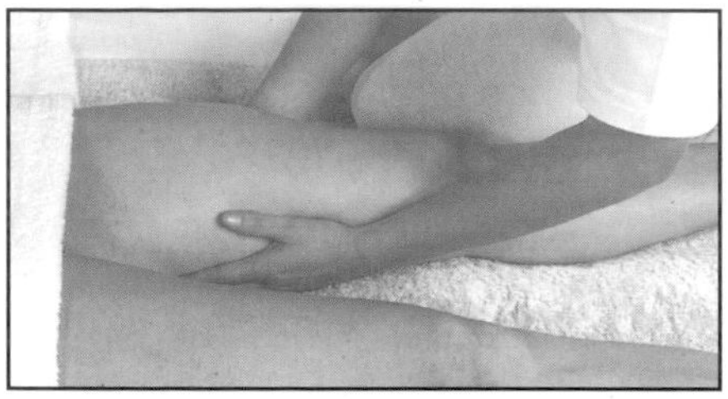

2 At the top of the thigh separate the hands and, using lighter pressure, come down either side of the leg to the knee.

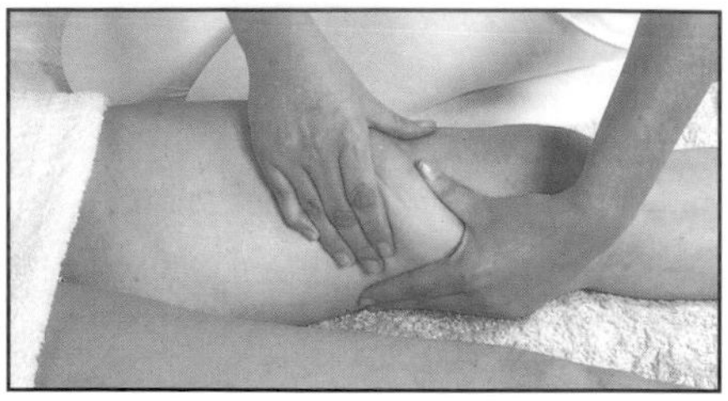

3 Begin kneading the inner thigh with both hands. Squeeze, then release the muscles, picking up and rolling them as you do so. Continue the kneading action over the top and outside thigh.

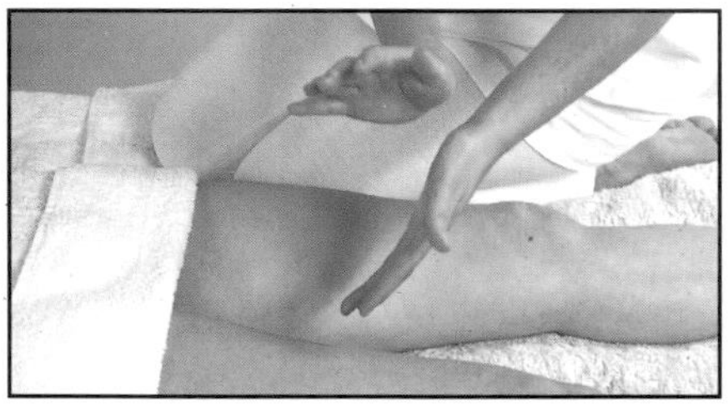

4 Now use a hacking movement all over the thigh. Briskly strike the area with the outside edge of one hand after another, using short, sharp movements. Keep a fast repetition going.

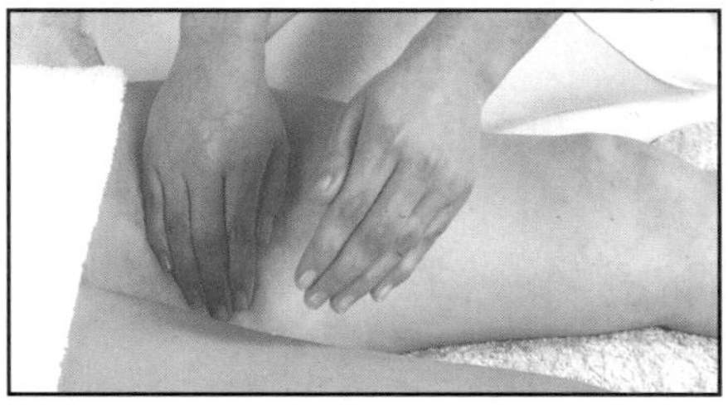

5 Continue with cupping all over the thigh, working quickly. Expect quite a loud cupping sound, but check with your partner that the strokes are not too powerful.

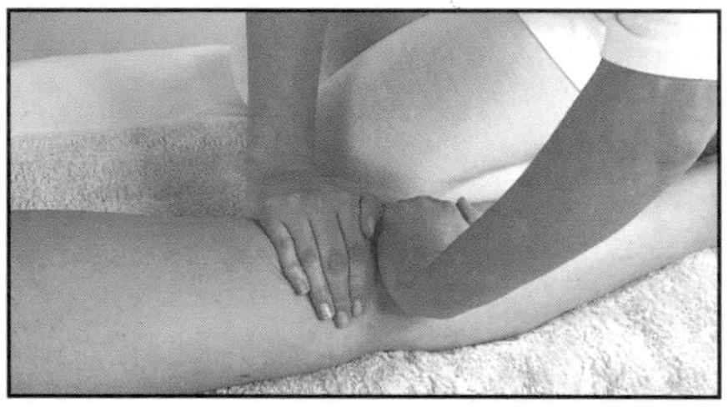

6 Begin at the knee and do some *effleurage* strokes up to the top of the thigh, sweeping the hands outward and back down to the knee, to soothe the area after the stimulating movements.

KNEES

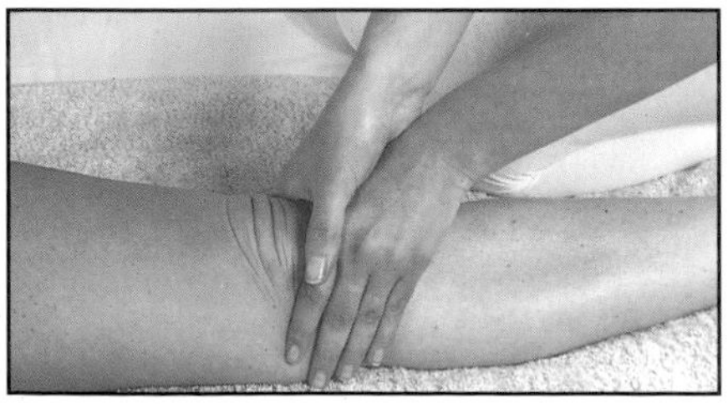

1 Place both hands just below the knee. Lightly massage around the kneecap, using your fingertips to work gently into the muscles. Repeat three times.

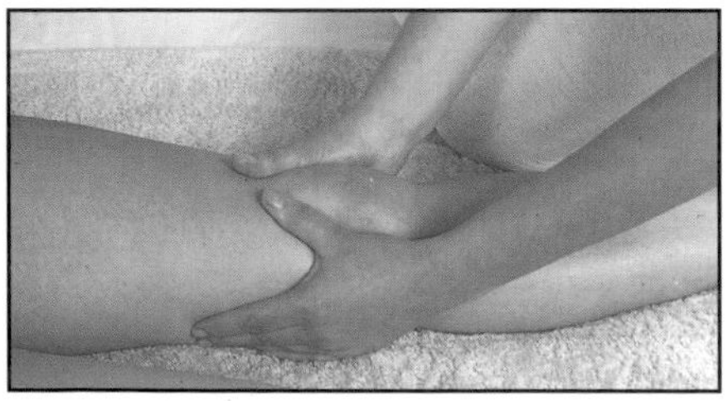

2 Starting with your thumbs above the kneecap, with your hands under the knee for support, slowly draw them lightly around the outside of the kneecap and release. Repeat three times.

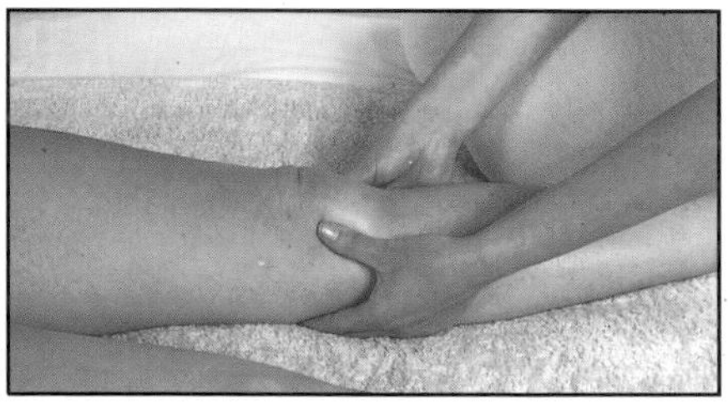

3 Support the back of the knee with your hands and use your thumbs to circle gently around the kneecap, working downward. Return to the top of the knee and repeat three times.

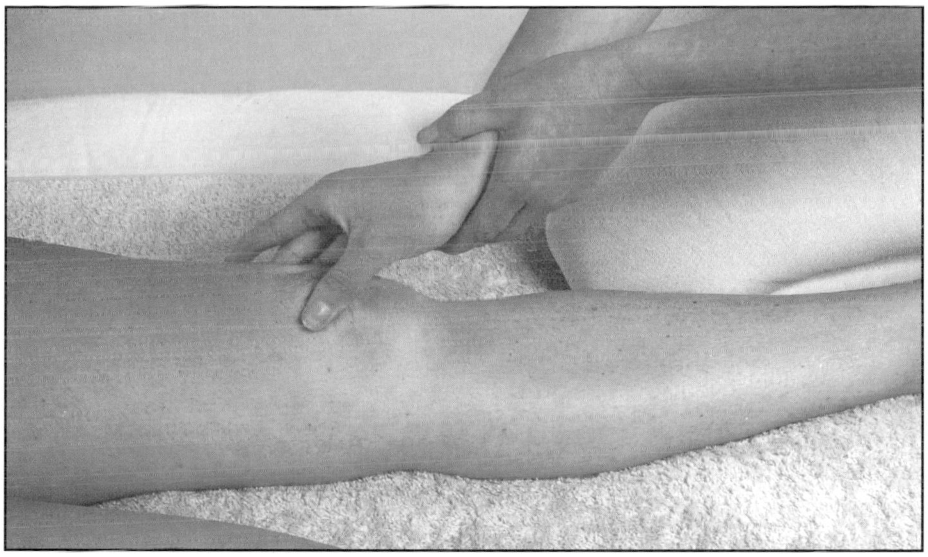

4 RIGHT: Raise the height of your hands above the knee. Work around the kneecap with one hand, loosening the muscles with your thumb and fingers. Use gentle, circular rotations to cover the area thoroughly.

You may find it easier to support your wrist with the other hand.

Do some more *effleurage* strokes, sweeping them up from the ankle to just below the kneecap and back down to the ankle. Repeat this several times.

CALVES

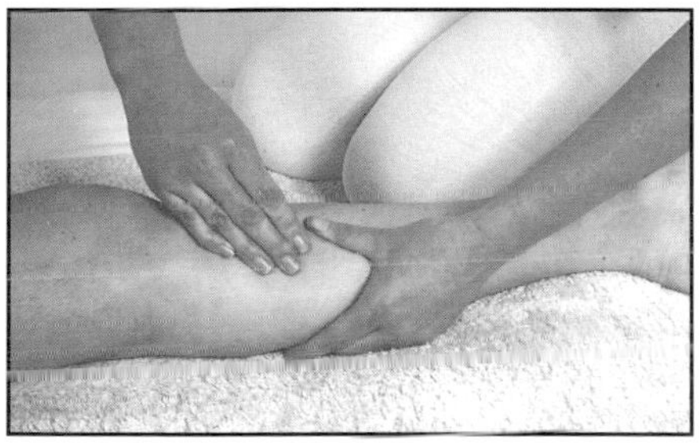

1 Knead the calf muscles. Squeeze and release them, working from the ankle up to the knee.

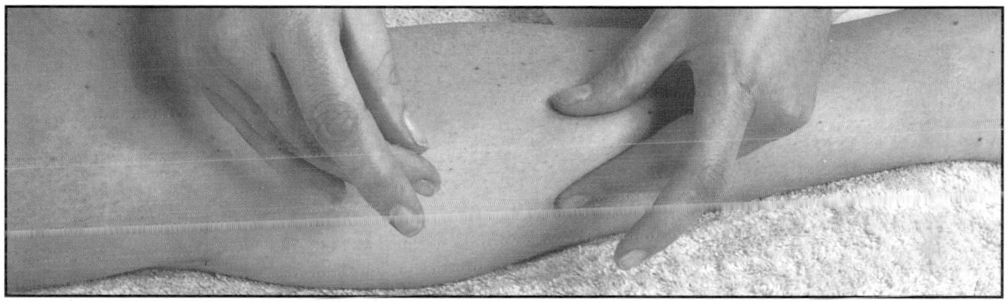

2 Lightly and quickly pinch the fleshy part of the calf with the fingers and thumbs, one hand after the other.

Check with your partner that you are not pinching too hard, although this needs to be felt to be effective.

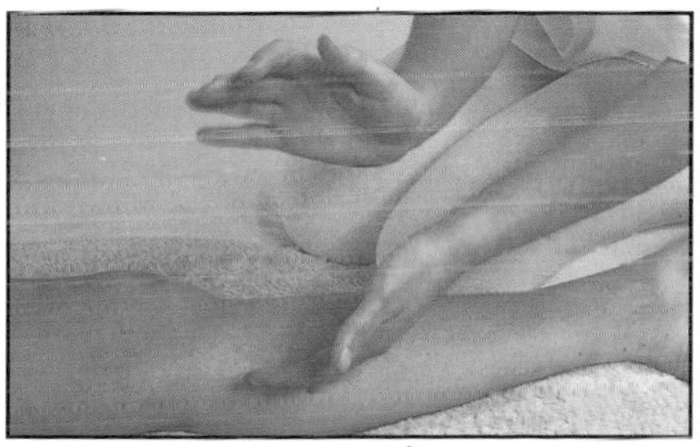

3 Using the outside edge of both hands, alternately and rhythmically strike the calf muscles, working up and down the entire length, but keeping away from the shin area itself. Keep the hacking action short and brisk.

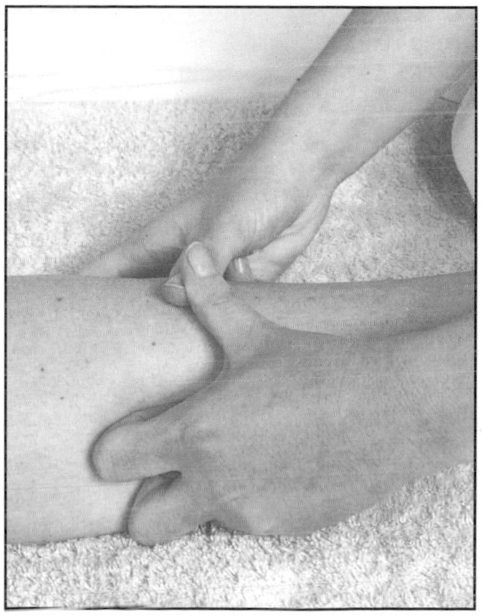

4 LEFT: Starting at the ankle and crossing your thumbs on top of the shin for support, with loose knuckles make semi-circular kneading movements, working up and down the calf.

Finish the leg with some *effleurage* movements from ankle to thigh.

FEET AND ANKLES

A foot massage is particularly relaxing after the legs have been worked on. It can alleviate anxiety and stress, stimulate the circulation and nervous system, help insomniacs to sleep, and energize anyone feeling tired and lethargic. There are thousands of nerve endings in the foot, particularly on the sole. Try to include the ankles to improve their flexibility.

Change the pressure of the strokes to suit your partner, remembering that deeper pressure tends to revitalize whereas gentle strokes increase relaxation throughout the entire person. When working on the feet it is best to use only a very little oil, otherwise your hands will slide around and tickle. If your partner's feet are hot, use talcum powder instead.

Before starting, you may wish to raise your partner's knees slightly with a rolled towel under them, to relax the muscles around the knees and in the lower back.

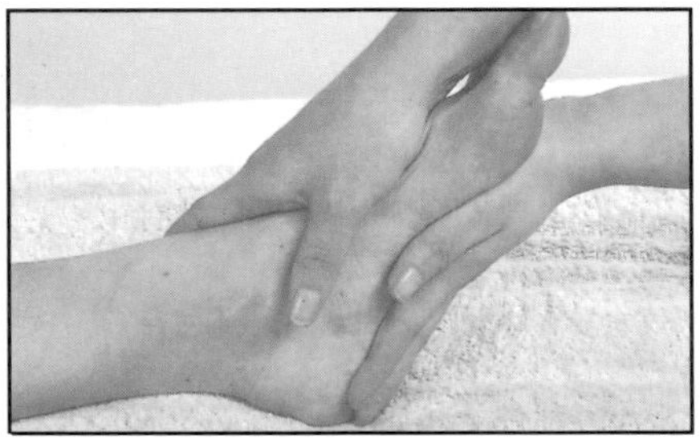

1 Kneel at your partner's feet. Starting with the hands at the ankle, gently slide your hands toward the tips of the toes and then release them. Repeat several times. If you are using oil, apply it with this stroke.

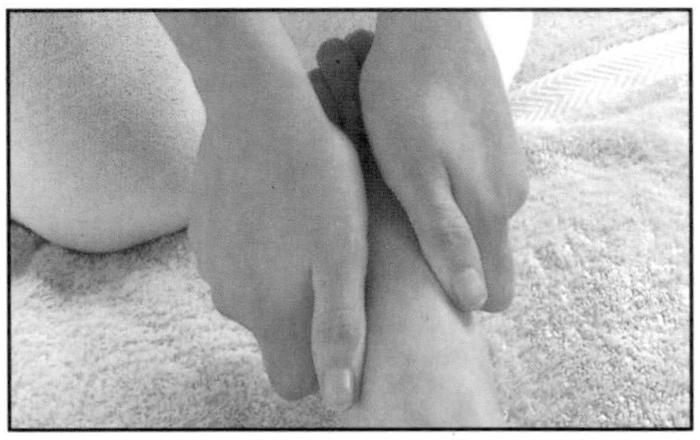

2 With the heels of your hands, give a good stretch to the top of the foot. Draw the heel toward the sides of the foot to give the stretch. Repeat a few times, working slightly further down the foot too.

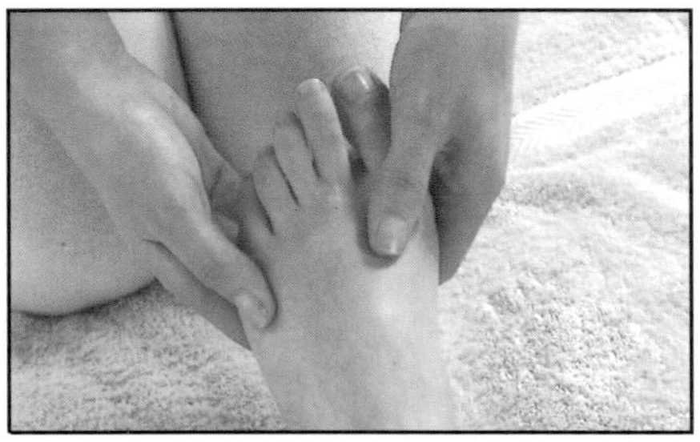

3 Supporting the foot in both hands, find the furrow between each tendon and, using small, circular movements, work both thumbs up the tendons toward the ankle. Repeat three times on each tendon.

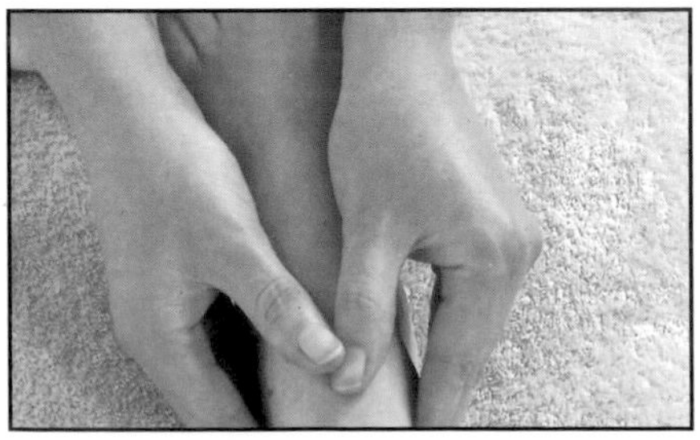

4 Resting the thumbs across the top of the ankle, work the fingers right around the ankle bone using light, circular movements.

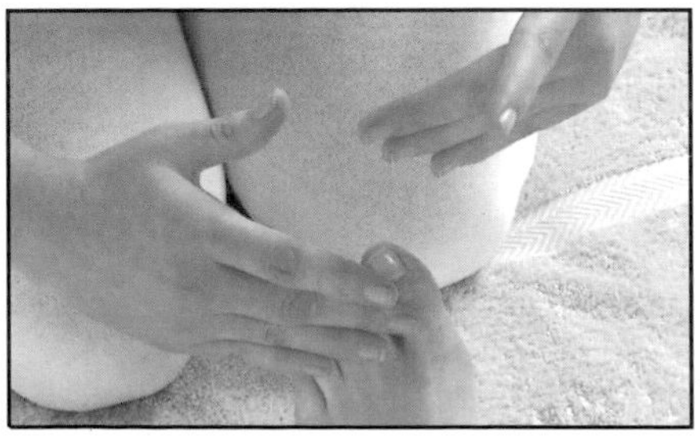

5 Lightly tap the toes with your fingers to build up some gentle friction.

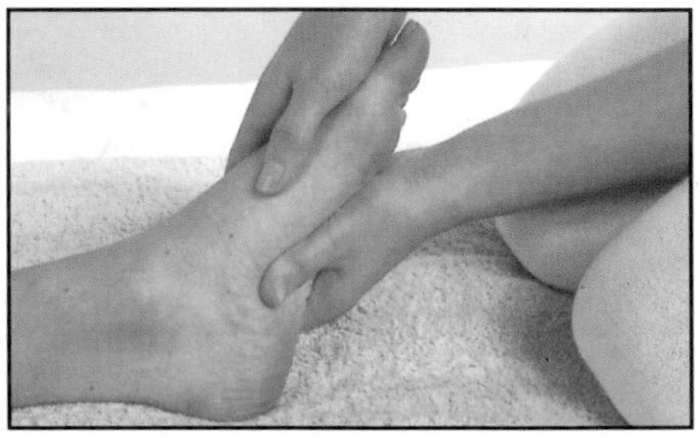

6 Now knead the foot firmly, working particularly well into the arch. You will need to use different parts of the hand, such as the heel, knuckle and thumbs.

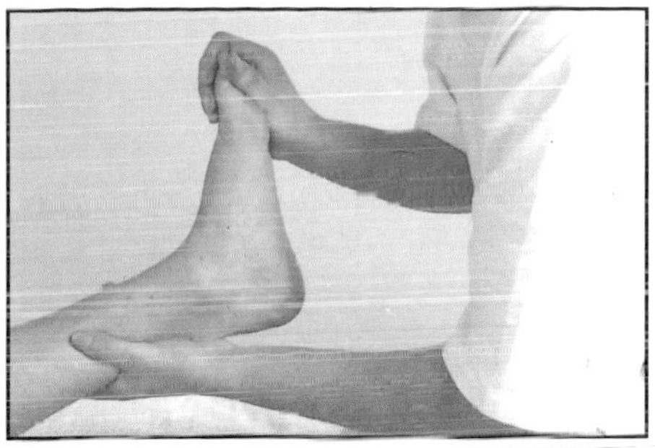

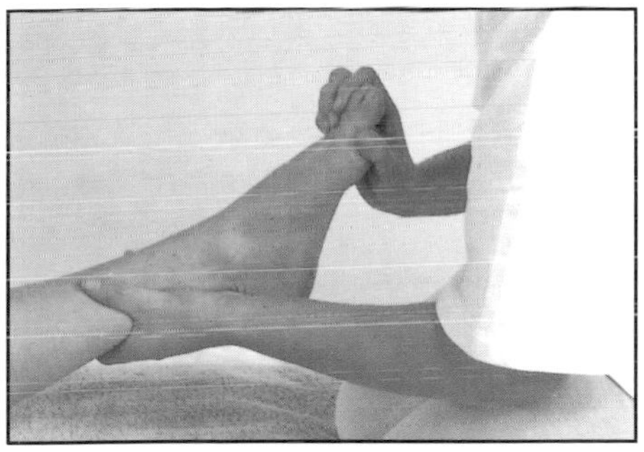

7, 8 Supporting the lower leg with your left hand, gently rotate the ankle three times in each direction, without forcing.

9 RIGHT: Give the foot a gentle stretch backward and forward, to relax and flex the tendons. Supporting the back of the lower leg, use your other hand at the toes to push the foot gently away from you. To reverse the stretch take the hand over the top of the foot, and press the foot down, still supporting the lower leg with the other hand.

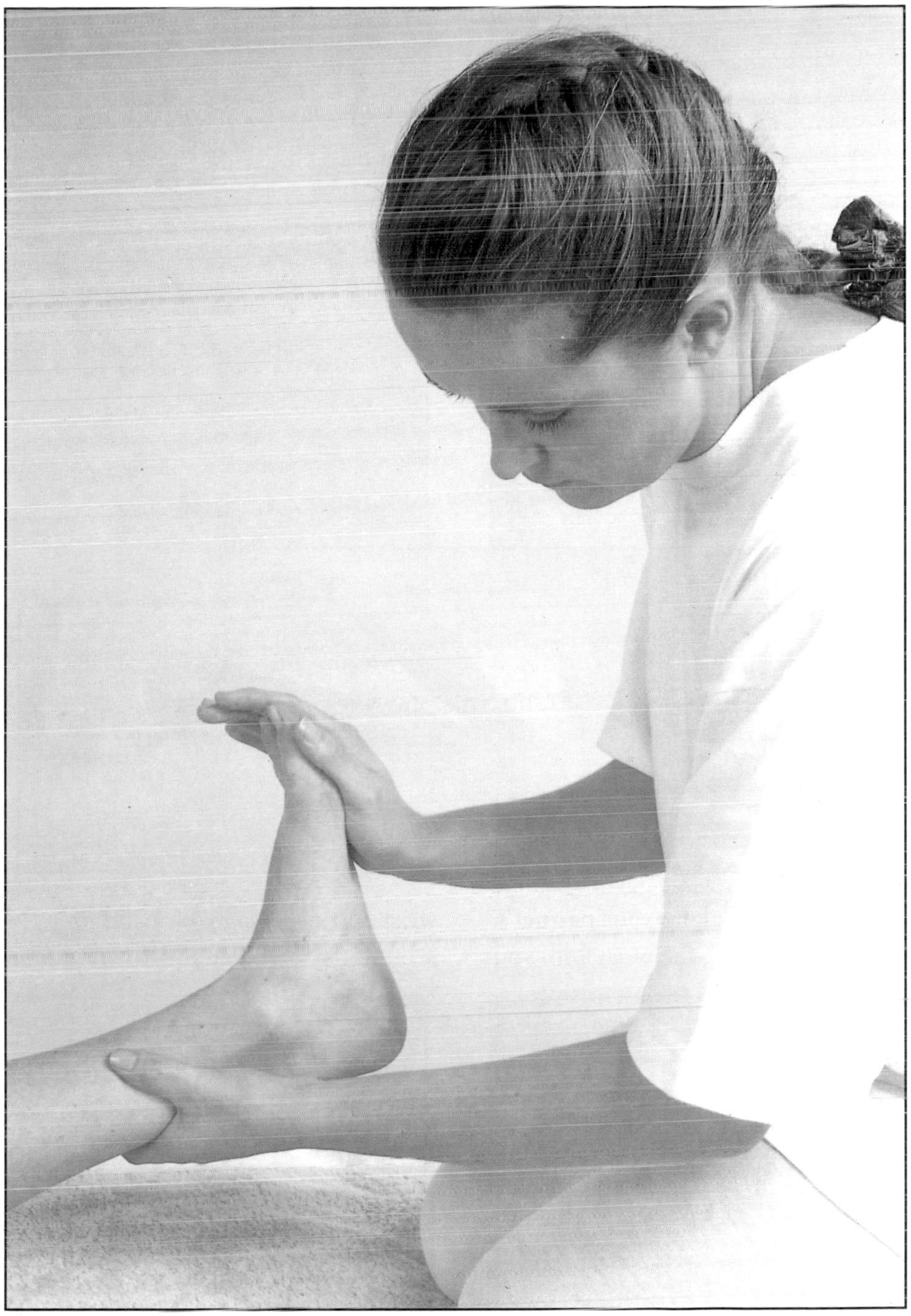

10 Finish the foot and ankle sequence with some long sweeping, *effleurage* strokes from the top of the foot up the lower leg and back down to the foot, to help reintegrate the foot and the leg. Repeat several times, varying the pressure.

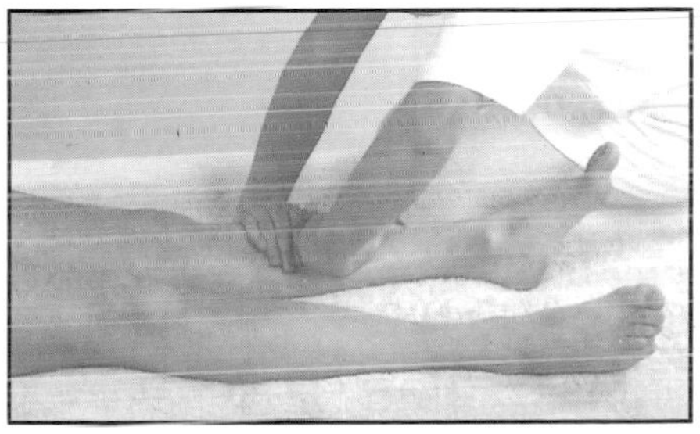

Move around your partner to kneel on the other side.
Repeat the entire sequence on the front of the other leg and the other foot.

SPINE

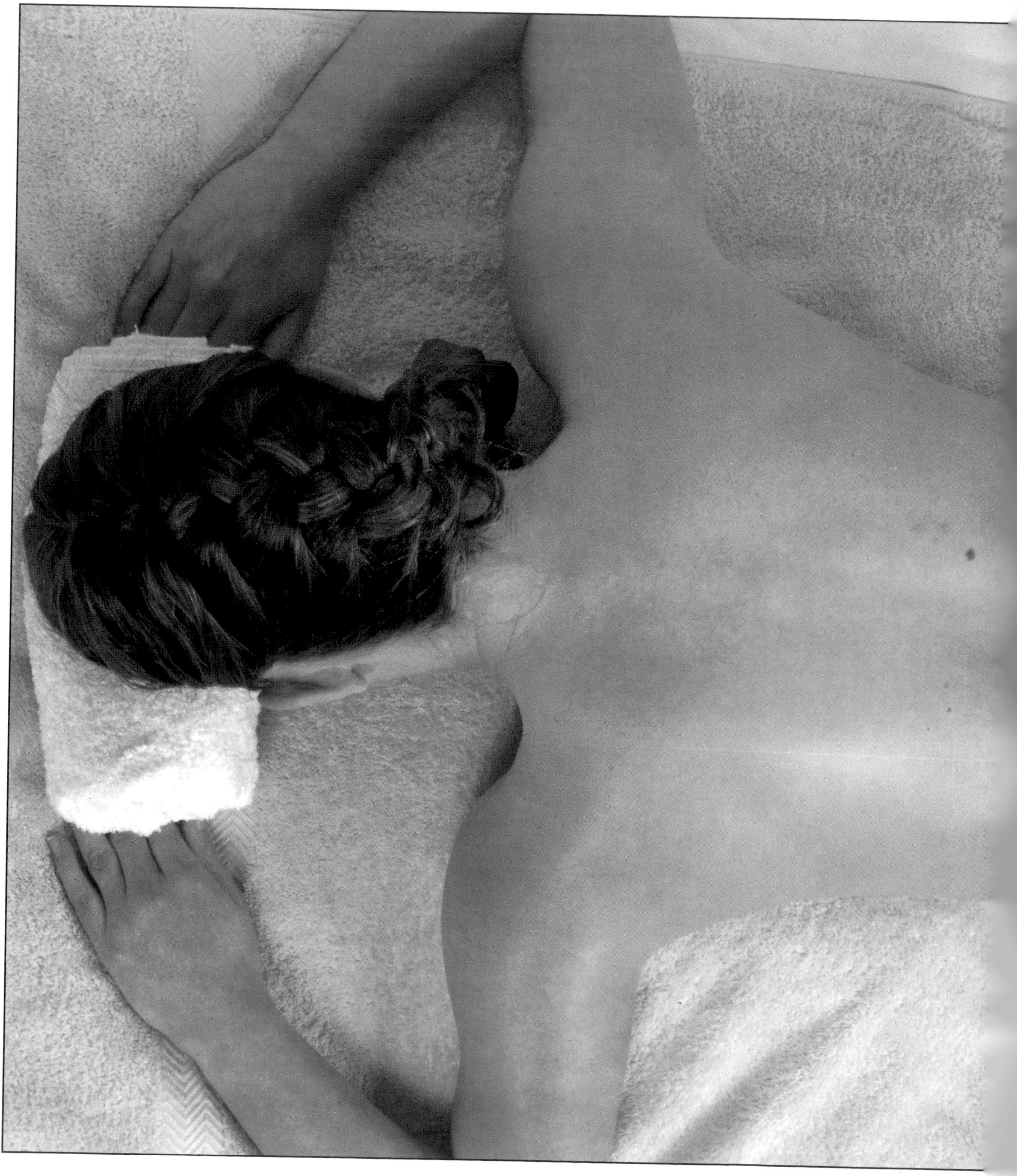

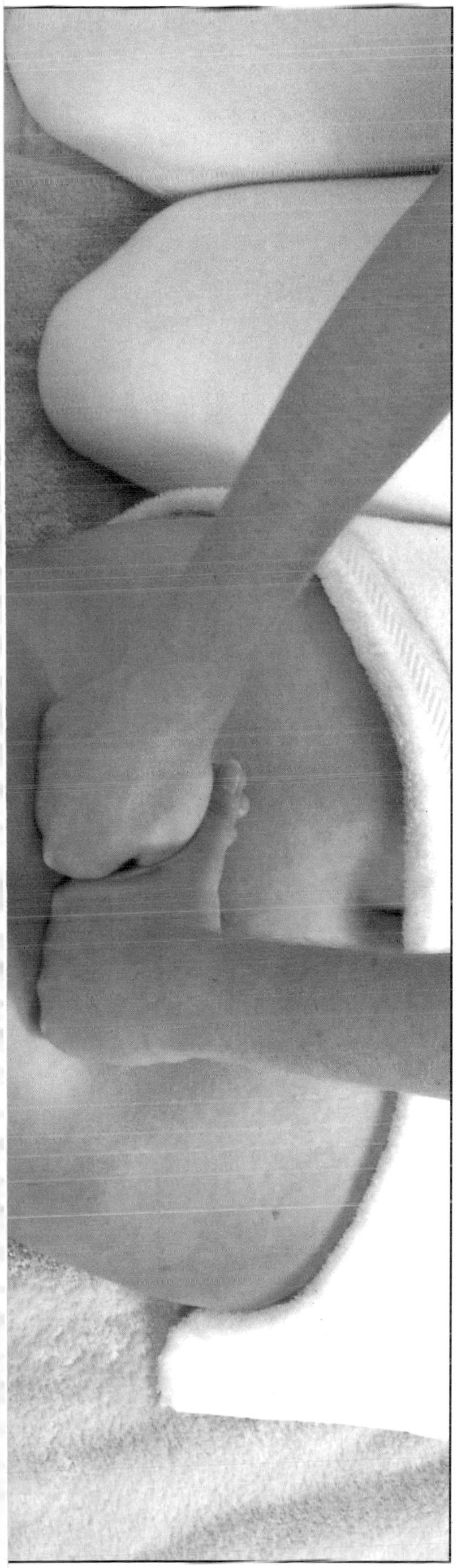

1 LEFT: With loose fists, and thumbs crossed for support, push the top of the hands up each side of the spine to the nape of the neck.

2 RIGHT: Uncurl the fingers when you get to the nape and sweep them back down the sides of the back. Repeat three times.

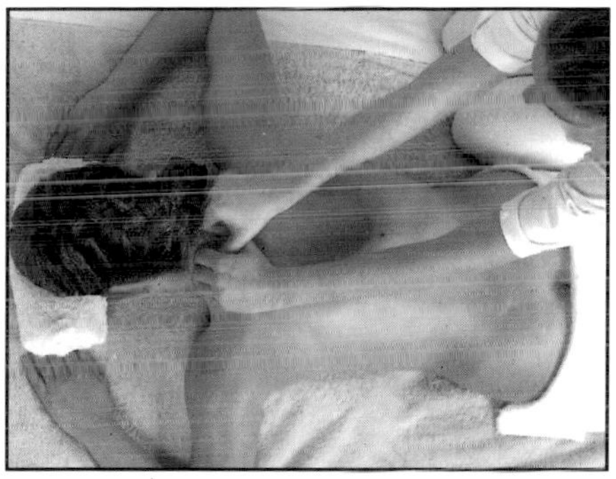

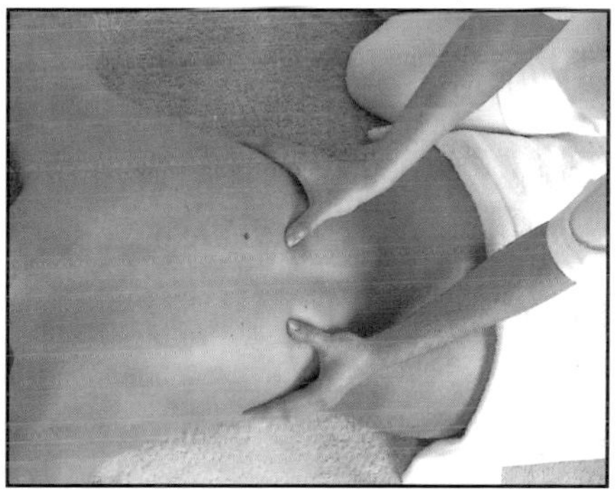

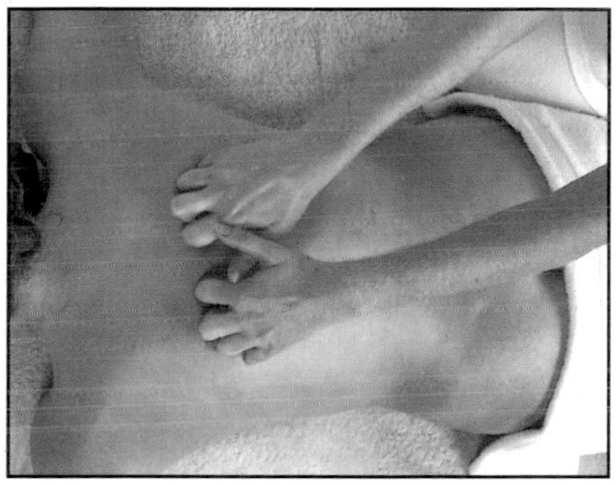

3 Starting at the lower back, place the thumbs on either side of the spine, resting your hands either side of the back. Rotate the thumbs in small circles, travelling up the sides of the spine until you reach the hairline. Use firm pressure. Reverse the movement, circling your thumbs back down each side of the spine.

4 Starting at the lower back, use loose knuckles, crossing your thumbs over each other for support, to work up either side of the spine and back down again. Repeat twice.

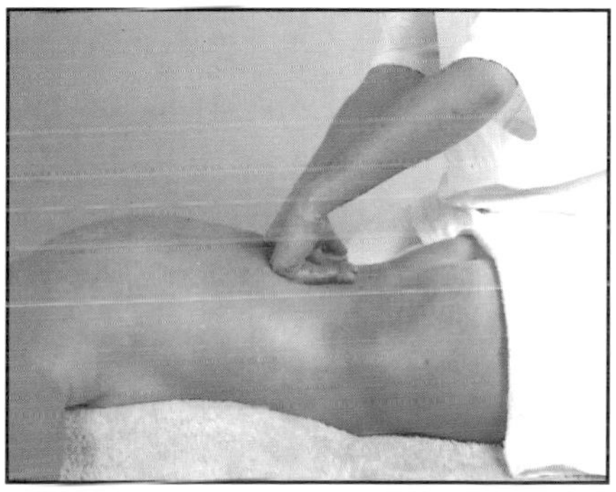

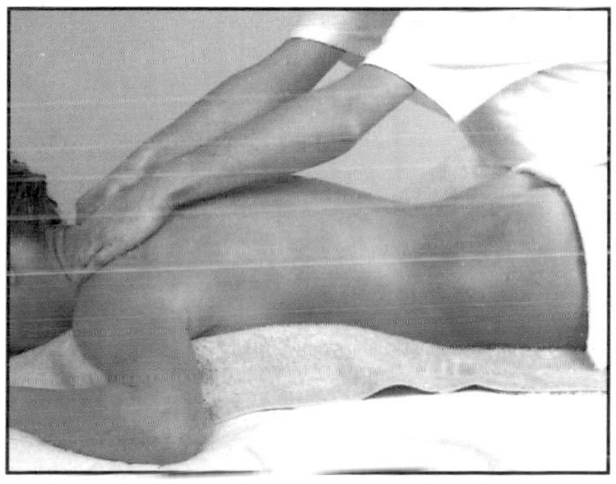

5 Using the backs of your hands and starting at the lower back, push up either side of the spine to just above the waistline. Then sweep your hands outward and back down around the hips. Repeat three times.

6 To finish the massage, repeat the *effleurage* strokes from the beginning of the sequence, starting at the lower back, up the back, around the shoulders and down again to the lower back, in a continuous sweeping movement.

BACK AND ABDOMEN

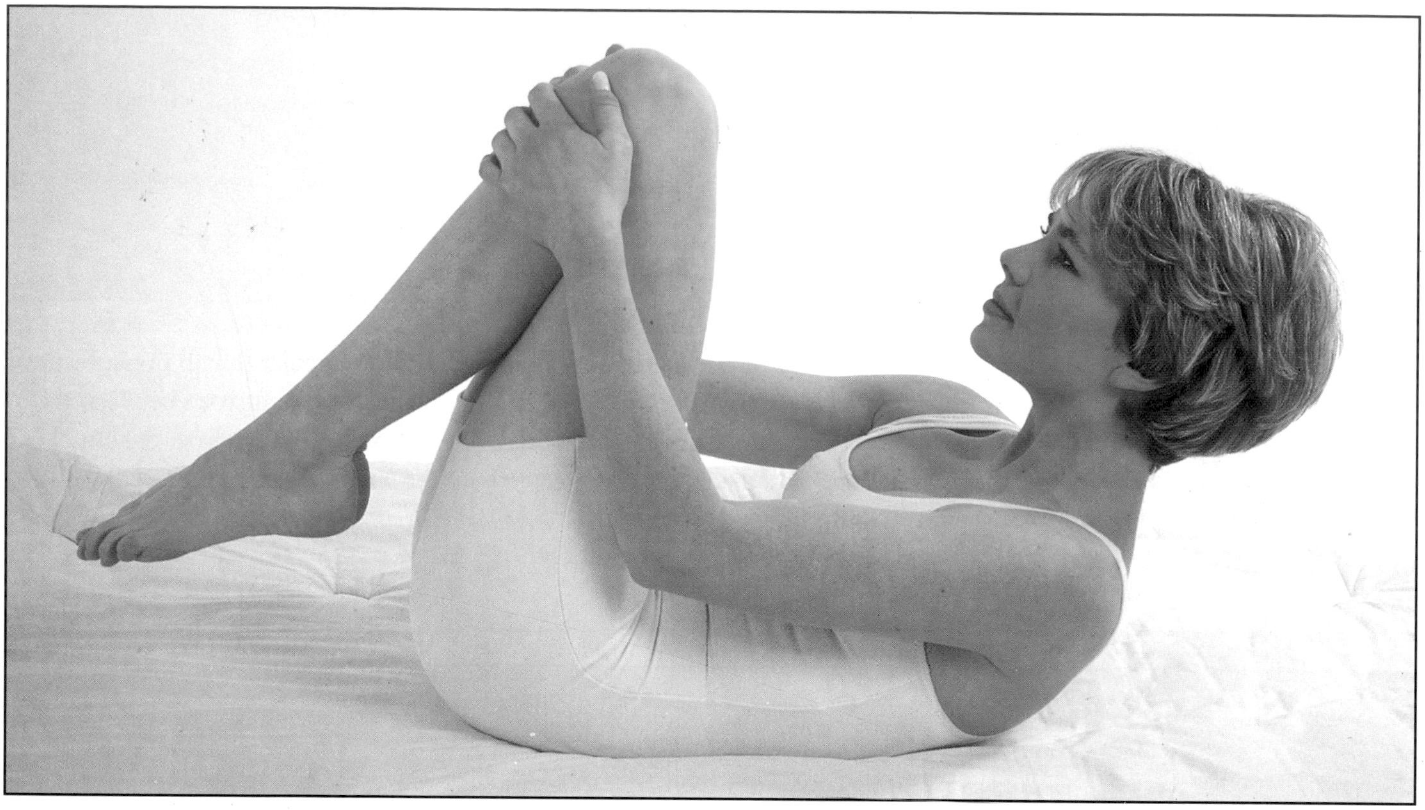

1 Lie on your back, clasp your knees and gently rock backward and forward to massage the lower back, buttocks and hip joints and gently stretch out the vertebrae.

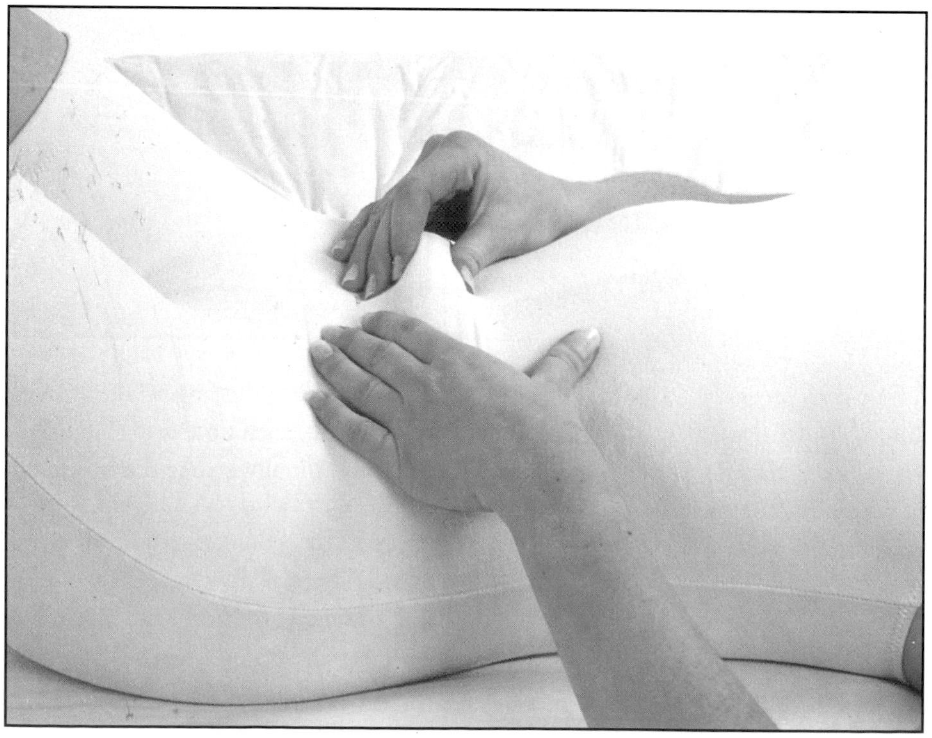

2 LEFT: Bend your knees up and use some gentle *petrissage* to knead the whole of the abdominal area. When you have finished kneading, place both hands flat on the centre of the abdomen, fingers pointing slightly together, and pause for a few moments. Then smooth your hands outward over the hips and thighs in a long, slow, moulding movement.

BUTTOCKS, HIPS AND THIGHS

1 Kneel up and pummel your hips and buttocks, using a clenched fist and keeping your wrists flexible.

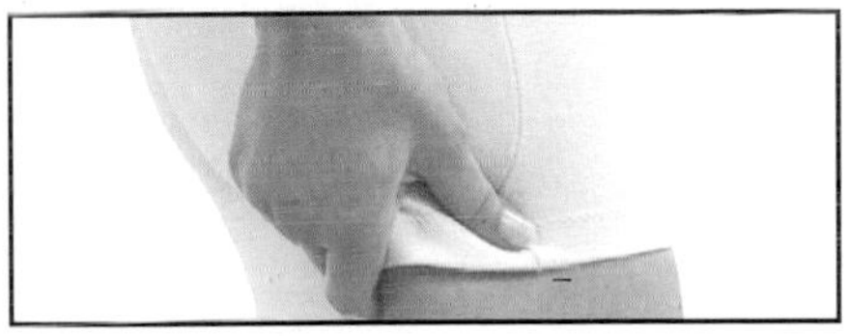

2 With the thumb and fingers, squeeze and release the muscles firmly and slowly, working from the top of the thigh over the buttock. Repeat on the left side.

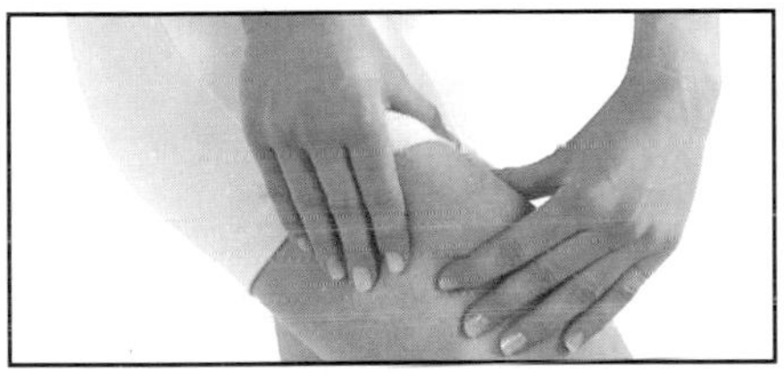

3 Use both hands to squeeze and release the muscles on the front and side of the thigh, kneading the entire upper leg. Repeat on the other side.

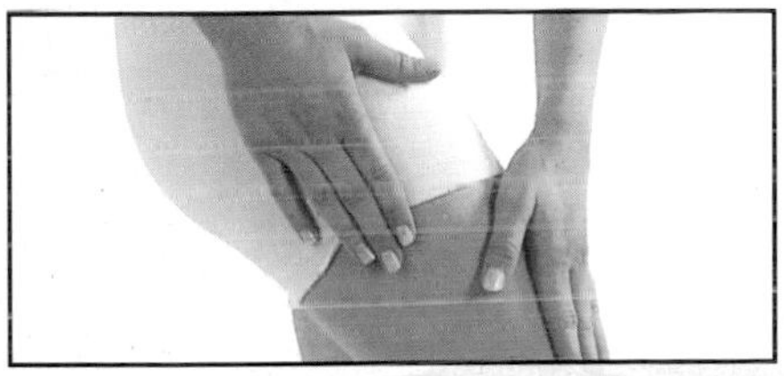

4 Starting at the knee, stroke up the thigh with both hands to soothe the leg.

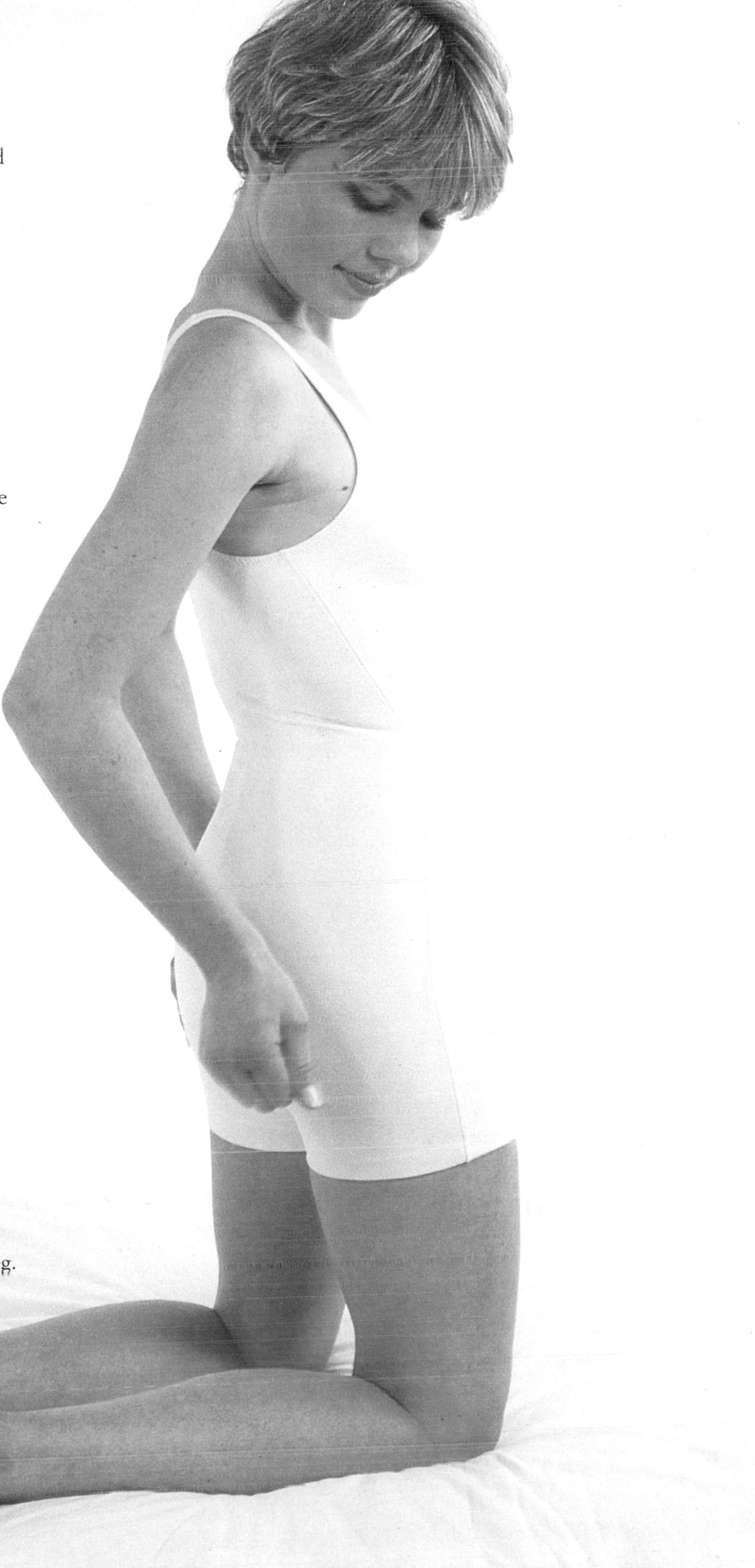

LEGS

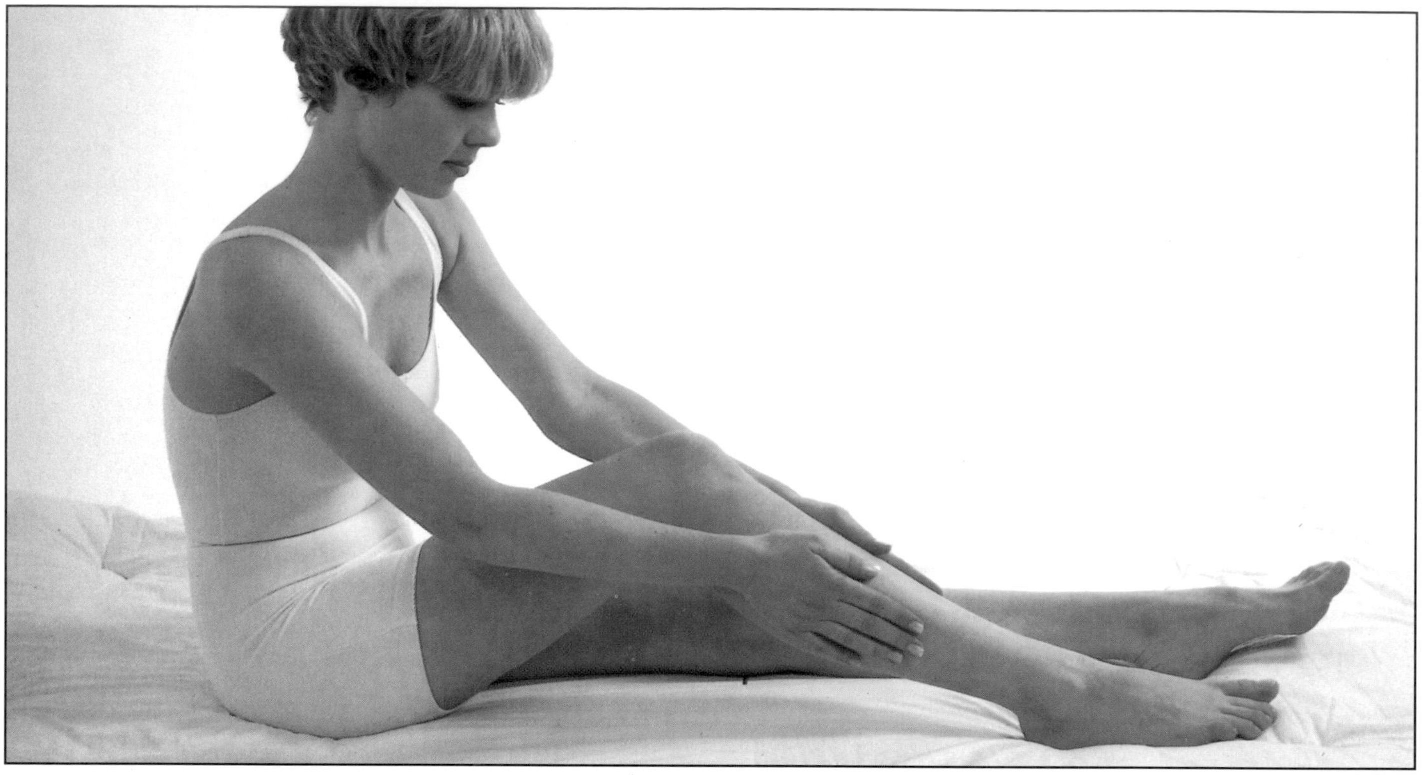

1 Sitting down, with one leg raised slightly, stroke the leg with both hands from ankle to thigh. Begin the stroke as close to the ankle as you can reach. Repeat several times, moving around the leg slightly each time to stroke a different part.

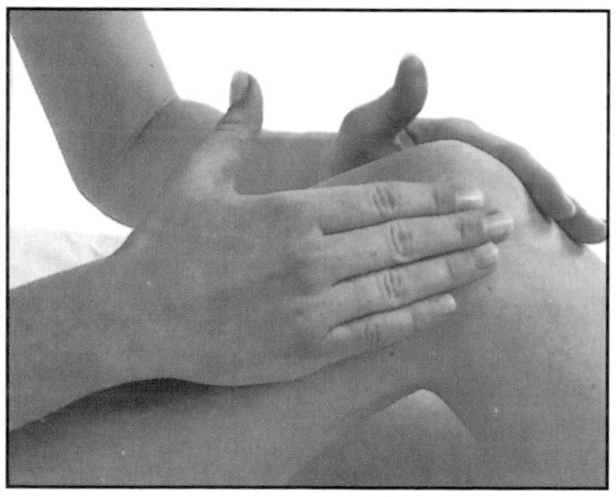

2 Massage the knee, stroking around the outside of the kneecap to begin with, then using circular pressure with the fingertips to work around the kneecap more firmly.

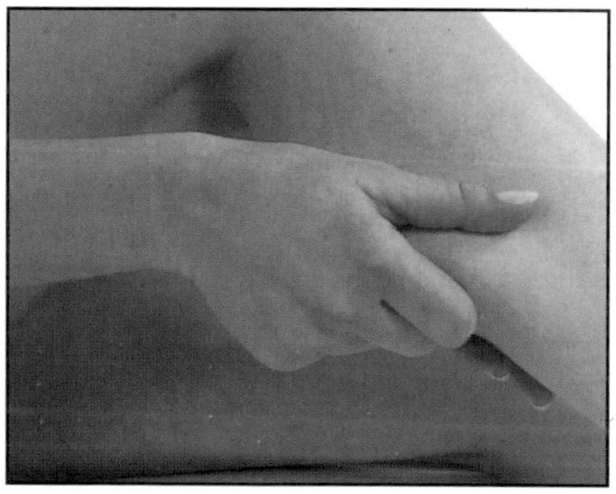

3 Knead the calf muscle with both hands, using a firm *petrissage* to loosen any tension in the muscle.

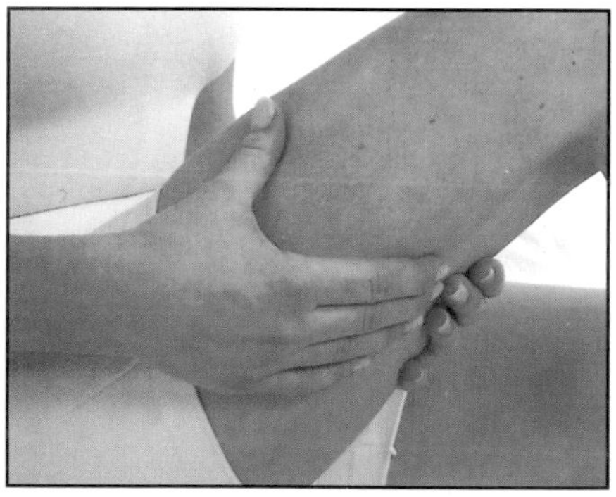

4 Continue the kneading on the thigh, working over the top and outside areas with alternate hands. Whilst the leg is still raised, do some soothing *effleurage* strokes up the back of the leg from ankle to hip.

Continue with the foot massage (opposite) before repeating all the steps on the other leg.

FEET

1 Sitting down and leaning back, raise a leg, supporting the weight with your hands. Rotate the right ankle five times in each direction.

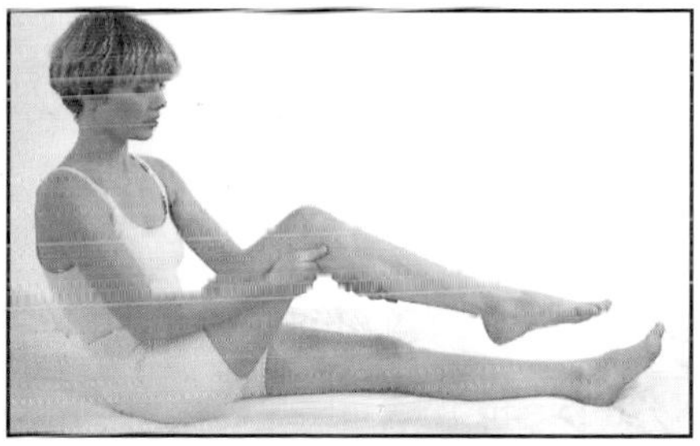

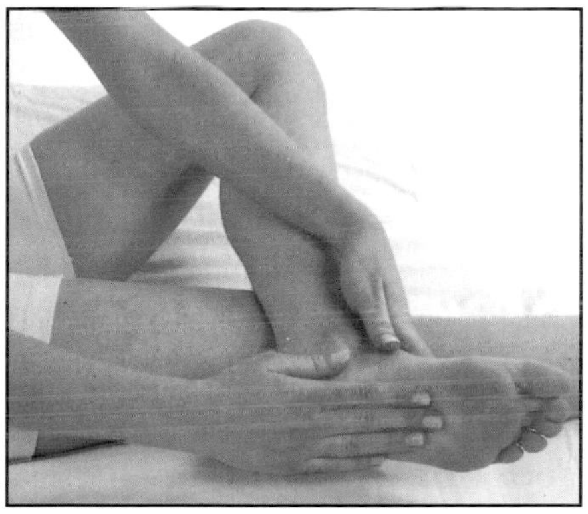

2 Gently bring your foot over the other leg. With one hand on top of the foot and one underneath, stroke up the foot from toes to ankle. Repeat three times.

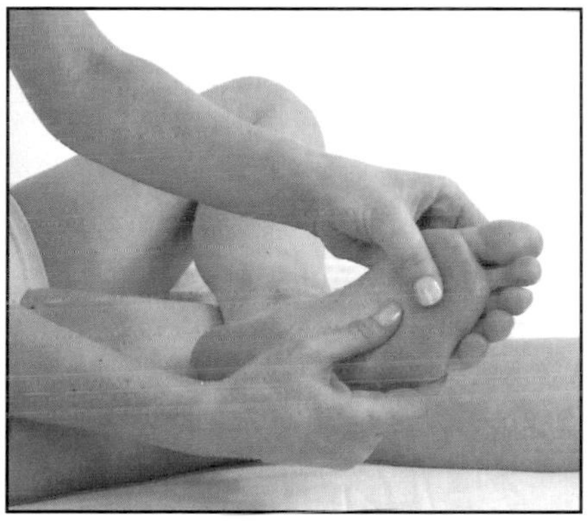

3 With the thumbs, apply circular pressure over the ball of the foot. Work in lines from the inside of the foot to the outer edge. Repeat three times.

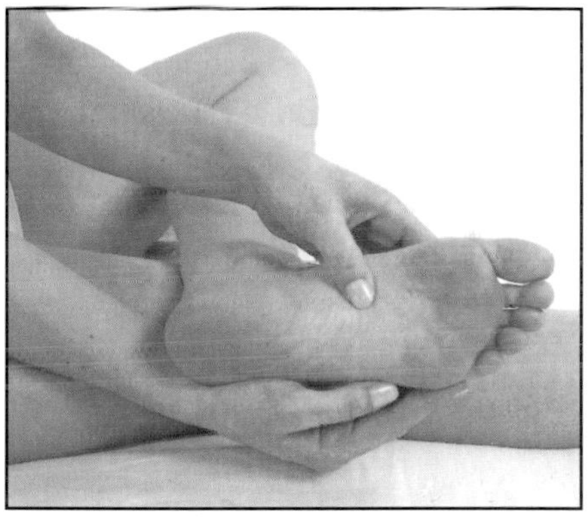

4 Supporting the foot with one hand, continue the circular pressures over the raised instep, working from the inner to the outer edge. Repeat three times.

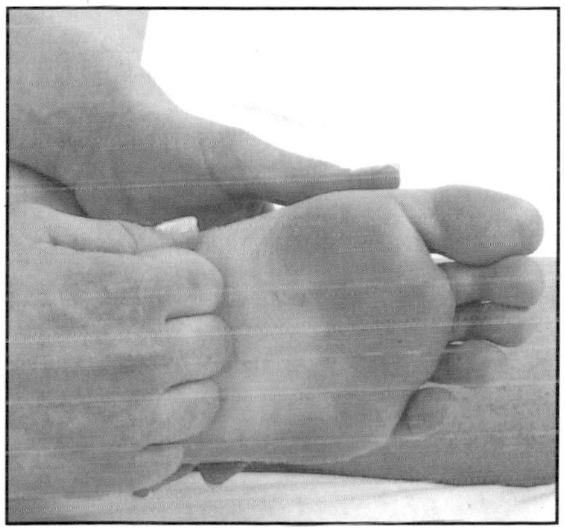

5 Still holding the foot with one hand, make a loose fist with the other and firmly rotate your fist over the instep. Work thoroughly into the arch.

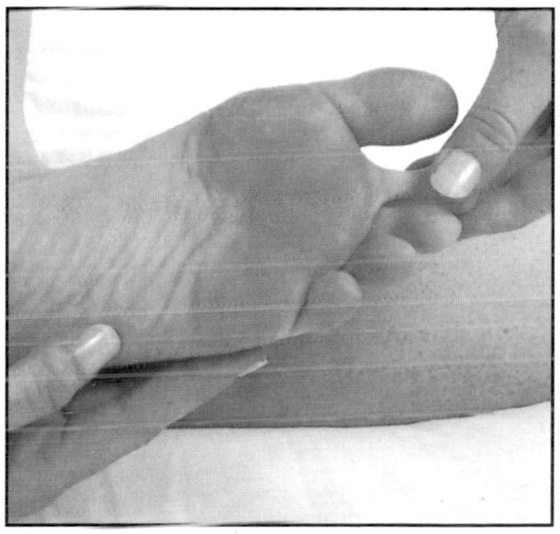

6 Massage each toe individually. Slowly stretch the toe between the thumb and finger, and pull gently, moving your fingers up the toe each time, until you reach the tip.

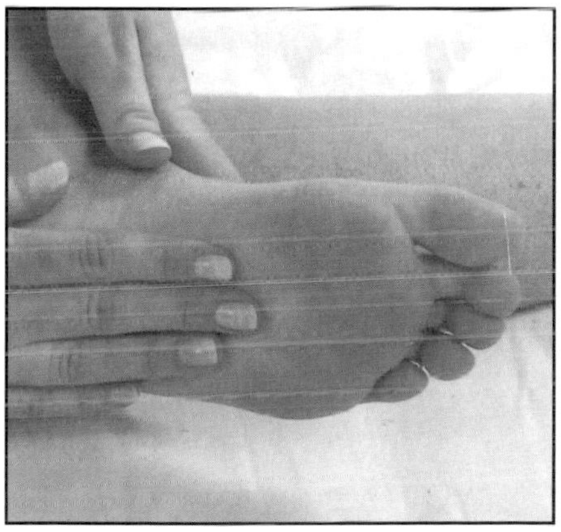

7 Repeat the *effleurage* strokes of the foot, with one hand over and one under the foot, working from toes to ankle, several times.

Repeat the leg and foot massage sequence on the other side.

BABY MASSAGE

A newborn baby instinctively responds to touch, and massage between mother and baby is a marvellous way of enhancing the natural bonding. All babies have this powerful sensitivity to being caressed and cuddled. Watch how a baby tightly curls its hands or toes as soon as something touches them.

There is no fixed sequence for massaging a baby. Keep the movements gentle and flowing. The simple action of gently stroking a baby will strengthen the natural bonding, and soothe and reassure the baby too. Massage has been shown to help calm difficult or colicky babies, and alleviate wind and other digestive problems. It may also build resistance to coughs and colds. Use a little light vegetable oil which is easily absorbed, such as sweet almond or sunflower, taking care to avoid the eyes.

GETTING COMFORTABLE

Lay the baby gently on the back on a warm, soft towel between your legs, or on your lap, whichever is most comfortable. Pour about 5 ml (1 tsp) sweet almond oil into a small dish. Make sure your hands are warm and that the room is quiet, very warm and there are no draughts. After a baby's bathtime is ideal.

WORKING ON BABY'S FRONT

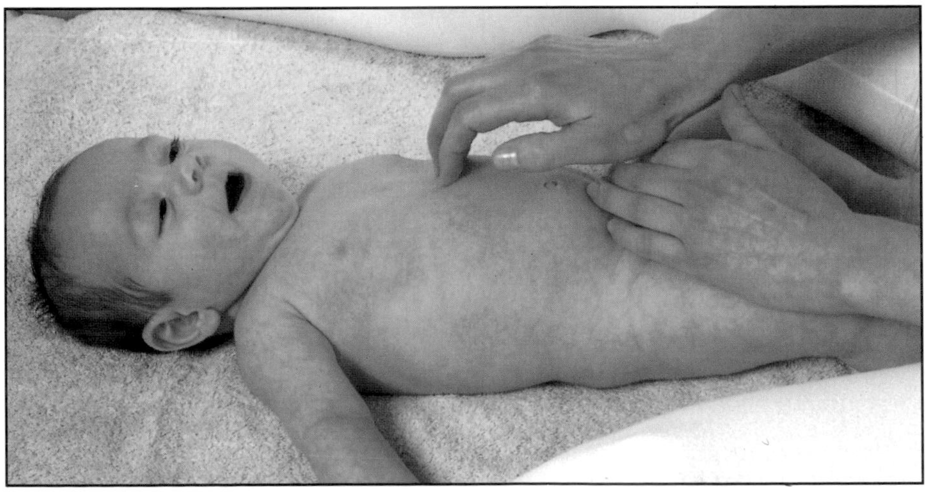

1 Slowly and gently, smooth a little of the oil all over the front of the baby's body, shoulders to feet, avoiding the face. Lightly stroke down the chest and abdomen, with the tips of your fingers. This is a delightful stroke which can be used to calm a baby at anytime.

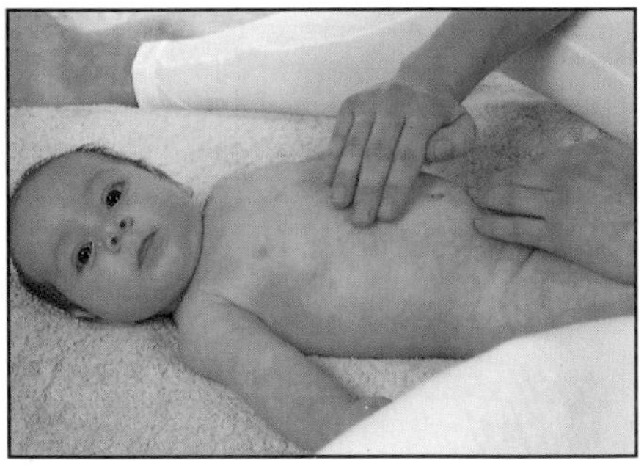

2 Keeping the pressure very light, smooth both hands over the abdomen in continuous, circular strokes, working up the baby's right side, across and down the baby's left side. Keep the movement continuous by lifting your left hand when your arms cross. Repeat these circular strokes several times.

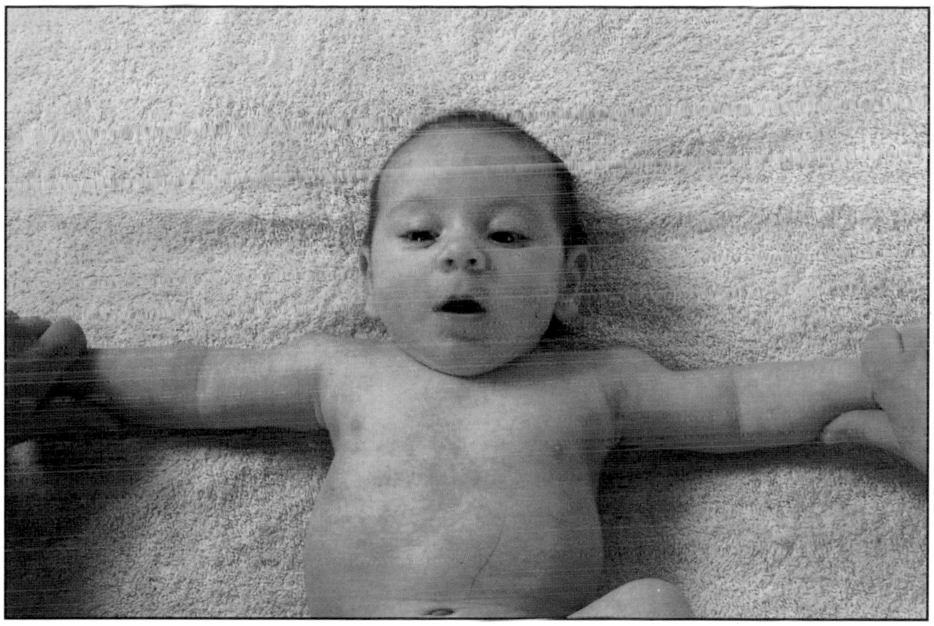

3 LEFT: Gently stretch out both arms to the side, spreading the hands and fingers if the baby will let you. Gently squeeze out along the arms, then massage the wrist and palms with light, circular thumb movements. Finish by stretching out each finger with a slight pull.

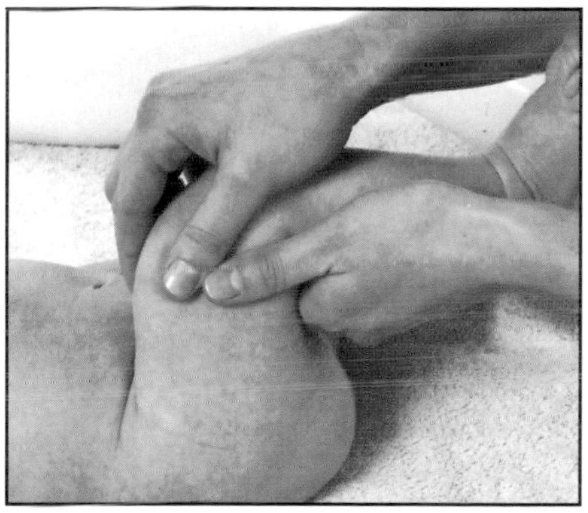

4 Move on to the legs and feet, working on one leg at a time. Support the leg with both hands and gently squeeze and release the fleshy part of the thigh. Then, supporting the leg with one hand, stroke the leg from the knee to the thigh and back down again.

5 RIGHT: Move your supporting hand down to behind the ankle. Gently smooth the palm of your other hand over the top of the foot from toe to ankle and back again. When you get to the toes, very gently stretch each one in turn.

Repeat steps 4 and 5 on the baby's other leg.

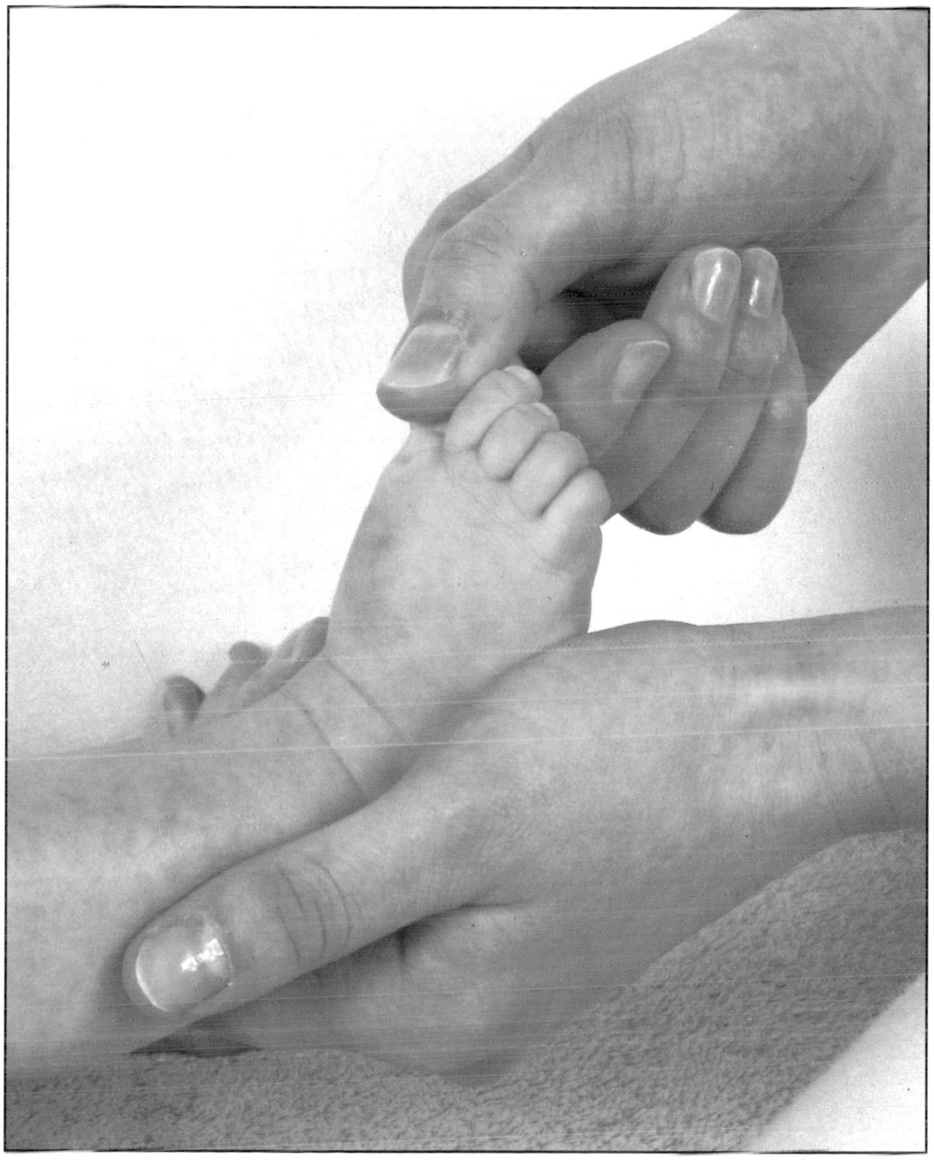

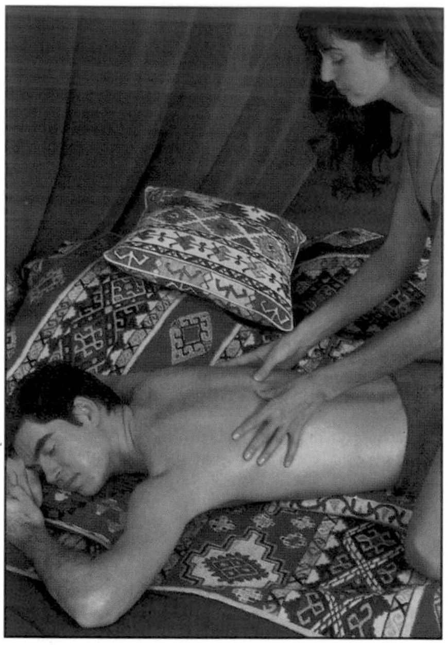

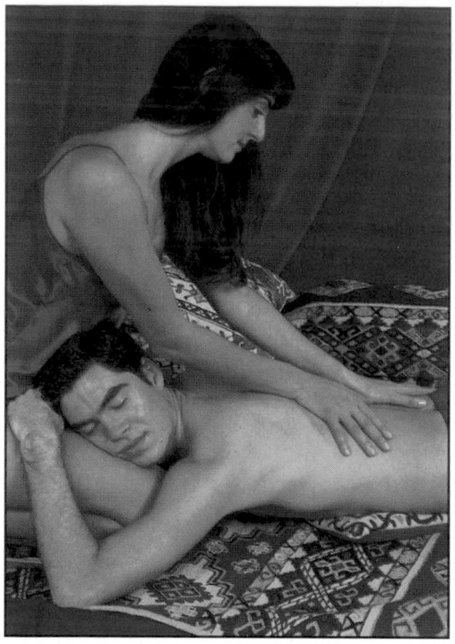

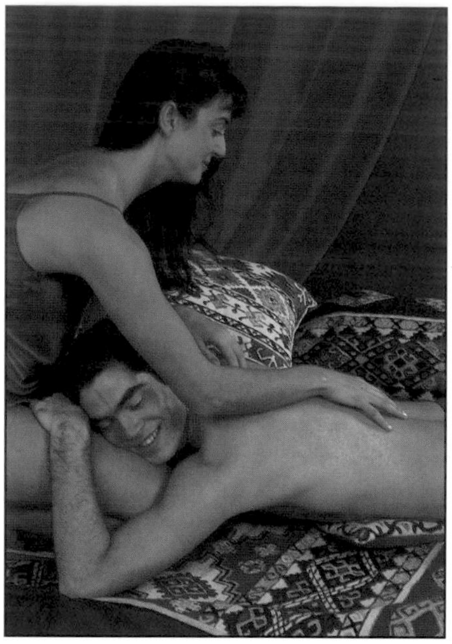

3 Check that your partner's head is still comfortable then, beginning at the nape of the neck, let your thumbs gently stroke down each side of the spine. When you get to the lower back return up each side of the spine, this time working with slightly more pressure and rotating the thumbs to release muscular tension. Work up and down the spine two or three times.

4 Move round so your partner can rest their head on your thighs, and with long, *effleurage* strokes, massage the length of the back from the neck right down to the buttocks and back up the sides of the trunk. Repeat three times.

5 Starting at the lower back, gently stroke up either side of the spine, making light feathery strokes with your fingertips. Repeat three times, making the strokes lighter each time, until they can barely be felt.

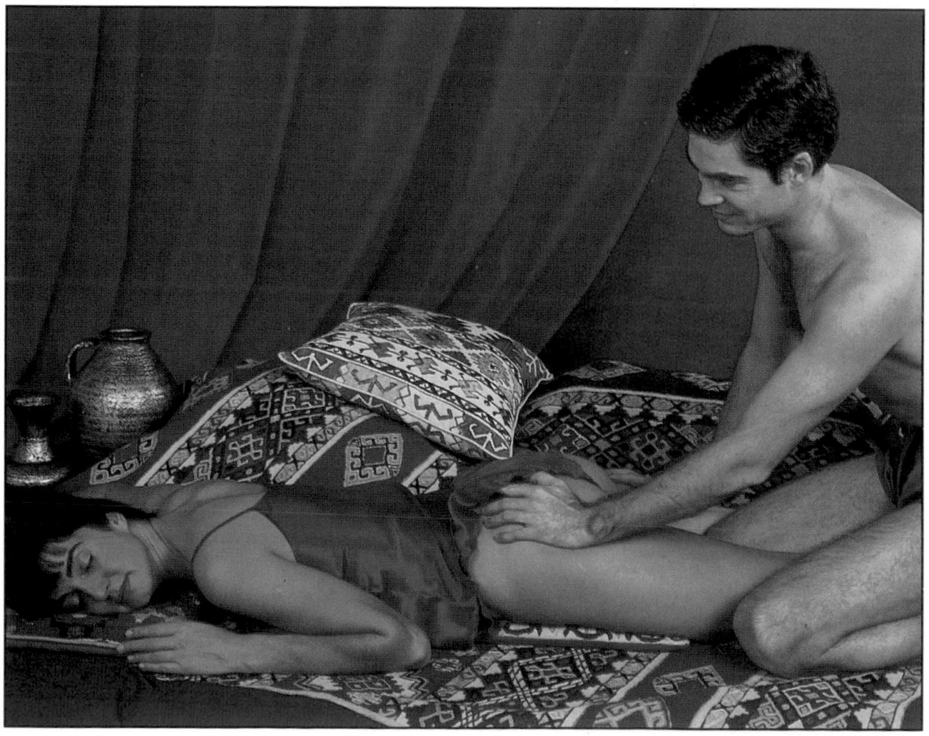

6 LEFT: Massage the lower back with some kneading. Using the flat, and in particular the heel, of the hand, knead the buttocks, then come back to the start and work over a different area. The nerves that cross this area relate to the man's groin, and the woman's uterus. The buttocks themselves are highly erogenous areas.

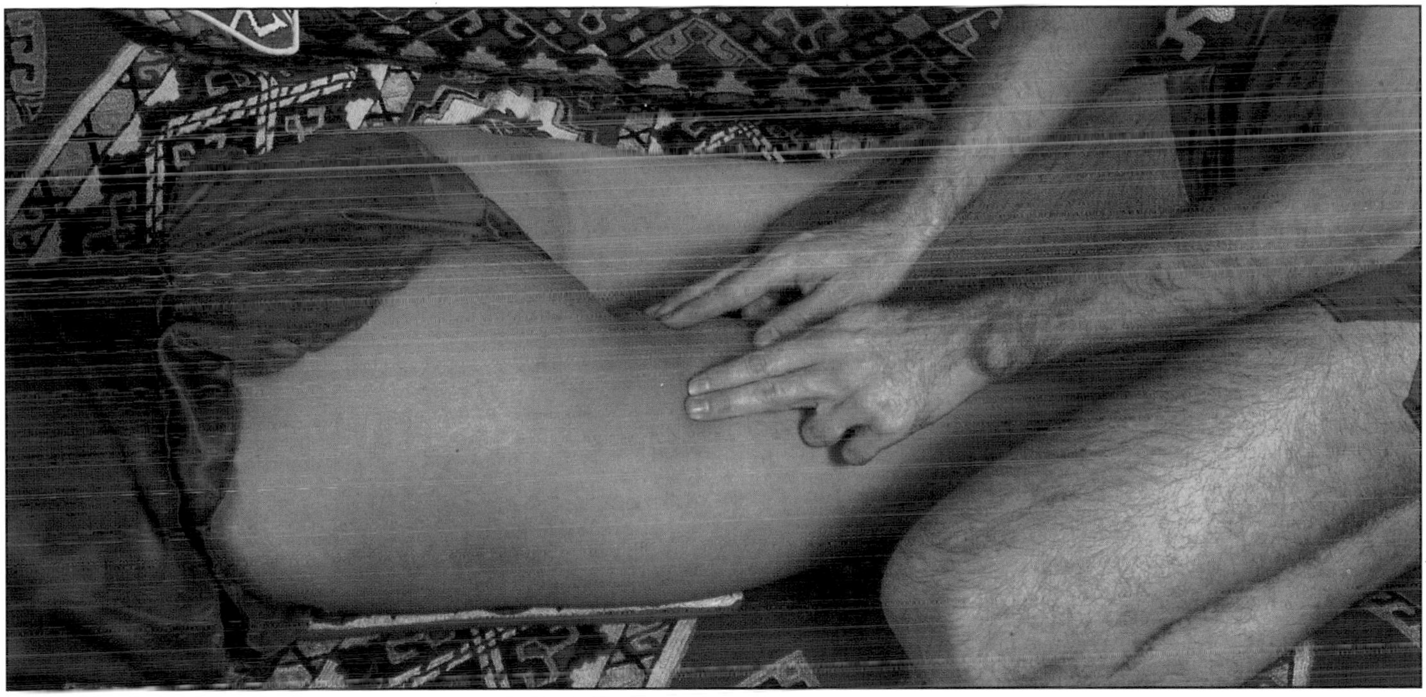

7 Curling your third and fourth fingers under, place your hands toward the top of the upper legs and circle your first and second fingers outward, one hand alternating with the other. This should be a slow, leisurely stroke with varying pressure.

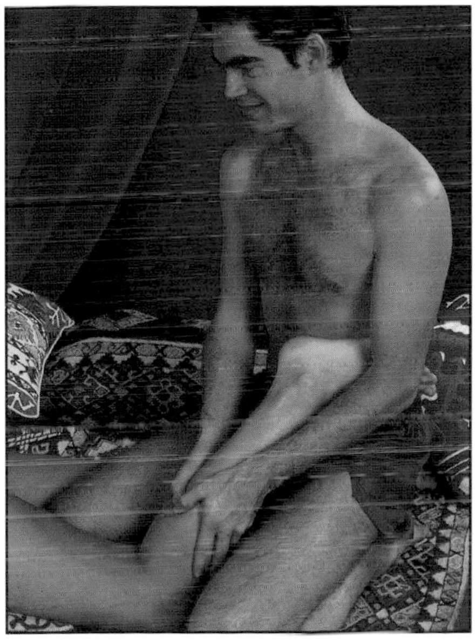

8 Support your partner's leg across your thigh and circle your thumbs over the calf, alternating the thumbs and applying firm pressure.

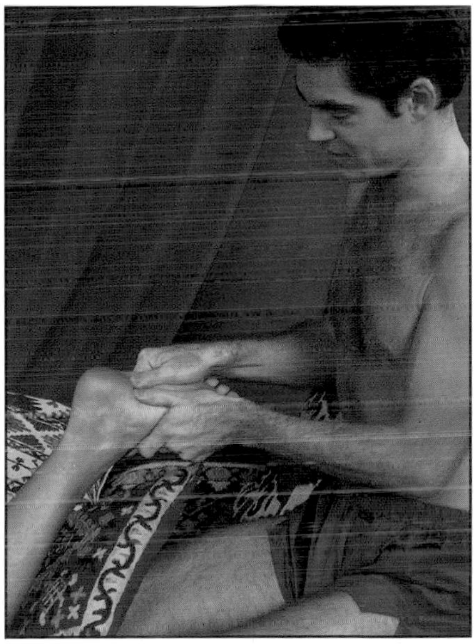

9 Raise your partner's foot, supporting its weight in your hands. Knead the instep firmly, using the thumbs to apply the pressure. Work all over the ball of the foot up toward the big toe.

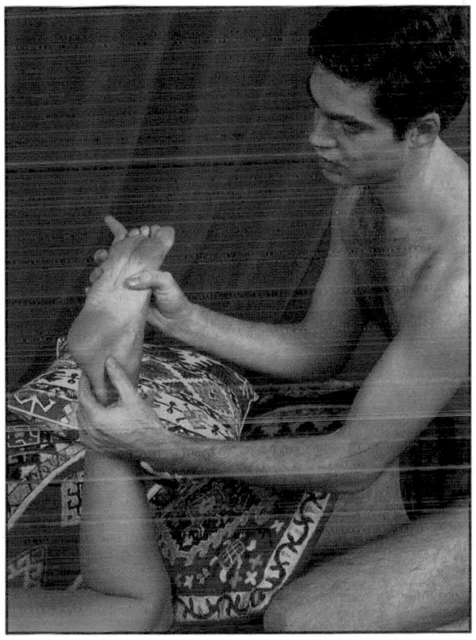

10 Support your partner's foot in one hand, and place the thumb of that hand firmly over the centre of the instep. This has a wonderful, calming effect. With the thumb and first finger of the other hand, stroke around the ankle using circular movements.

REFLEXOLOGY

Most people enjoy massage to the feet – one of the most sensitive parts of the body. All foot massage is beneficial and relaxing, but reflexology provides a more specific method of working to diagnose problems and stimulate health in the whole body. It is based on the principle that the body can be divided into ten vertical zones, each corresponding to an area of the foot, so that the feet are, in effect, a map of the body. Reflexology can be an effective way of relieving pain and helping to restore the body's natural well-being.

Foot Charts

The foot charts are only guidelines for interpretation. When you find a tender or congested part of the foot you may look for that part on the charts and see approximately which reflex the tenderness lies on. This is only a rough guide because every pair of feet are different and will not be the same shape as your chart. Also, the charts are two-dimensional and your body is three-dimensional and therefore the reflexes on your feet reflect this. In reality your organs overlap each other, whereas the charts are much simplified for clarity, to give an idea of where things are.

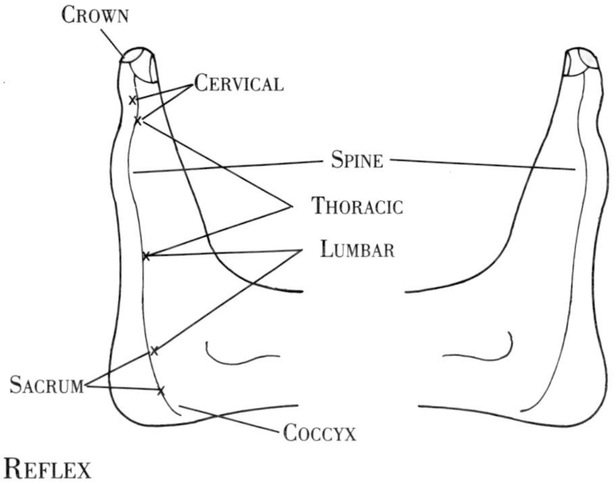

Spinal Reflex

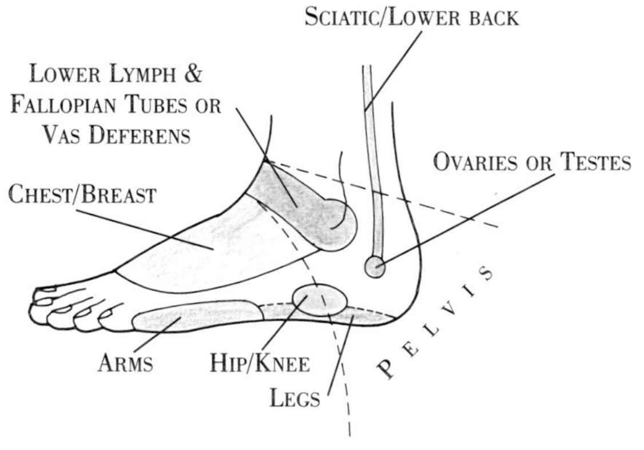

Outer Foot

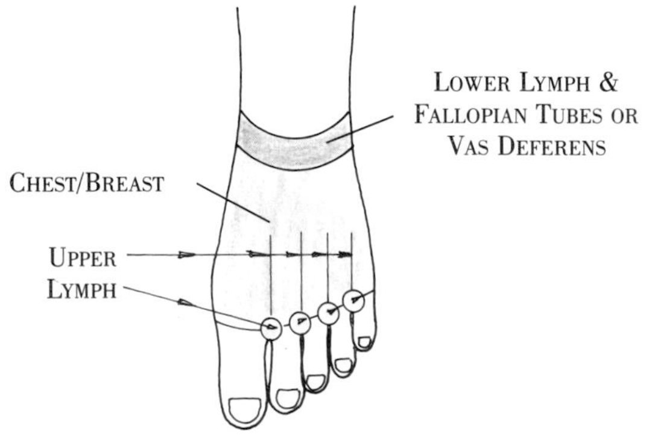

Top of Foot

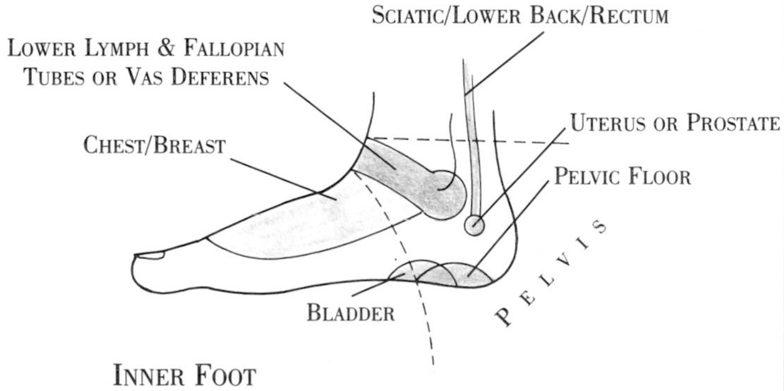

Inner Foot

THE BACKGROUND

The concept of using the body's reflexes for therapeutic purposes is not new – the early Chinese developed the technique of acupressure thousands of years ago. This provided the basis of knowledge about reflex zones and points and connections between different parts of the body. We know that the early Chinese, Japanese, Indians and Egyptians worked on the feet to promote good health, and many of the long-established principles developed by these civilizations are used today.

Reflexology as it is known today is based largely on the work of Dr William Fitzgerald and Eunice Ingham. Dr Fitzgerald devised his own system of acupressure points which produced an analgesic effect when stimulated. He found that the body could be divided into ten zones running from the top of the head to the tips of the toes, and that everything occurring in a specific zone of the body could affect the organs and other parts of the body in that zone. The theory was refined in the 1930s by a young physiotherapist called Eunice Ingham, who introduced a special grip technique and the action of the thumb on the foot and developed a more intricate zone system. The system has been further refined into the internationally recognized method now practised.

Modern reflexology offers tremendous health benefits: it reduces stress, improves circulation, cleanses the body of impurities and toxins, and can revitalize energy levels.

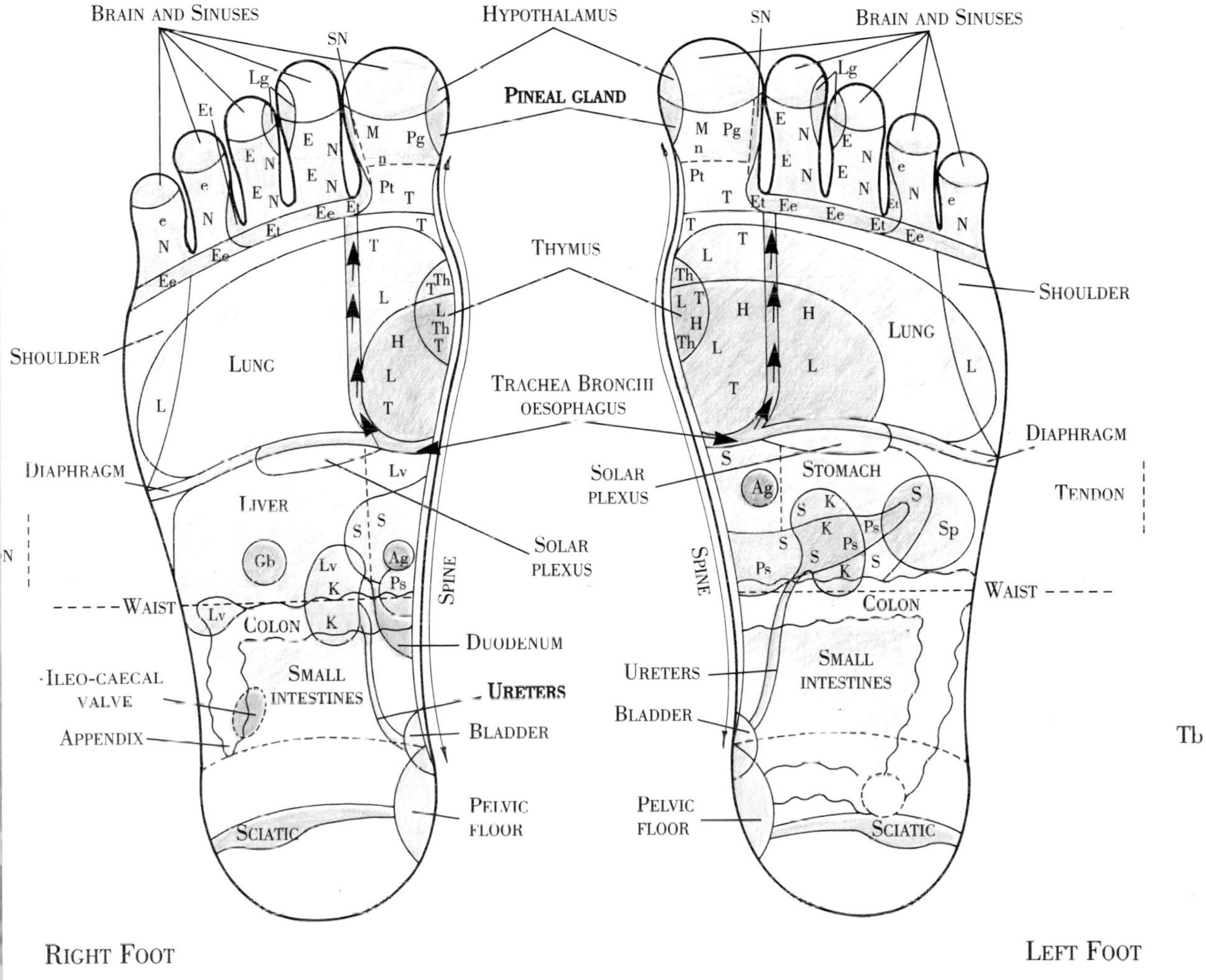

KEY

Ag Adrenal glands
e Ears
Et Eustachian tubes
Ee Eye/Ear helper
E Eyes
Gb Gall bladder
H Heart
K Kidneys
Lg Lachrymal glands
Lv Liver
L Lungs
M Mouth
N Neck
n Nose
Ps Pancreas
Pt Para-thyroid
Pg Pituitary glands
SN Side of neck
Sp Spleen
S Stomach
Tb Trachea bronchi oesophagus
th Thymus
T Thyroid

the alexander technique principles

Once you start studying the technique, it quickly becomes clear that it helps you in all kinds of ways that other alternative remedies do not. That is not because it is superior, but because of its key agenda. As shown here, it helps us focus on our minds and bodies in new ways, and on aspects of our being that we might take for granted. The technique gets us back to basics.

Primary Control

"Misuse" occurs by contracting the muscles of the neck and pulling the head back and down into the shoulders. This has the twin effect of actually compressing the spine and narrowing and shortening the stature, creating tensions throughout the body. It is definitely something to be avoided.

Frederick Matthias Alexander discovered that the relationship between the head, the neck and the back, or "primary control", mechanically controlled movement and co-ordination in the whole body. To make ourselves aware of this consciously in our daily activities is the basis of good use.

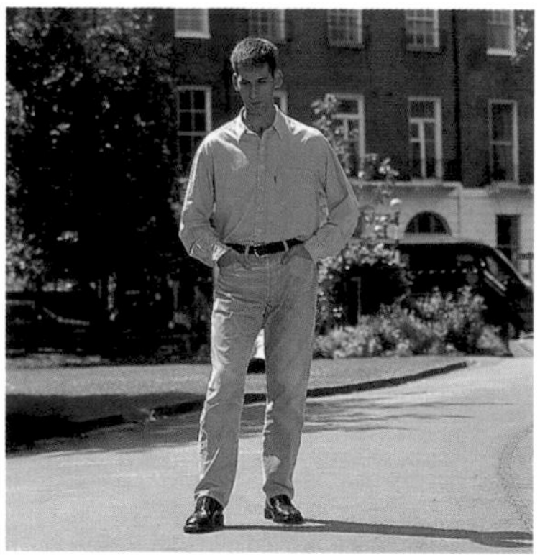

See how this model is misusing himself. He is leaning over to the right, shortening and creating an imbalance in his body.

Inhibition

In its psychological-physiological sense, inhibition means a fast-moving yet natural control of your reactions, suppressing and smothering any possible spontaneity.

However, Alexander discovered that if he managed to stop himself from behaving in his habitual way, he could choose how he wished to respond to a stimulus. If someone rings the doorbell, your immediate response may be to go straight to the door. In doing so, you will be responding habitually. If you stop yourself from responding automatically, you then choose exactly how you will approach the door with the minimum effort.

Concepts

The concept of end-gaining is extremely important in the work of Alexander technique teachers. Alexander realized that the habits he was encountering were far more deep-rooted and powerful than he had at first thought. The most serious of these was the tendency to try to react impulsively – end-gaining. End-gaining means reacting immediately and too quickly to a stimulus, without thinking. You respond by wanting something to happen, and become interested in the end result instead of being in the present. A typical example is if you are going to be late for an appointment and start to worry about the consequences. You get worked up during this process, forgetting that you might be sitting on a train, and that things are happening around you. In effect you are letting your thoughts take the situation into the future, instead of being in the "here and now", in the present.

Cutting yourself off from your environment has inevitable consequences for body positioning. It tends to lead to a pulling back of the head, a rounding of the back, a tightening of the legs and a loss of connection between the arms and the back. The gaze becomes fixed, the breath held. Essentially, the whole person is affected, both in mind and in body.

Alexander suggests you should use your "means-whereby". To put Alexander's conclusion into context, if we accept that we cannot change circumstances, we can change our approach to our bodies and allow ourselves to experience the new. It is then possible to learn to be in the moment rather than the past or the future, and to maintain a sense of inner balance and unity.

Direction

Directions are signals given by the brain to parts of the body prior to or during physical action. It is possible to alter these signals to promote a positive change. You will find that the combination of direction and inhibition enables one to transform habitual ways of moving and eliminate old patterns of misuse.

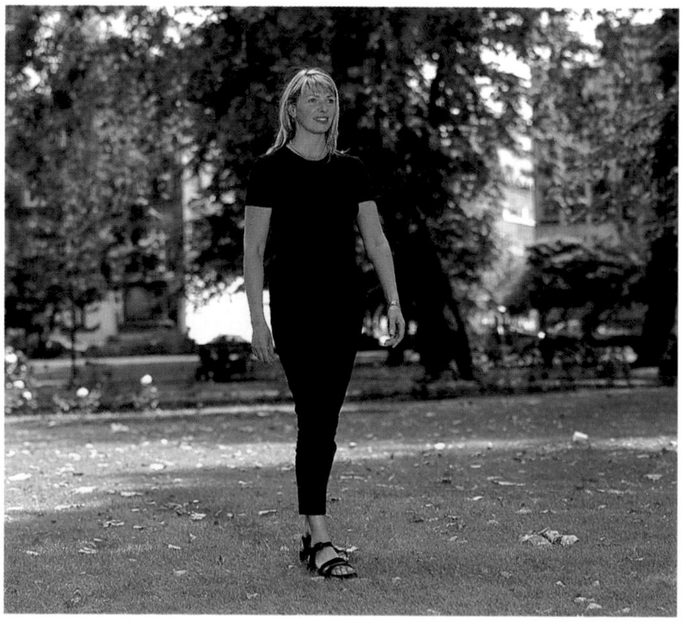

Note how this model is walking. Her head, neck and back are all correctly aligned. Her arms are free to move in a relaxed way.

Natural Poise

Nothing is more elegant and enviable than someone with perfect poise. It is something most of us have when young, but sadly it can be quickly lost to laziness and bad postural habits. In fact, it is quite easy to be totally unaware just how bad our posture is. At various times during the day it is worth freezing your movements, and taking a good look at yourself. You will be surprised at how often you fall well short of the ideal. Sitting at work is probably the one situation when your back is almost always wrongly positioned, becoming increasingly hunched, tense and stiff. Once you have ascertained exactly when and how you are going wrong, you can start putting matters right. If in any doubt, just look at young children. They instinctively know how to move gracefully and effortlessly without strain. That is something we should all try to emulate.

The Human Skeleton

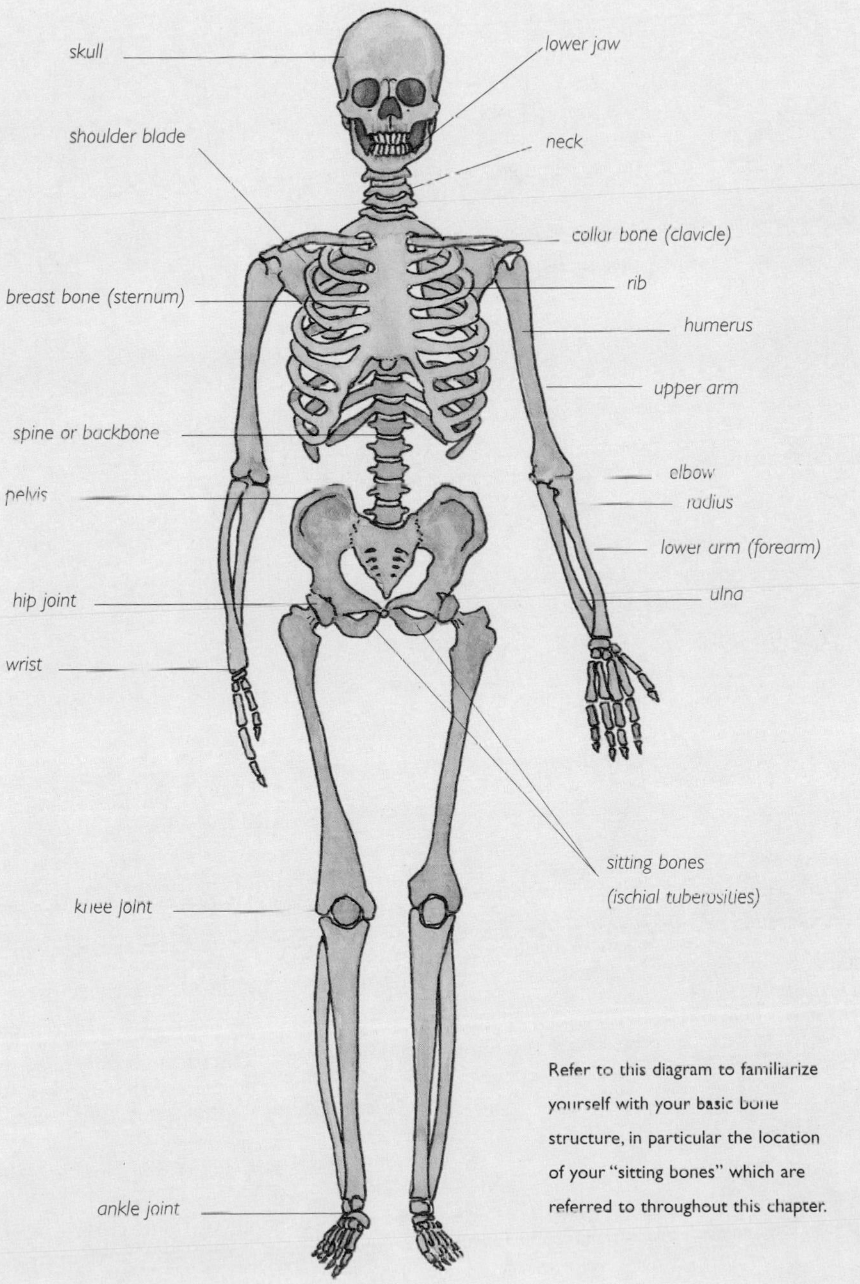

Refer to this diagram to familiarize yourself with your basic bone structure, in particular the location of your "sitting bones" which are referred to throughout this chapter.

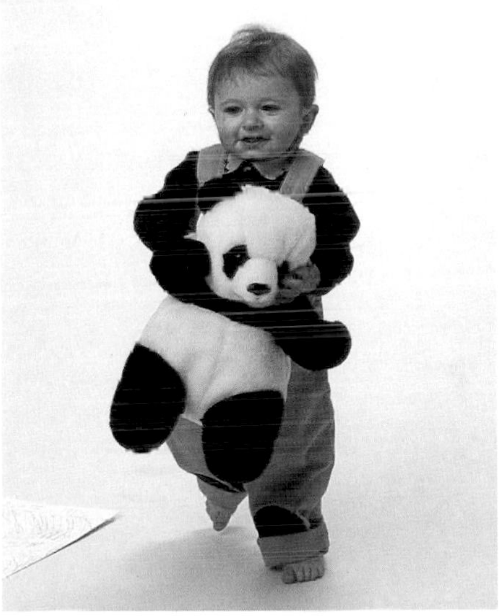

This child carries his toy close to his body., allowing it to lengthen and relax. This ensures good nervous energy and blood flow and allows full expansion of the lungs for breathing.

Primary Directions

- Think of freeing the neck.
- Let the head go forward and up.
- Let the back lengthen and widen.

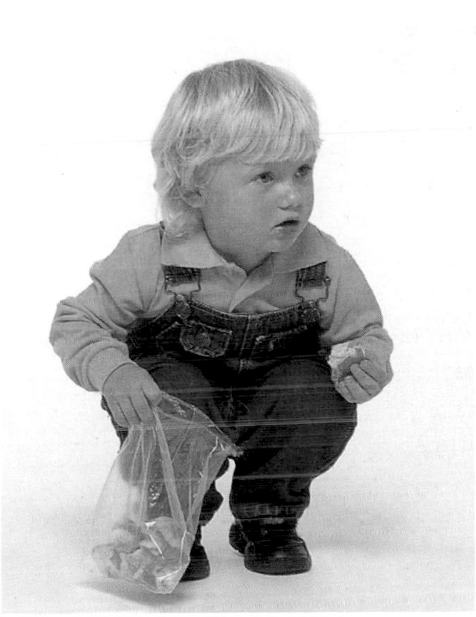

Note how this child is using his joints to squat, and how he simultaneously holds the plastic bag quite effortlessly.

"Possession of property … a means to happiness not an end."
Thomas Jefferson

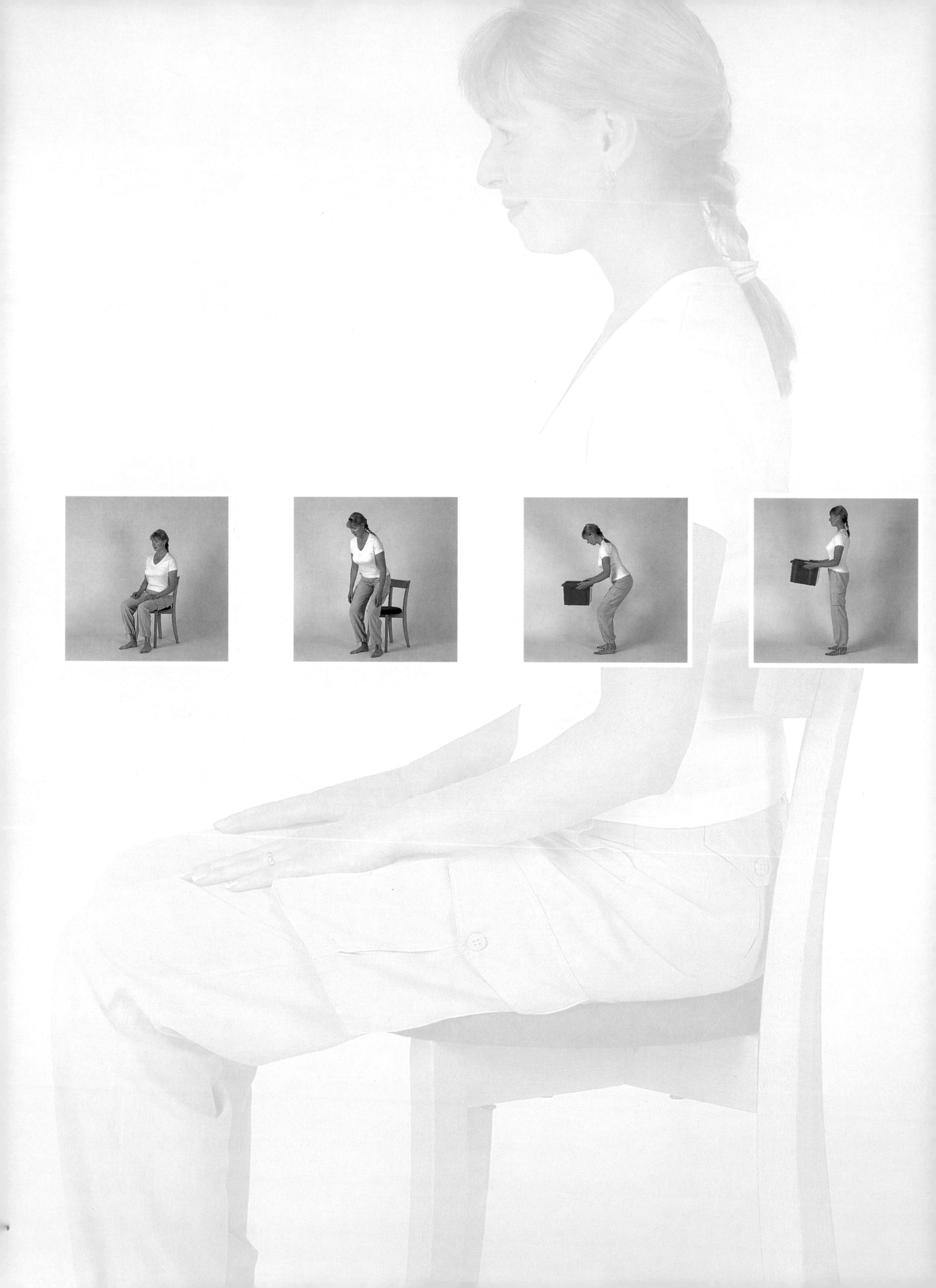

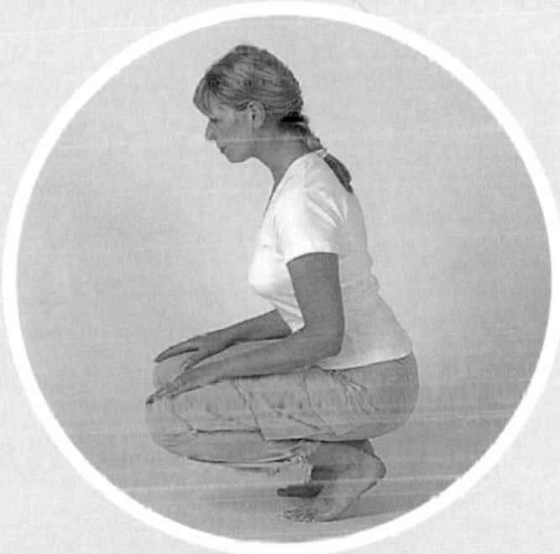

putting the alexander technique into practice
putting the alexander technique
into practice

putting the alexander technique into practice

A certain, rightful degree of commitment is paramount during a course of lessons because the older and more set in your ways you are, the longer it can take to change, to release unnecessary muscular tension, and to re-educate the system. Success, however, is not hard to achieve but note that it will not happen overnight, and that some slight pitfalls are always going to be inevitable, so do not be put off.

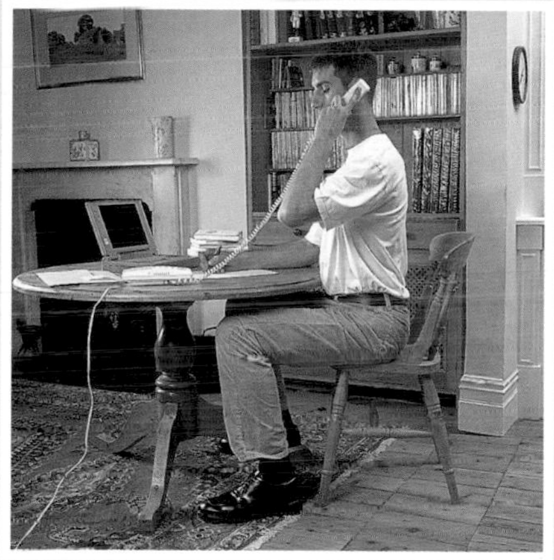

For example, you may well find yourself trying to do the directions as a routine mechanical exercise when in reality success lies in the power of the body and mind uniting as one, and in the power to think about what you are doing. Do not imagine there are any short cuts, there are not. There is also the distinct possibility that you might be tempted to give up out of sheer frustration because your time scale is too unrealistically short and limiting, and you have not allowed sufficient time for a significant, quantifiable improvement. Do not be hard on yourself, and do not imagine that you can become an expert in a ridiculously short space of time. The technique deserves more respect.

What therefore follows is the identification of the main procedures that we use most often in daily life, the areas that most concern us. In fact, the use of the word "procedure" is quite deliberate because it totally avoids the suggestion of a mind-body split and maintains a sense of psycho-physical unity. The emphasis throughout is on the means of achieving these procedures, but with the minimum of muscular tension and effort. Many students have said that a course of lessons in the technique could be compared to learning to drive or learning a new language. Dedication and determination are a sure basis for total success.

use of the eyes

If you want to know something about someone, just look straight into their eyes. They reveal an amazing amount about their current frame of mind. You can easily spot the depressed, dull and lifeless by their deadpan, almost one-dimensional eyes; the totally alert looking for a lively reply; the sad; the plaintive; the cheeky; and the happy. The technique reminds you how to stay lively and alert, and in touch with the rest of the world.

STAYING ALERT

If you observe people when they are either standing or walking, they often seem to be completely locked in a private world of their own, totally unaware of their own surroundings. They have stopped communicating with that is out there. When the gaze is fixed, the breathing also tends to suffer. It becomes rather restricted and there is less freedom in the body. The gaze should therefore be directed towards the outside world, taking in information so that you are not exclusively concentrating on what is happening within.

One of the strongest habits that a teacher perceives is the tendency of certain pupils to look down, not with their eyes, but by a general collapsing motion from the neck. This is the result of a fundamental misunderstanding of the alignment of the head, the neck and the back, and the position of the joints in the body.

Note how the models in this sequence of photographs (*below*) are using their eyes. Which do you think is the correct position? Can there be any doubt?.

"It's no good shutting your eyes if you're crossing a busy road."
F. M. Alexander

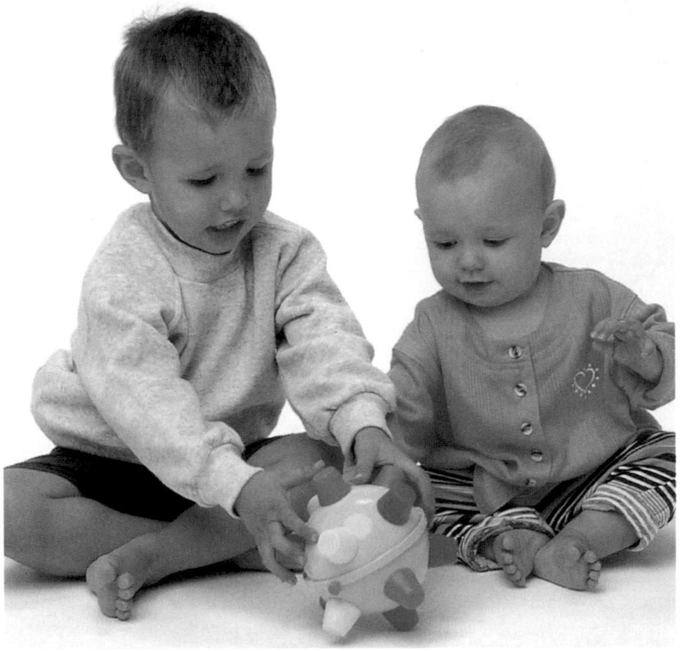

Here children are using their eyes to look at their toys. They have not disturbed the alignment between their heads, their necks and their backs, thus maintaining their good use.

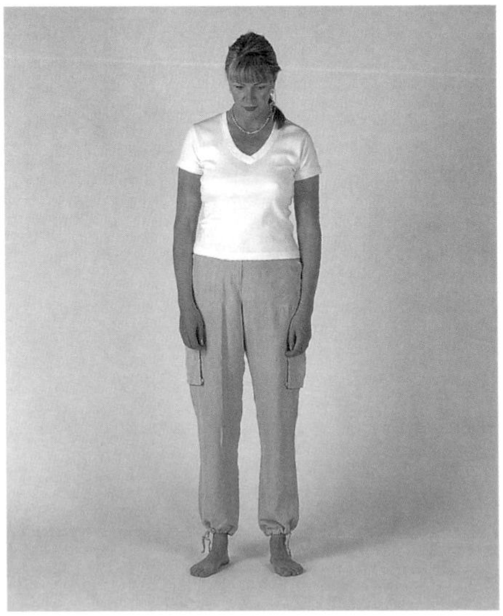

In this position, the model is breaking the alignment between her head, her neck and her back as she looks down, thus using her neck inappropriately.

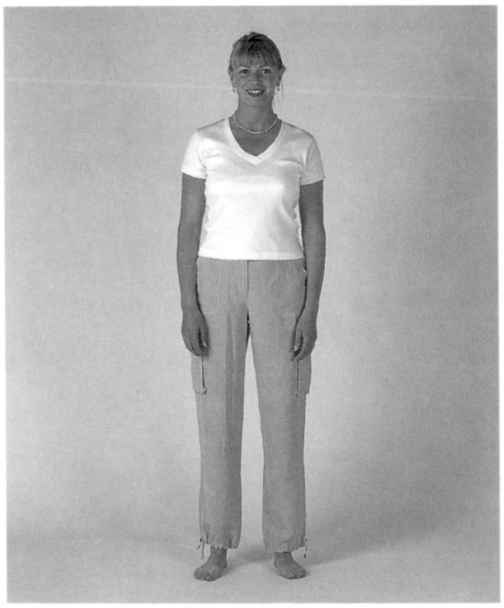

Note how the model is correctly aligned. She is maintaining her length and her width. Her eyes are alert and taking in her surroundings.

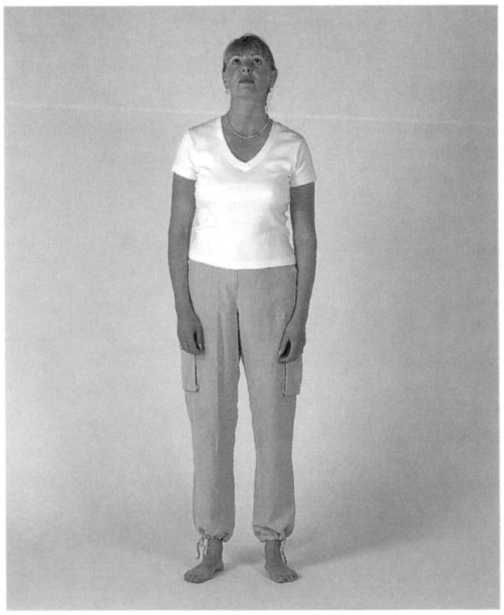

Here the model is breaking at the neckline and pulling her head back to look up, disturbing the alignment between her head, neck and back.

the semi-supine position

Standing for long periods easily compresses the spine. Lying down in a semi-supine position is a way of alleviating unnecessary tensions in the muscles and joints, and should be practised every day for at least 20 minutes. It encourages a better awareness of the head-neck-back relationship. This position does not necessarily need monitoring by a teacher, and it also gives you much needed time for yourself.

THE POSITION

Try to keep your eyes alert and open. It is preferable to avoid closing them because you will probably find it quite difficult not to fall asleep, which is definitely not the point of the exercise!

During your daily 20-minute session try and give yourself the time to practise some sharp, well directed thoughts to avoid your mind from wandering and spreading out, covering other possible important issues. This session can also encourage you to put into practice your excellent skills of observation. A good practice is to go over the primary directions, and to notice if you are aware of any tension in your body and to address it without trying to correct it. That is the secret of success.

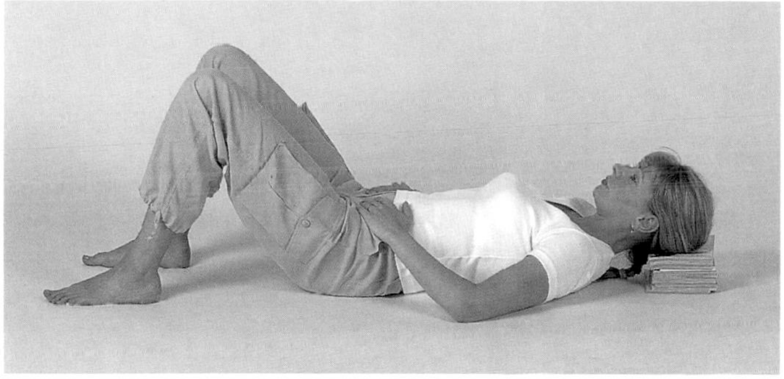

Books are used to support the head. If you have too many, however, your chin will drop and you will feel pressure on your throat.

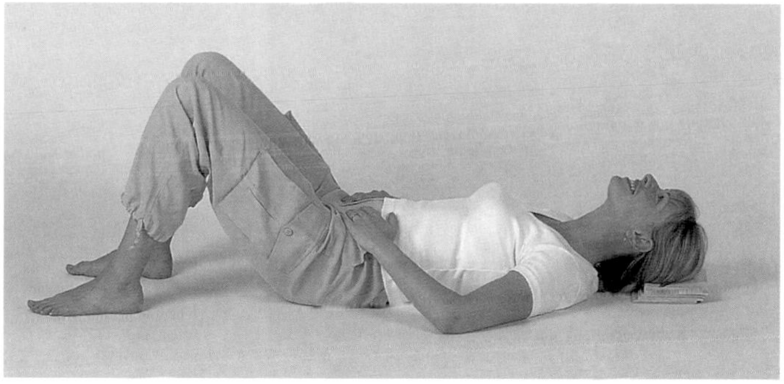

Correspondingly, if you do not have enough books your head will tilt back and will not be properly supported.

MOVING INTO THE SEMI-SUPINE

It is preferable to lie down on a hard, carpeted surface or alternatively on a rug on the floor. Avoid beds as they will not offer you adequate support. The number of books you need will depend on their thickness, and will also vary from person to person.

To lie down on the floor, place the books far enough behind you to give enough space for the whole of your torso and your bottom. When sitting, you can place your hands palms down on the floor behind you to help you lower your back. Take care not to stiffen the arms or to hold your breath in the process. To get up, it is preferable to roll over to one side, leading with your eyes rather than your head, and following with your torso and legs. Then place the free hand flat on the floor and go on to all fours. Be careful to maintain the alignment between your head, your neck and your back and not to hold your breath. Walk your hands back so that you move your bottom back towards your heels.

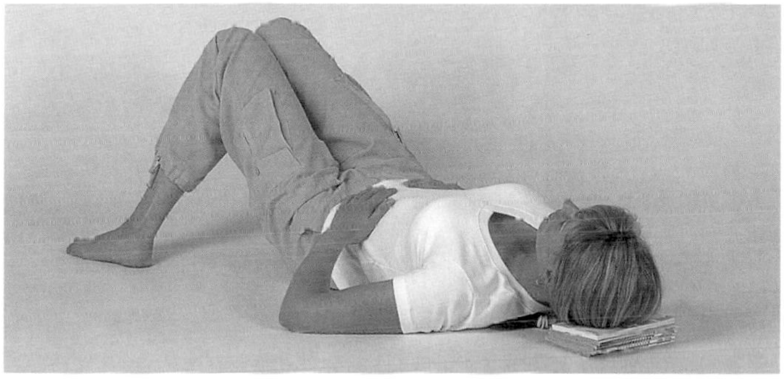

Make sure that your legs are about hip width apart and that your knees are directed towards the ceiling.

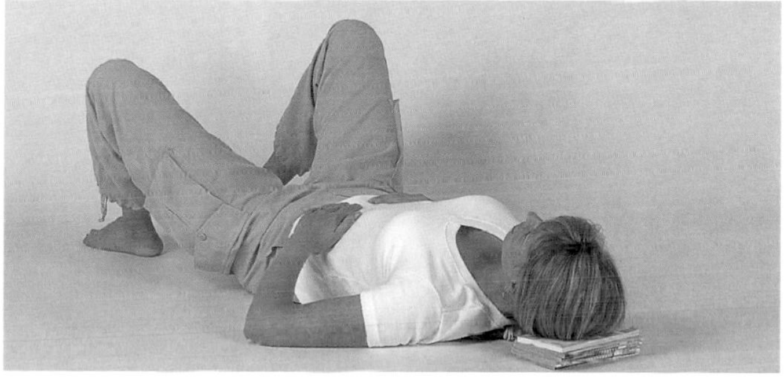

If your knees are falling out, you will probably lose the contact between the inner side of your foot and the floor.

"monkey" or bending

The position known as the "monkey" enables us to move with more flexibility in our daily activities. It is a useful means of moving from standing to sitting or squatting, as well as helping with lifting, picking things up, working at a desk, washing, ironing, and participating in sports such as skiing and golf. The "monkey" respects the relationship between the head, neck and back.

THE POSITION

The "monkey" position might sound tricky, but it really is not. Try it slowly, see how it works, then try it again at a more natural speed. It basically involves the head moving forwards and up, and then the knees moving forwards and away over the feet to counterbalance the bottom going back over the heels, enabling the arms to move freely. It is also important to remember that when you go into "monkey" you must review your primary directions. What is more, stay alert at all times, and avoid fixing your gaze or holding your breath. Such moves will quickly undermine the marvellous effects of the "monkey".

To be more precise then, stand with your legs hip-width apart, with the feet slightly turned outwards. Your weight should be evenly distributed, neither too far forwards nor too far back on your feet. To start going into the "monkey", allow the knees to bend slightly over your feet as you tilt forwards from your hip joints, making sure your head, your neck and your back are aligned. Avoid collapsing over yourself!

One final point is to make sure you think of widening and lengthening your back as you widen across the shoulder girdle, to allow free movement and your arms to hang freely. This extra tip will ensure you enjoy the full effect of "the monkey".

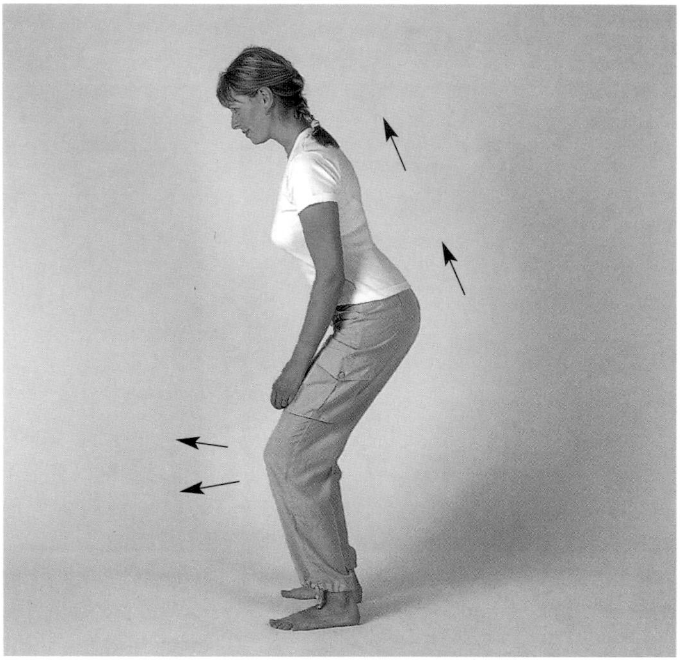

This model is in the correct "monkey" position. Her head, her neck and her back are aligned. Her knees are bent forward and away from her hips.

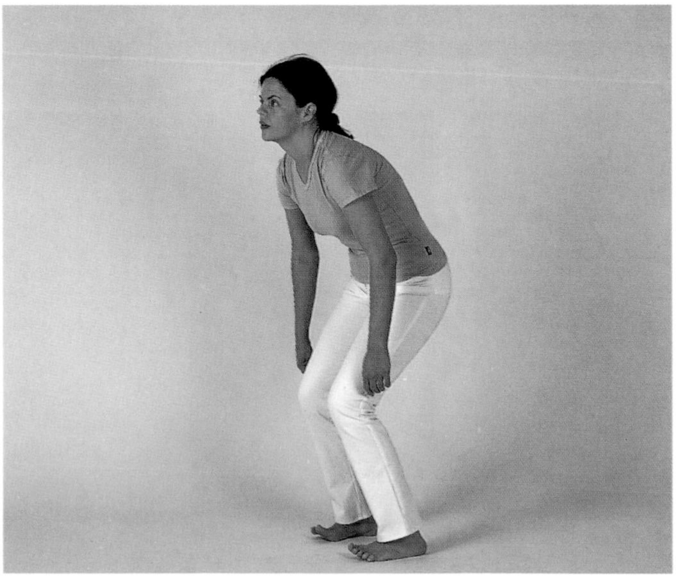

When going into the "monkey" avoid retracting the head back and down into the spine. Note how the model has rounded her shoulders and pulled in her knees.

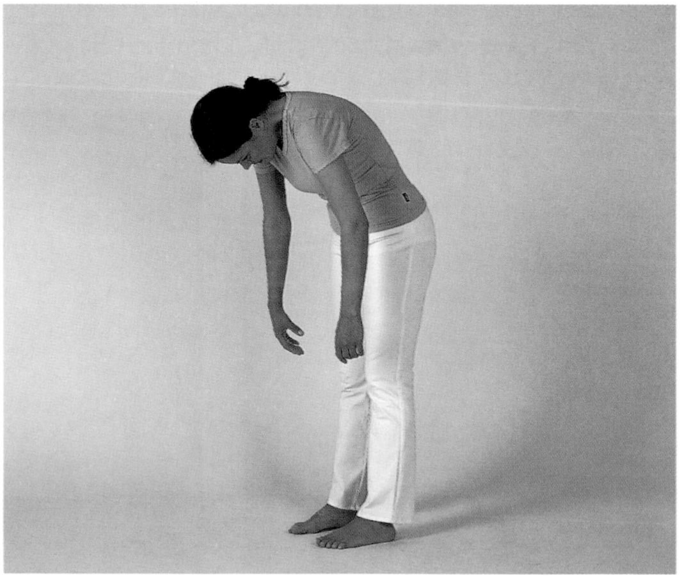

Here the model is not bending her knees as she bends forwards. Her back is collapsed over her body, and her legs are straight and braced.

everyday situations

In everyday situations it is important to pause before reacting, to make sure you are so positioned that you do not misuse yourself. The more aware you are, the more likely you will encourage muscular release through your whole system. Equally, the more at peace you are, the easier it is to apply the principles of the Alexander technique. The following excellent examples show how the "monkey" can keep you healthy.

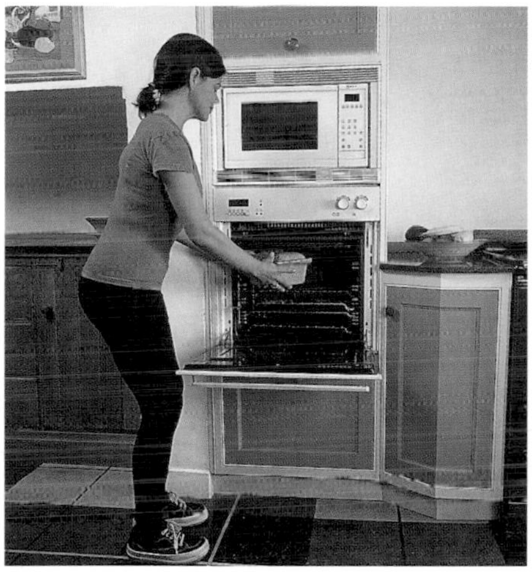

Note how the model's back is correctly aligned, keeping to the head-neck-back principle. See how she is using her joints and allowing her widening arms to handle the dish.

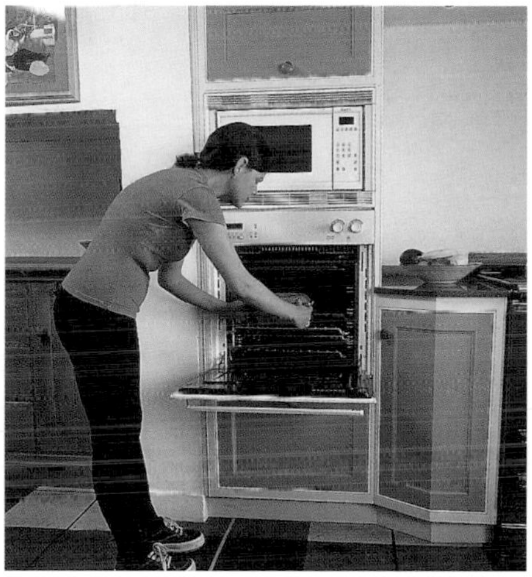

How things can go wrong. Here the model has started pulling her head back. Also, her back is rounded, her legs are braced and her arms have become much too tense.

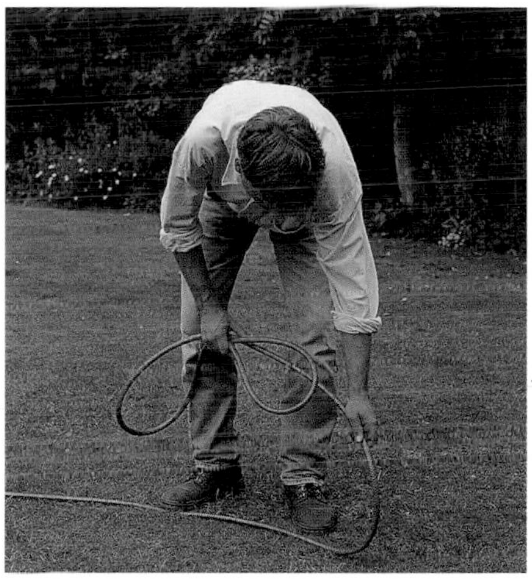

In this highly incorrect stance, the man is collapsing from his waist down as he begins works in the garden. His shoulders are far too rounded, and his head is being pulled back.

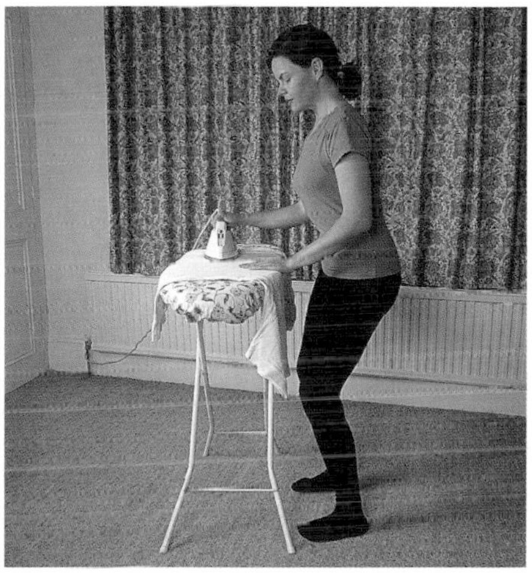

In this correct procedure, the model is neatly poised and balanced, and she is well aligned to begin her ironing. Her hand, wrist and arm are also free as she holds the iron. The other crucial point to note is how she is widening across her upper arms. It is clear that she looks balanced and feels alert.

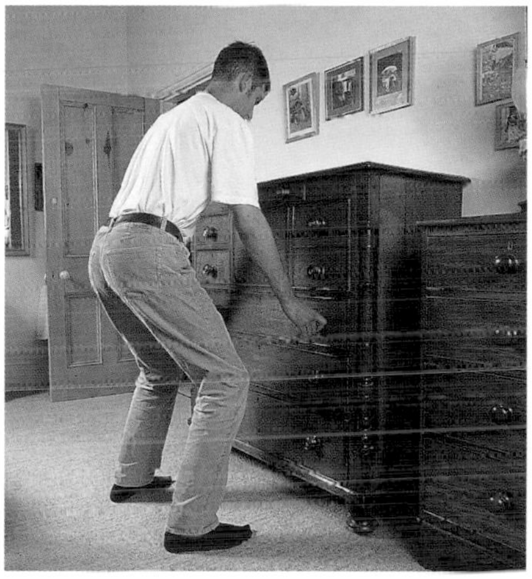

See how the model is using the whole of his back quite correctly. He is sensibly allowing his weight to come back on to his heels, and his knees go forwards and away over his feet.

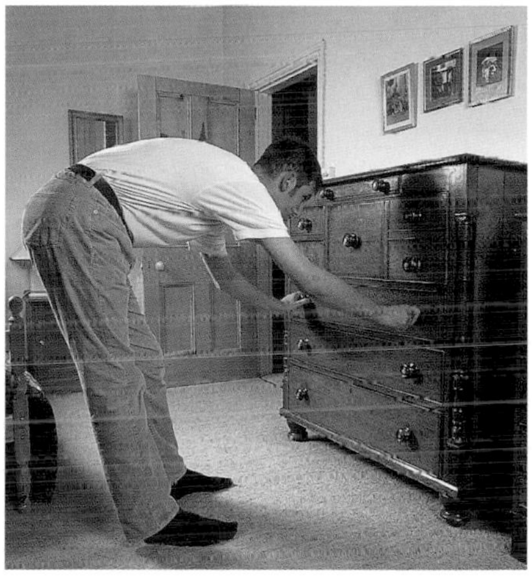

An example of how not to do it. Here he is completely out of alignment. You can sense it is not right, but why? He is actually pulling his head back, rounding the back, and holding in the arms. This position is entirely the result of bad habits. Without the Alexander technique, he would never know how to right this.

"lunge monkey"

The "lunge monkey" is similar to the "monkey" because the knees go forwards and away, and the torso tilts slightly forwards from the hip joints. Also, one foot is placed behind the other, and the legs are placed hip-width apart, enabling you to balance the upper part of your body on to the forward or the back leg whenever the need arises. In this way, your weight is placed forwards or backwards according to your activity.

BENDING

The "lunge monkey" is extremely useful when you need to lift something heavy from the floor; when you need to move an object from one side of a surface to another, for example during cooking; or when you need to push or pull something rather heavy into place.

When you adapt the "lunge monkey" it is important to remember to keep your head, your neck and your back correctly aligned. The legs must be hip-width apart, with the arms hanging freely on either side of your torso.

Also, allow your weight to move to the right on to the right foot (or to the left, as the situation demands). If moving to the left, reverse the instructions.

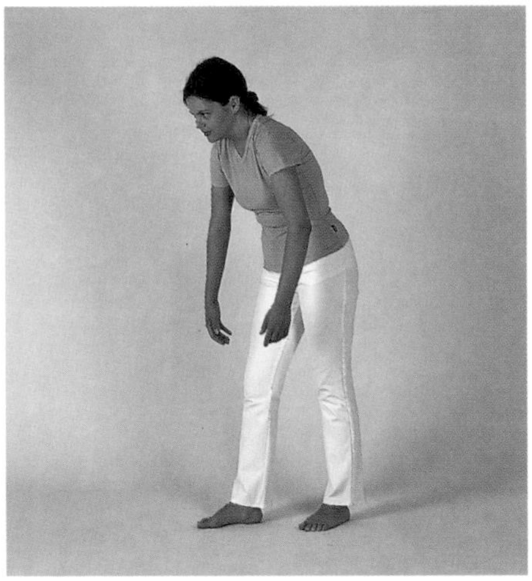

See how the model has collapsed badly from the waist down. Her shoulders are rounded, the legs are straight and the knees are braced, causing tension.

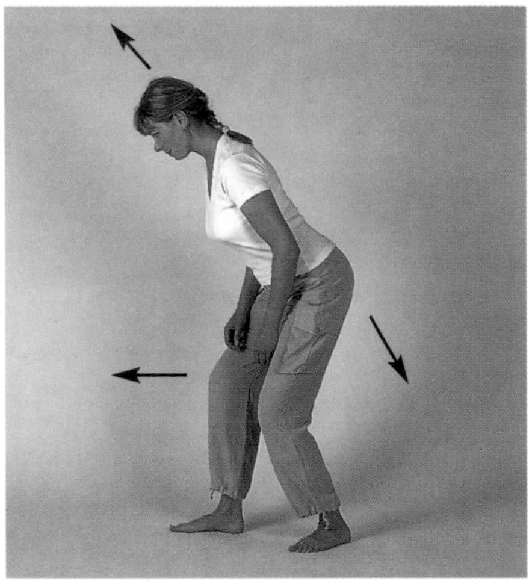

Observe how the model has gone into the "lunge monkey". Her head, neck and back are neatly aligned, and her knees are going forward away from her hips.

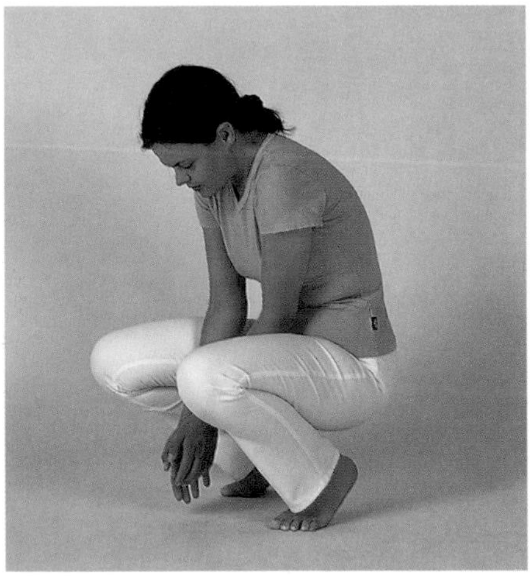

Note how the model has completely lost the correct alignment with her back as she squats. Her head has dropped, and her shoulders are hunched and rounded. Furthermore, she looks ill at ease and uncomfortable. There is no poise or grace. This position is definitely one to avoid.

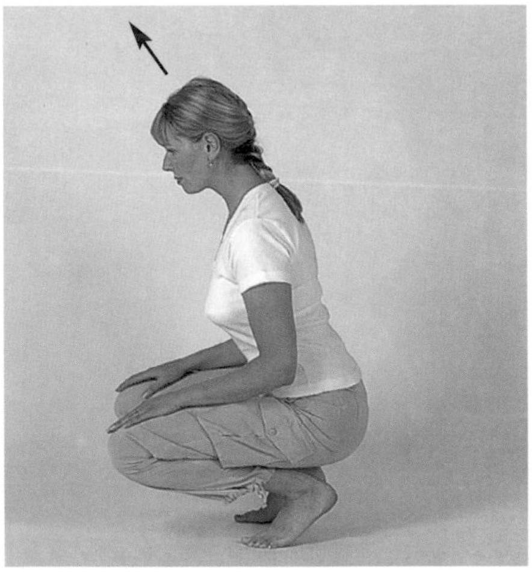

In this correct procedure, observe how the model's head, neck and back are correctly aligned. Her shoulders are widening across her upper arms. She looks well balanced, and fully in control of her movements. Also note how her heels are tucked in under the bottom. The position is also easy to get into.

SQUATTING

In Western societies most people find it difficult to squat in their everyday lives. Young children have very little difficulty in doing so, but as we grow older we lose the necessary flexibility to squat as our joints become less mobile.

A low "monkey" or semi-squat is the best way that an Alexander teacher can re-introduce a student to squatting over a series of lessons. To squat, follow the same guidelines as for the "monkey", but with a wider stance. Remember to maintain the alignment between the head, the neck and the back, and to allow the joints in the hips, the knees and the ankles to be free. As you go into a deeper squat you might find that your heels come off the ground. This does not present a problem as far as the technique is concerned, so long as you keep your balance. As a general rule, go only as far as you feel comfortable.

the technique in the home

The key point to note about the Alexander technique is that it is not an abstract theory that you can apply when the mood takes you. It is a specific, practical everyday guide that will help you enormously whether you are bending, squatting, lifting or carrying. It gives you terrific control whatever you are doing, injecting extra confidence that will keep you alert and relaxed.

BENDING

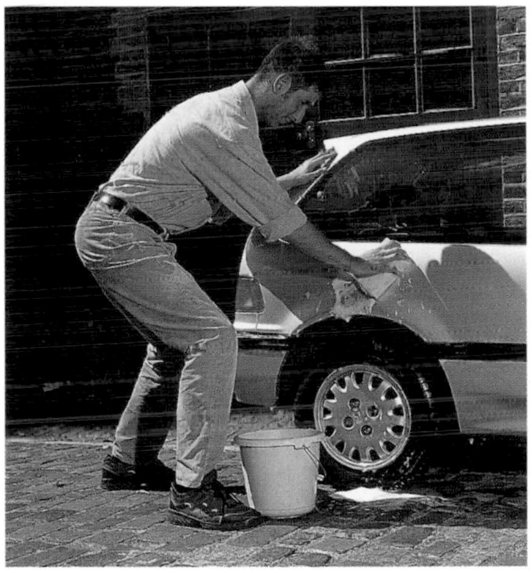

Note how the model is tilted forwards to get a greater range of movement. His arms are free, supported by his back.

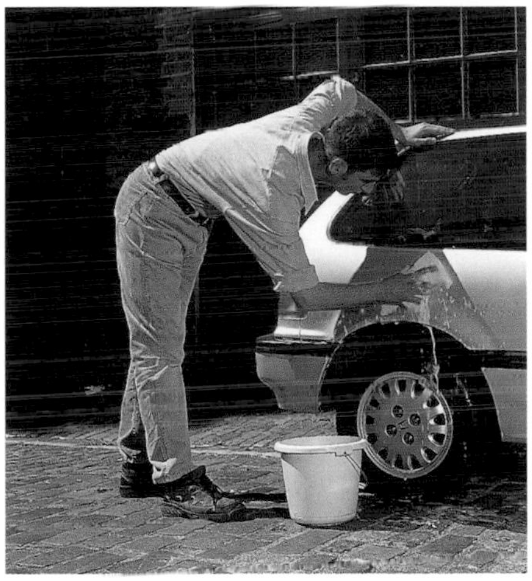

Now he is incorrectly bending forwards from the waist. His legs are braced, and his head is pulled back.

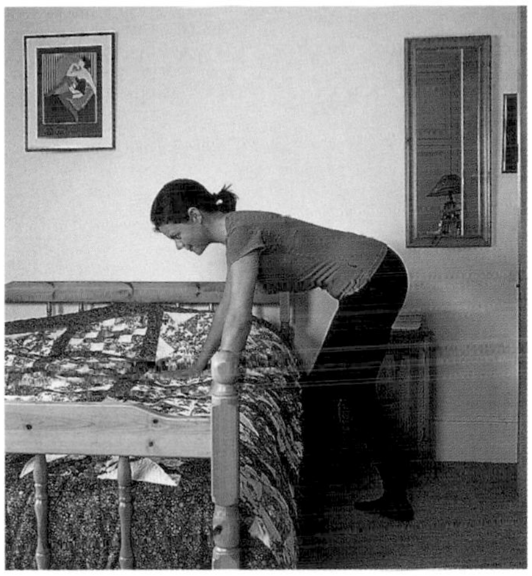

Here the model has aligned herself nicely to make the bed. Her legs are bent, creating a greater range of movement.

SQUATTING

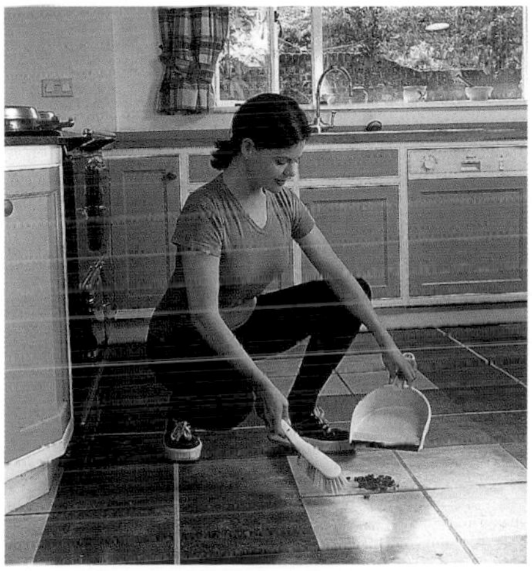

This model is lunge squatting to brush up dirt from the floor. She has maintained her good use, giving herself a maximum range of movement. She looks good and feels good.

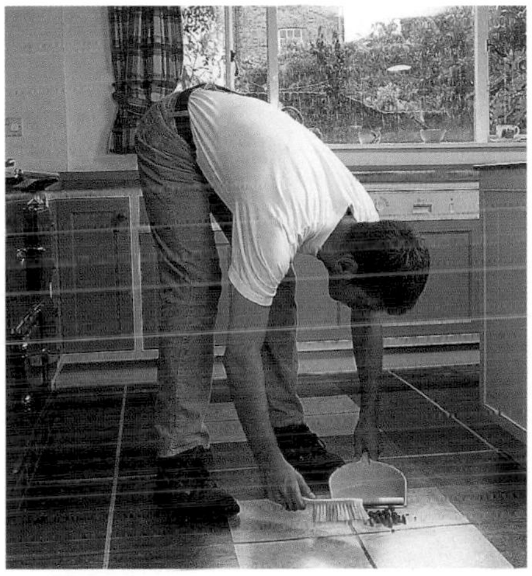

Here, in an incorrect example of how you should sweep the floor, the model is badly restricting his range of movement. He is quite clearly unbalanced, and feels totally uncomfortable.

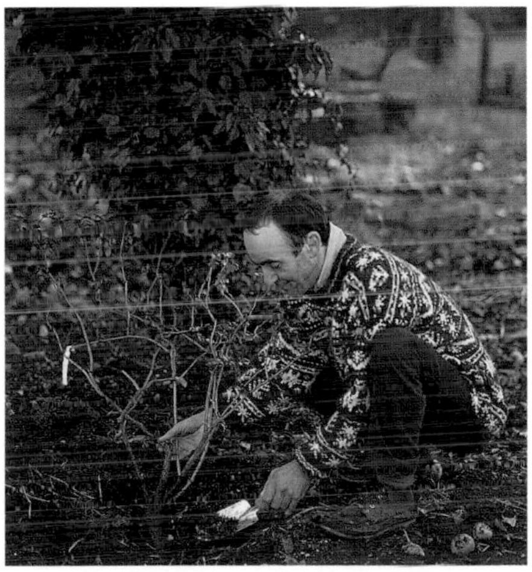

Note how this man is squatting sensibly to plant a rose bush in his garden. By placing himself at the same level as the rose, he is allowing himself a greater range of movement.

lifting and carrying

A lot of back pain is the result of lifting heavy weights. To avoid back strain, stand near to the load by placing your feet either side of it, and maintain the alignment between head, neck and back. Go into the "monkey" or "lunge monkey" and squat. Then bend your arms so that your elbows are close to your body. Make sure that you widen out across the upper arms, and avoid tension in the arms and wrists.

LIFTING

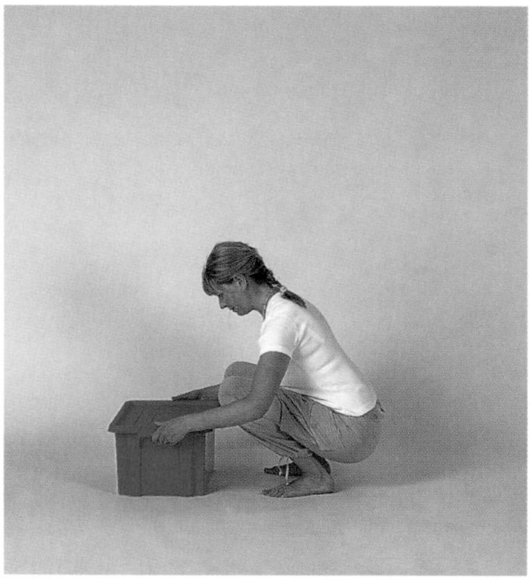

1 Once you are holding the load as closely to your body as you can, come out of a squat or lunge squat into a "monkey" before standing.

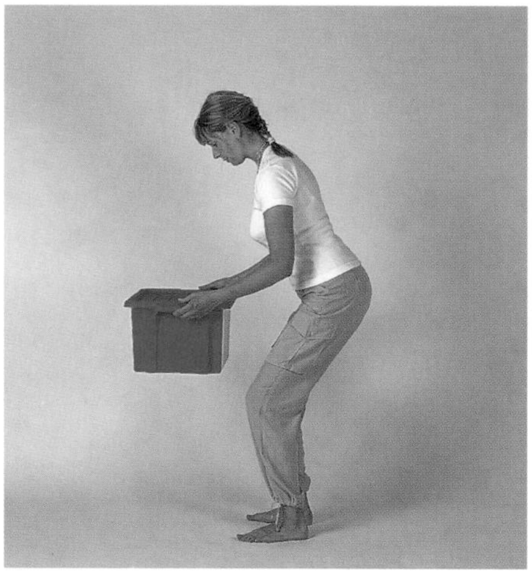

2 Lift the weight in a flowing action, that does not jar or suddenly pull against the back. If the weight proves too heavy, it is easy to bend and put it down.

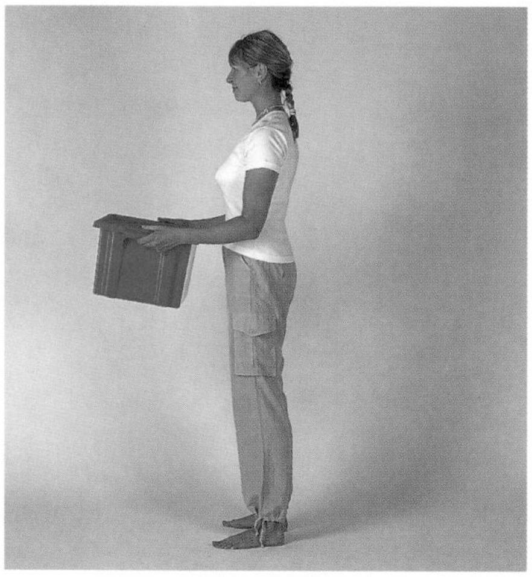

3 To place the load back on the ground, reverse the process and apply the same principles, making sure that your head, neck and back are aligned.

CARRYING

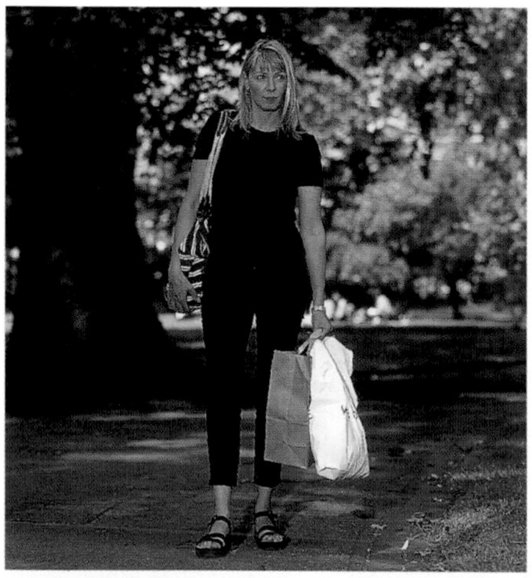

Here the model is carrying all her shopping bags in one hand, creating an imbalance as she is pulled down to the left. She is raising her right shoulder in an attempt to support her handbag.

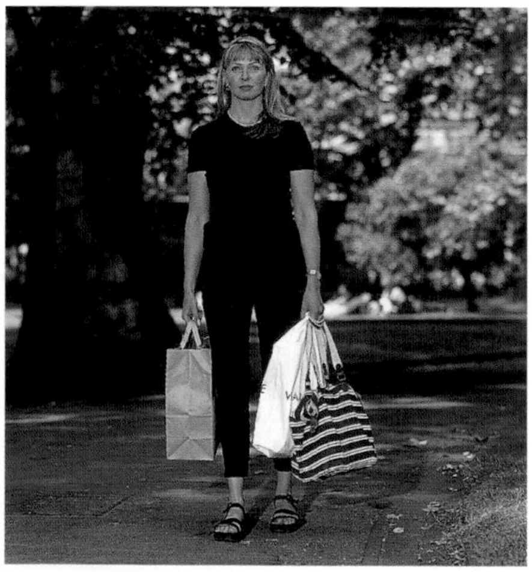

This model is carrying her shopping bags sensibly and correctly so that they are evenly distributed on both sides. She is well balanced and able to walk freely. She looks content.

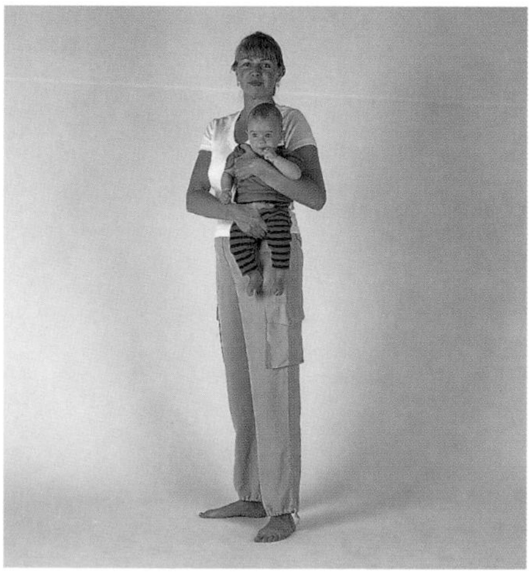

Look at the excellent way this mother is carrying her child. Her weight is evenly distributed and she is holding the child close to her body, firmly supporting his upper and lower body.

daily routines

The most surprising point about the Alexander technique is that it is not just for big, set piece movements such as lifting heavy weights, when doing it incorrectly can obviously lead to back problems. The technique even extends to the minutiae of life, routines that we completely take for granted, such as eating, drinking, and driving. If you had always wondered how they should be done, read on. These tips will make all the difference.

EATING AND DRINKING

If you are standing upright while you are drinking remember that you still need to be fully alert at all times. Therefore, make sure that you do not fix your gaze rigidly and thereby lose all communication and contact with the outside world. You also need to ensure that your head leads you away from your heels (see the section on Standing for further guidance). You will find that your shoulder girdle brings mobility to your arms, and that the pelvis provides stability which simultaneously facilitates mobility in your legs.

The very same principles also apply to eating. Whether you are going to eat something from your hand or use a fork, it is all too easy to forget your posture completely. Remember that you should not totally focus on the matter in hand, but that you must also consider your stance, alertness and poise.

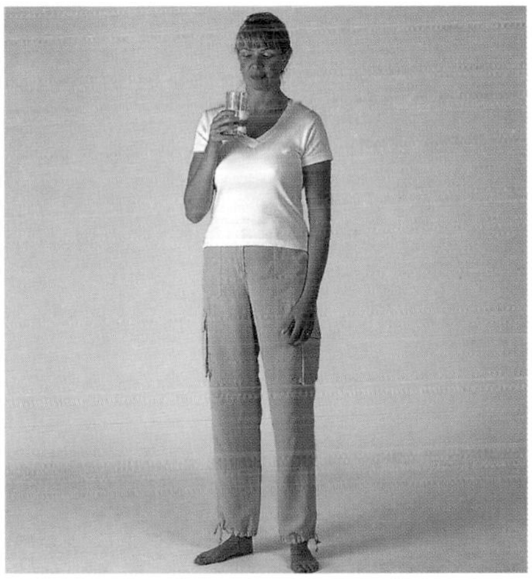

Avoid gripping or clutching your glass. Be aware of the connection with your arm, which links to your back and then into your heels. As you raise the cup to your lips, bring your weight back on to the heels, so as not to pull in your lower back. Also, bring the glass to the lips, rather than leaning down into it.

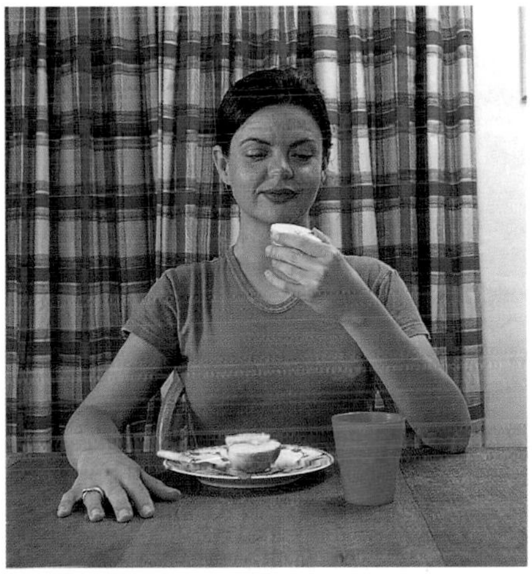

Take some time to consider how you are seated at the table and then bring the food up to your mouth, rather than the reverse. Your feet should be correctly positioned on the floor. You should also be aware of both your sitting bones, and how your back should be lengthening and widening. This position also aids digestion.

DRIVING

Most of the problems experienced by drivers are due to fixed postures, long journeys and poor seating support.

Too many people who spend huge amounts of time driving find themselves constricted by the position of the steering wheel and the pedals. Such a cramped environment is bound to lead to stress and strain on the back, and equally on the arms and legs.

When choosing a car take time to see whether the seat is firm and supportive. If you already own a car and it does not have a lumbar support adjustment, you can use a wedge-shaped cushion to give you adequate support in the lumbar area and the pelvis. It makes a vital difference.

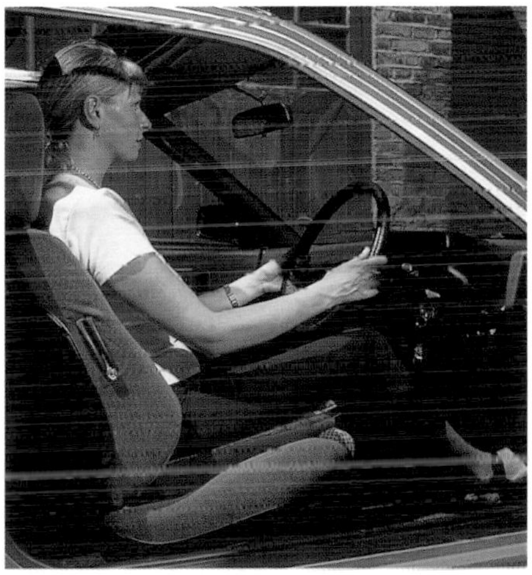

You should be able to reach the pedals quite easily. A wedge-shaped cushion is extremely useful to avoid a poor, slumping position.

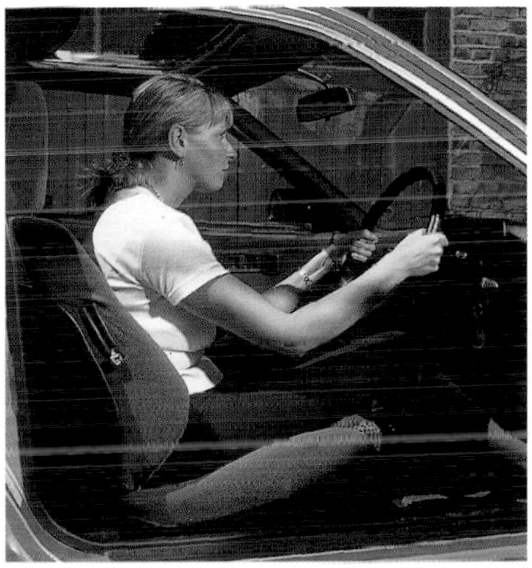

See how the model is badly collapsing forward, how the neck is being strained and the arms are rigidly tense. Such a position will cause lots of discomfort.

t'ai chi for health or self defence

If you simply want to go out and strike a pose, jumping about like Bruce Lee, t'ai chi is not for you. It is a very serious, highly regarded ancient technique that has two major qualities. It improves your health, and teaches you how to overcome stronger hostile forces when you are under attack. The most amazing part of t'ai chi is the way its movements are almost balletic.

The Benefits of T'ai Chi

Although t'ai chi can eventually be used in self-defence, and most classes do incorporate some of its practical applications, it is initially practised mainly for its health-giving benefits. It is particularly useful for increasing alertness and body awareness, and for developing concentration and sensitivity. It helps with balance and posture, and enhances a sense of "groundedness". However, all the postures can also be used when defending yourself against an attack by an opponent. Its gentleness and subtlety do not preclude its use as a very effective form of self-defence.

It is not easy to separate the physical and mental aspects of t'ai chi, as they are closely interrelated. In Chinese medicine, the interdependence of mind, body and spirit is seen as integral to well-being.

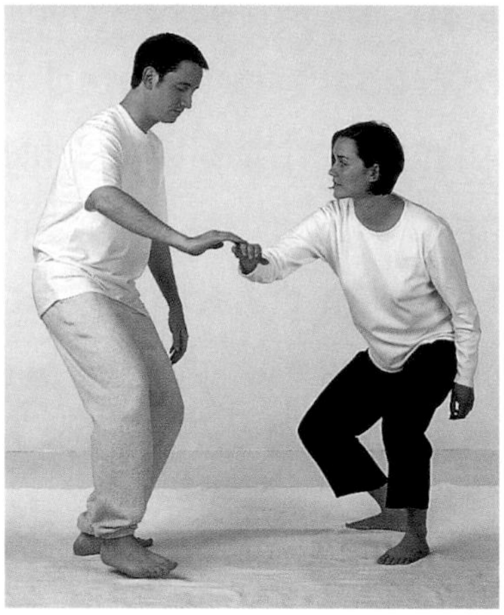

The ancient art of t'ai chi instills enormous grace and confidence.

The Theory of T'ai Chi

Like music, t'ai chi cannot be appreciated purely on an intellectual level. It also has an enormous spiritual side, and when you watch any highly experienced t'ai chi practitioners you will see how they are almost in a kind of trance, in a separate world where they cannot be touched. Correctly done, it is quite hypnotic.

For now, we must look at some of the concepts that are fundamental to the martial arts, as well as to medicine and philosophy. Although these disciplines are all treated quite separately by those in the West, they are all inseparable in the Eastern view. From thousands of years of close observation of patterns of energy, the Chinese successfully evolved a way of life that actually ropes all three ingredients together.

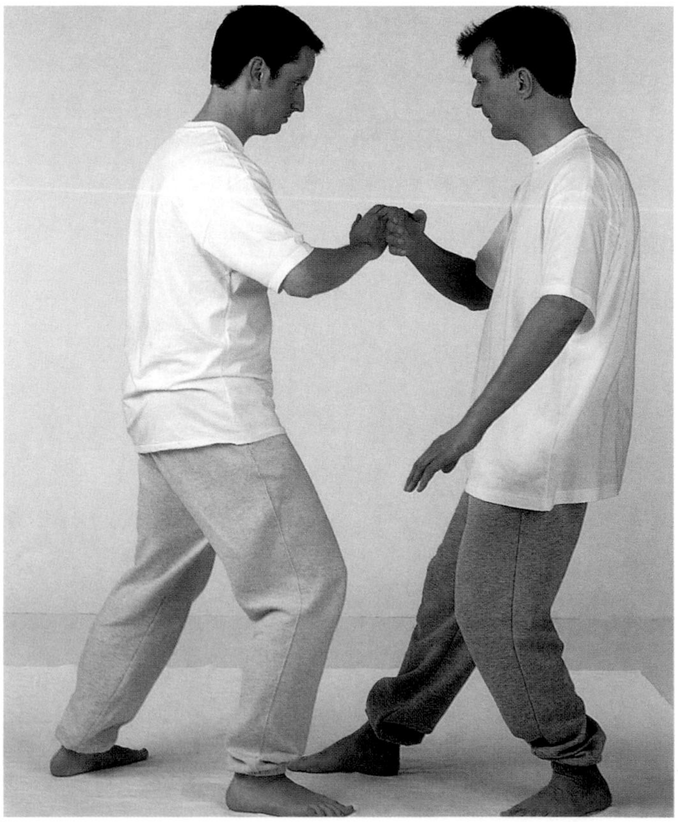

Chi

Chi is the prime driving force of human life, the spark behind thought, creativity and growth which maintains and nurtures us. It can be felt as movement of energy in the body, like the ceaseless flow of an electrical current. Chi flows through the body along channels called meridians.

The Tan Tien

The Chi is stored in the Tan Tien. This is an area about the size of a golf ball, located four finger-widths below the navel, and about one-third of the way from the front to the back of the body. It is the centre of gravity of the body, and in t'ai chi all movement emanates from it. Try to let the breath and the mind sink to the Tan Tien.

Yin and Yang

Yin and Yang describe the complementary yet opposing forces of nature. Their relationship has a harmony and balance: both Yin and Yang are necessary, are constantly moving and balancing each other, and this interaction creates Chi. The Chinese observed that when the balance of Yin and Yang is disrupted so too will be the body's Chi, leading to ill health.

One of the key requirements for t'ai chi is excellent balance.

warm-up exercises

Perform these exercises slowly and gently, with the mind and the breath focused in the Tan Tien. Notice any differences between the right and left sides of your body, and between the upper and lower parts. The object is gradually to enter the world of t'ai chi, and to warm up all your muscles so that you do not get any strains. The more you warm up, the better your technique will be. The movements will flow like a stream.

CIRCLING HANDS

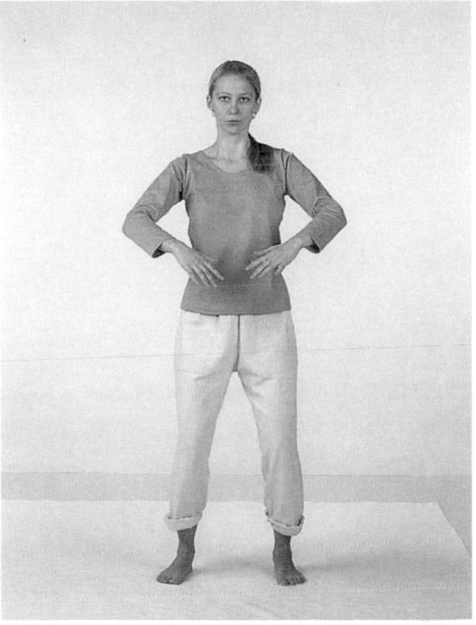

1 Inhale and allow both hands to float upwards a comfortable distance in front of your body, palms facing downwards.

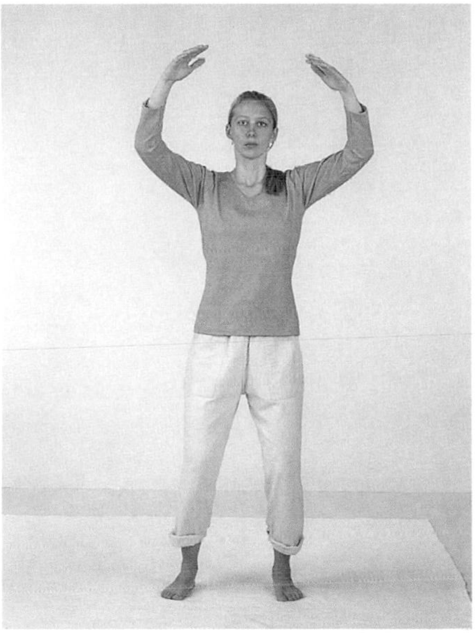

2 As your hands rise above your head, relax the wrists and begin to open the palms outwards. Begin to exhale.

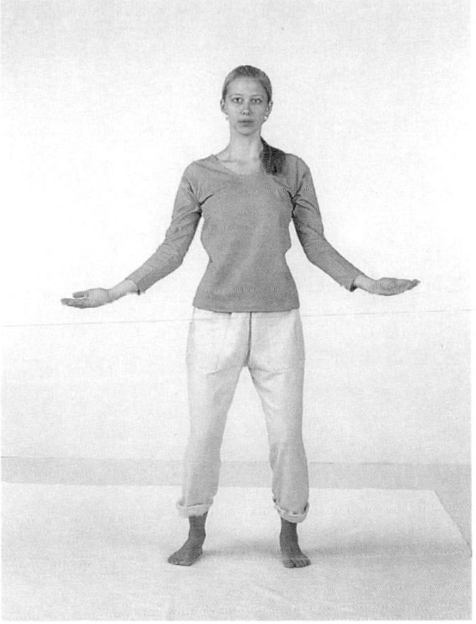

3 Open out your arms to your sides. Draw your hands inwards at the bottom of the circle and smoothly begin again.

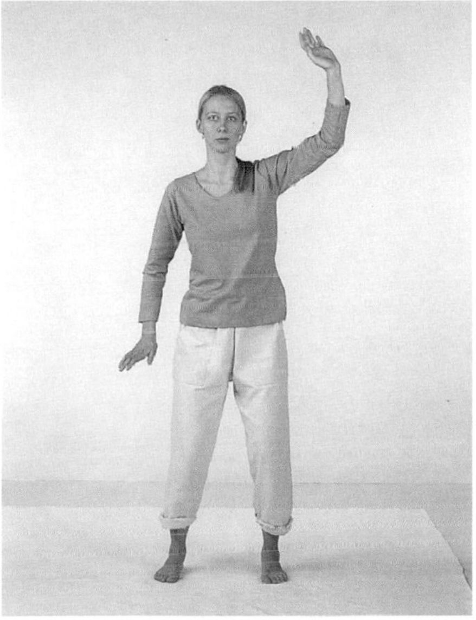

4 Inhale as your palms, facing upwards, float in front of your body. Exhale and push your right hand down by your hip and your left hand up by your temple.

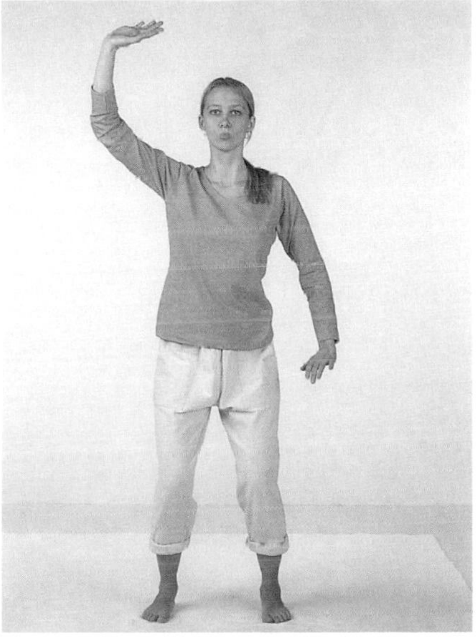

5 Breathe in again, relax your palms which now turn to face each other and begin moving them towards each other in front of your body.

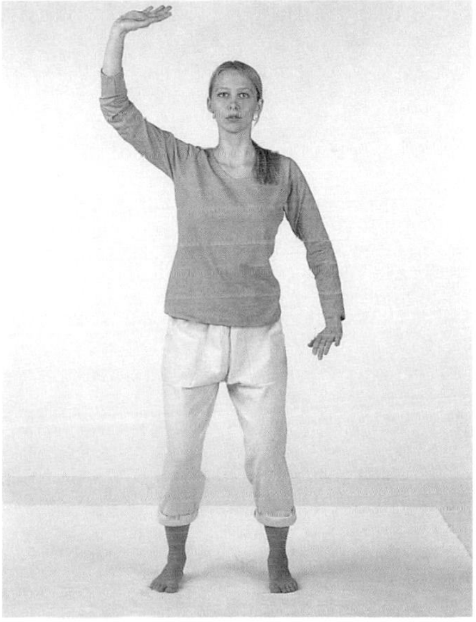

6 Repeat step 4 in reverse as you exhale. Breathe in again and bring your hands in front of your body in a mirror image of Step 5.

SHAKING OUT SHOULDERS, ARMS AND HANDS

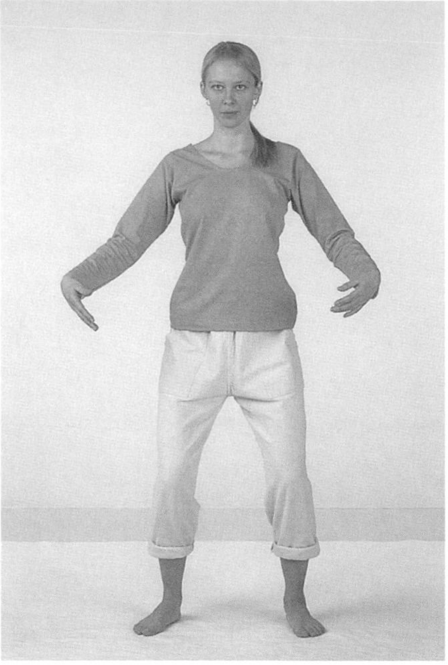

1 Gently shake out any tension in your wrists and hands. Gradually work up to include your shoulders. This exercise is especially useful before, during and after long periods at a keyboard, or repetitive work with the hands.

LOOSENING SHOULDERS

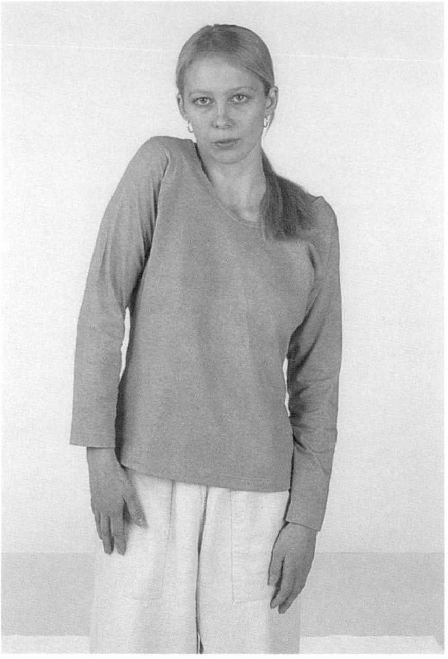

1 Make increasing circles with one shoulder. Change direction and decrease the size of the circles. Repeat for the other shoulder. Rotate your shoulders alternately.

ROTATING WAIST

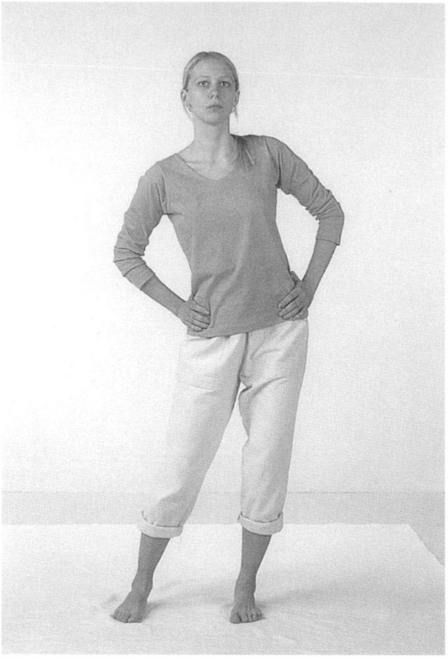

1 Place both hands lightly on your hips. Keeping your head up, begin by spiralling your hips slowly outwards, feeling for any restriction, tightness or lack of ease. Change direction and spiral back in slowly.

KNEE ROTATIONS

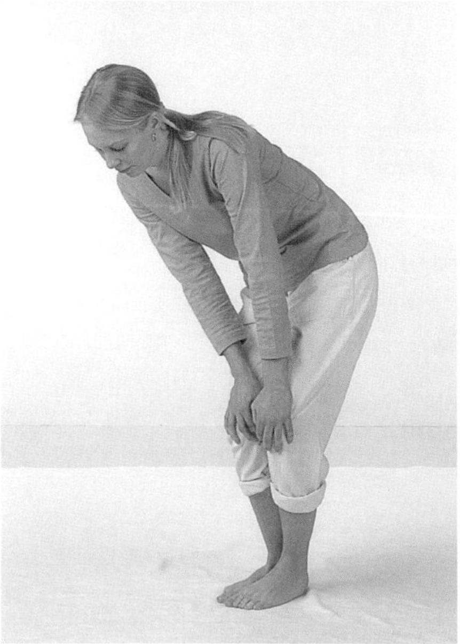

1 Bring your feet together and place your palms lightly on your upper kneecaps. Feel the Chi from your palms radiating deep into your knee joints. Circle your knees clockwise several times, then change direction.

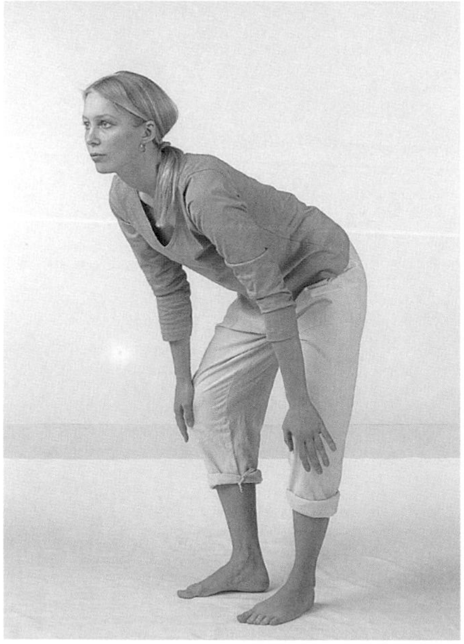

2 Keep your legs and hands in the same position. Rotate your knees in opposite directions – one circles clockwise while the other circles anti-clockwise (counter-clockwise). Change the direction of each knee and repeat the rotations.

CALF STRETCH

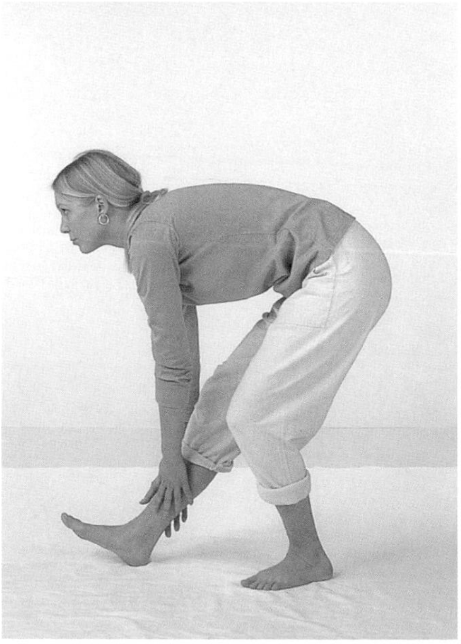

1 Step forward with your right foot. Keeping the heel on the floor, pull up your toes towards the knee. Drop your body forward, keeping your right leg straight. Hold for a few breaths and release. Repeat for the other leg.

FOUR-DIRECTIONAL BREATHING

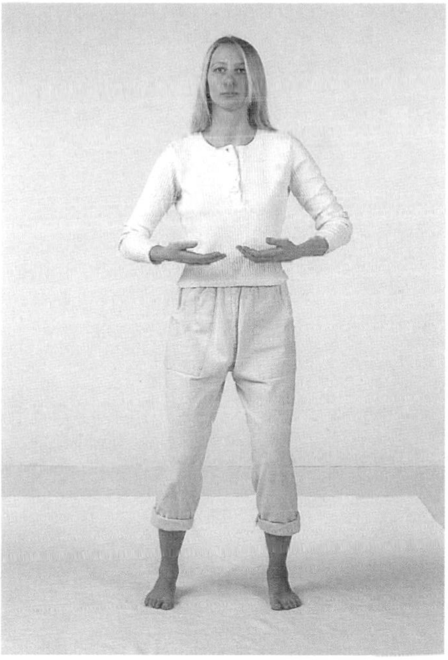

1 As you inhale, bring your hands up to chest height, palms facing upwards.

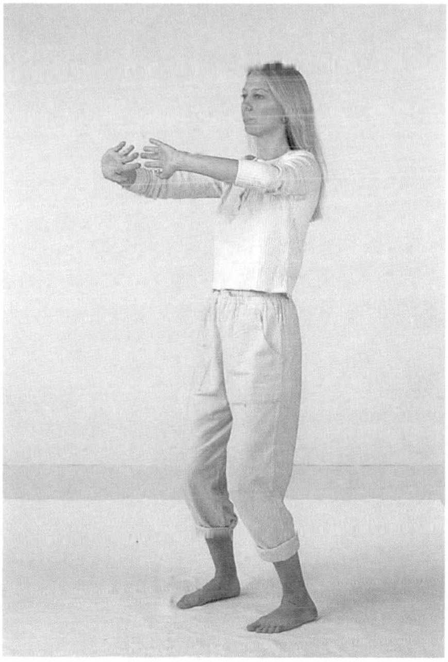

2 As you exhale, turn the palms to face away and extend your arms as if pushing something away. On the next inhalation, turn your palms back to face your body, softening your arms and drawing them back in towards your chest.

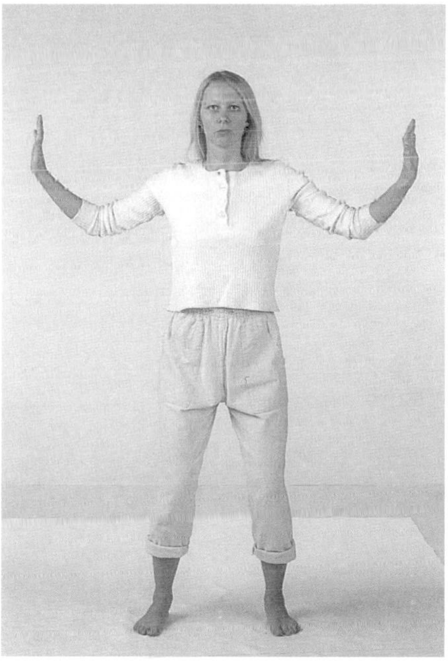

3 Exhale again, turn the palms out and extend your arms out to your sides.

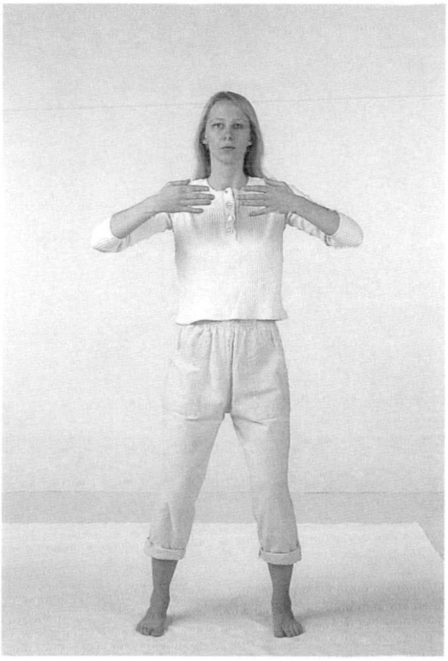

4 Relax and bring your arms in towards your chest as you inhale.

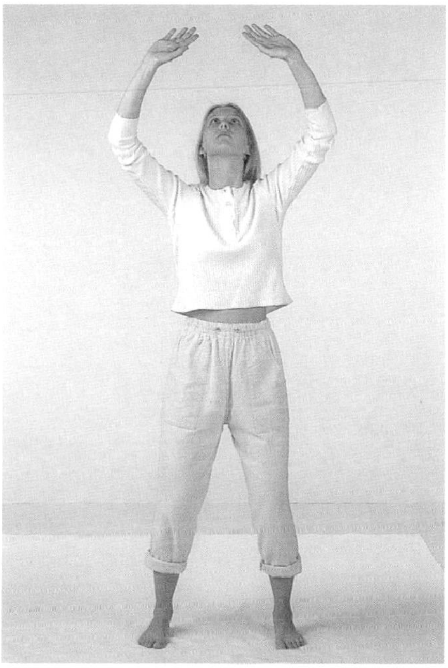

5 On the next exhalation turn your palms upwards and extend your arms towards the sky.

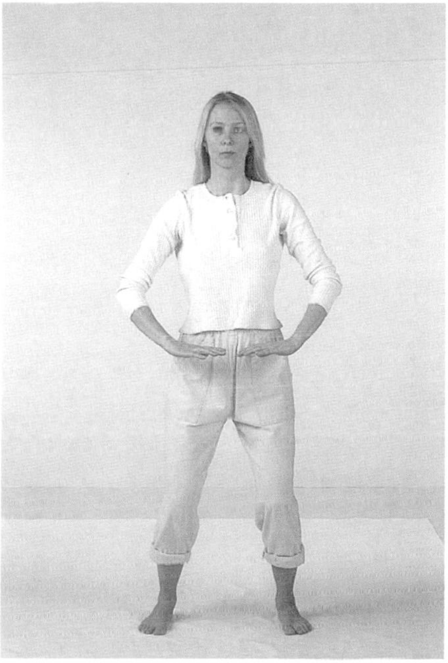

6 Inhale and let your arms descend, palms facing downwards. As your arms pass the solar plexus, exhale and push down towards the earth. Repeat this sequence several times.

SHIFTING WEIGHT

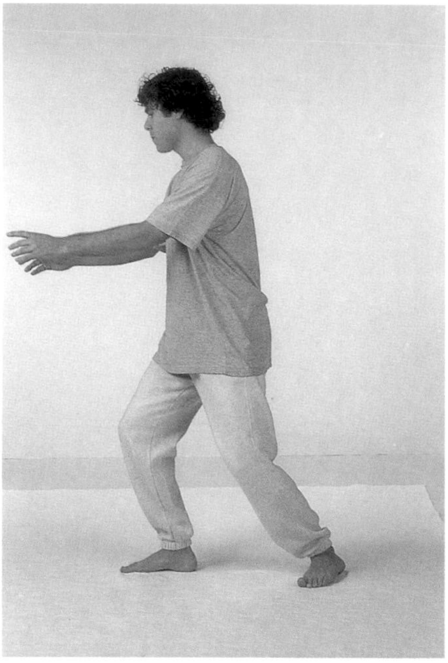

1 Place your left foot at 45° and your right foot forward, heels shoulder-width apart. Shift your weight from one leg to the other – do not tip your pelvis forwards or backwards.

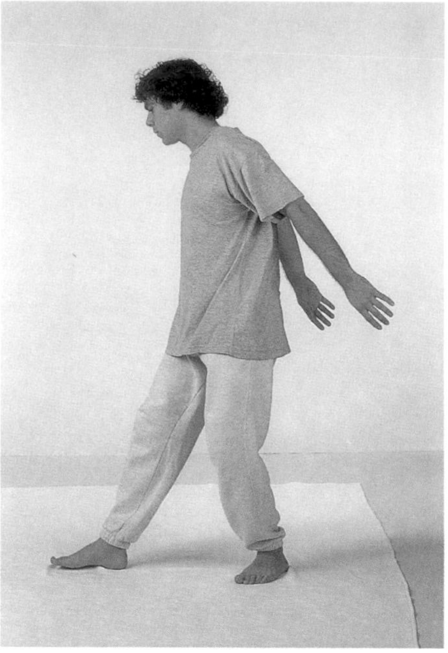

2 Let your arms swing naturally. Continue for about 1 minute, then change legs and repeat the sequence again. Feel a strong root developing through your feet into the centre of the earth.

ROTATING WHOLE BODY

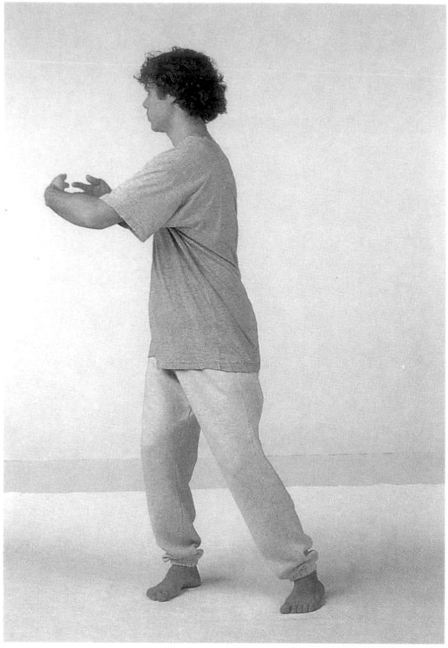

1 Hold both arms in front of the chest, palms facing inwards, fingertips almost touching. Turn your waist and arms and shift your weight to the right. Repeat to the left.

WAVING HANDS IN CLOUDS

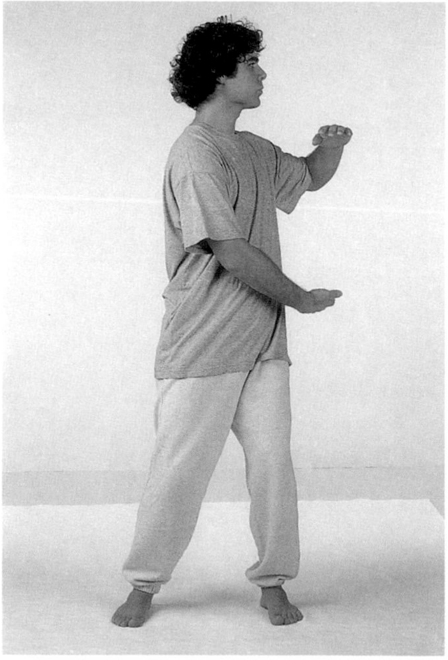

1 Begin with your right hand facing the Tan Tien, your left hand directly above it, facing your chest. Turn your waist to the left, shifting your weight into your left leg. Turn your palms towards each other.

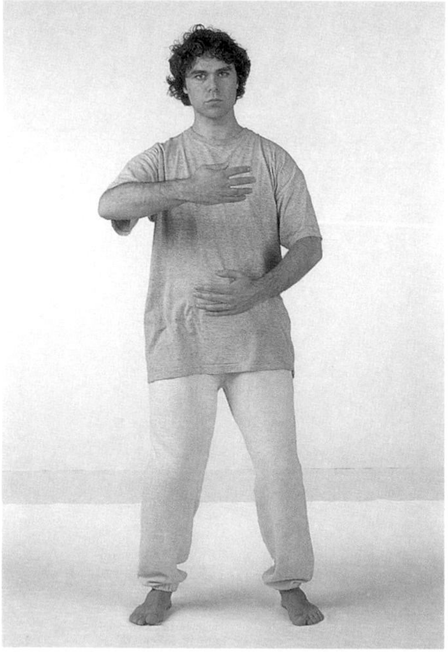

2 Bring your waist back to the front. As you do so, lower your left hand until it is opposite the Tan Tien and raise your right hand to the level of your chest, with your palms facing your body.

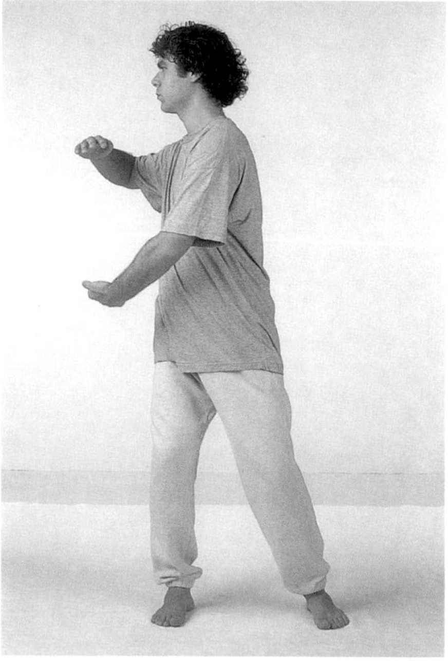

3 Now turn your waist to the right, shift the weight across to your right leg, and turn your palms towards each other in a mirror image of Step 1. Repeat the entire sequence several times.

PUSH TO CENTRE, PUSH TO CORNER

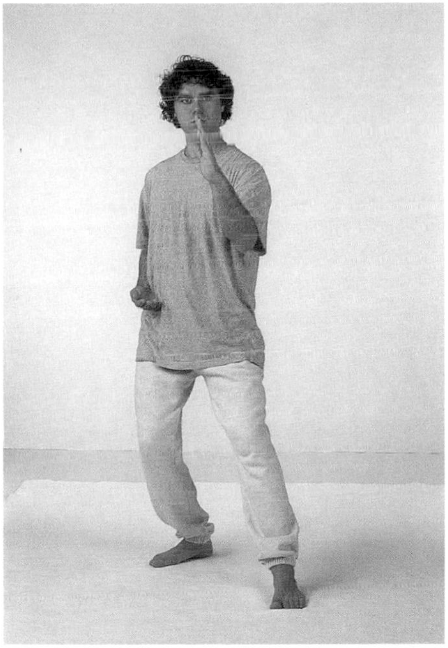

1 Place your right foot at 45° and step forward with your left foot. Begin with all your weight on your right leg, right hand resting palm upwards on your right hip, left fingertips in line with your mouth, palm facing diagonally forwards and to the centre.

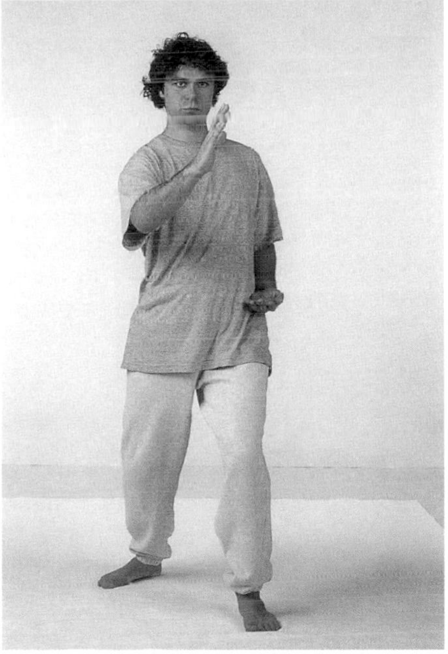

2 Bring your weight forward on to your left leg. Your right hand turns diagonally forwards as it comes to push towards the centre of your body; your left hand turns palm upwards as it draws back to rest on your left hip.

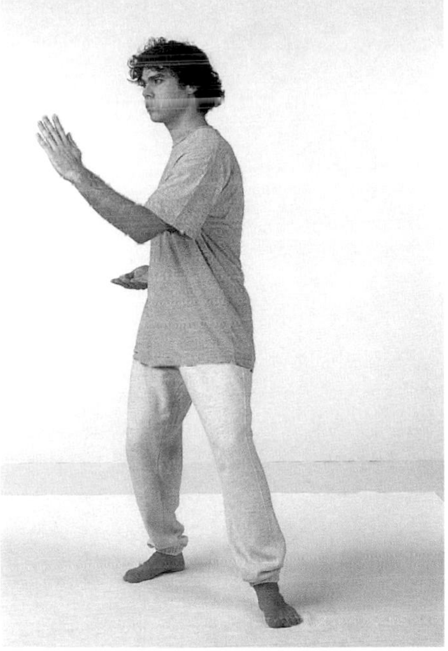

3 Shift your weight back on to your right foot, turning your waist 45° to the right. At the same time draw your right hand back to your right hip and push your left hand towards the corner until it is in line with the centre of your body, fingertips opposite your mouth. Repeat steps 1, 2 and 3 for about 1 minute.

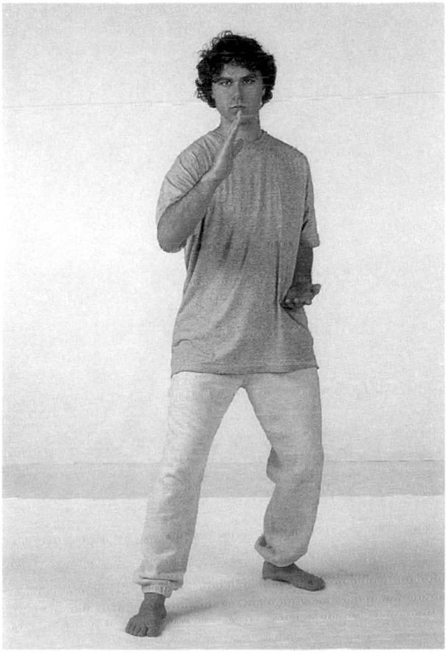

4 Repeat the sequence in mirror image as it is shown above. Make sure that all your movements are smooth and flowing and that the weight is gently shifted between your feet.

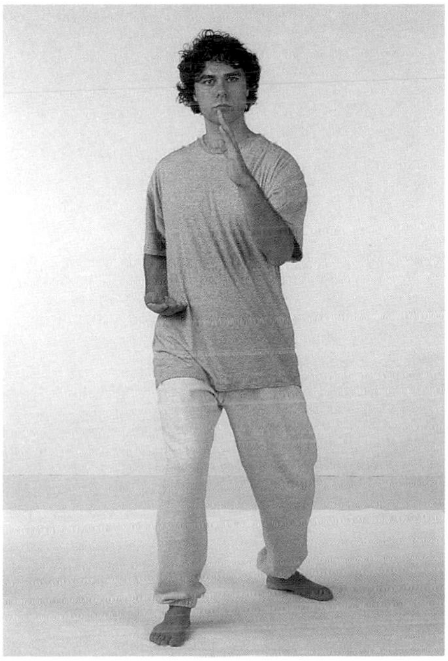

5 Bring your weight on to your right leg. Your left hand turns diagonally forwards as it comes towards the centre of the body, your right palm turns upwards as it draws back to rest on the right hip.

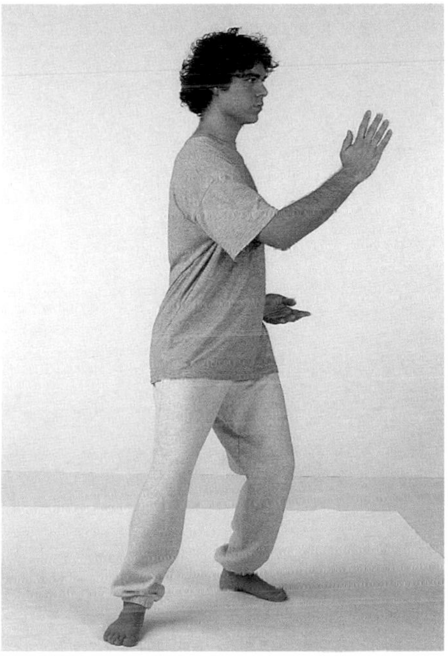

6 Shift your weight to your left foot, turning your waist 45° to the left. At the same time, draw your left hand to your left hip and push your right hand to the corner. Repeat the cycle in Steps 5 and 6.

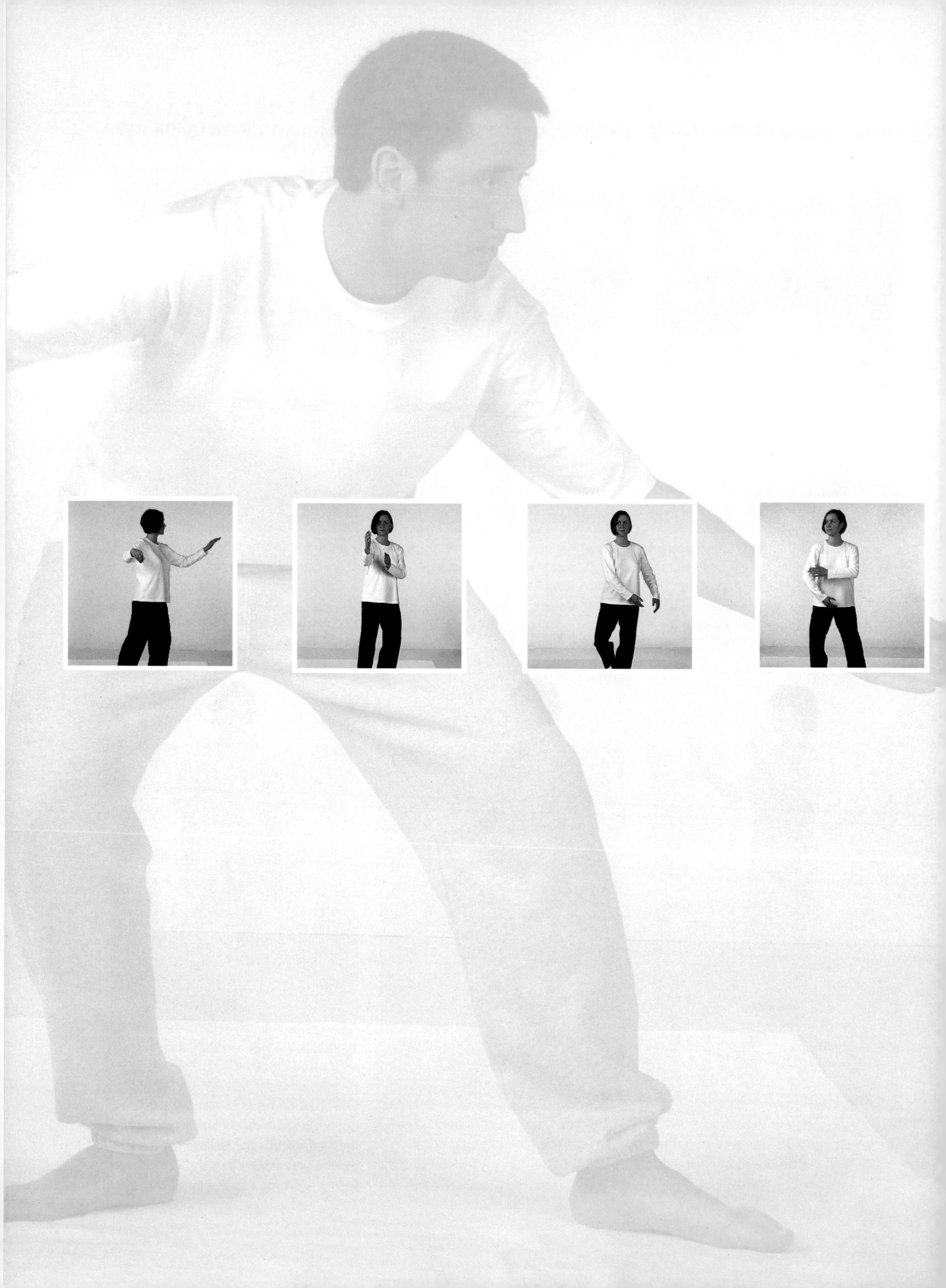

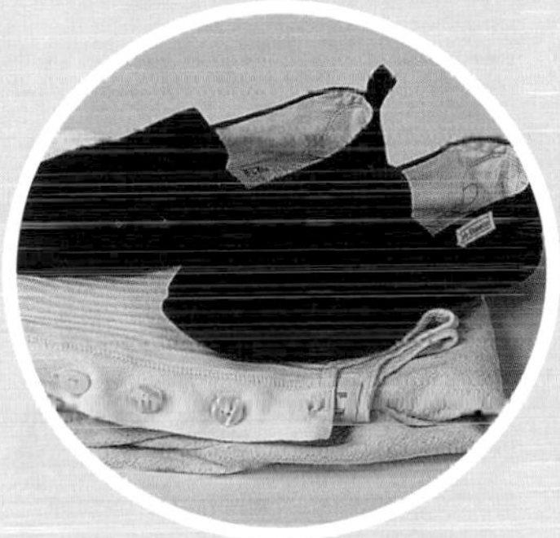

yang-style short form
yang-style short form

yang-style short form

After completing all the warm-up exercises, and having a moment or so quietly standing to see if you can find a point of equilibrium, a few minutes of t'ai chi walking may now follow. This is known as walking with an "empty step", rather in the manner of a cat tentatively putting out its paw before committing its full weight on to the front leg.

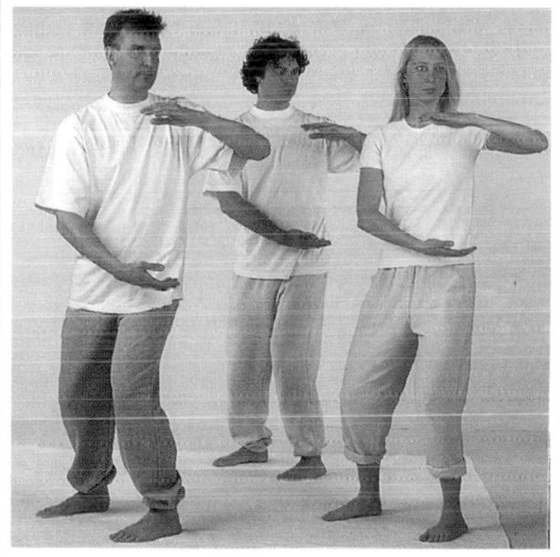

In fact, it is well worth studying an adult cat that is gracefully walking, or gliding forwards when it has spotted its prey. Its whole movement is one of ceaseless flow, of elegant, unforced movement when every part of its body seems to be an extension of another part, and nothing is hurried or rushed.

As you progress through the form, use the following pages as an aide-mémoire for your practice, especially for the transitions from one posture to the next. Remember to keep your movements slow and smooth, like clouds drifting gently by on a summer's day, and relax. If you worry about this new exercise, you will not succeed.

In many ways that is the key problem for the new Western practitioner. Doing these exercises initially means that you will be highly self-conscious because there is nothing like it in our culture. Yet gradually, after a few lessons, and above all after watching expert t'ai chi practitioners, it becomes clear that this is something which you can do successfully, and without having to worry about what you look like.

Once you launch into the first few movements, the rest follow, and you find that an awkward state of self-consciousness is quickly replaced by an inner calm as you become less aware of the outside world, and more aware of inner ones. The key to t'ai chi is being able to make seamless flowing moves, with the emphasis not so much on specific poses as on the linking means of getting there. Ultimately, you too may be able to go into a park in the early morning, as they do in the East, and carry out t'ai chi utterly unself-consciously, gaining spiritual refreshment.

FAIR LADY WEAVES SHUTTLES (RIGHT AND LEFT)

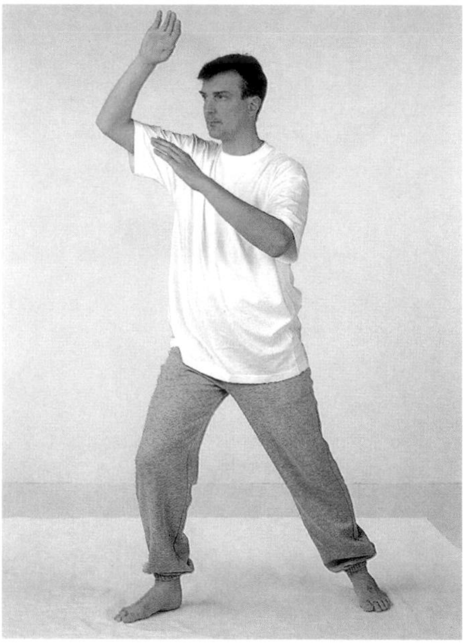

6 Turn a further 135° right, to the corner. Step to shoulder width with your right foot, and shift 70% of your weight into it, pushing towards the centre of your mouth with your left hand. Bring the right hand up to guard your forehead, palm facing diagonally.

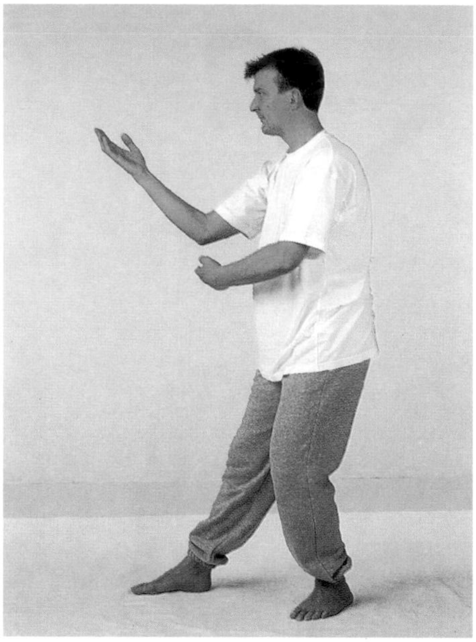

1 Turn to the left, sinking all your weight into your left leg. Pick up your right foot and draw it in. Transfer all your weight to your right foot, then step to the left (45°) with your left foot. Turn your palms in and draw your right arm across the left palm, left arm in a ward-off position.

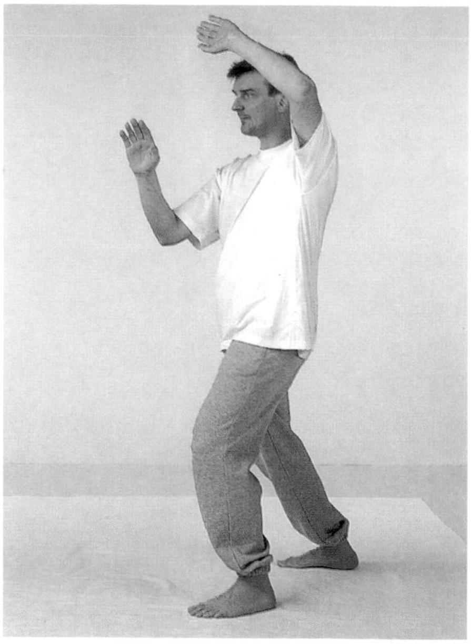

2 Your left hand then moves up and turns outwards by your head, while the fingers of your right hand come into the centre in line with your mouth. Now repeat the postures described in Steps 4, 5 and 6 of the previous exercise.

WARD OFF LEFT. WARD OFF RIGHT. ROLL BACK, PRESS AND PUSH. SINGLE WHIP

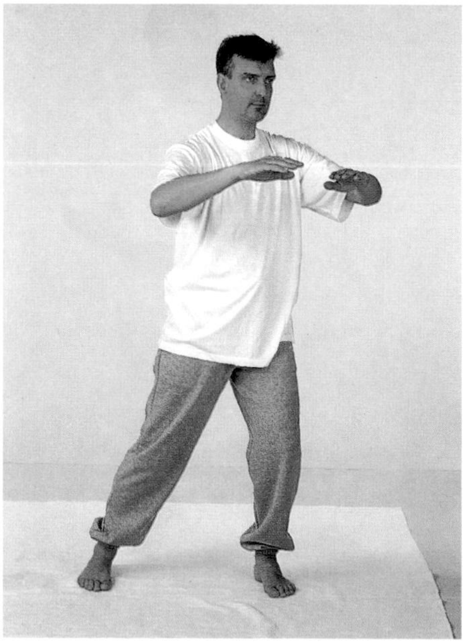

1 Sink your weight into your left leg as your waist turns to the left. Both arms come round with the movement of your waist, the left hand lower than the right. The right toes come round to the front.

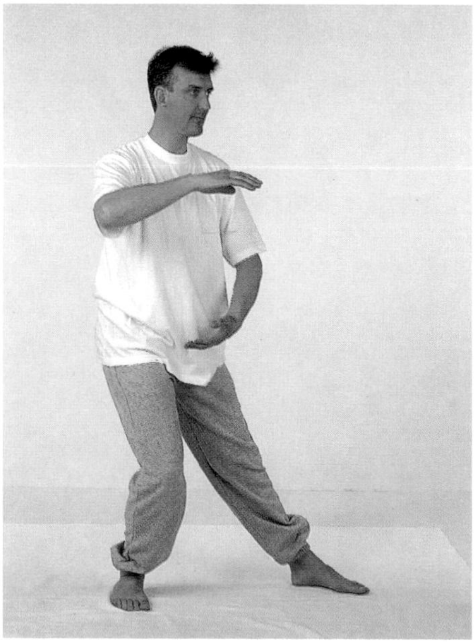

2 Sink your weight into your right leg as your left hand presses down, palm facing downwards. Take a shoulder-width step with your left foot.

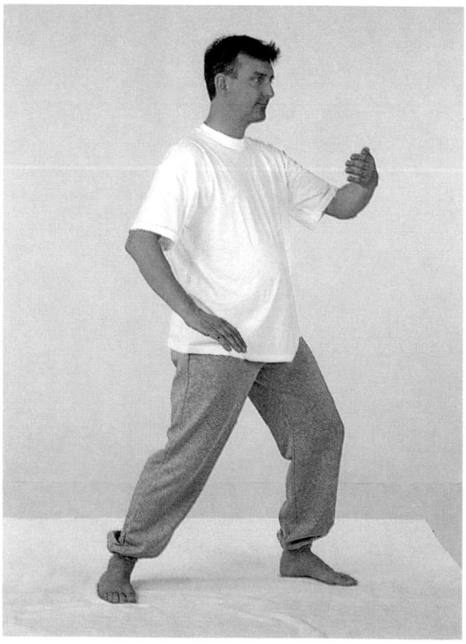

3 Transfer your weight 70% into your left foot. Your left hand comes up in front of your chest. Your right hand floats outside your right thigh. Repeat previous step.

SQUATTING SINGLE WHIP. STEP FORWARD FOR SEVEN STARS

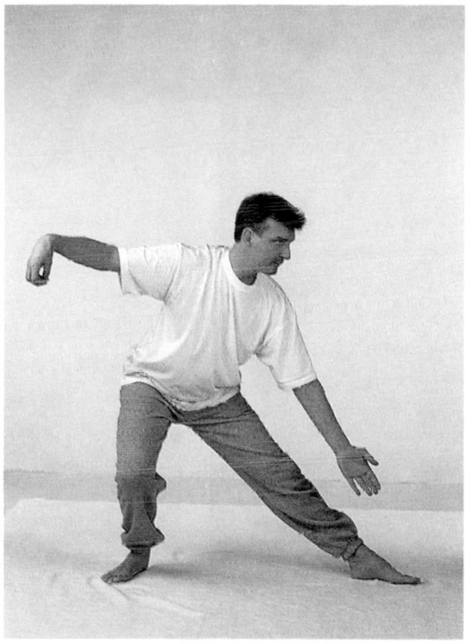

1 Repeat the postures described in Steps 1, 2 and 3 of "Golden Rooster Stands on One Leg (Left). Squatting Single Whip", ending by brushing open the left knee.

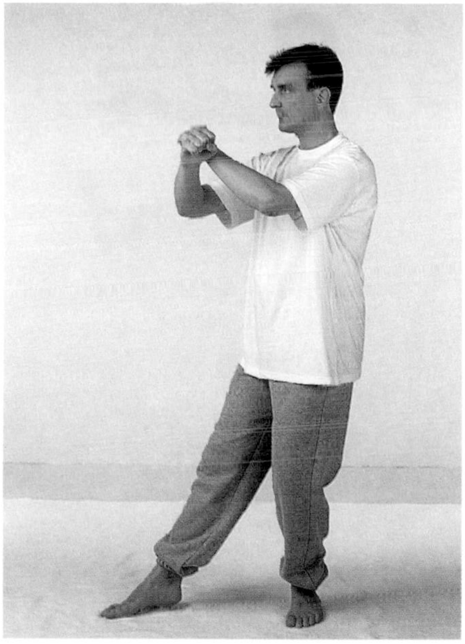

2 Transfer all your weight into your left leg. The right hand hook opens and the hand descends, then comes up in front of your neck, where it forms a loose fist. At the same time, your left hand rises up to form a loose fist, and connects at the wrist inside your right hand. Move your right toes forward to touch the ground without any weight whatsoever.

RIDE TIGER

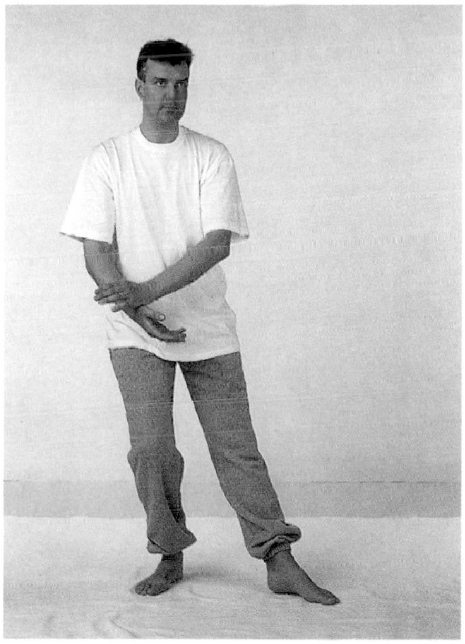

1 Keep your weight in your left leg and step back with your right foot, toes touching the ground first. Sink your weight into it and turn your waist to the right. The fists open and then move down by your right hip, with the wrists still connected.

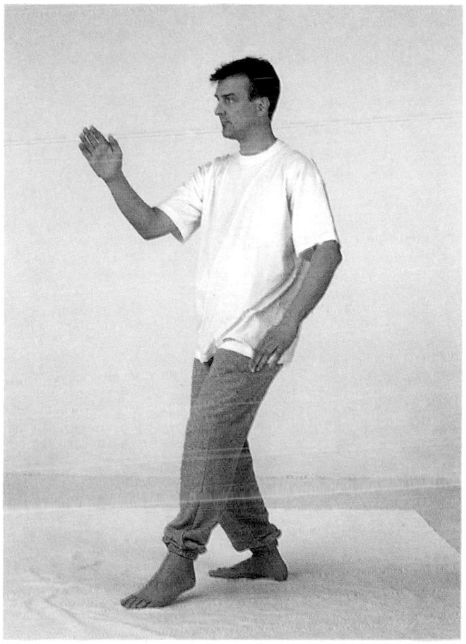

2 Pick up your left leg as your waist turns right, then place your toes down as your waist turns back to the left. Your right hand comes round to the front, fingertips level with your right ear, and your left hand rests by your left thigh.

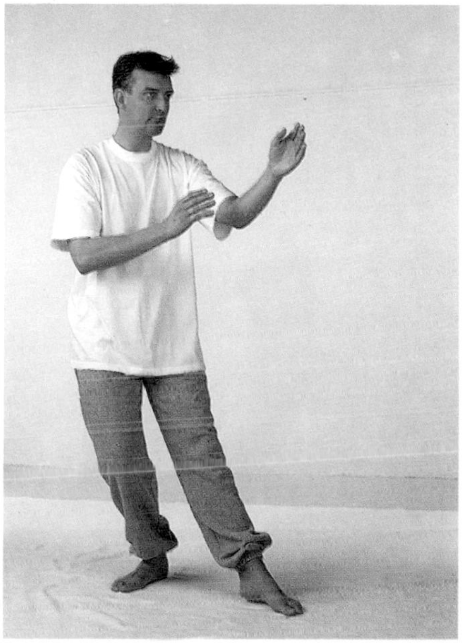

3 Pick up your left toes, turn your waist to the left corner and place the toes down empty of any weight. Your right palm faces your inner left elbow. Your left hand is at the height of your left shoulder, elbow relaxed.

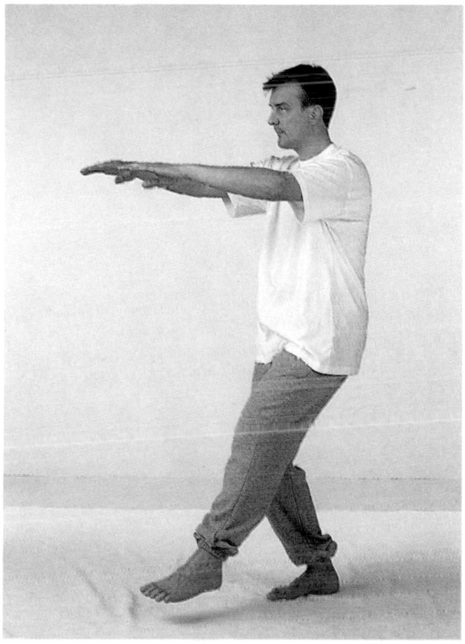

4 Lift your left toes and swing your waist clockwise, pivoting on the ball of your right foot. Your arms swing to the right with the movement of your waist.

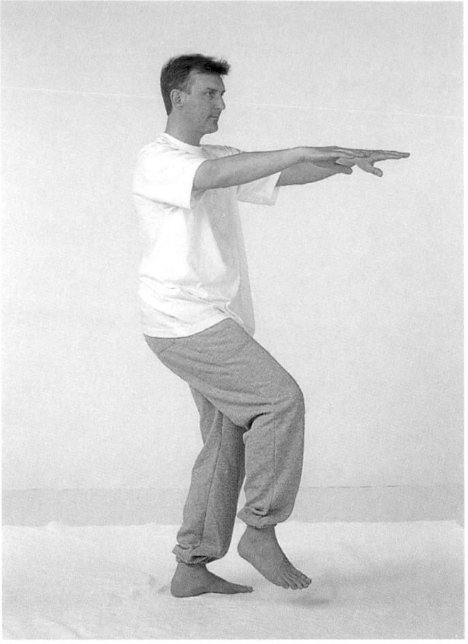

5 Drop your left foot and transfer all your weight into it straight away. Look closely at the photograph above to check how you should be standing.

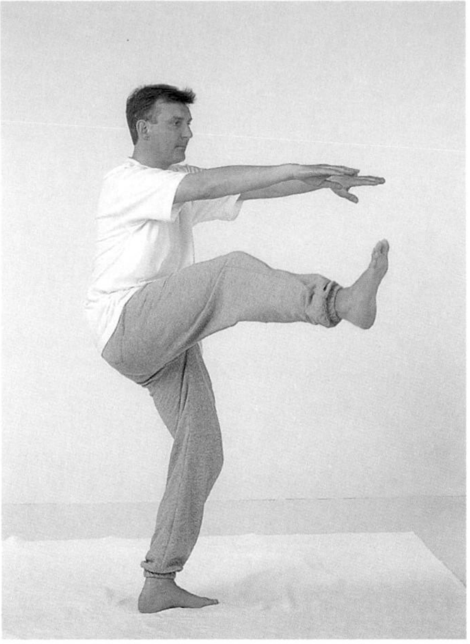

6 When your arms and waist reach the front (the arms at shoulder height and shoulder width with the palms facing downwards), your right foot lifts up and circles clockwise.

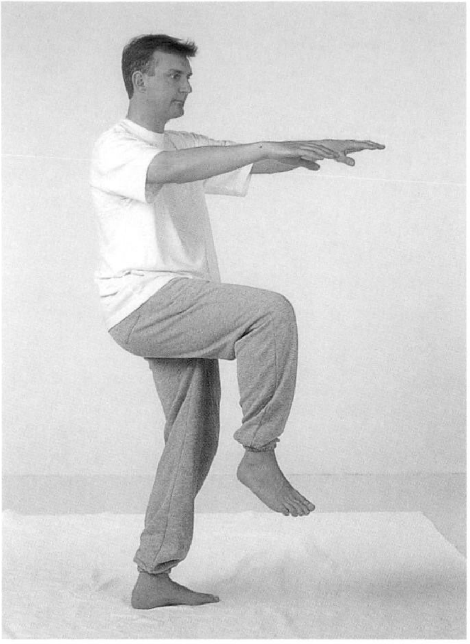

7 After circling, your right leg comes to rest with the upper leg parallel to the ground and the foot comfortably relaxed. Your left leg is bent while the arms are still pointing ahead.

BEND BOW TO SHOOT TIGER. STEP FORWARD, DEFLECT DOWN, INTERCEPT AND PUNCH

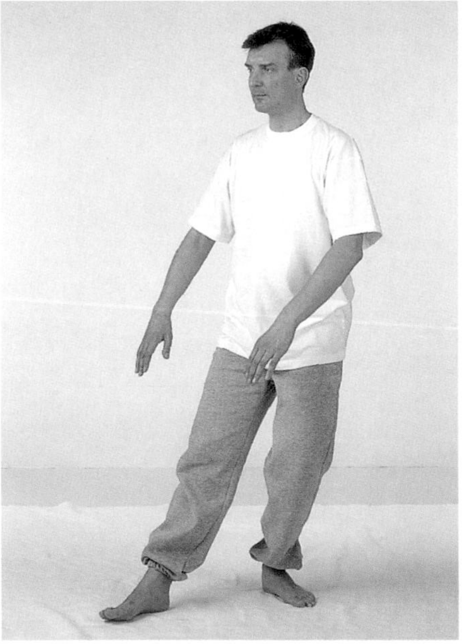

1 Turn your waist to the right. Your arms follow your waist, dropping down parallel, and your right foot is placed facing the right corner.

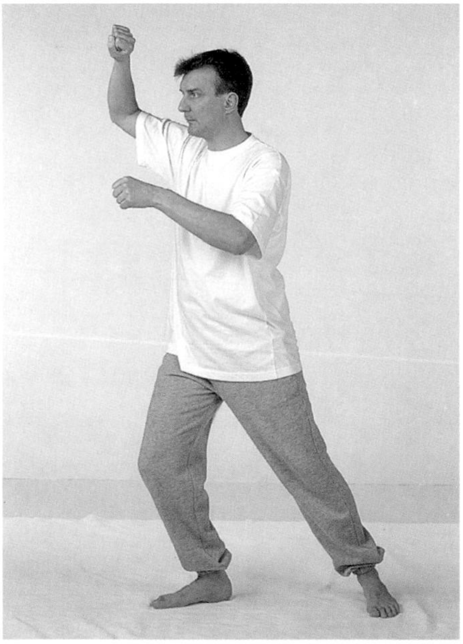

2 As your waist turns to the right, shift the weight into your right leg and circle your arms round to the right. As your waist turns back to the left, raise your arms and circle round with the waist. Form loose fists. Bring the right hand up to the right of your forehead, knuckles facing the right eyebrow. The left hand is at shoulder height.

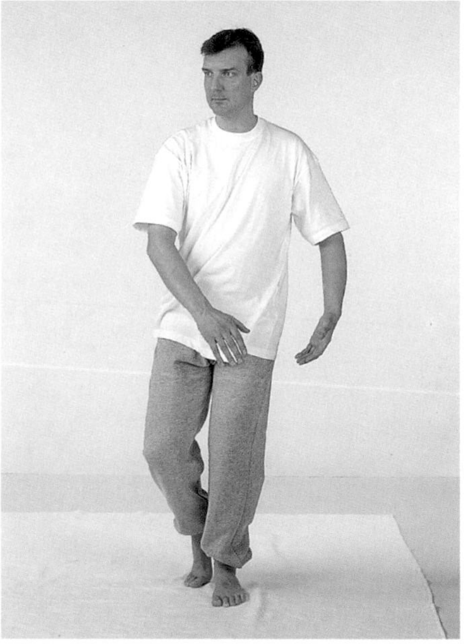

3 Sink your weight into your left leg and pick up your right foot, placing the toes by your left heel. Open the left fist as your arms move across your body following the waist movement.

WITHDRAW AND PUSH. CROSSING HANDS. CONCLUSION.

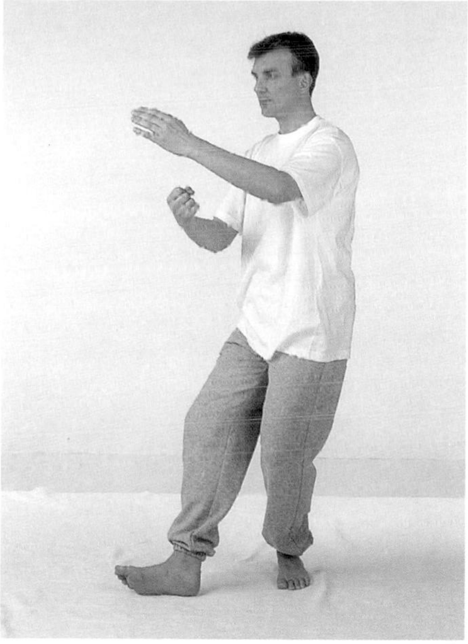

4 Both hands and your right foot simultaneously arc in towards the centre line, as your waist turns to the right. The right foot lands "empty", completely in line with the left instep.

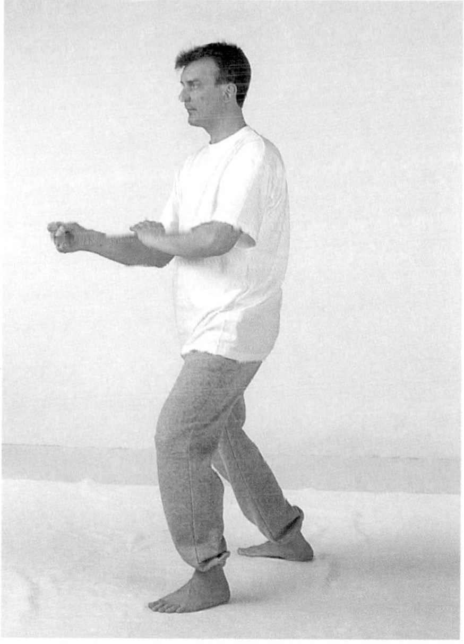

5 Continue to turn your waist, bringing the right fist palm upwards to rest on your right hip and shifting your weight to the right foot. Step through at shoulder width with your left foot. Shift 70% of your weight to the left and bring your right fist forward to punch in a corkscrew. Your left arm comes across your body.

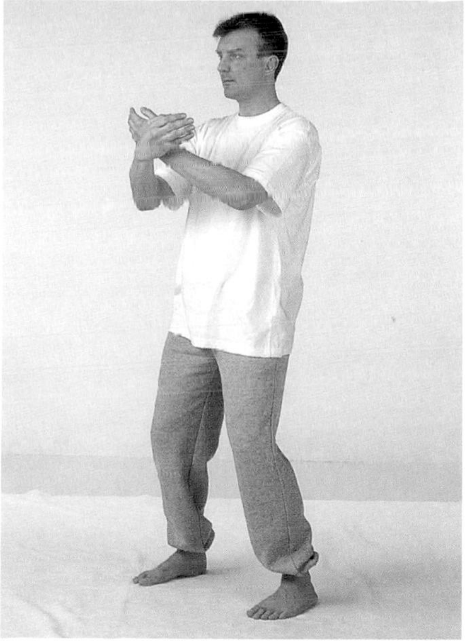

1 Repeat the postures described in "Withdraw and Push. Crossing Hands". Ensure your weight is 70% in your left leg when crossing hands.

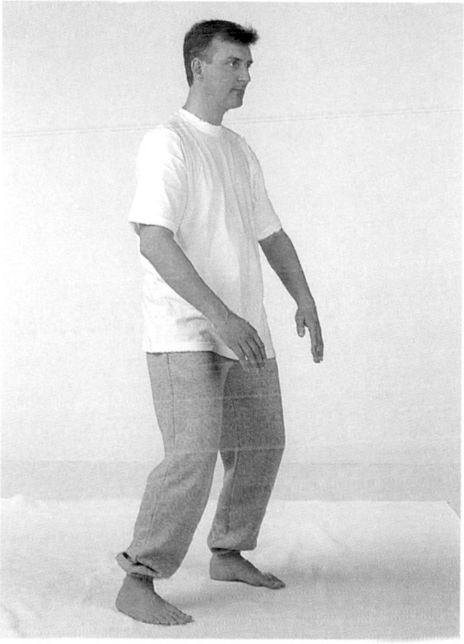

2 From crossing the hands, turn both palms down to face the ground as your body now rises up.

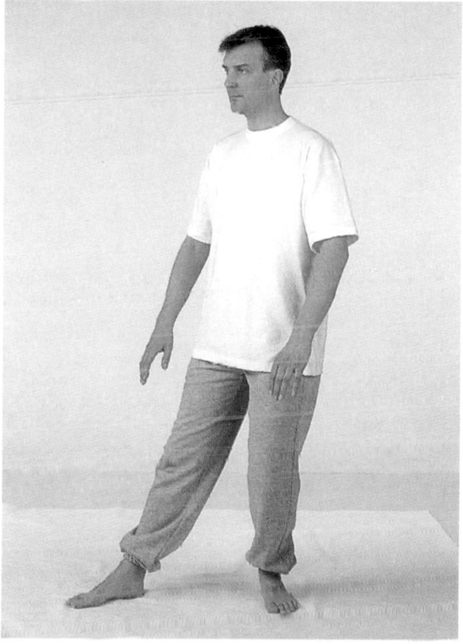

3 Bring all your weight into your left leg, turn your waist to the right and pivot on your left heel, turning the foot out to an angle of 45°.

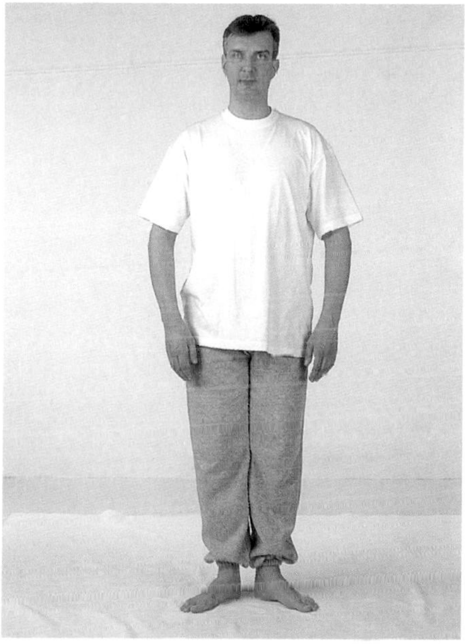

4 Move all your weight into your right leg. Step in with your left foot so that the feet make a right angle. Bring half your weight to the left foot. Rest your arms and hands by your side with shoulders relaxed. You may now begin again.

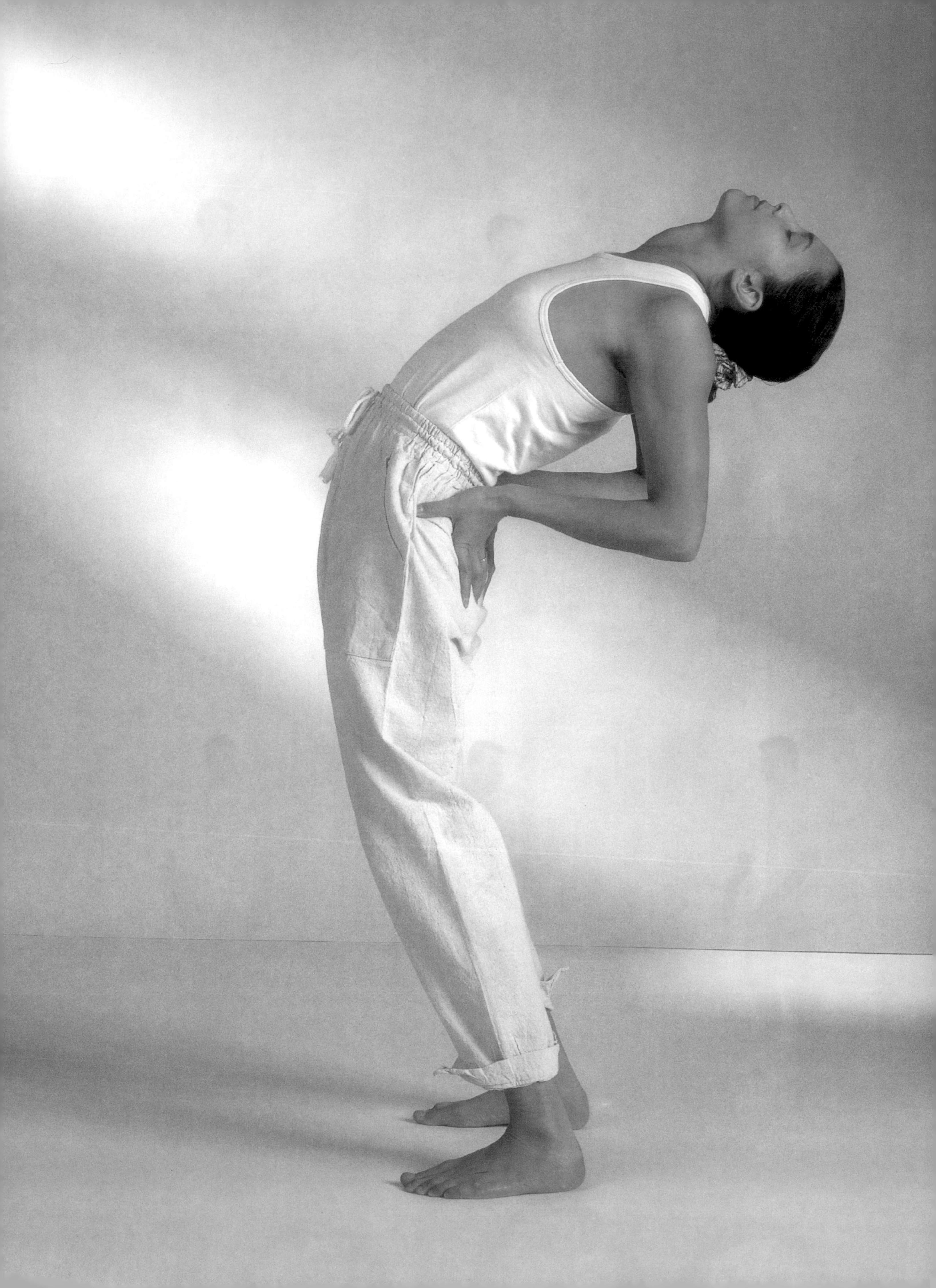

yoga stretches
yoga stretches

yoga stretches

Have you ever watched a cat waking up? More often than not, it will give an exaggerated yawn, then arch its back until stretched to its limit, before loosely letting go and gracefully moving off on its way. Have you ever stopped to wonder why it makes these movements? The cat knows instinctively the value of stretching in maintaining flexibility and improving circulation to the muscles; you too can become stronger and more flexible with regular stretching exercises.

Most of us tend to hold in patterns of tension arising from everyday cares and worries, bad posture, lack of exercise and so on. These patterns make us feel stiff and unbending, and directly interfere with our movements. Inflexibility within our bodies can in turn affect mental flexibility, and we can become stuck in thought as well as in action. Regular stretching exercises not only free our bodies, allowing us to move easily, but can also help us to think and act without being so restricted. They are excellent improvers. In fact, by stretching muscles, ligaments and tendons, we make them much more efficient and stronger. The lengthening actions also help us to stand and walk taller, and even with added grace. The joints are better supported and are more able to go through their full range of movements, while the muscles are better nourished from the increased blood supply. The stretches give you that extra edge.

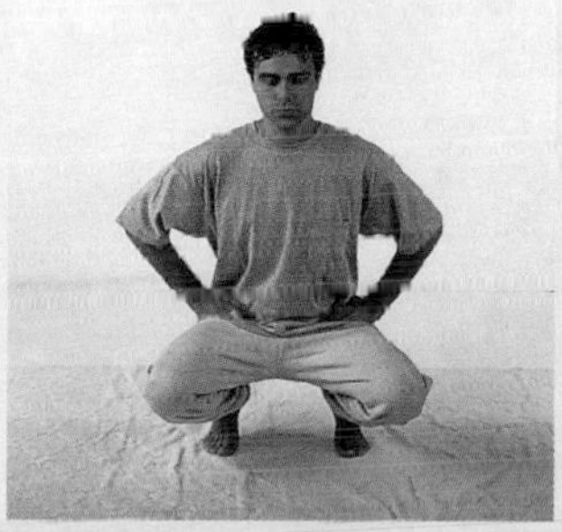

warm-up exercises

As any athlete will tell you, before starting to do any serious stretching or exercise, such as tennis, it is important that you first do some gentle warm-up exercises. They ensure that your muscles are nicely warmed and loosened, and will help to prevent any sudden strain or injury. The best thing is they only take a few minutes, and they can also be practised at any time if you are feeling stiff and need to loosen up.

SHRUGGING SHOULDERS

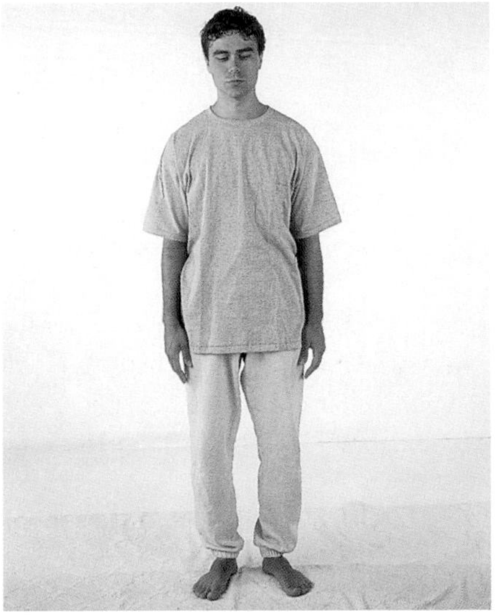

1 Stand upright with your feet slightly apart and your shoulders relaxed.

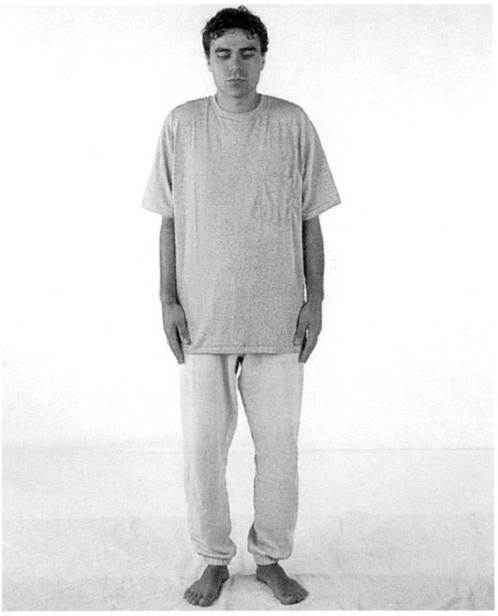

2 Lift your shoulders up as high as they will go, then let them fall down again. Stay relaxed and repeat a few times.

ARM CIRCLING

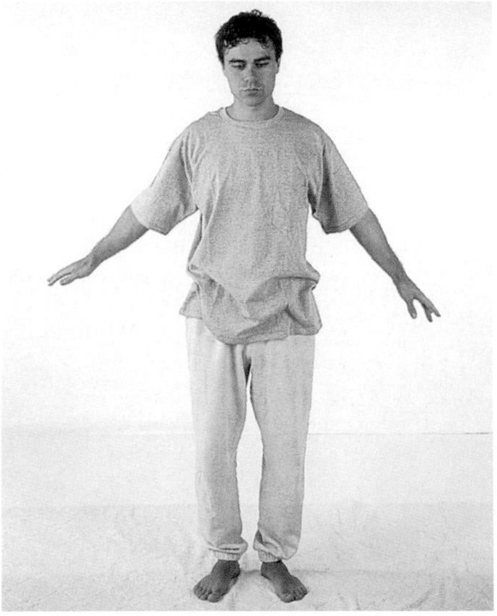

1 Wheel your arms around from the shoulders in slow, large circles.

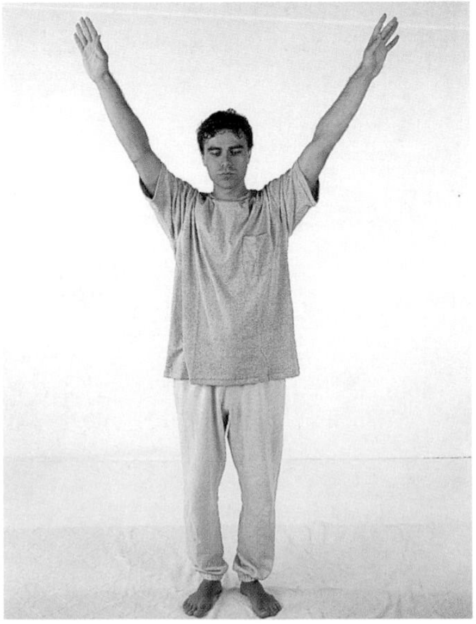

2 Do this a few times going backwards, then repeat circling your arms forwards.

SQUATS

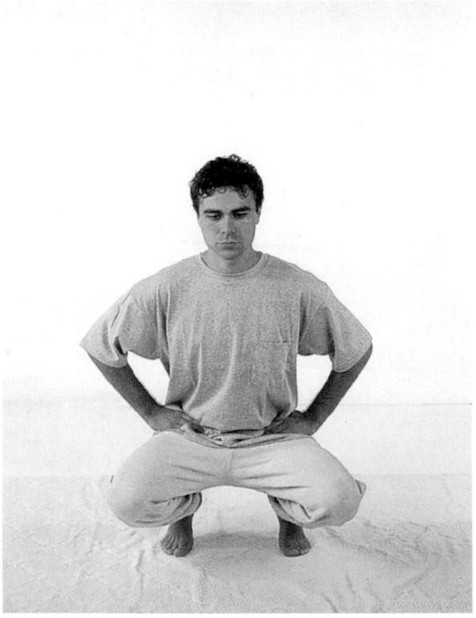

1 Stand with your feet slightly apart, hands on hips. Go slowly into a squat.

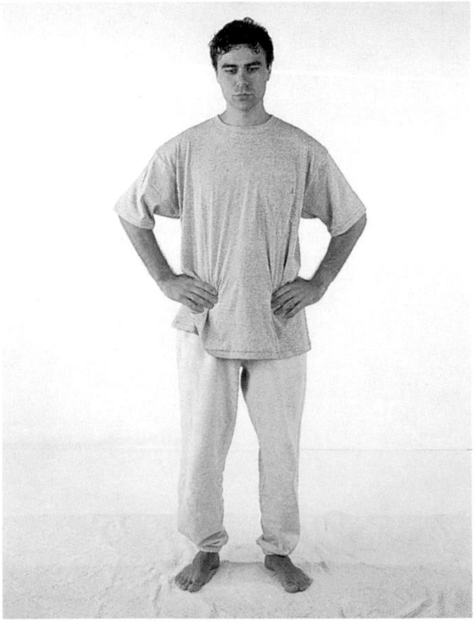

2 Slowly return to a standing position, then repeat. Your back should be upright.

LOOSE TWISTS

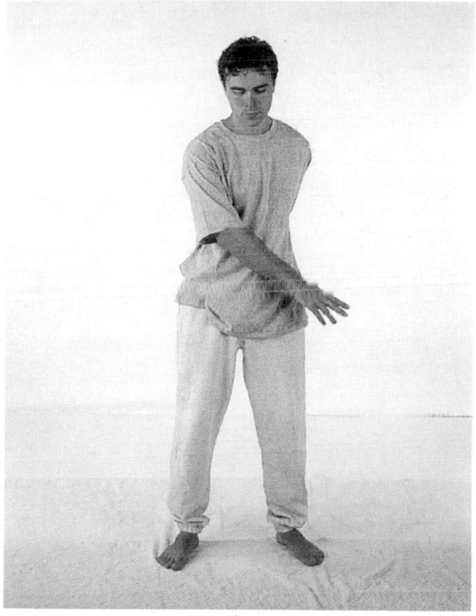

1 In a standing position with feet comfortably apart and knees relaxed, swing your arms loosely backwards and forwards around your body. Keep your head and body facing forward all the time, and keep your feet and pelvis still. Repeat a few times to loosen your arms and shoulders.

ARM STRETCHING

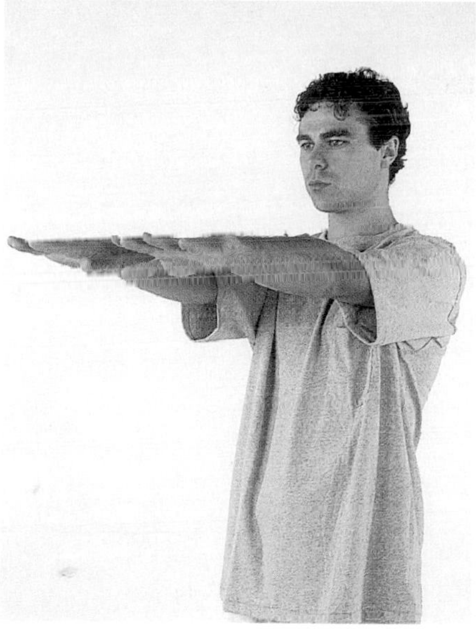

1 Stand with your arms straight out in front of you, at chest height. Take in a deep breath and exhale.

SIDEWAYS BEND

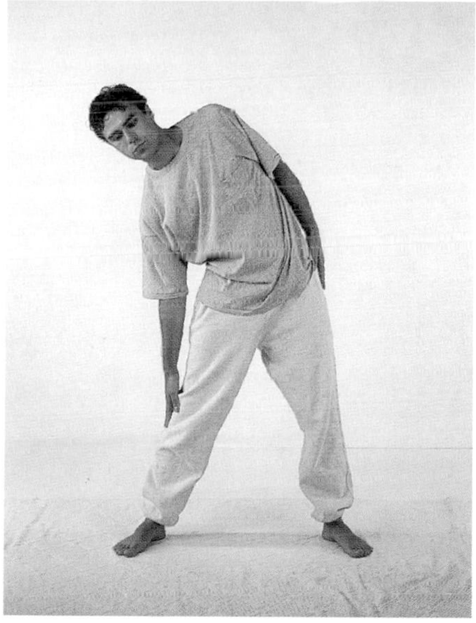

1 Stand with your feet at least shoulder-width apart and your arms hanging down at your sides. Bend down to one side, trying not to twist. Slowly return to the upright and then bend to the other side. Straighten up and now repeat.

SHAKE

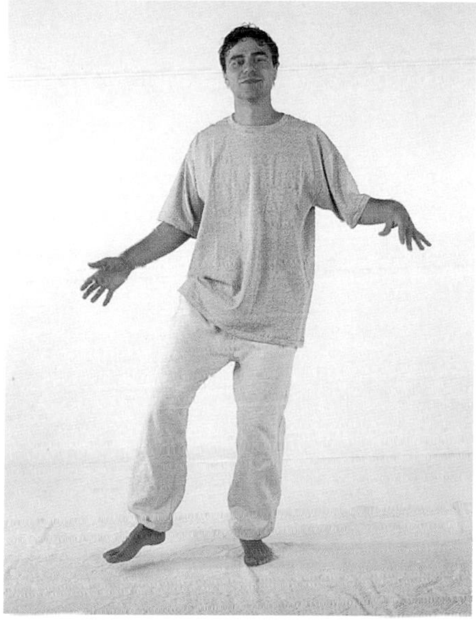

1 Try to relax and let your whole body go completely floppy. Shake your limbs to release any tension. Continue for as long as you feel comfortable. If you prefer, shake each limb in sequence, starting with your right arm.

CAT STRETCH

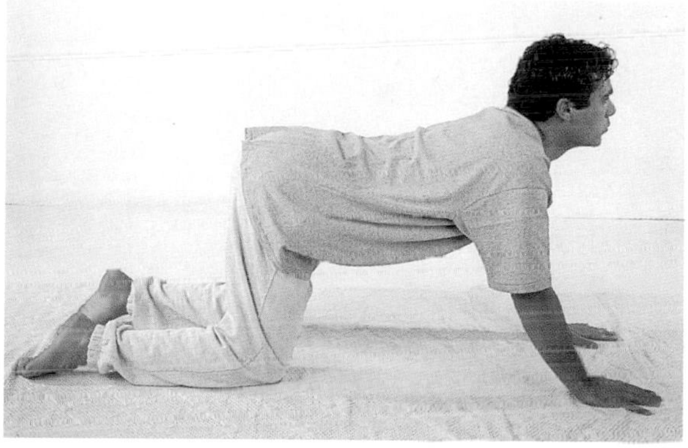

1 Kneel on all fours, with your hands and knees shoulder-width apart. As you start to inhale, bring your head forward and slightly hollow your back.

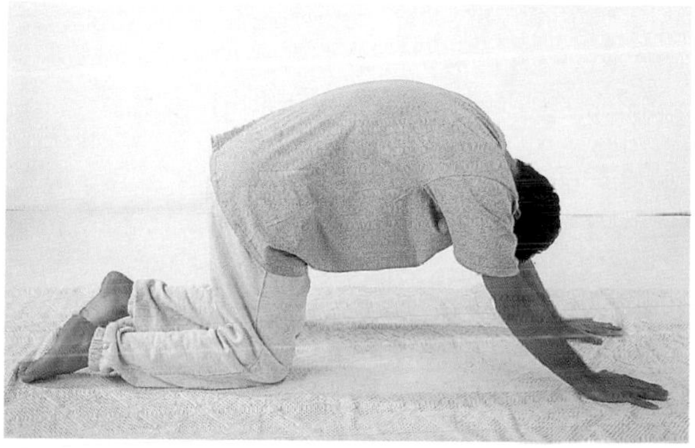

2 Now breathe out and, as you do so, arch the back upwards like a cat, allowing your head to drop down. Repeat a few times.

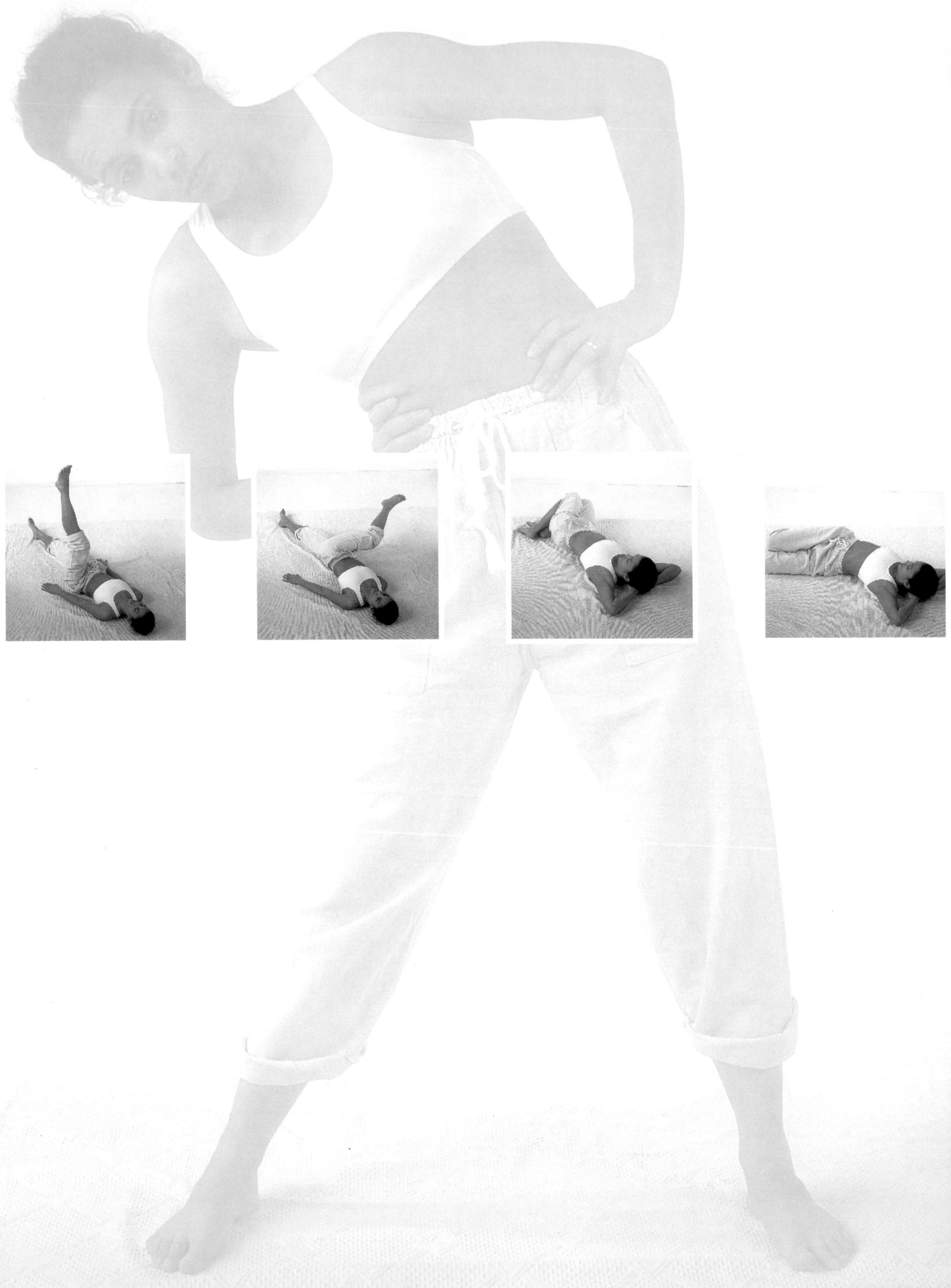

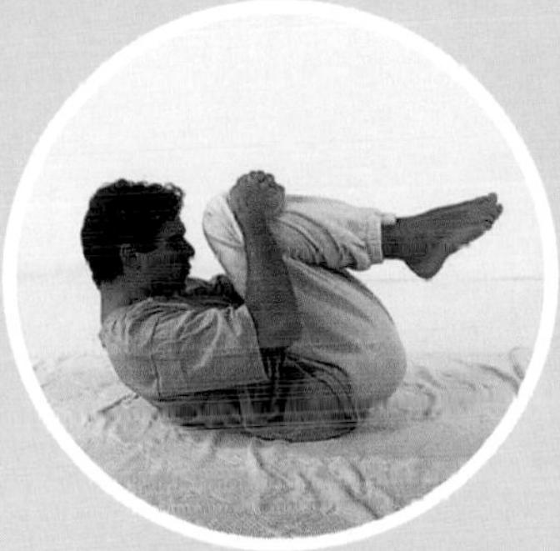

therapeutic movements
therapeutic movements

therapeutic movements

One of the best things about stretches is that you can do some simple, straightforward exercises anywhere, at any time: at home, in the office, standing in a queue or even sitting in the car; there are no restrictions. However, in order to get the most benefit from regular stretching, and particularly from doing yoga practice, it is important to create a quiet, comfortable space and to give yourself plenty of time to do the movements without any pressure or interruptions from the telephone or colleagues. In fact, making this space is in itself a relaxing, unwinding step, and will enhance the effectiveness of the actual exercises.

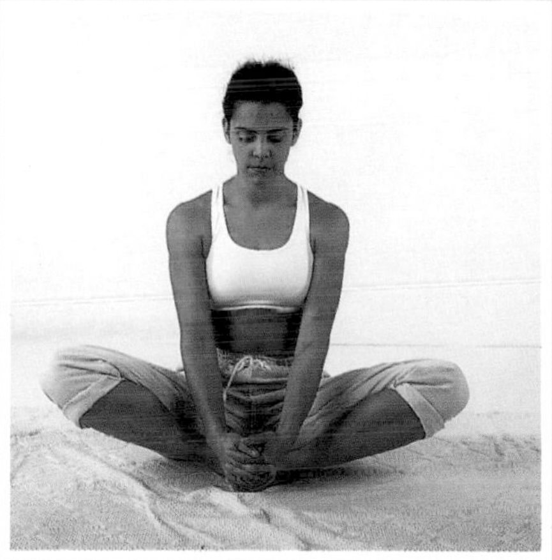

Ideally, make an area that feels quiet and calming to you, perhaps with softer lighting if it is needed, maybe with a thick, soft mat for the floor-based stretches. If you have any back discomfort, or just need extra support when lying down, then a couple of cushions may be extremely useful. It is helpful to wear loose fitting, airy clothing so that you can move freely and easily. If the weather permits try to let in some fresh air, but do not risk getting cold. These exercises are not intended to work up a good sweat or strain the heart, but to make you feel altogether less stiff and tense, and generally much more flexible. They are great for loosening you up, releasing tensions, improving circulation, toning the body, and generally making you feel much freer and more confident with your own body. They can really perk you up. After each exercise you will also need time to relax quietly, before you plunge back into everyday life.

If you find them an enormous benefit and become inspired, and want to try out more exercises, then do find a good, local class. Yoga exercises are generally best learnt in such a class, with a skilled, experienced teacher for maximum benefit. Alternatively you could create your own class at home, inviting a yoga teacher, friends and family on a regular basis.

tension and backache relievers

In the great majority of cases back trouble is the result of chronic tensions which can build up around the spine. Tired, tight muscles are also much more prone to strain or injury. The stretches that are shown here are intended to aid flexibility of the spine, and to make you feel much more supple, but if you already suffer from back pain or an injury then you must seek professional advice.

COBRA

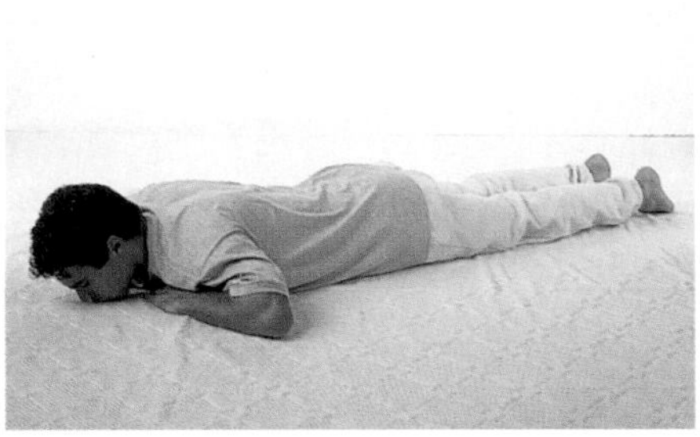

1 Lie on your front, with your arms bent and your hands under your shoulders.

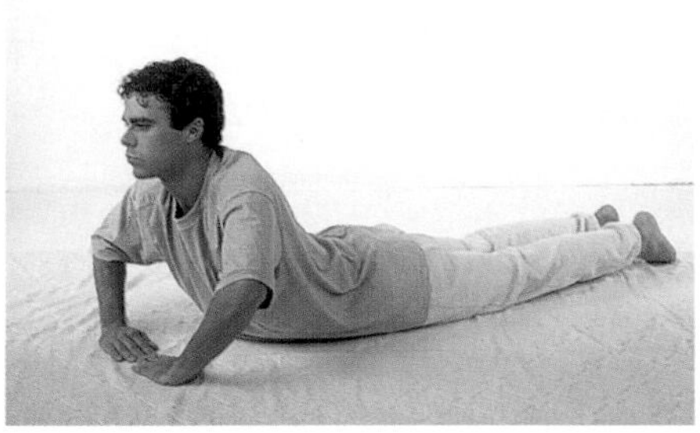

2 Slowly lift your head and push down on your arms to help raise your trunk.

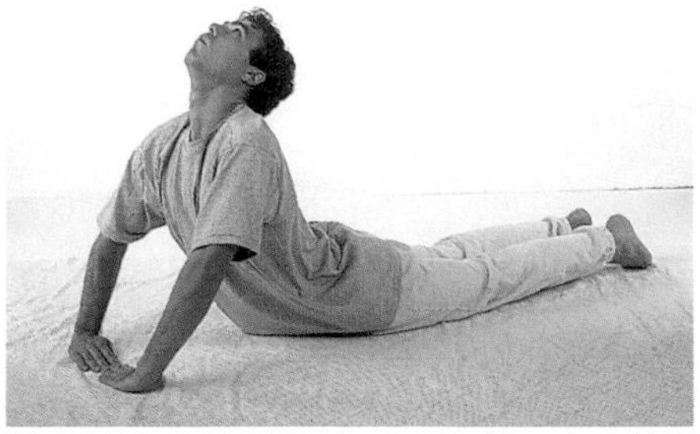

3 If you can, tilt your head backwards and stretch up and back, then relax.

SIMPLE TWIST

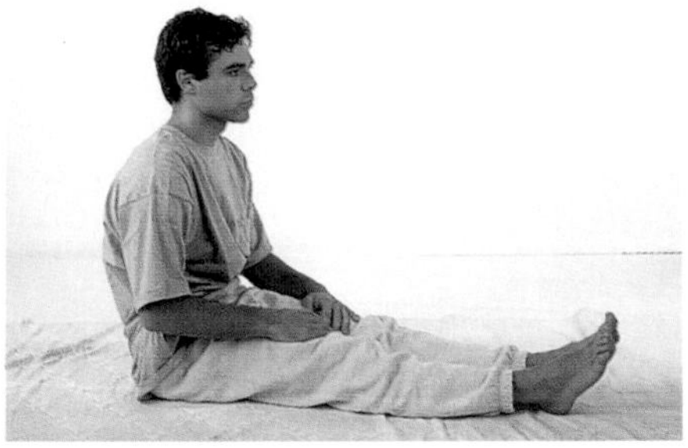

1 Sit on the floor with your legs stetched straight out in front of you.

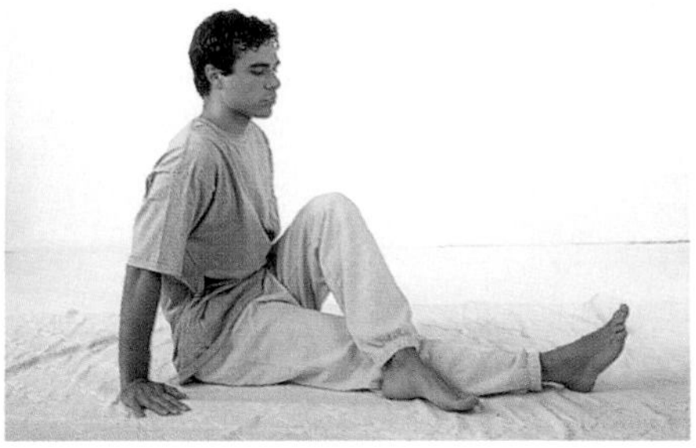

2 Bend one leg and place the foot on the floor across the other knee.

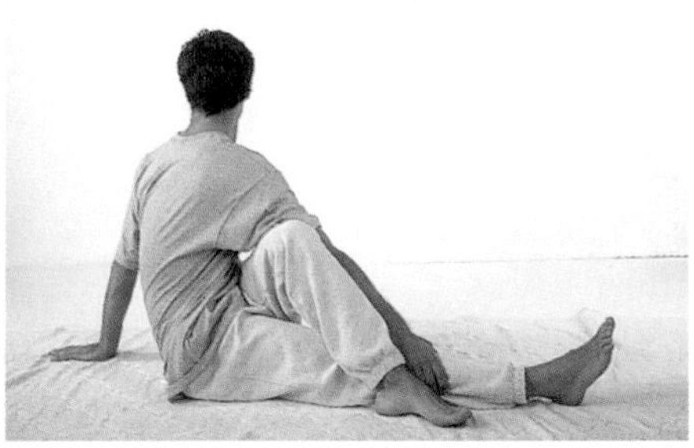

3 Place your opposite arm in front of your bent leg and twist to look over your shoulder.

FULL TWIST

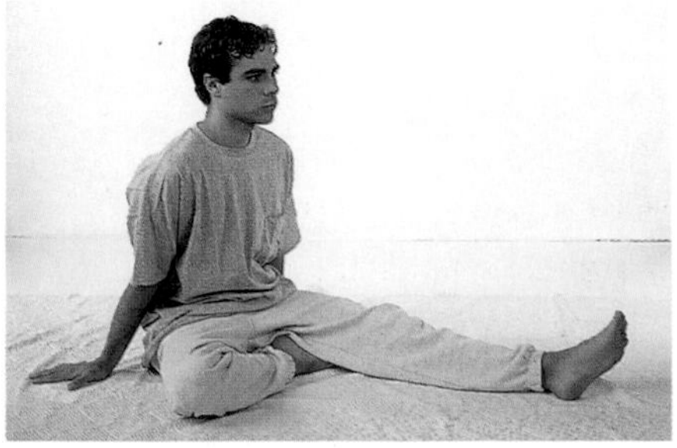

1 Bend one leg so that the foot rests on the inner thigh of the other leg.

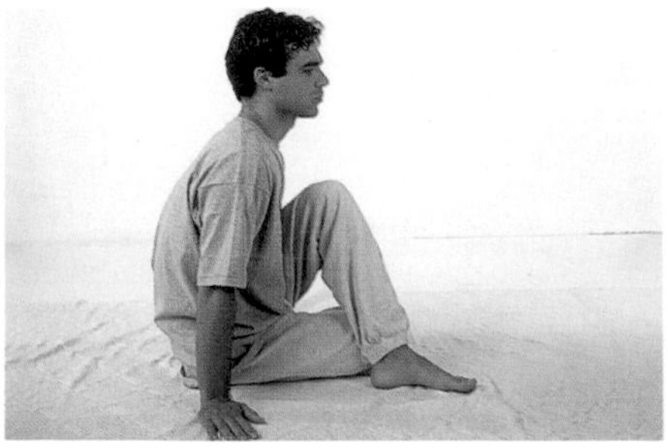

2 Bring this leg over the first one, then grasp your foot with the other arm.

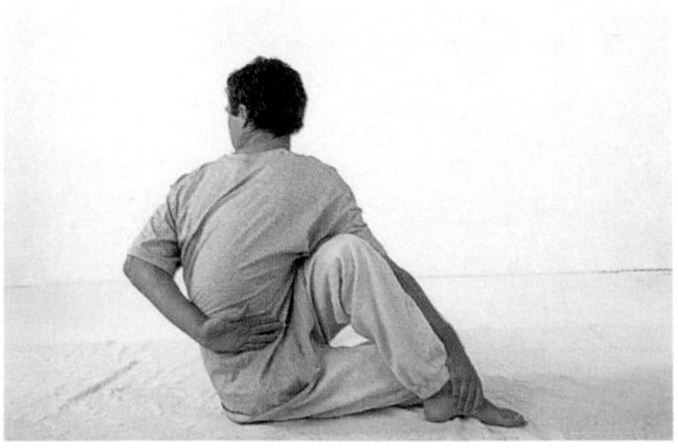

3 Twist as far around as you can, hold, then relax. Swap over your legs. Repeat.

TRIANGLE

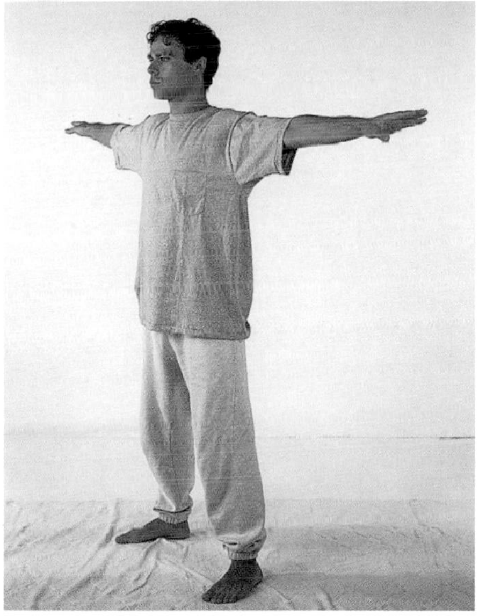

1 Stand with your feet shoulder-width apart and your arms straight out to the sides. This should be a well-balanced, easily held position. Your head should feel like a ball balancing on your neck. Stare straight ahead.

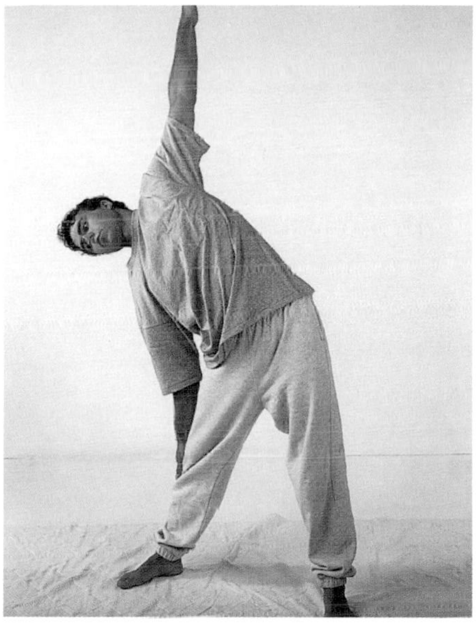

2 Bend down to one side without twisting your body, letting the opposite arm rise in the air. If you find this awkward or uncomfortable, do not strain yourself. The object is to loosen the body, not injure it.

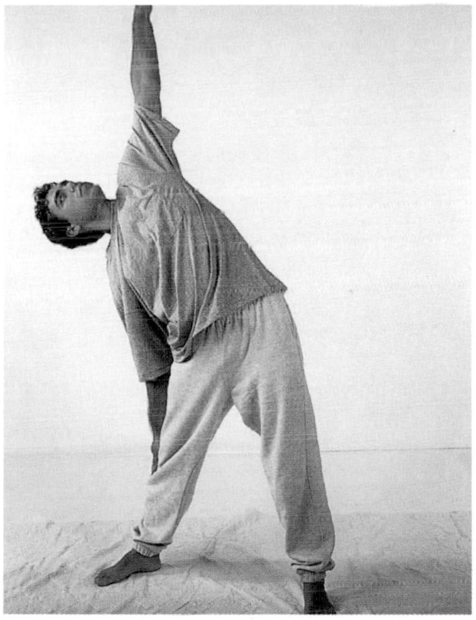

3 Stretch the raised arm, look up and hold. Slowly straighten and repeat on the other side. If you can, repeat several times, but be careful to move slowly into position to avoid a strain.

BENDING TWIST

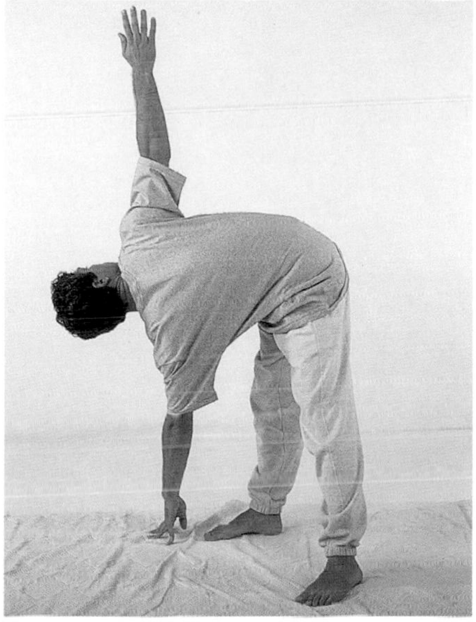

1 Stand with your feet shoulder-width apart and your arms straight out to the sides. Bending forward, try to touch your foot, or the floor in front of it if you can, with your opposite hand. Slowly uncurl and return to the starting position. Repeat on the other side.

SLOUCH STRESS

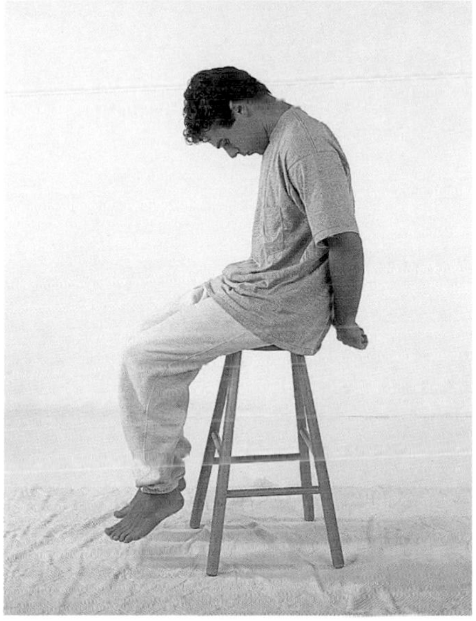

1 Sit on a tall stool so that your feet are just off the floor. With your hands behind your back, slouch so that your back is rounded, with your head now lowered down towards your chest.

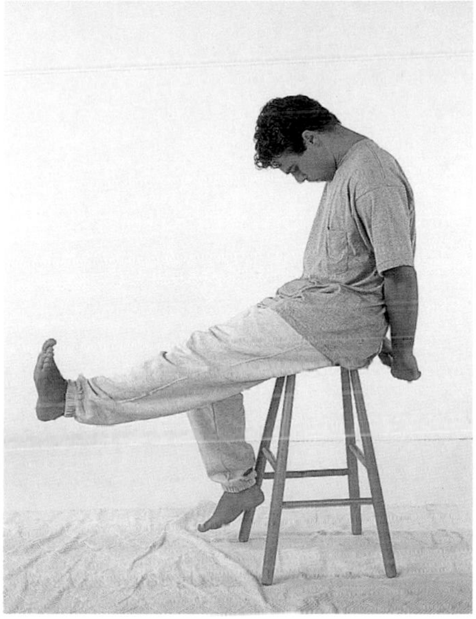

2 Flex one foot, and lift the leg to straighten it if possible. Release the leg, relax, then repeat a few times. Repeat with the other leg. Note that the object is to build up a slow pace, not to go fast.

soothing and removing tension

Many of us suffer at some time from tension headaches and know that they begin with a gradual feeling of pressure in the head or neck, or a taut sensation in the facial muscles. Once you are aware of such tension, tackle it immediately. A few simple stretches can help to relieve these muscular spasms and prevent them leading to a severe headache. They can be done almost anywhere.

SIDEWAYS NECK STRETCH

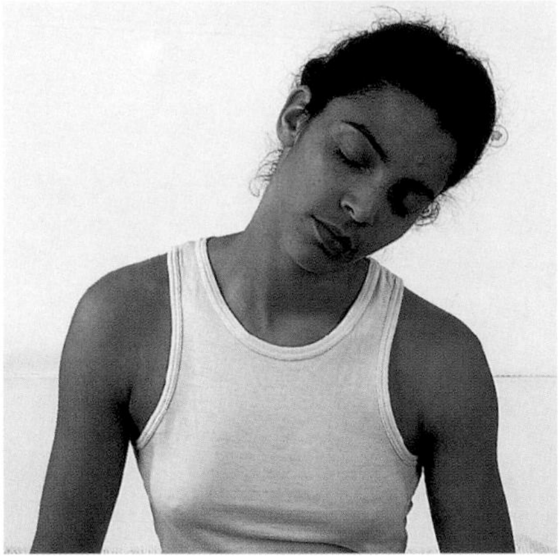

1 Slowly stretch your head down to one side, feeling the pull in the neck muscles. Return the head to the upright position and repeat on the other side.

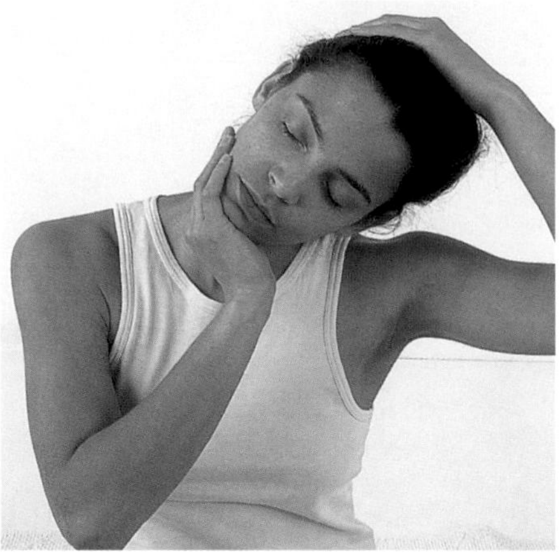

2 To make this stretch of the neck muscles more effective, use your hands to give extra leverage. Place one hand under your chin and the other on top of your head; repeat the other side.

HEAD TO CHEST

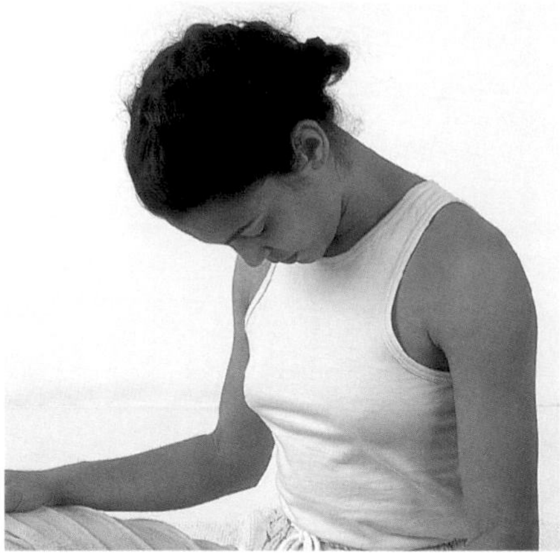

1 Lower your head towards your chest, feeling the pull on the back of the neck. Hold at your furthest stretch before slowly raising the head again. Repeat two or three times.

LION POSTURE

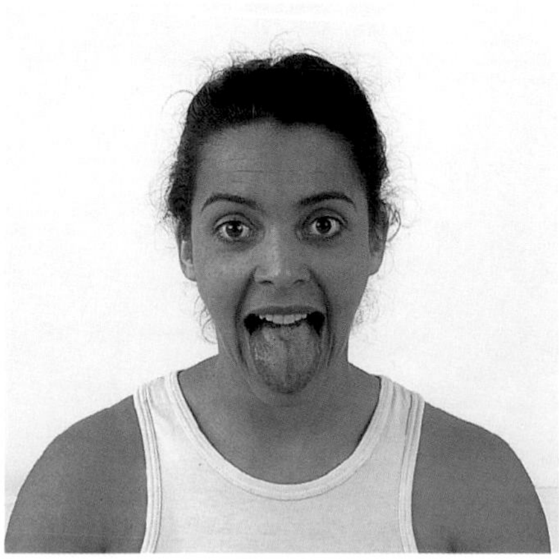

1 To stretch the facial muscles and release tension, open your mouth as wide as possible and push out your tongue. At the same time, open your eyes into as wide a stare as you can manage. Repeat a couple of times.

SEMICIRCLE ROTATION

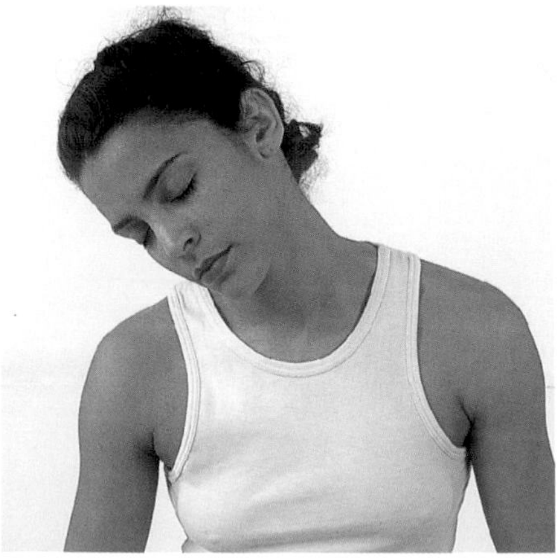

1 Turn the head to one side, then steadily rotate it in a semicircular movement, letting the chin drop down across the chest.

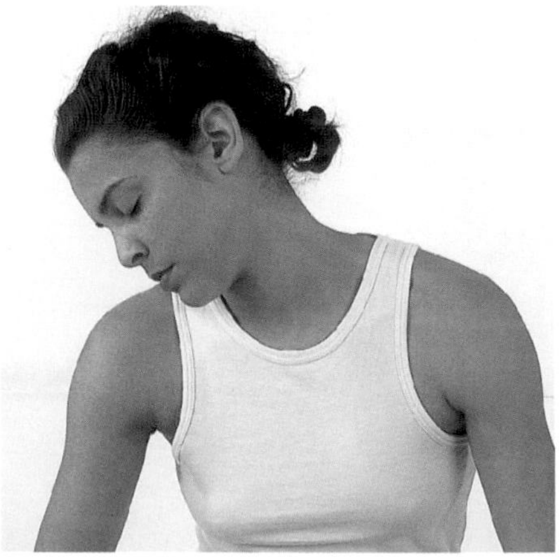

2 Dropping the head backwards compresses the neck, so it is best not to make this a full circle rotation. Repeat, going back in the opposite direction.

posture enhancers

One of the great benefits of an exercise system such as yoga is the fact that it gradually and increasingly gives you considerable grace and poise. In addition it will make a huge difference to your overall posture. If it was previously a bit lax, and you ended up slouching, you will really notice the difference. In fact, learning to hold yourself properly can help you to look and feel much younger, and reduce muscle strain.

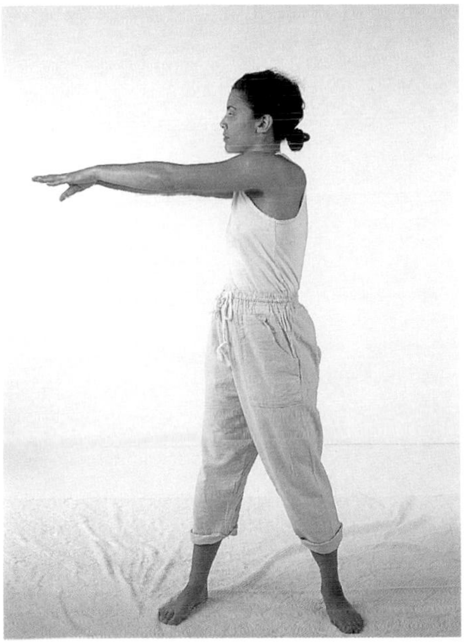

1 Stand with feet slightly apart and arms raised in front. Slowly twist to one side. Repeat on the other side.

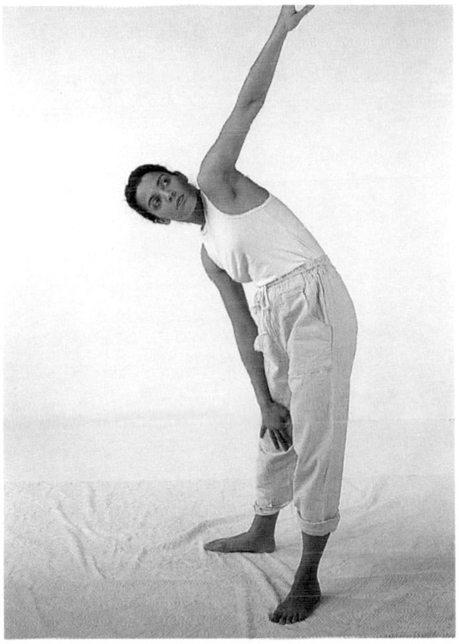

2 Stand with your feet apart, and hold your arms out. Bend over, sliding one hand down the inside of the same leg.

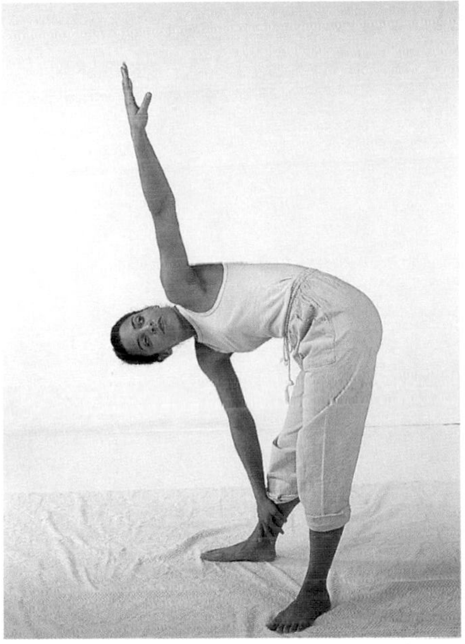

3 Reach as far as is comfortable, then slowly return to the upright and repeat on the other side.

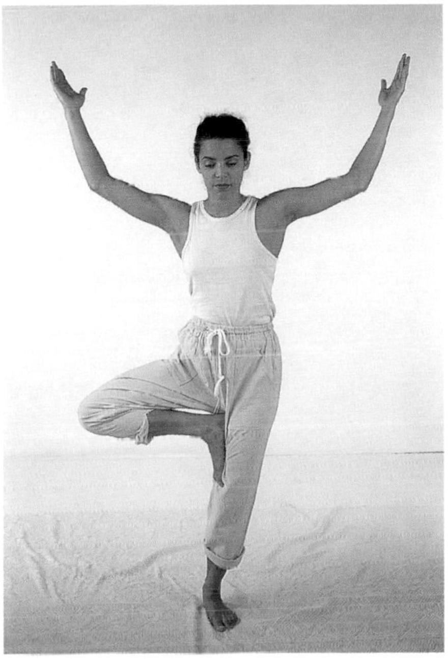

4 For the tree routine, stand on one leg and bend the other knee, as shown.

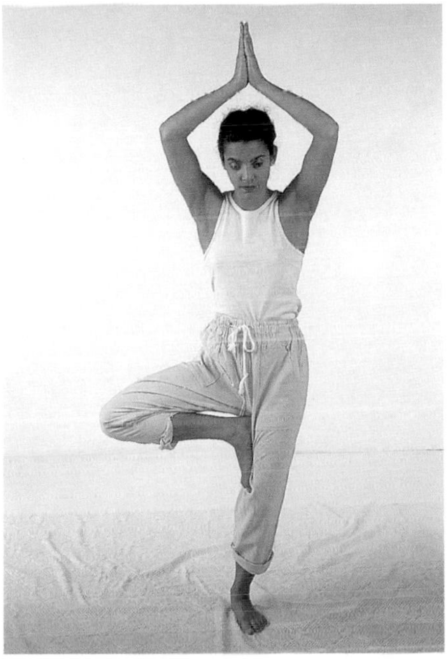

5 Either place your palms together above your head, or raise the hands.

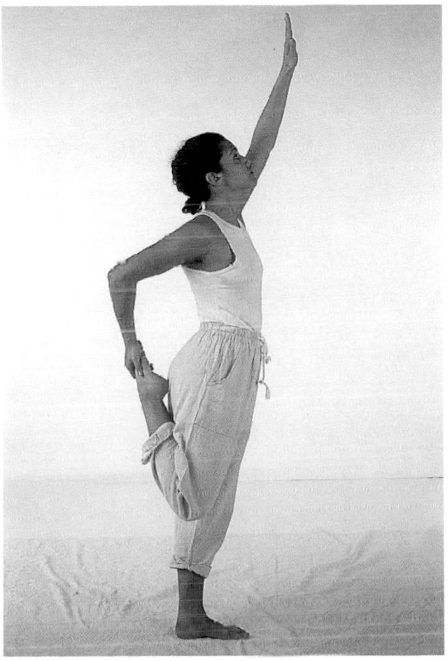

6 For the arm and leg stance, stand on one leg and hold the other foot behind.

tired and aching leg revivers

Most of us spend too long each day with our legs stuck in fixed positions, and stiffness of the lower limbs from inactivity or tension can make you feel quite tired. Legs benefit from being stretched, keeping them toned and supple. These exercises prevent the legs, thighs and lower back from getting too tense. Since some of these positions are quite difficult, do beware of straining yourself.

ALTERNATE LEG PULLS

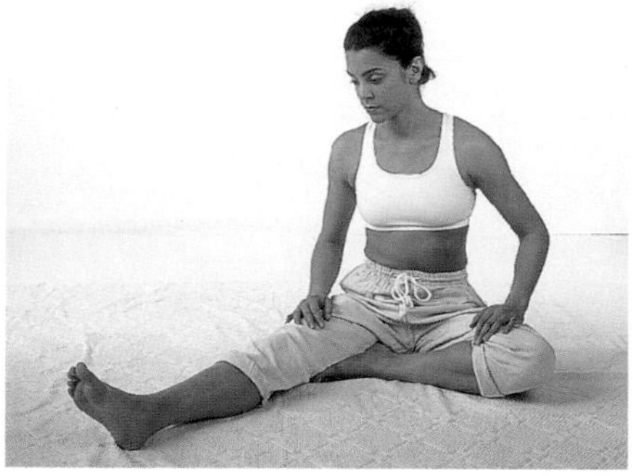

1 Sit on the floor, with one leg out straight and the other bent so that the foot rests on the inner thigh of your extended leg. Do it with care.

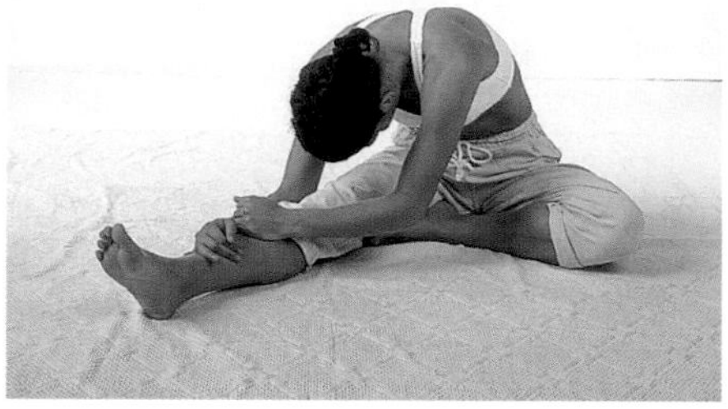

2 Lean forward and clasp the straight leg as far down as is comfortable; pull your chest down a little further and hold for a moment. Change legs and repeat.

FULL LEG PULLS

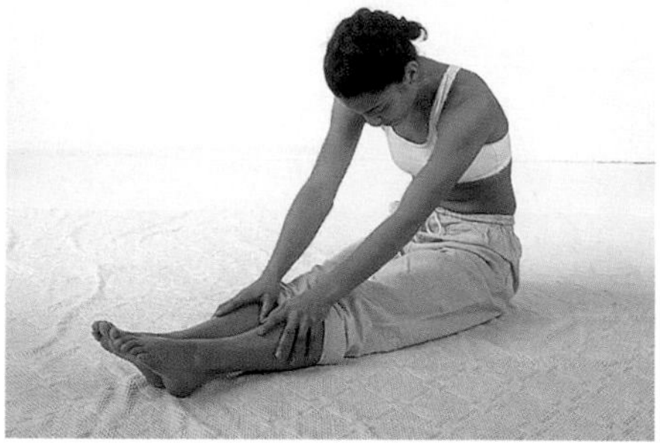

1 The previous stretch can be extended by starting with both legs straight out in front of you. Repeat as described.

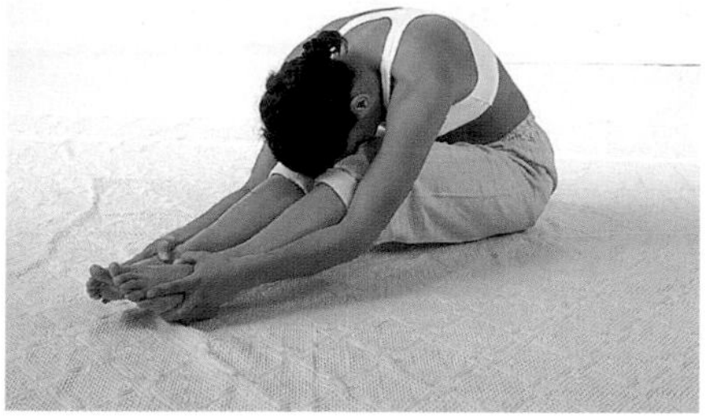

2 Lean forward and hold the legs with both hands; pull yourself down a little further and hold for a moment. If this is difficult, bend the legs slightly.

SIDE LEG RAISE

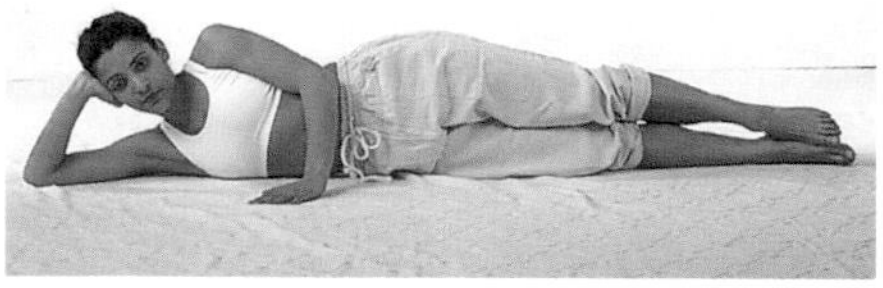

1 Lie on your side with your legs and body in a straight line. Support your head with one hand and place your free hand on the floor for balance.

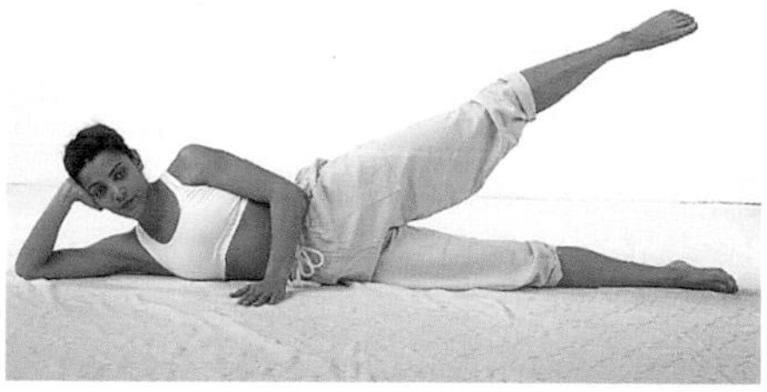

2 Without twisting your hips, steadily raise the upper leg as far as is comfortable. Hold, then lower slowly. Repeat with the other leg.

CAT STRETCH

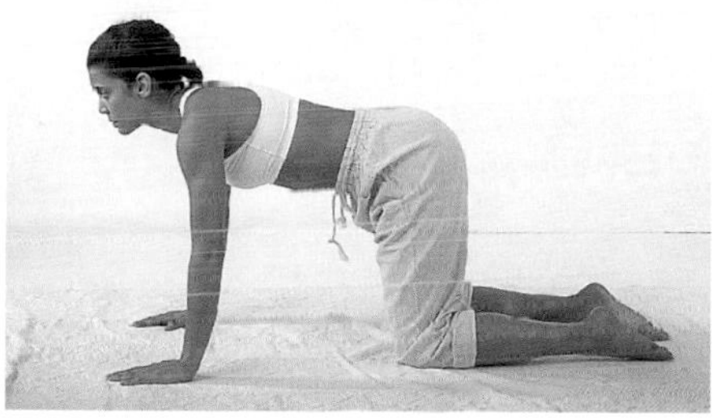

1 Kneel on all fours with your hands and knees shoulder-width apart. Raise your head and look straight ahead.

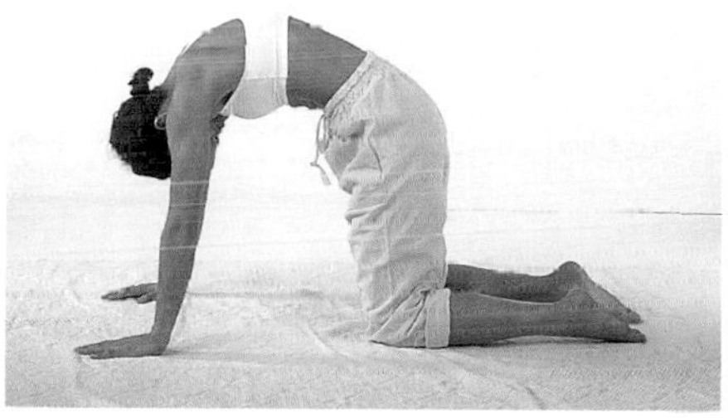

2 Breathe in, and as you exhale lift and arch your back. Hold for a moment before relaxing back into the original position. Inhale, then repeat.

BACK PUSH-UP

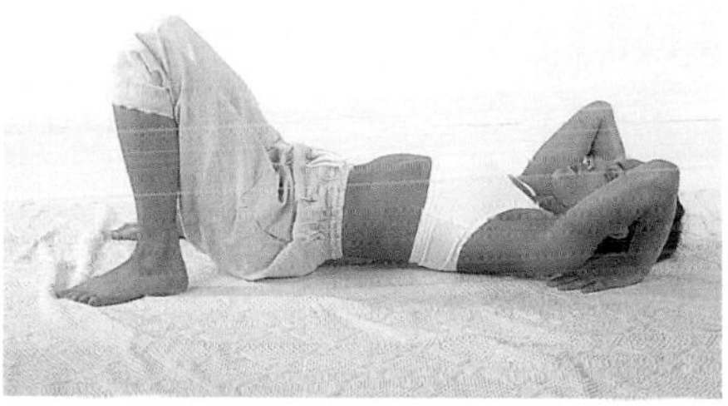

1 Lie on your back with your knees bent and your feet on the floor, hip-width apart. Now place your hands on the floor by your shoulders.

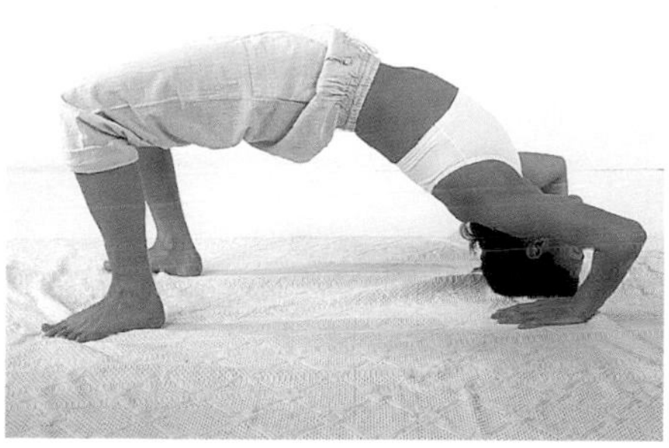

2 Push up with your hands and feet, arching your back at the same time. Hold for a moment, then lower your body back to the floor. Do not strain yourself with this movement – it works on lots of muscles at the same time.

SIT UP/LIE DOWN

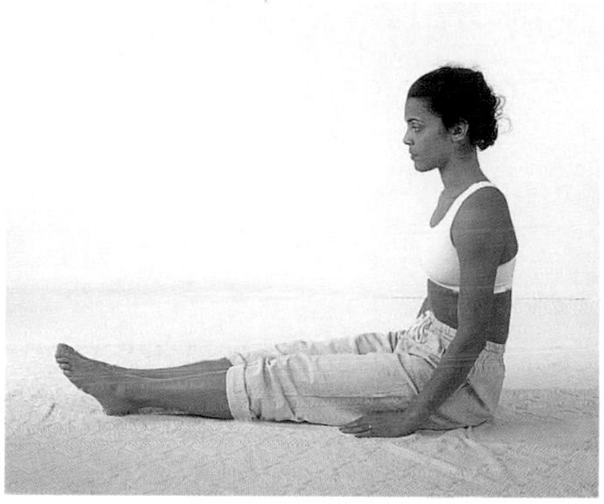

1 Sit on the floor with both legs straight out in front of you. Your torso should be at right angles to your legs, with your eyes looking forward.

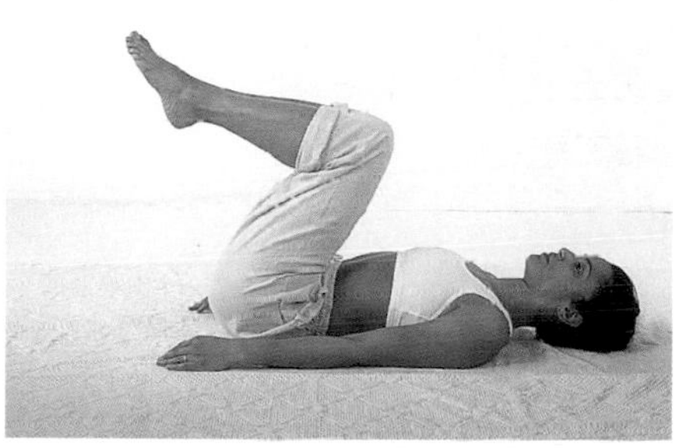

2 Slowly lower your back to the floor, then start to bend the legs and raise them off the floor.

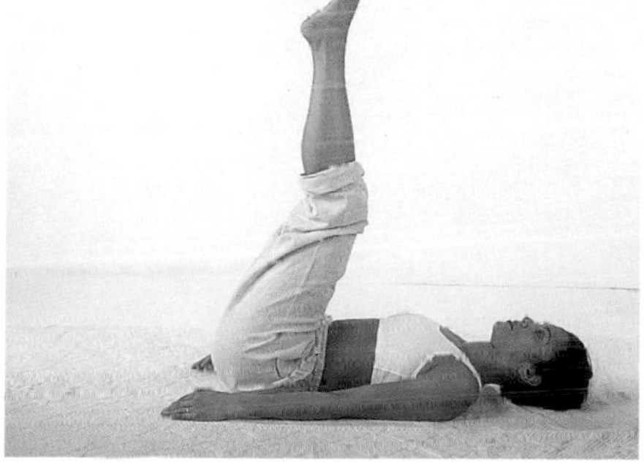

3 As you raise the legs, slowly start to straighten them until they are as close to the vertical as you can manage. Again, take care not to strain yourself.

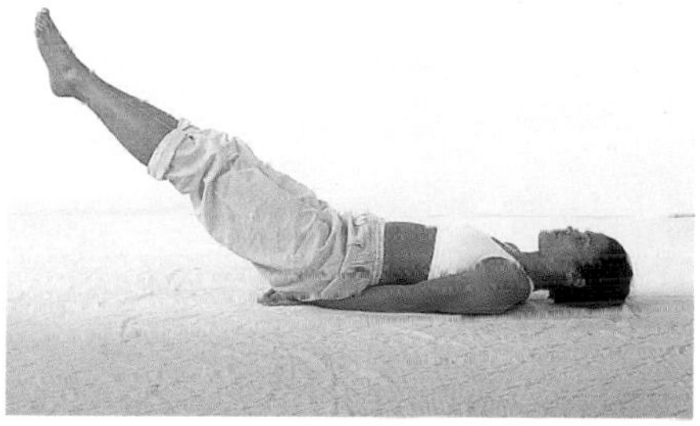

4 Keeping the legs straight, slowly lower them to the floor.

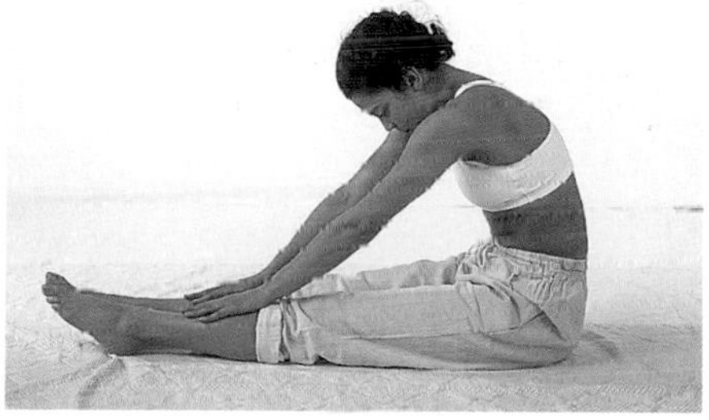

5 Continue the movement by sitting up and clasping your legs with your hands to bend forwards. Slowly return to the original sitting position.

abdominal tension relievers

We tend to hold and lock up too much tension in our abdomen, especially if we are the kind of people who always bottle up our feelings. Even simple muscular tension can leave us feeling stiff and rather uncomfortable, and much less flexible around the waist. Consequently exercises aimed at reducing stiffness and increasing flexibility in the abdominal region are extremely useful.

LOTUS

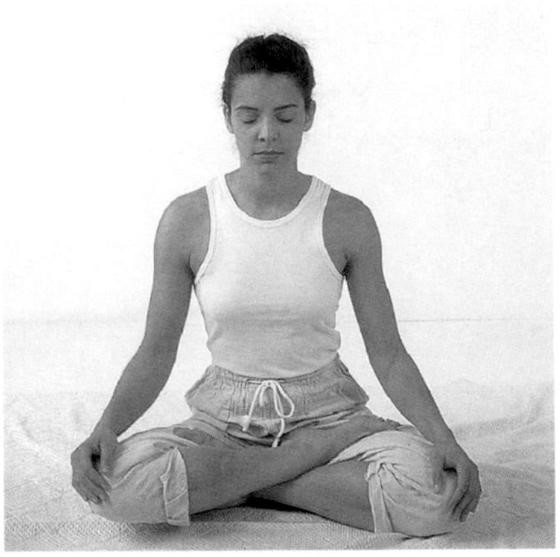

1 For the full lotus, the first leg should be bent with the foot on top of the other thigh, and the second leg bent so that the foot goes over the other leg on to the opposite thigh. Hold if possible.

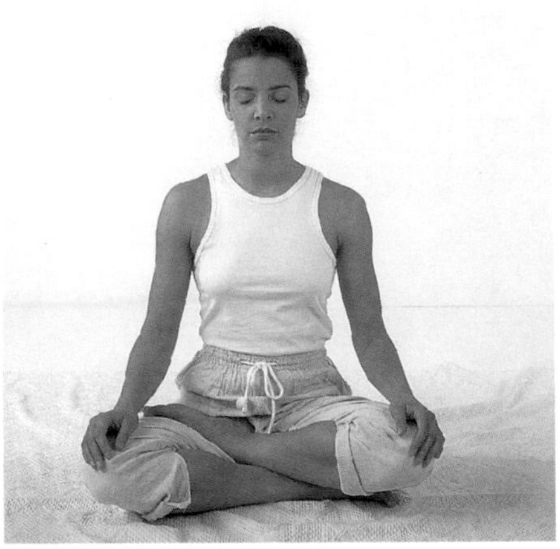

2 For an easier version bend one leg and rest the foot on the inner thigh of the other leg. Bend the second leg and place the foot on top of the opposite thigh. Keep the spine upright.

ABDOMINAL MOVEMENTS

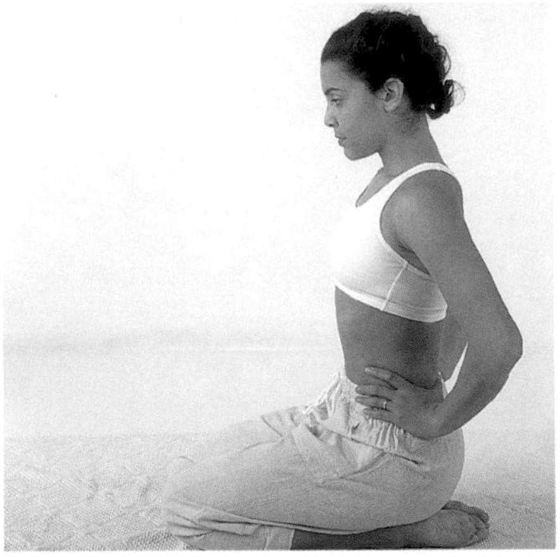

1 Either sit cross-legged or kneel, and place your hands on your waist or thighs. Breathe out completely.

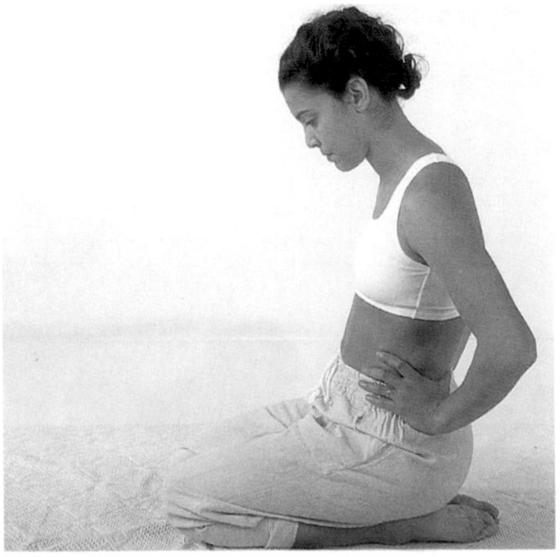

2 Without inhaling, pull in your abdomen as far as you can, then "snap" it in and out up to five times before taking a breath. Relax for a few moments, breathing freely, before repeating.

LEG OVER

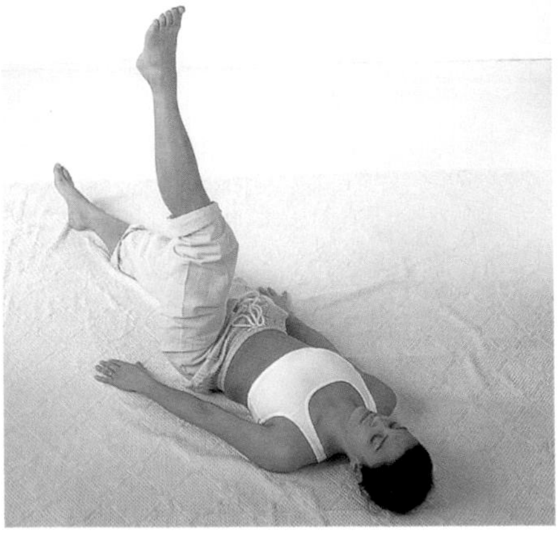

1 Lie on your back, with your legs out straight. Raise one leg as close to the vertical as is comfortable, then move it across the body, keeping your hips in contact with the floor.

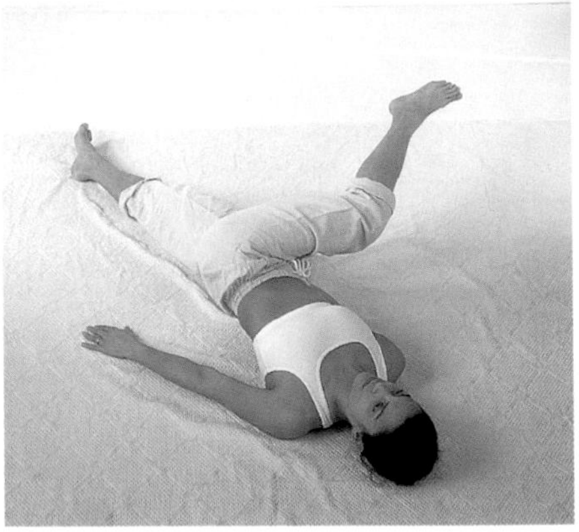

2 Push the leg as far over as possible, then slowly return to the original position. Repeat with the other leg.

LYING TWISTS

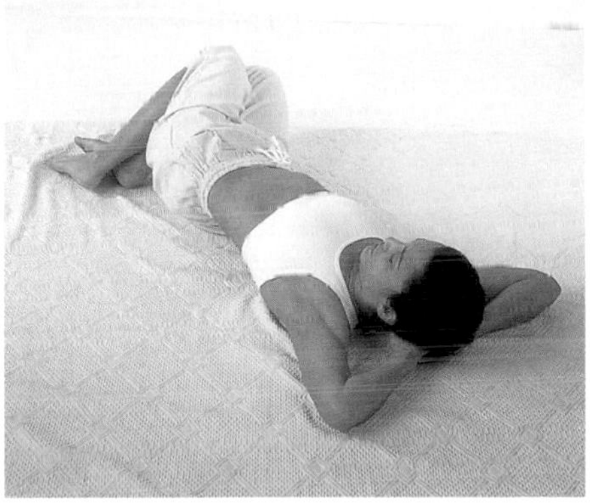

1 Lie on your back, hands behind your head and legs together, knees bent.

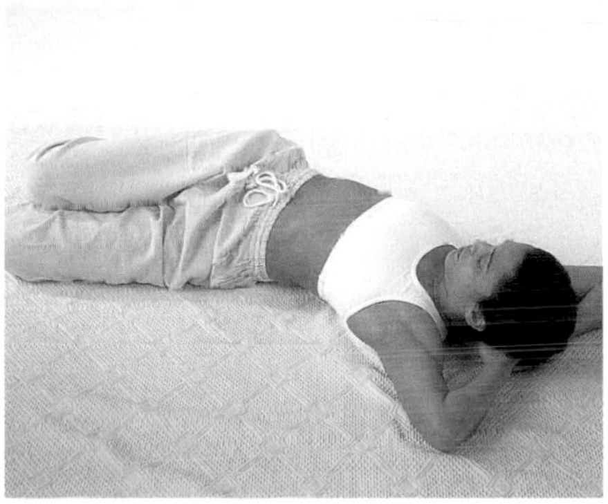

2 Twist the legs from side to side, keeping the back and hips on the floor.

SIDE BENDS

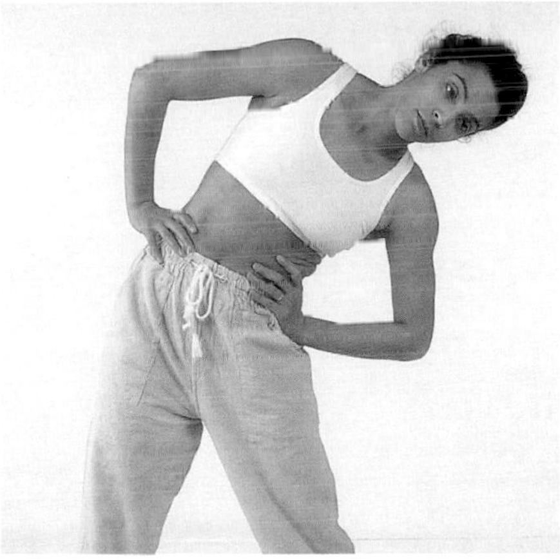

1 Stand with feet apart and hands on hips. Bend down to one side.

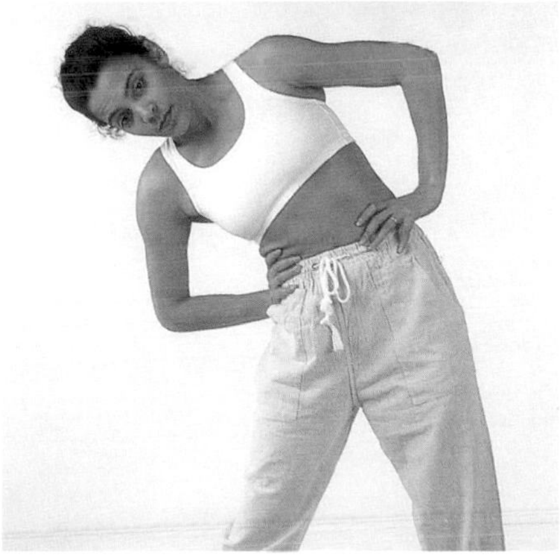

2 Slowly return to the upright position and bend to the other side. Repeat.

ROLL TWIST

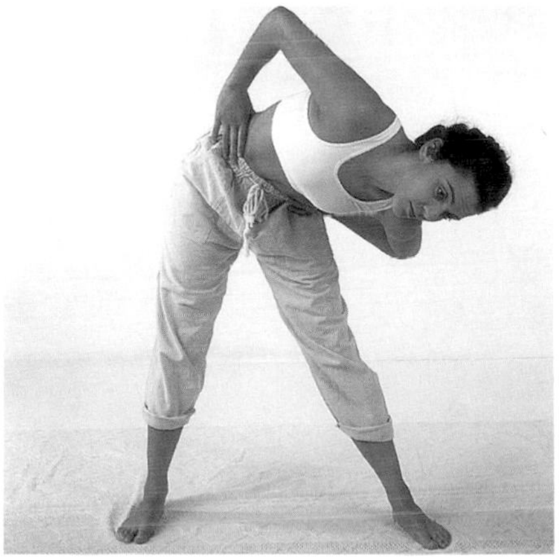

1 Keeping the legs and hips still, roll your upper body around in a clockwise circle.

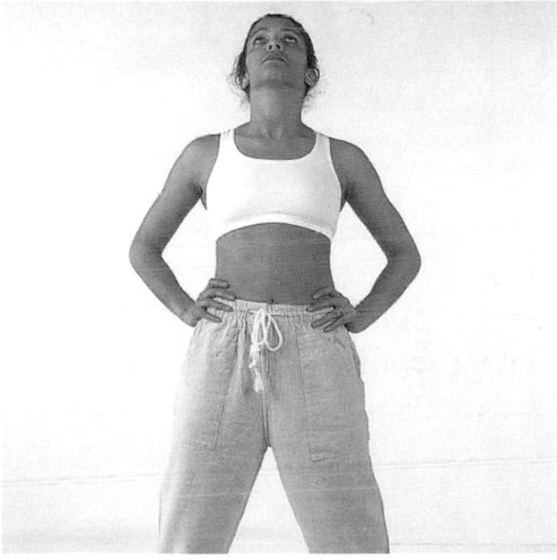

2 Move slowly and carefully, and bend only as far as is comfortable.

SIT UP/LIE DOWN

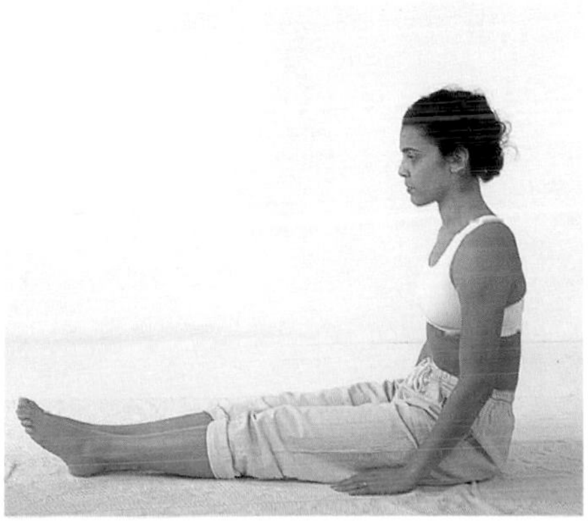

1 Sit on the floor with both legs straight out in front of you.

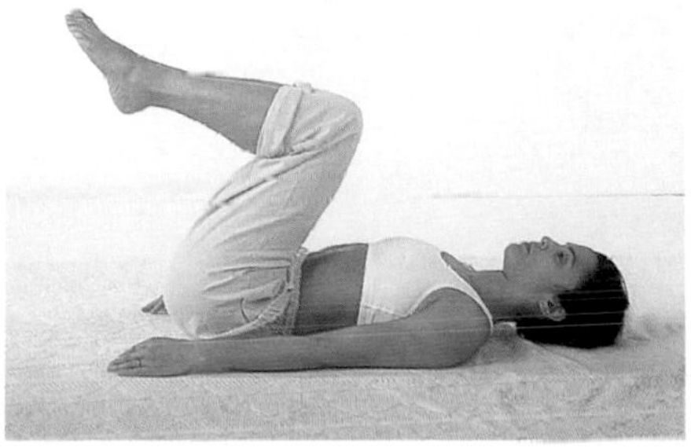

2 Slowly lie back, then start to bend the legs and raise them off the floor.

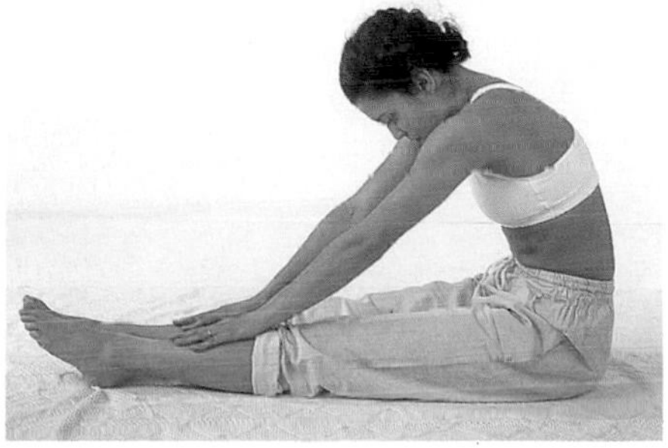

3 Sit up, bend forwards, clasp your legs and slowly return to the sitting position.

office tensions and stiff muscles

For people who spend their working day sitting at a desk it is very easy to get stiff, aching muscles. Badly designed chairs do not help, and as you get tired, so posture suffers and you can end up getting round-shouldered. It is therefore absolutely essential that every now and again you get up and walk around, relax your body, and try some of these excellent loosening-up exercises.

SEATED CAT STRETCH

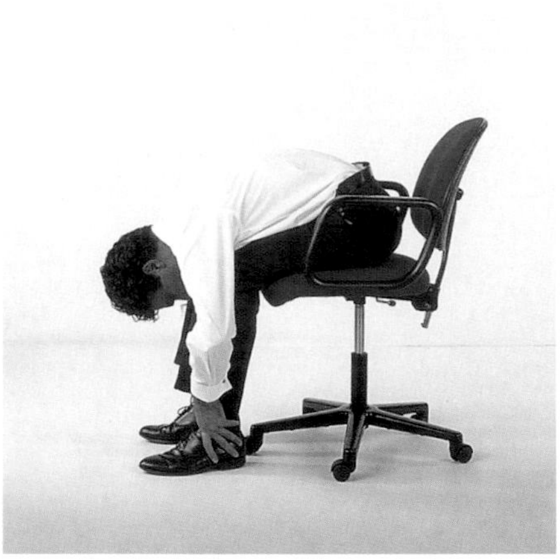

1 Pull the chair back from the desk slightly to give yourself more room, then bend forward and clasp your ankles.

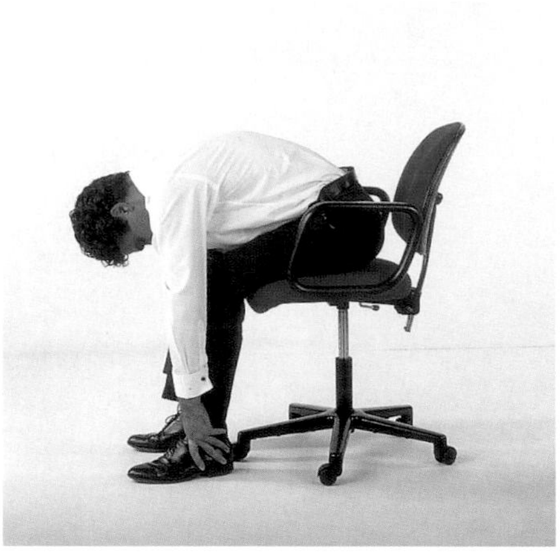

2 Carefully arch your back to stretch, then relax back and repeat.

CALF STRETCH

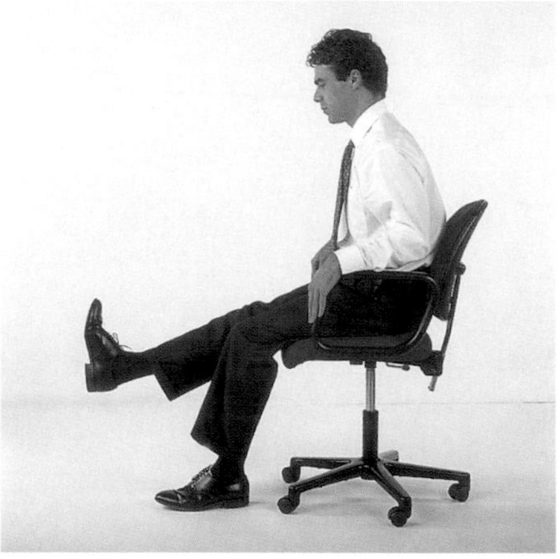

1 Sit fairly upright, then lift and straighten each leg alternately. Repeat a few times.

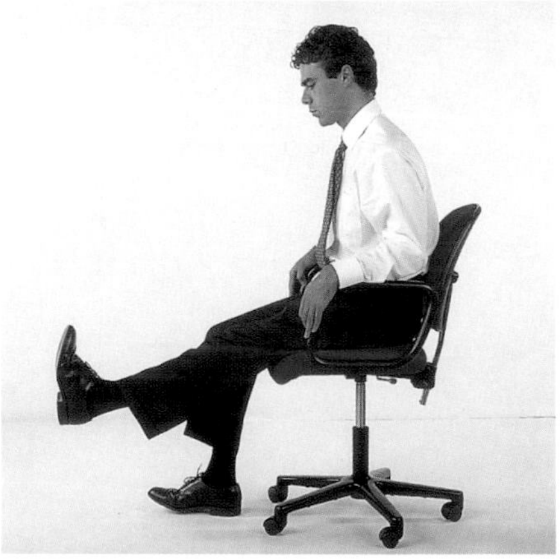

2 Flex the foot to stretch the calf muscle. Repeat a few times.

NECK TWISTS

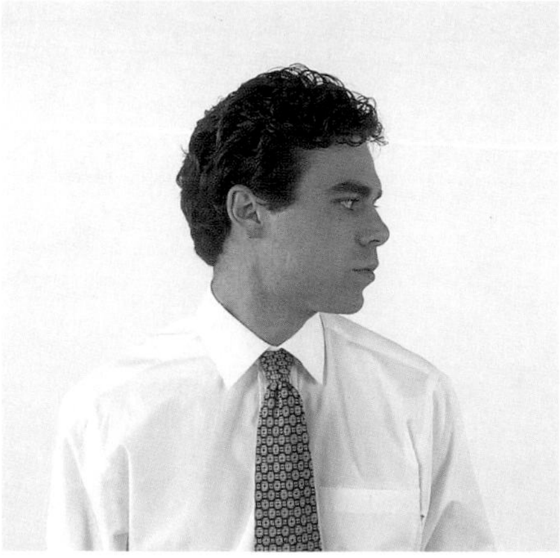

1 Turn your head to one side, feeling the extension in the neck muscles.

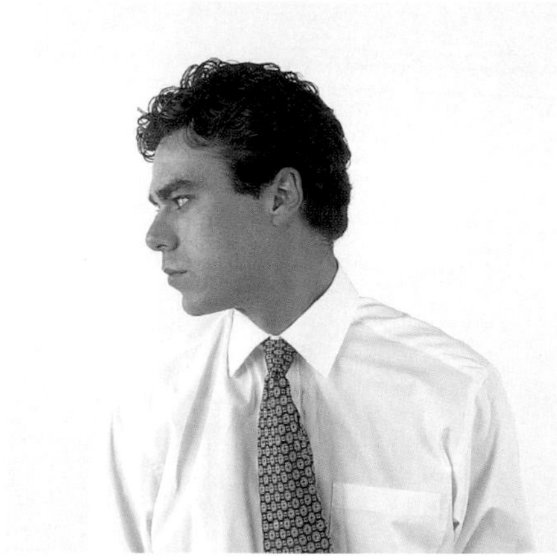

2 Repeat, turning the head from side to side. Do both steps quite slowly.

ARM AND CHEST STRETCH

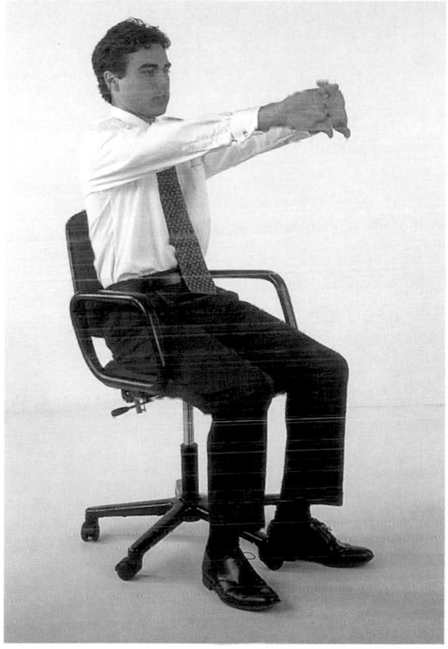

I Sitting upright, link your hands together, palms away from your body, and push your arms straight out in front of you. Hold for a couple of seconds, relax and then repeat.

ARM AND BACK STRETCH

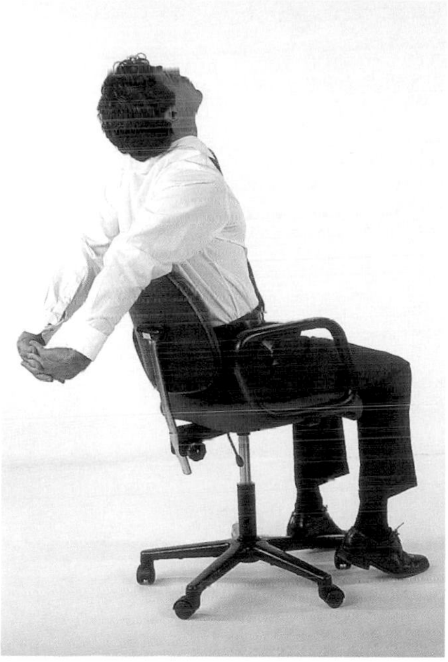

I Link your hands together behind your back, over the top of the chair, and lift your arms slightly. Do not strain yourself. Push away from your body, hold, then repeat the exercise.

FOREARM STRETCH

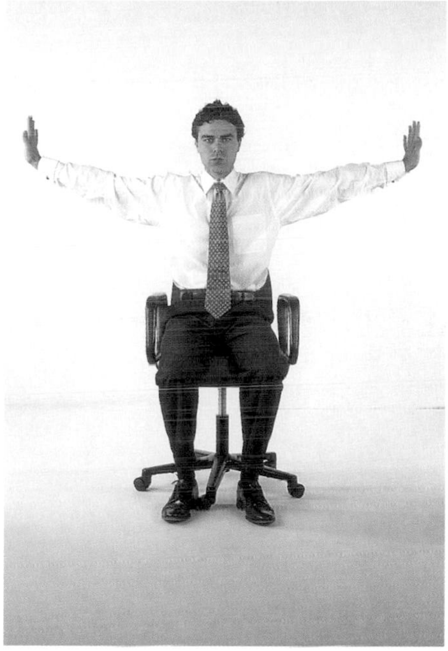

I Hold your arms straight out to the sides and stretch them. Alternately flex and extend your hands. Feel the pull on the upper and lower sides of your forearms as you do so.

BACK/SHOULDER STRETCH

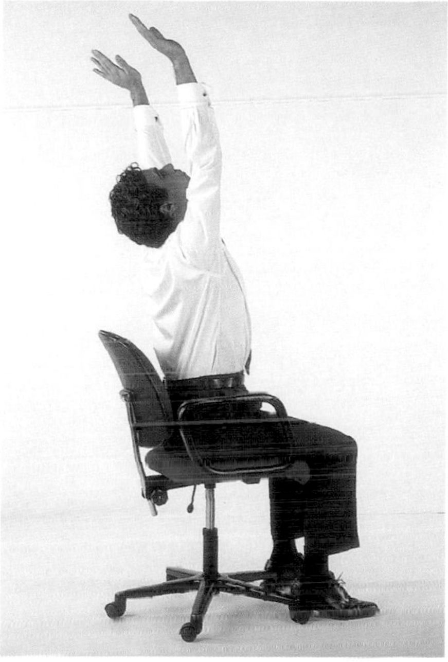

I Stretch your arms up in the air over your head. As you breathe in, arch your back ever so slightly. Relax with the exhalation and repeat the exercise a couple of times.

POSTURE CLASP

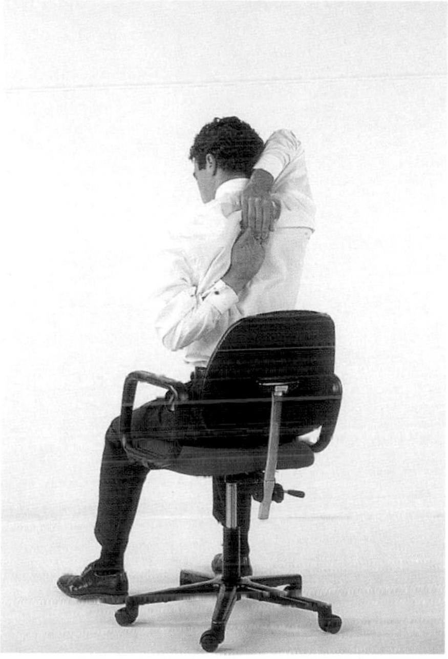

I Put one arm behind your back and bend it up, with the hand reaching the other shoulder. With your other arm raised and bent down over your shoulder, try to clasp your fingers.

SHOULDER RELEASE

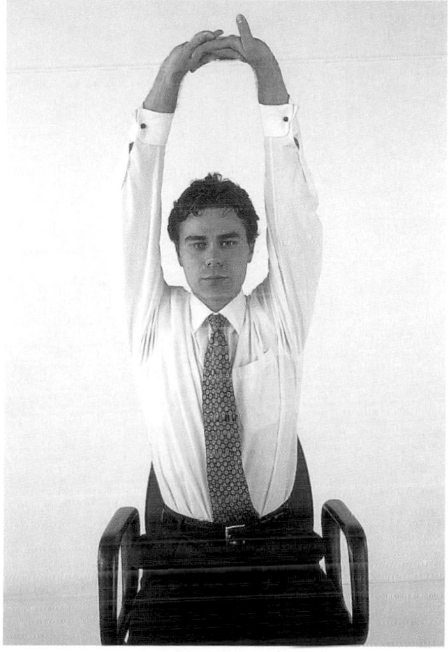

I Link your fingers together and stretch your arms high above your head. Repeat several times.

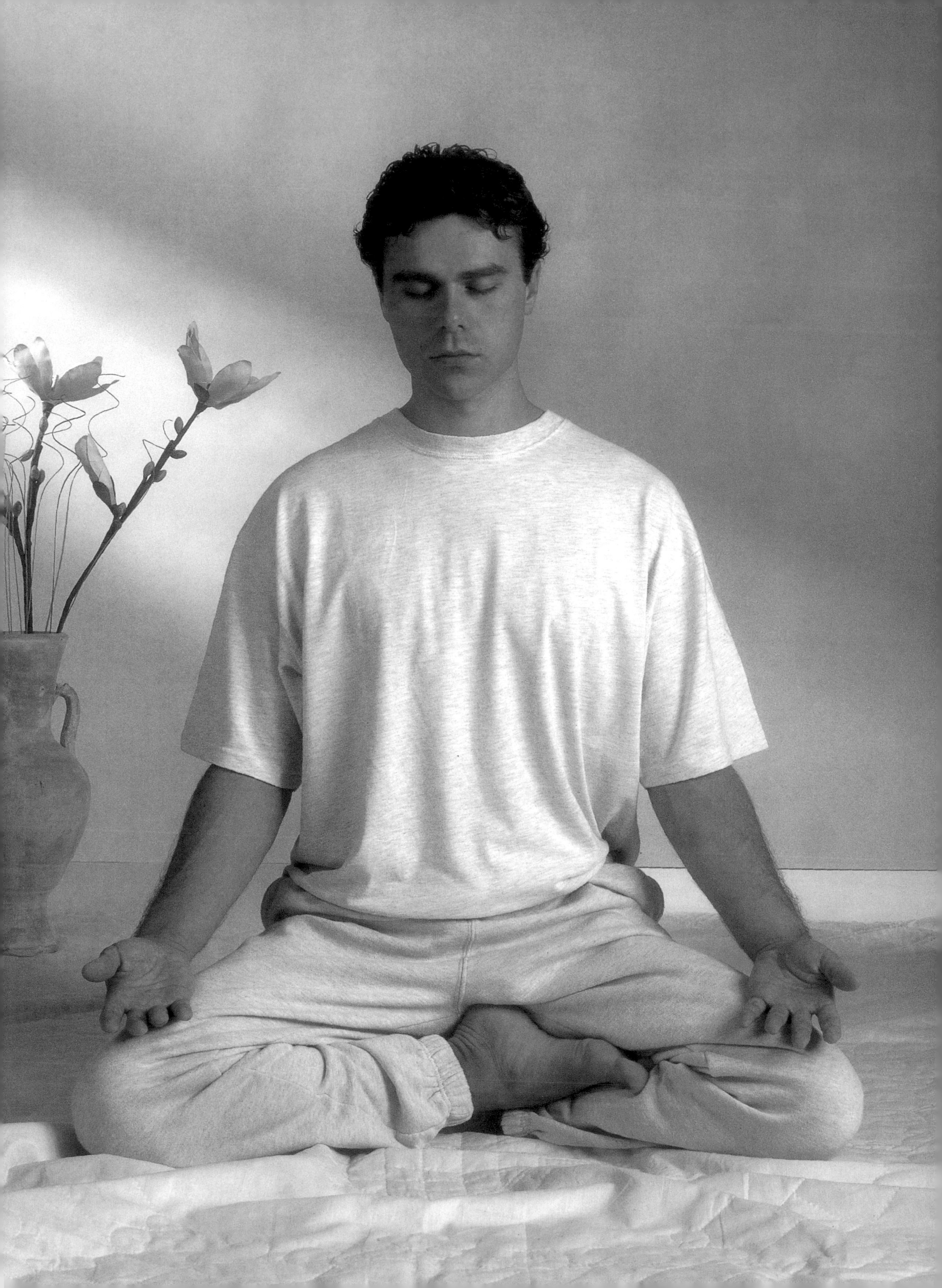

meditation
meditation

meditation

Meditation has been in use from the beginning of time: people have always sought inner quiet and physical relaxation, whether for reasons connected with the spirit, self-realization or health. You do not have to be a physical contortionist to achieve and enjoy the benefits of meditation at both physical and mental levels.

What, then, is meditation? It has been described as just sitting and relaxing. Many people find that their lives are so full of the demands of work, family, friends and organized leisure pursuits that they have no time to "stand and stare". Many are so caught up in planning and working towards the future that they take little pleasure from the here and now. In their bustle to "get on" they miss out on the simple pleasures of life. But beauty and joy are there to be seen and experienced, even in industrial cities.

The benefits of meditation come from regular use. If you are under stress, you may find that meditating twice daily will be effective in restoring composure. Make a time and space you can call your own, and use breathing and relaxation exercises to ease yourself into the meditative state. The more you practise meditation the less time you will need to spend on these, but they remain useful in calming and preparing you. Allow at least 10 minutes, ideally 20, for meditation in each session.

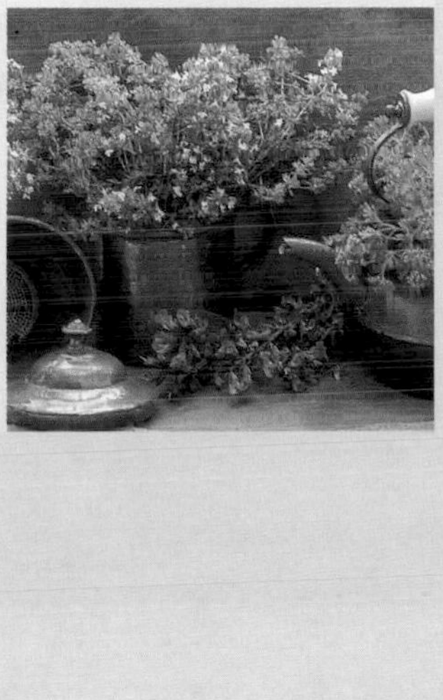

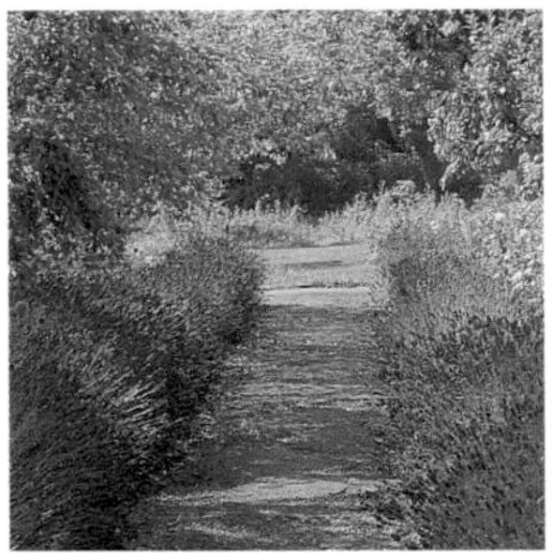
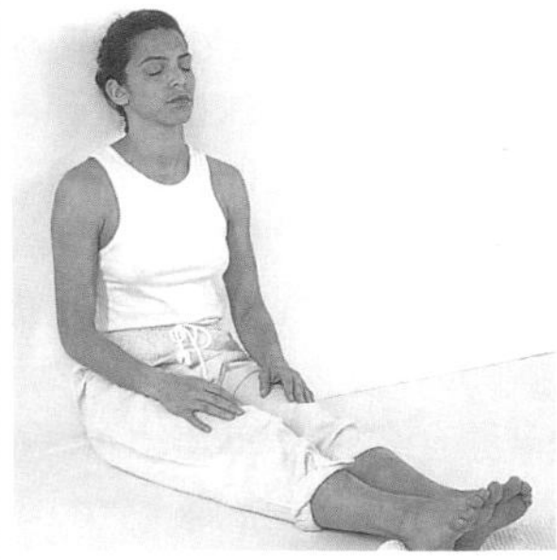
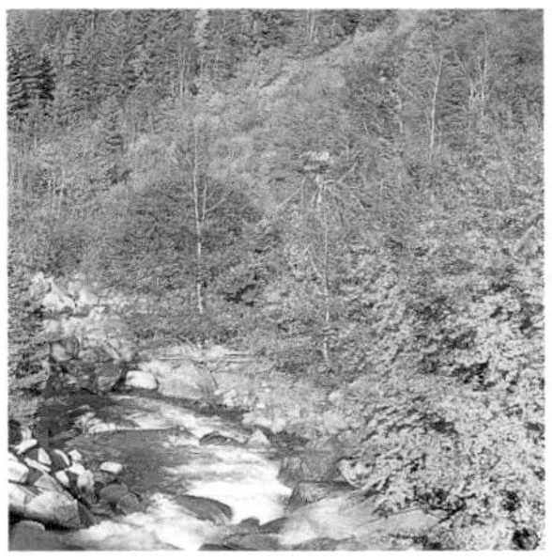
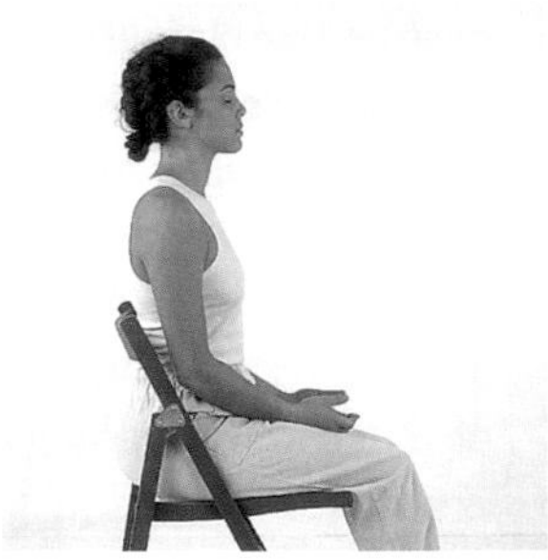

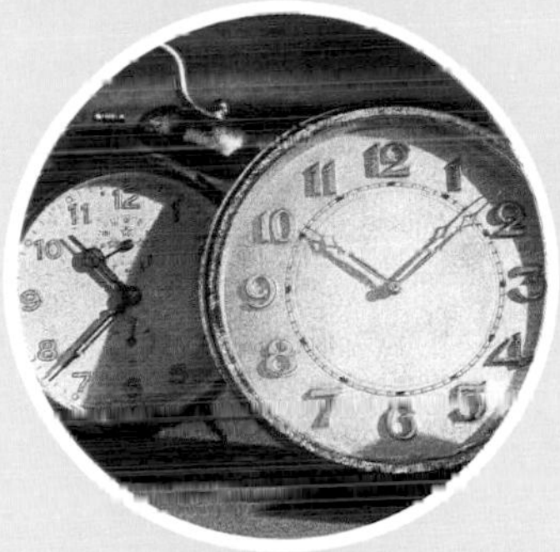

how to use meditation
how to use meditation

how to use meditation

The key to using meditation lies in recognizing that you actually need it. Once you get into the whirlpool of work and stress, they can both all too easily become an integral part of your lifestyle. In fact, they can be such a formidable cornerstone that you cannot imagine what life could possibly be like without them. But once you stand back and see clearly and exactly what is happening to you, what your life has become, then suddenly you see you actually need a way out. One of the best ways involves deep meditation.

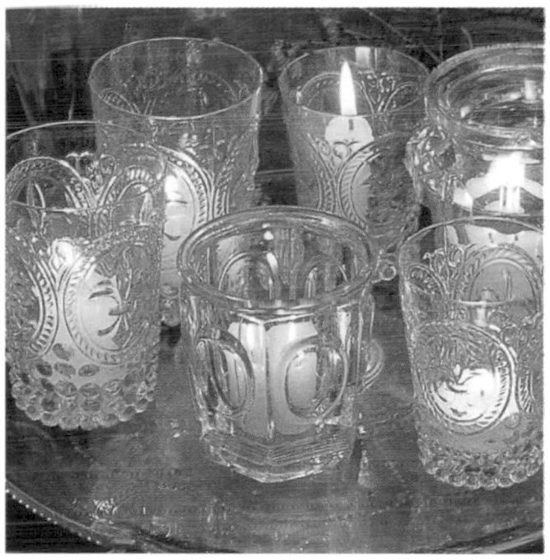

Meditation needs to be done like regular exercise. In fact you might say you are exercising the ways in which you relax. The very first step involves switching off, like switching off a light in a room, and concentrating on what could be called the "Inner Other", that is to say the marvellous, relaxed, empty inner spaces inside your head and body. This stage, put crudely, means sweeping out all the noise and mayhem and chaos of everyday life and getting ready to enter another world.

The second stage involves being carried along what one expert teacher calls "a moving but going nowhere sound that coils round and even through itself in a perpetual state of being". Perhaps the best way of evaluating it is by hearing what people have to say after meditation. "As good as a holiday" or "like a wonderful deep refreshing sleep" is what most people say. If you are to get its full, continuous benefits then you really must make sure that meditation is something that you do regularly every day, at certain times, because like almost all forms of exercise the more often you do it, the better you are at it; the quicker you can switch off and tune in, and enter that fantastic deep state of total energizing, refreshing relaxation.

You must use meditation with care though. It is not like switching on and off a tap. It needs to be respected. Few people who meditate try, even if they could, to describe its ultimate power. That would be like divulging a wonderful private secret; to have it is quite enough.

simple meditation techniques

If you want to learn to meditate seriously, you would do well to find an experienced teacher to guide you. However, there are many simple techniques that you can practise alone, often with quite powerful effects. Try the ones described here, and see which you feel in tune with. The more you practise, the easier it will become to reach a deep meditative state.

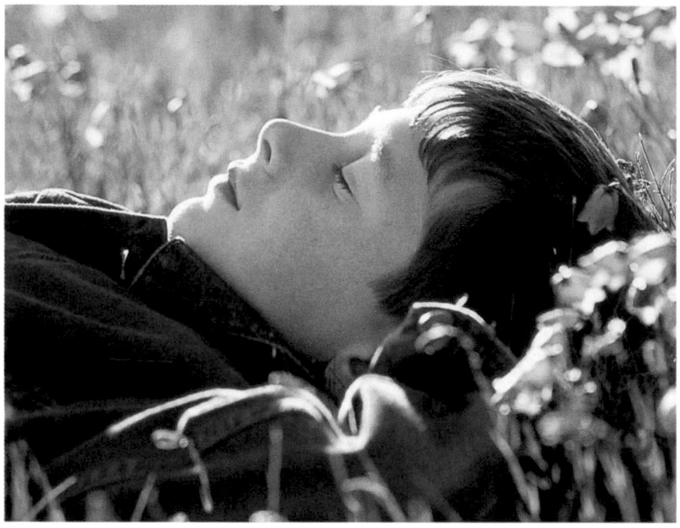

Introduce a child to meditation by using the Numbers Game.

THE NUMBERS GAME

This is a very simple form of meditation using a blackboard, real or imaginary. It is a good "game" to use with children (or adults), giving them a taste of meditation, and they really enjoy it. It is described here as if you are leading a group, but it can be easily used on one person, and provides an excellent way to clear the mind through concentration, imagination and patterns: all wonderful ways of gaining a real experience of deep meditation.

What you must do is this …

1 Get the children to sit or lie comfortably. Once they have found a really comfortable position ask them to remember it.

2 With chalk on the blackboard, draw a diagram of numbers, making sure that there are no mathematical links, like this:

3 1 5
8 6 9
4 7 2

3 Give the children one minute to memorize this sequence.

4 Ask them to return to their relaxed position, eyes closed, and concentrate on the numbers alone.

5 Rub out the numbers, telling them to do the same in their minds. Do this slowly saying "That leaves just four numbers", etc.

6 Then rub out the last number, saying "Now concentrate on what is left" … Let them remain in silence until you notice a restlessness – this is often three or more minutes.

7 Wake them gently with an instruction to "Sit up". Ask them what the last number was and for their reactions.

THE HAVEN

Once you have managed to achieve complete physical relaxation and calm, gradually allow your mind to enter a place, whether real or imaginary, that is quite special to you. Now you can allow your mind to drift … drift to a pleasant, peaceful place. A place that you know and where you always feel able to relax … completely. A safe … secure … place … where no one … and nothing can ever bother you.

It may be a place you have visited on holiday, a beach or a place in the countryside. Or it may be a room … a room you have had … a room you do have … or a room you would like to have … an imaginary place. But it is a place where you can always feel able to let go … completely … a haven, a haven of tranquillity, unique and special to you.

In order to help you imagine this place … notice first the light: is it bright, natural or dim … is there any particular source of light … natural or man-made? Notice also the temperature level … hot, warm or cool … and any particular source of heat. Be aware of the colours that surround you … shapes … and textures … the familiar objects that make that place special. Begin to see it in all its detail. You can just be there … whether sitting, lying or reclining, enjoying the sounds … the smells … the atmosphere … with nobody wanting anything, nobody needing anything and no one demanding anything from you. Relax.

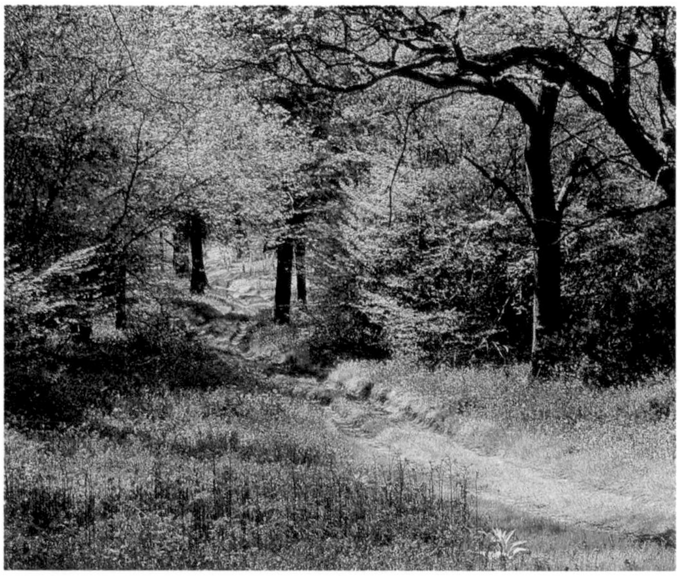

Everyone has their own haven, a quiet magical place like this.

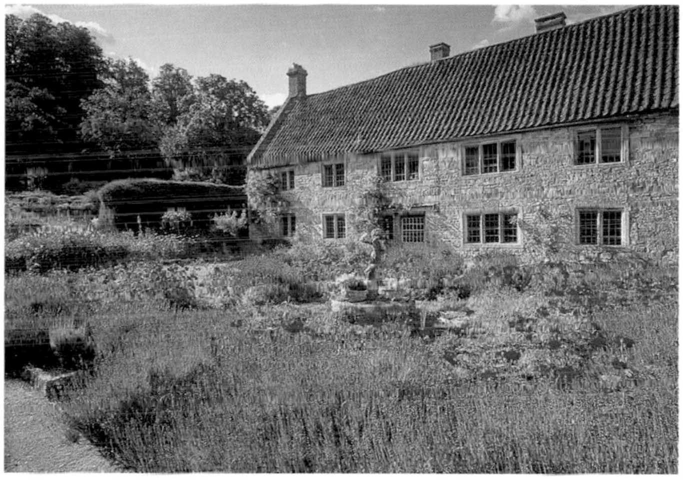

Try to imagine your perfect country house.

A GUIDED VISIT TO A COUNTRY HOUSE

Imagine that you are visiting a beautiful country house ... a really beautiful old country house or a stately home with magnificent sweeping lawns on a warm, sunny, summer's afternoon. You are standing on the staircase that leads into the entrance hall, one of those wide ceremonial types of staircase. And as you look down across the entrance hall you can just glimpse, through the open doors opposite, a gravel drive, and the sunlight on the gravel. It is a beautiful, sunny, summer's afternoon and there is no one around to trouble or bother you as you stand alone on that staircase ...

Now you are moving down the last ten steps to the hallway, relaxing more and more with each step down.

10 Taking one step down, relaxing and letting go ...
9 Taking another step down, feeling at ease ...
8 Becoming more relaxed, letting go even more ...
7 Just drifting deeper ... and deeper ... everything is getting darker and darker, and even deeper down still ...
6 Becoming calmer ... and calmer ... even calmer still ...
5 Continuing to relax, continuing to let go and feeling good ...
4 Relaxing even more ... letting go even more ...
3 Sinking deeper ... drifting even further into this welcoming, relaxed state ...
2 Enjoying those good feelings, all those feelings of inner peace and relaxation ...
1 Nearly all the way down now, feeling very good ... beautifully relaxed ... and **0**.

You are wandering across that hallway now, towards the open doors and the gardens beyond, soaking up the atmosphere of peace and permanence in that lovely old building. You wander out through the doors and down the stone steps outside ... and find yourself standing on the gravel drive outside, a wide gravel drive that leads down to the entrance gates.

As you stand there you notice the lush green lawns, so flat and well-clipped ... and there are shrubs and trees, different shades of green and brown against a clear, blue sky ... and you can feel the warmth of the sun on your head and shoulders as you enjoy this beautiful summer's afternoon in this lovely old garden ... There are flowerbeds with their splashes of colour so carefully arranged and neatly tended. And there's no one else about ... nobody needing anything, nobody wanting anything and nobody expecting anything from you, so you can enjoy the peace and serenity and solitude of this afternoon in this beautiful garden that's been so well looked after for so many, many years.

A little way down on the right-hand side of the driveway, you notice an ornamental fish pond. So you decide to wander down and have a look at those fish. Sometimes they seem almost to disappear behind the weed and shadows, but always they reappear, with their scales catching the sunlight, red, gold, silver or black. And as you watch those fish your mind becomes even more deeply relaxed ...

THE WELL

This continues from the previous visualization of the beautiful country house and is intended to take you to even deeper levels of meditation.

... As you watch those fish you notice that the centre of the pond is very deep. It could be the top of a disused well. You take from your pocket a silver-coloured coin, and toss that coin so that it lands over the centre of the pond, and then you watch as it swings down through the water. The ripples drift to the edges of the pond, but you just watch that coin as it sinks deeper and deeper through that clear water, sometimes it seems to disappear as it turns on edge, at other times a face of the coin catches the sunlight and it flashes through the water ... sinking, drifting deeper and deeper, twisting and turning as it makes its way down ... Finally it rests at the bottom lying on a cushion of soft brown mud, a silver coin in that still, clean water on its own cushion of mud ... And you feel as still as that coin, as still and cool and motionless as that water, enjoying that feeling of inner peace and stillness.

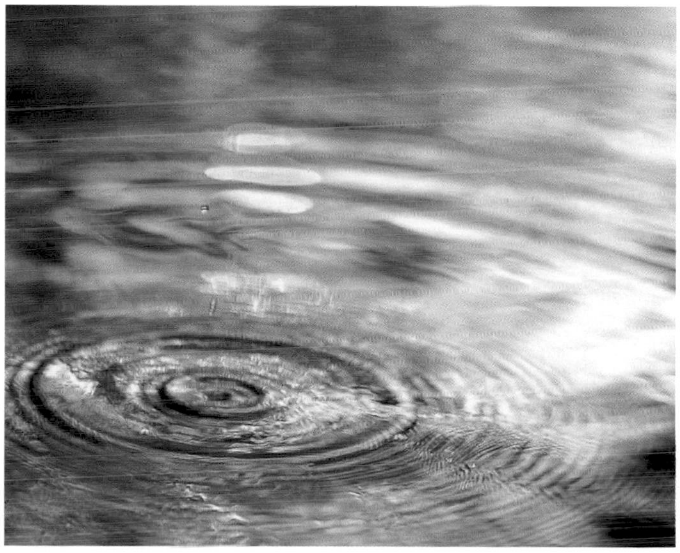

Watch the ripples as the coin lands in the very centre of the pond. Look even more closely as it tumbles down through the water ...

personal development

Affirmations are a deceptively simple device that can be used by anyone and they are remarkably effective. Try to use this method while in the meditative state, having planned and memorized the affirmations involved. These powerful, positive phrases will improve communication with all parts of your mind. All you need is a simple phrase summing up how you want to be.

THE POWER OF WORDS

To make affirmations effective, they should

- be made in the present tense
- be positively phrased
- have an emotional reward.

Now contrast the power of such phrases with what happens if you are asked not to do or think of something. The words "no", "not", "never" and so on generally have the opposite effect to that intended, and why? Yours is the most influential voice in your life because you believe it. It comes live, straight out of the personality and intellect, and is fuelled by your dreams and language. The power you have over yourself is extraordinary. That is precisely why you must be careful to avoid any negative or demeaning statements you regularly make about yourself, either to others or to yourself – "I am shy", "I lack confidence", "I cannot", "I get nervous when" and so on – they are self-limiting beliefs that you are reinforcing each time they slip into your conversation or mind. You become what you say.

The point about affirmations is that instead of running yourself down, albeit in a subtle, insidious way, you actually start building yourself up. You start creating the inner psychological scaffolding to support the new you. Such affirmations are best used while in a wonderful state of meditation.

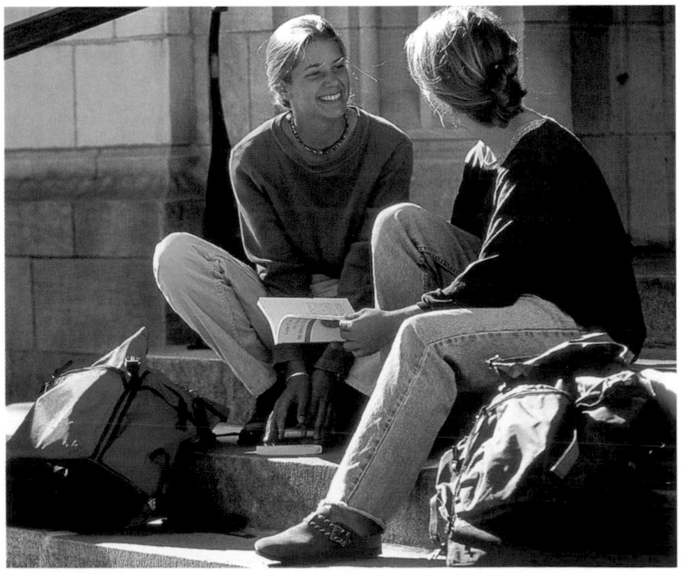

The difference affirmations can make is extraordinary. From shy and introverted to open, confident and winning.

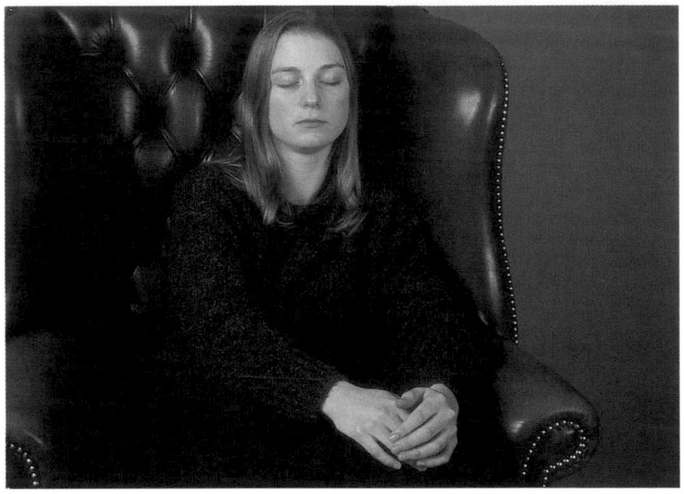

Thinking through what you want to be is the big key to success.

IMPROVED SELF-WORTH

We all have attributes and qualities in which we can take pride and pleasure. This exercise is about emphasizing these positive aspects to allay the doubts that only serve to limit our potential.

- I like my [physical attribute].
- I am proud of my [attitude or achievement].
- I love meeting people – they are fascinating.
- My contribution is valuable to [name person].
- I am lovable and can give love.
- Others appreciate my [opinions, assistance, a personal quality].
- I enjoy being a unique combination of mind and body.

Now imagine yourself speaking to colleagues, boss, employees or friends ... See yourself behaving and looking confident, standing and looking a confident person ... Notice how you stand ... your facial expression ... hear the way that you speak ... slowly, calmly, quietly, clearly and with confidence. You are communicating your needs ... ideas ... opinions in a positive way. Notice how your words flow easily, and how others are listening attentively to you ... valuing what you have to say. Now "climb aboard" ... be there – know how it feels to stand like that ... to speak like that ... and to have that positive reception from others. Get in touch with the stance ... expression ... and feelings ... and know that you can use these any time in the future to gain those same feelings or that inner strength in everything you do. See yourself in different situations: at home, in a social setting, in all the parts of your life, confident and assured, going from strength to strength.

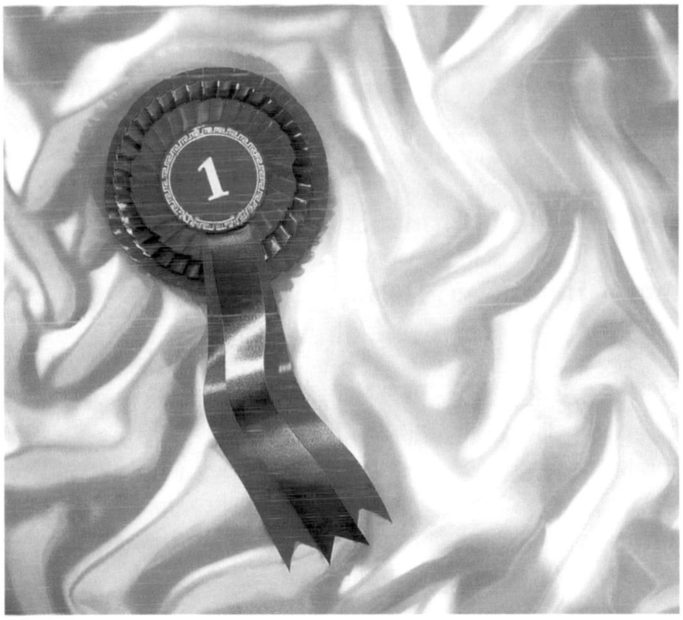

If you want to be No. 1, then take time to concentrate on seeing yourself as the best. Give yourself the power to come out top.

VISUALIZATION

In the same way that you can utilize your voice, so, perhaps more powerfully, you can use your imagination. The imagination can stimulate emotions, and they can register new attitudes in the mind. It can be a direct communication with the deeper levels of the mind, providing a powerful influence for improvements in your attitudes, behaviour patterns and overall confidence.

Visualization requires that you imagine yourself in a situation, behaving, reacting and looking as you would wish to do at an interview, an important meeting, a social gathering, a one-to-one situation, or perhaps a sporting event. Imagine what that will mean for you, your reactions, the reactions of those around you and, importantly, feel all the good feelings that will be there when this happens in reality.

It is like playing a video of the event, on that screen on the inside of the forehead, the mind's eye, from the beginning of the situation through to the perfect outcome. Should any doubts or negative images creep into your "video", push them away and replace them with positive ones. Keep this realistic, and base it upon real information from your past.

CONFIDENCE IN FUTURE SITUATIONS

The meditative state, affirmations and visualization can be a valuable rehearsal and preparation for a future event. Athletes and other sportsmen have proved that it actually does work. We can all use these extraordinary techniques to achieve our own optimum performance during any situation. Now consider the following phrases, and how they relate to you …

- I am quietly confident in meetings.
- I speak slowly, quietly and confidently so that others listen.
- My contribution is wanted and valued by others.
- I enjoy meetings, as they bring forth new ideas and help to renew my enthusiasm.

Imagine an important meeting that is about to happen, and see yourself there, filling in all the details that you know, and the people too; imagine yourself there looking confident and relaxed, concentrating on what is happening. Be aware of the acute interest you are giving to what is happening with complete, concentrated attention, and then imagine yourself speaking, to give information or to ask a question: hear yourself speaking quietly, slowly and calmly …

Notice people listening to what you are saying; they wish you well and support you, as you are expressing your viewpoint or raising a question they may well have wanted to ask, too. Notice how you are sitting or standing, how you lean slightly forward when speaking, that expression of calm confidence on your face. When this is clear in your mind, just like a film playing in your mind's eye, play it back and forth. When you are feeling comfortable with it, get into that imaginary you, "climb aboard" and be there in your mind, seeing things from that perspective, hearing things from that point in the meeting. As you speak, get in touch with those calm feelings, and the attitudes that allow you to feel calm, in control, and quietly confident … It is like a rehearsal; the more you manage to rehearse the better the final performance will be. You will acquire the right attitudes, stance and tone of voice, so that when you are in that situation all of these will be available to you, and it will be just as you imagined, as if you had done it all, successfully, before.

In short, what this technique does is take you step by step through a rehearsal. Imagine every possible scenario, and how you will deal with it. That is the key to a successful outcome.

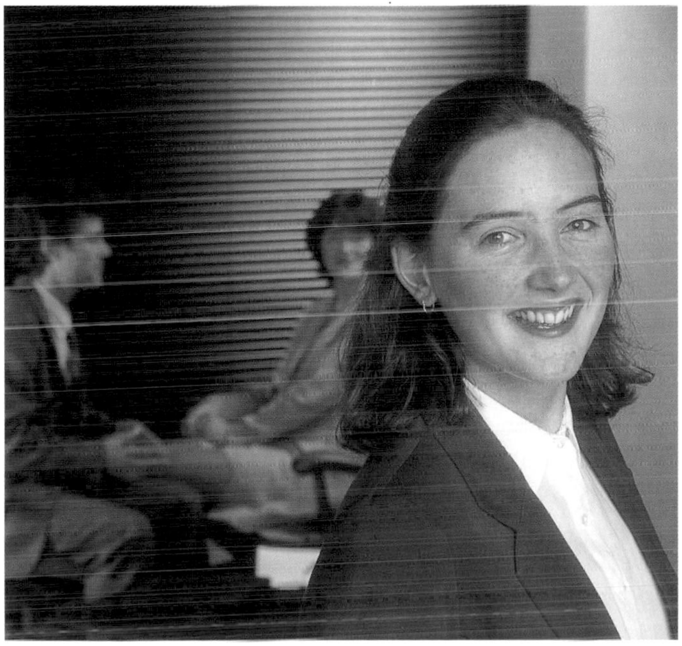

The preparation was worth it; you went into a meeting knowing you could do it, and that is exactly what happened.

GENERAL FITNESS

Fitness is the key to a healthy mind and body. It is based on stamina, strength, and suppleness – the three "S"s; better shape and self-esteem are two extra "S" bonuses. Being fit does not merely improve your physical prowess and grace, it also makes you feel better overall. But although we are more health-conscious about our diet nowadays, regular exercise is still not a part of most people's daily lives. Surveys always draw the same conclusion as to the reasons for this: lack of time, energy, interest, and confidence. Becoming fit is neither as difficult nor as time-consuming as it may appear to be: you can get fit – and get a better body into the bargain – more quickly, easily and enjoyably than you may think.

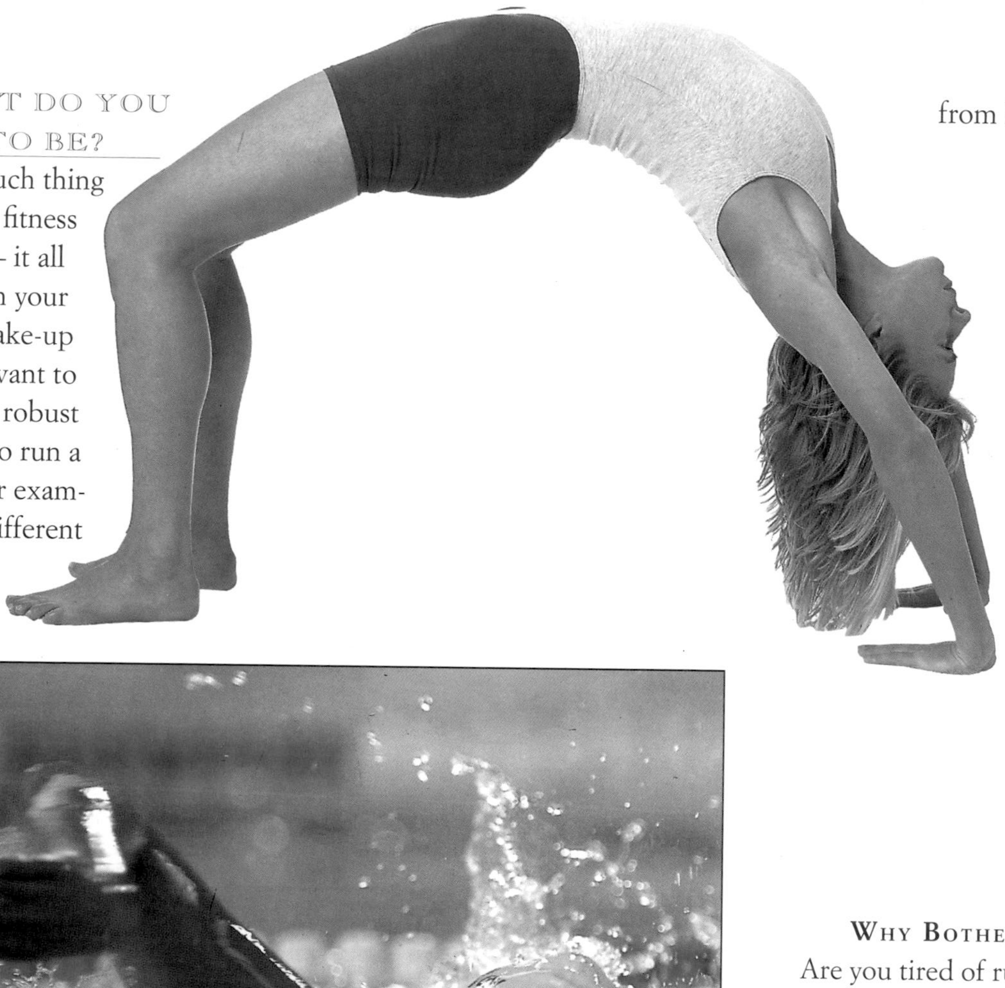

HOW FIT DO YOU NEED TO BE?

There is no such thing as a standard fitness gauge – it all depends on your personal make-up and why you want to be fit: being robust enough to run a marathon, for example, is very different from honing the three "S"s. For exercise to be of any help to you, though, it should boost your metabolism and improve your cardiovascular and respiratory systems.

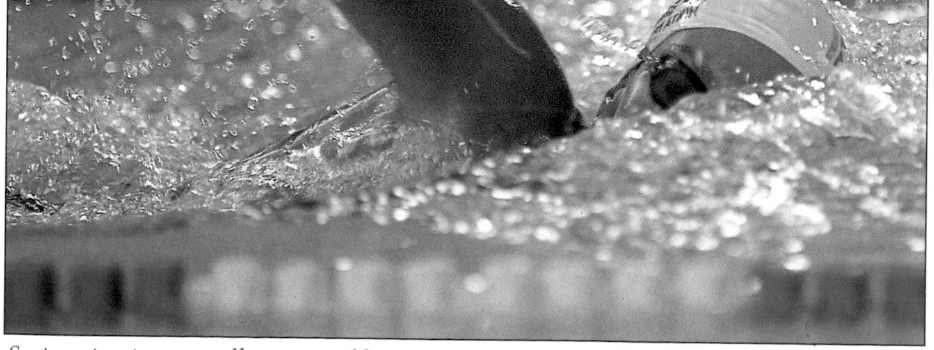

Swimming is an excellent way of keeping the whole body in good physical condition when done regularly and conscientiously.

WHY BOTHER WITH FITNESS?

Are you tired of running out of puff, being out of shape or always feeling under the weather? Do you often get colds, or suffer from pre-menstrual syndrome (PMS), stress, or sleepless nights? These are just a handful of the signs that could manifest themselves when you are unfit.

So exercise is worth the effort, because when you are fitter, problems such as these may ease or disappear.

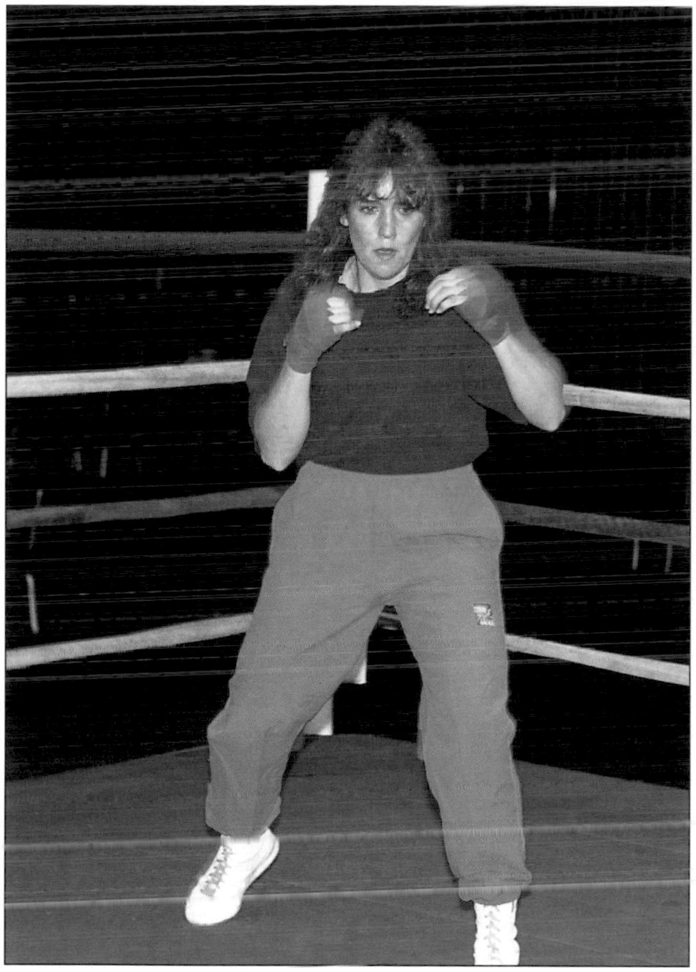

Women are increasingly attracted to strenuous sports such as boxing that until recently were considered to be solely a male preserve.

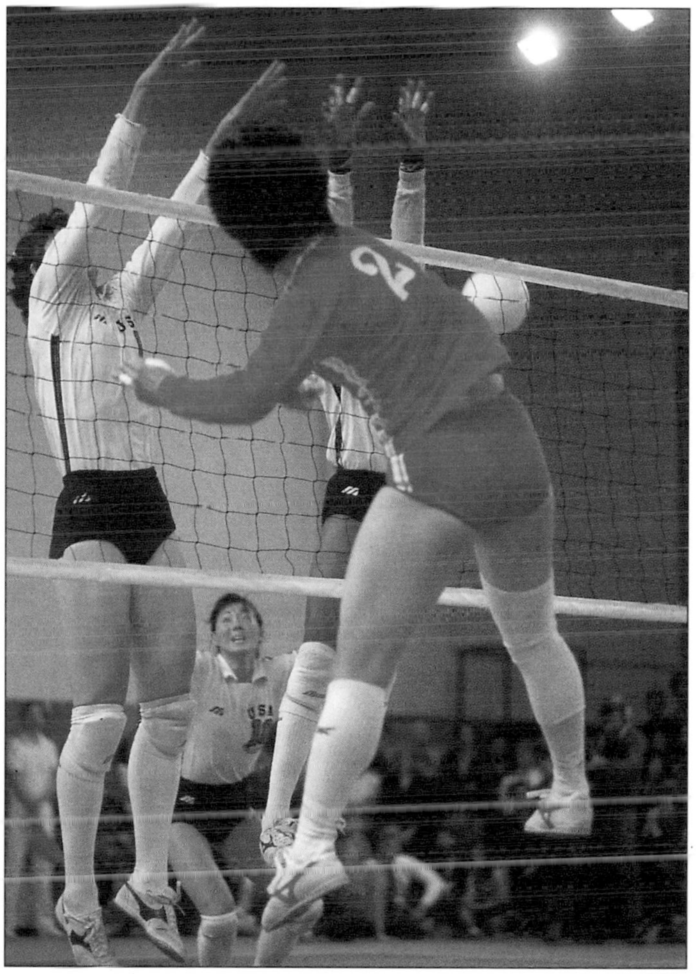

Competitive team sports such as volleyball not only provide an opportunity to improve physical fitness, they are also highly enjoyable.

YOUR GOAL

Finding a goal to inspire you is the secret of success. Set the deadline and stick to it. Depending on what you want to achieve, a three-week plan is ideal because it is not too long and if you persevere (take it week by week or day by day – whichever you find easiest), you will see results. Be realistic: if your goals are too high you are likely to fail: if they are too low, you will not have enough of a challenge.

Goals will inspire you, but speedy results are the key to keeping up regular exercise – it is natural to want to see rewards for all your hard work – although it is advisable to build up a pattern gradually.

The minimum amount of exercise you need to do to improve your personal fitness is 20 minutes, three times a week – the "3 × 20" maxim. This means three bouts of exercise vigorous enough to make you fairly breathless (but not gasping for breath). So if you do the general fitness exercises outlined in this book three times a week for 20 minutes you will get fitter. If you want to see fast results, though, you need to add extra activities – such as a couple of games of tennis, swimming, or brisk walking – to your exercise quota, so that you are actually exercising six days a week.

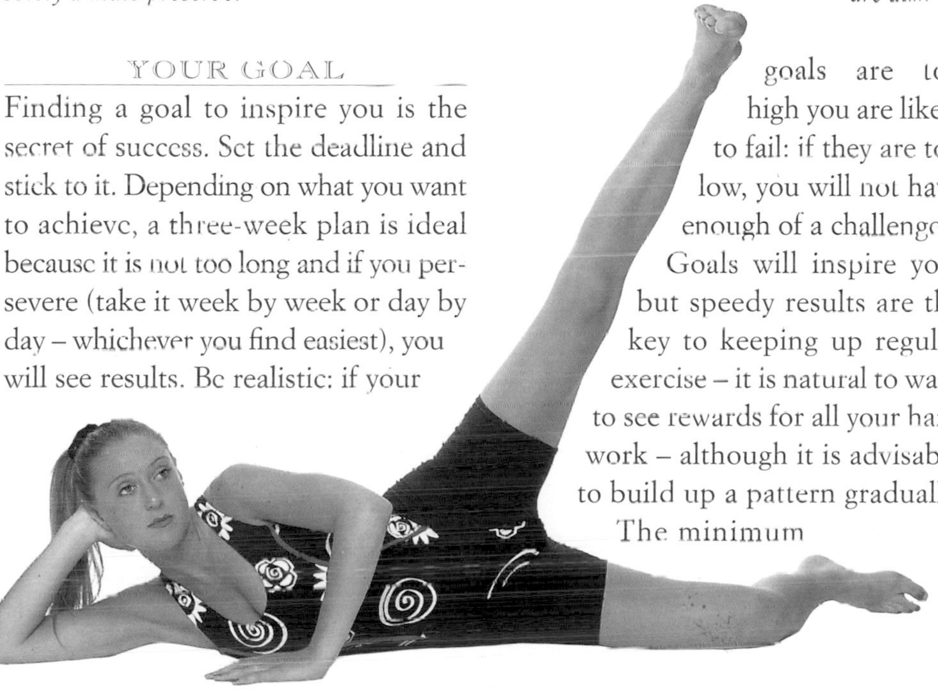

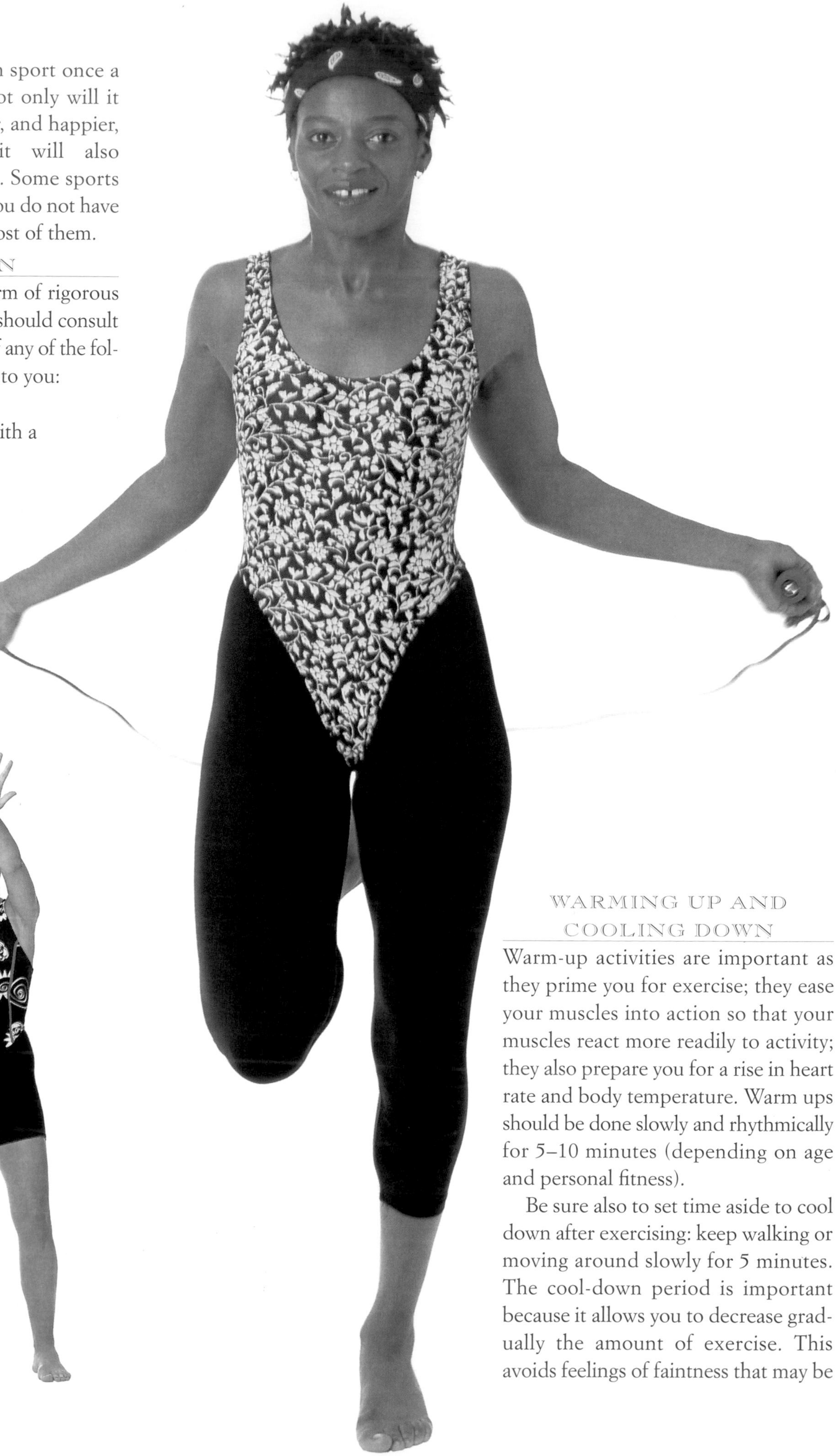

Taking part in a team sport once a week is a good idea: not only will it make you fitter, slimmer, and happier, the competitive spirit will also strengthen your resolve. Some sports need special skills, but you do not have to be an athlete to do most of them.

CAUTION

Before taking up any form of rigorous exercise or training, you should consult your doctor – especially if any of the following conditions apply to you:

- diabetes or epilepsy
- over 35 years of age with a long history of inactivity
- cardiovascular or respiratory problems
- severe illness and ensuing medication
- chronic joint or back problems
- obesity
- pregnancy
- heavy drinking or smoking

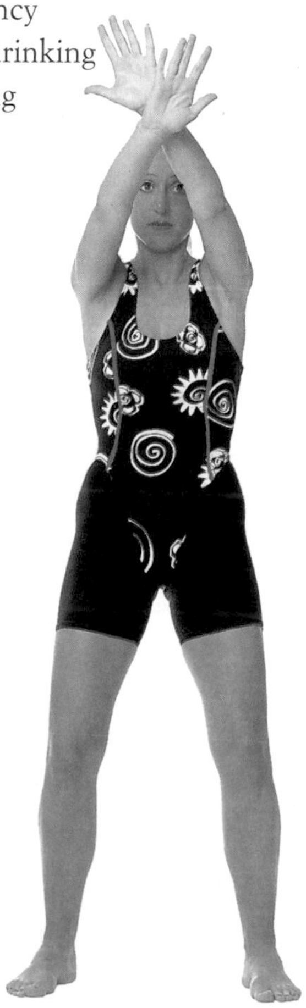

WARMING UP AND COOLING DOWN

Warm-up activities are important as they prime you for exercise; they ease your muscles into action so that your muscles react more readily to activity; they also prepare you for a rise in heart rate and body temperature. Warm ups should be done slowly and rhythmically for 5–10 minutes (depending on age and personal fitness).

Be sure also to set time aside to cool down after exercising: keep walking or moving around slowly for 5 minutes. The cool-down period is important because it allows you to decrease gradually the amount of exercise. This avoids feelings of faintness that may be caused by the pooling of blood below the waist that occurs during vigorous exercise.

YOUR PULSE RATE

Monitoring your pulse rate allows you to keep a check on whether you are exercising adequately. The maximum heart rate for an adult is roughly 220 beats per minute minus your age in years. The ideal heart rate during exercise is in a target zone of 65–80 per cent of this figure. The aim of exercise is to get your heart rate to within a certain range. These are the ideal exercise heart rates for the different ages:

Age	Pulse Range
20+	130–160
30+	124–152
40+	117–144

To find out your active pulse rate per minute, rest two fingers lightly on your pulse immediately after exercising, count the beats for 10 seconds and multiply by 6

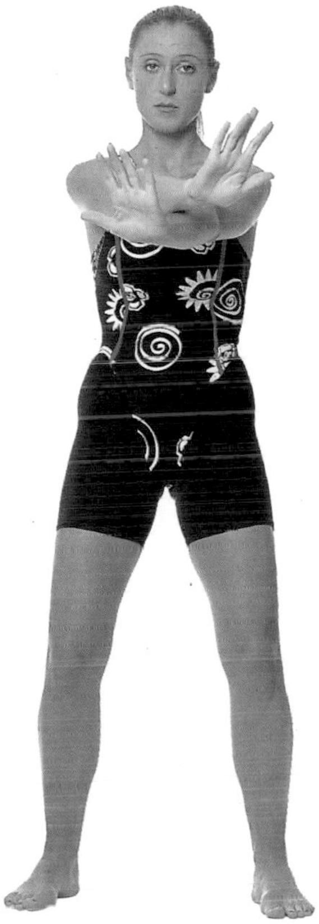

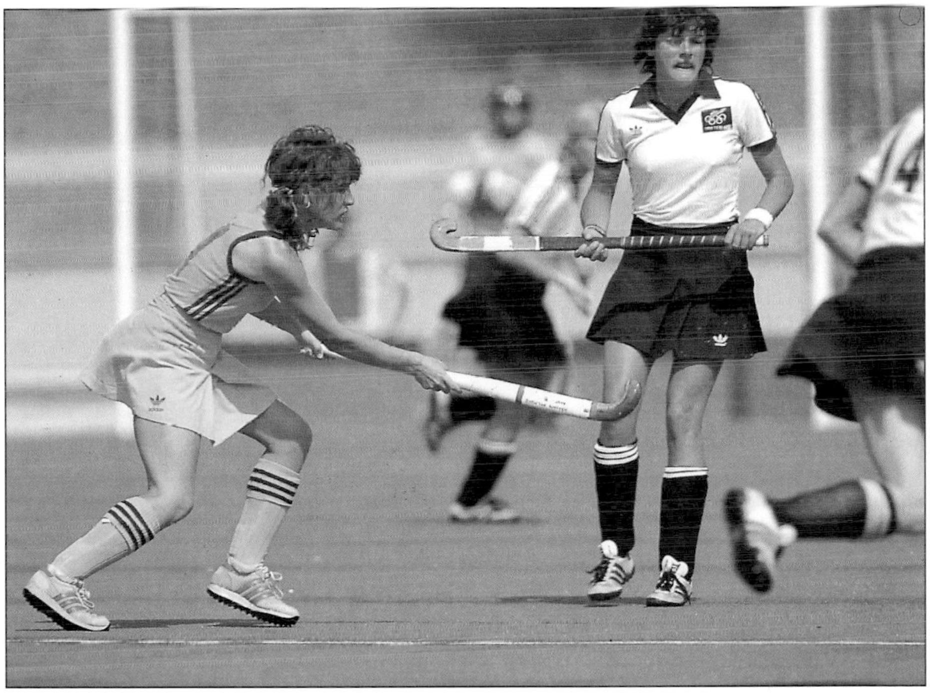

Hockey is a demanding sport that strengthens the legs, is beneficial to the heart and lungs, and significantly improves co-ordination.

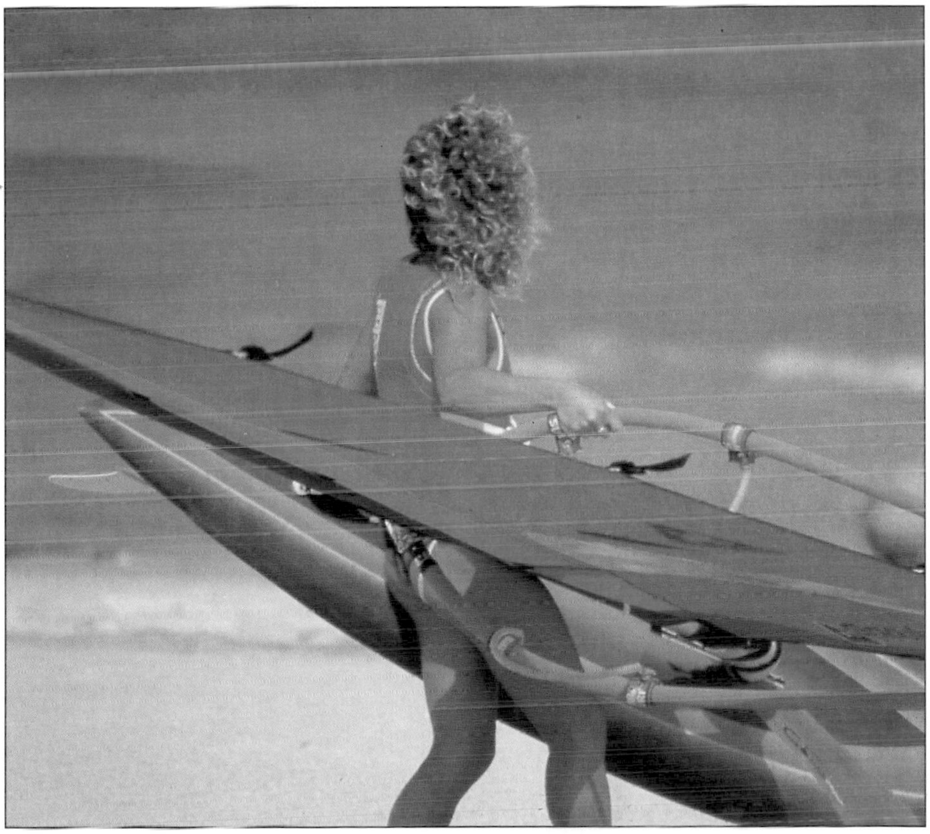

A good many water sports demand strength, stamina, and a fine sense of balance. Wind surfing is no exception to the rule.

EXERCISES FOR GENERAL FITNESS

This exercise routine helps to improve over-all fitness and should take you roughly 30 minutes to complete. Aim to do it three times a week and try to do extra aerobic exercise – such as swimming, walking or cycling – on the other days (aerobic exercises include any activity that can be done rhythmically and continually and that boosts the efficient uptake of oxygen). To warm up your muscles before exercising, either spend 2 minutes running up and down the stairs, walking briskly, cycling, or doing the special warm-up exercises outlined below.

WARM-UP EXERCISE A

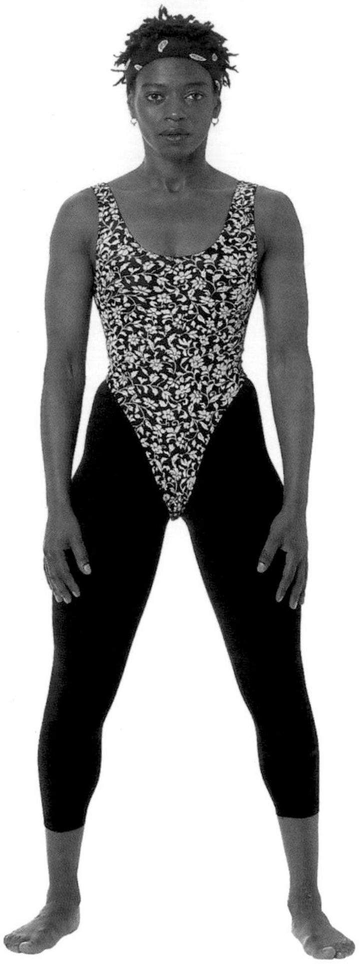

1 Stand upright with your feet apart and in line with your shoulders, with your arms hanging loosely at your sides and your shoulders down.

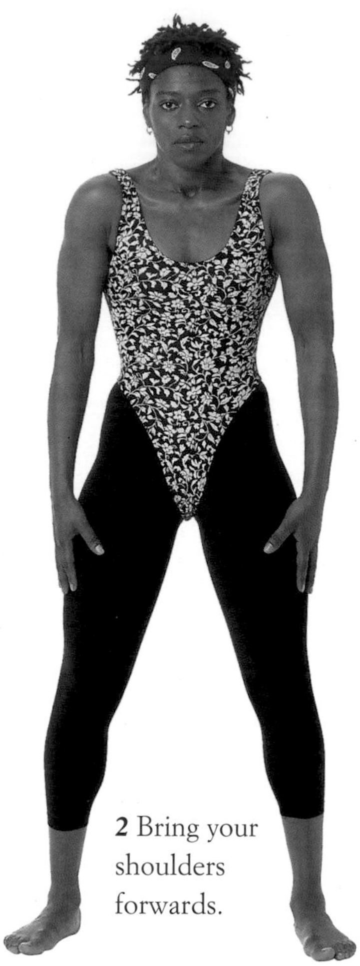

2 Bring your shoulders forwards.

❦ If you feel any pain – or experience anything other than the normal sensation of muscle fatigue – stop exercising. Always work out at your own pace; and skip exercise if you are ill.

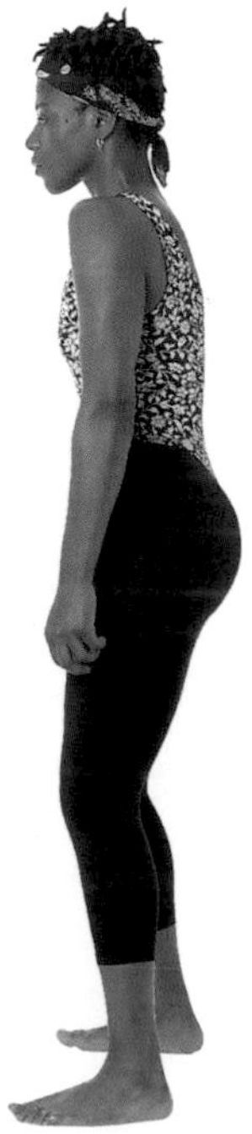

3 Raise them up high.

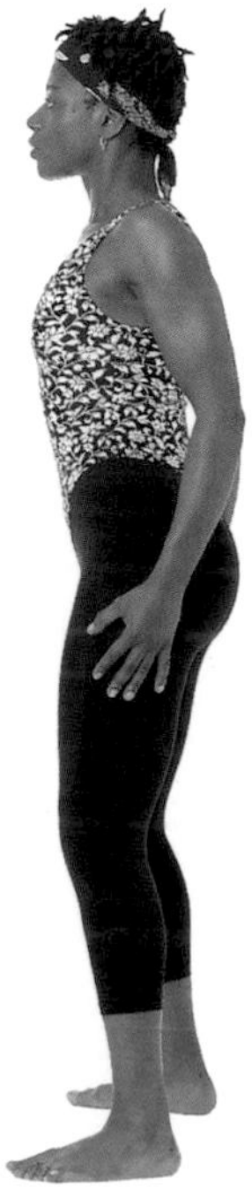

4 Move them back as far as possible, then back to the start position.

Toning Exercises	Repeats/Time Allowance
Warm-ups	5 minutes
Press-ups	10 repeats
Lying Flies	10 repeats
Reverse curls	10 repeats
Sit-ups	10 repeats
Squats	10 repeats
Cool Downs	3–5 minutes
Aerobic Exercise	20–30 minutes

The recommended 10 repeats are for beginners – you should aim to repeat each exercise 15 times. Start by doing this set of exercises twice a week, work up to three times a week and combine it with some other form of exercise – ideally aerobics – for the time suggested above.

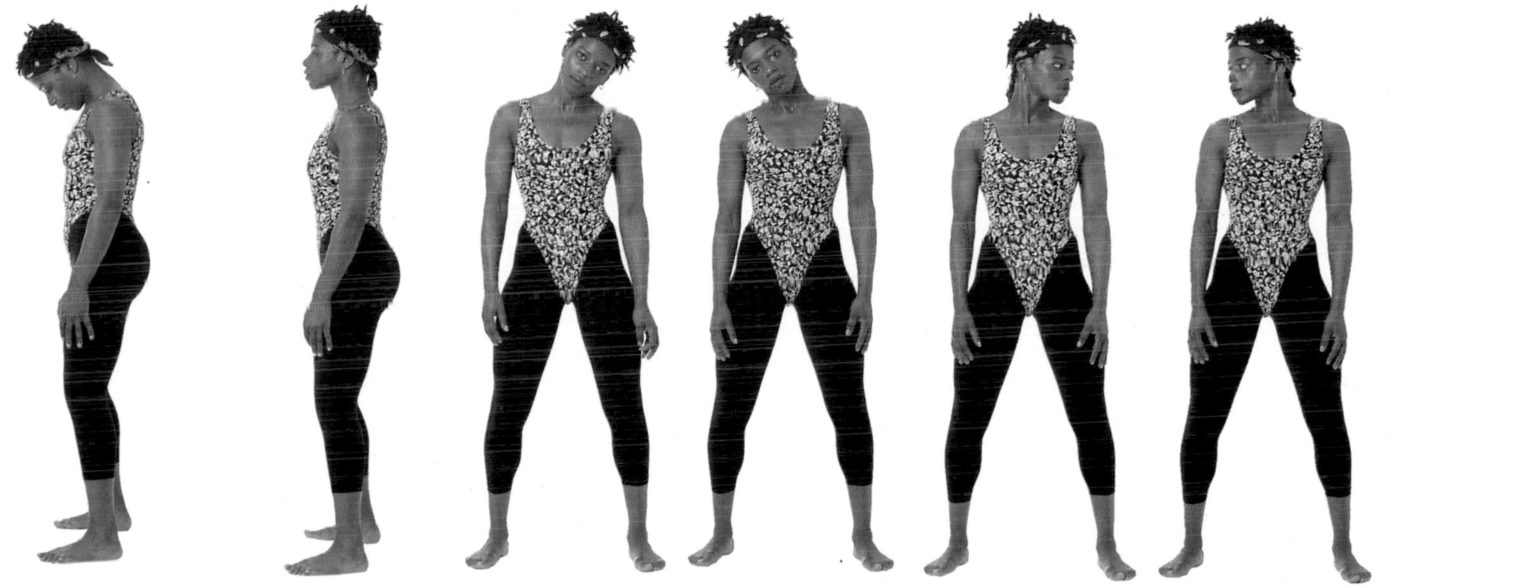

WARM-UP EXERCISE B

1 Maintain an upright posture as in Exercise A. Tip your head forwards so that your chin is almost resting in your chest.

2 Raise your head, stretching and lengthening your neck as you return to the upright position. Repeat four times.

3 Now tip your head to the left, keeping your shoulders down. Bring it back to the centre and then stretch and lengthen your neck.

4 Repeat step 3 but tip your head to the right side. Repeat four times on each side, remembering not to raise your shoulders.

5 Keep your head upright and turn so that you are looking over your left shoulder. Then face forwards again and stretch and lengthen your neck.

6 Now turn and look over your right shoulder. Face forwards again and stretch and lengthen your neck. Repeat steps 5 and 6 four times, then do the whole sequence again twice.

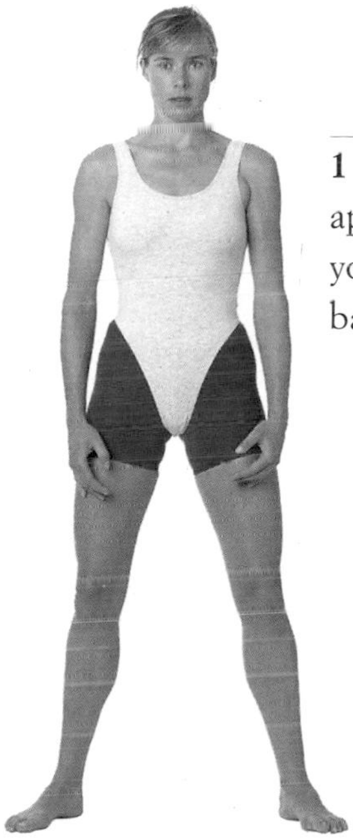

WARM-UP EXERCISE C

1 Stand with your feet apart; lean forwards from your hips keeping your back straight.

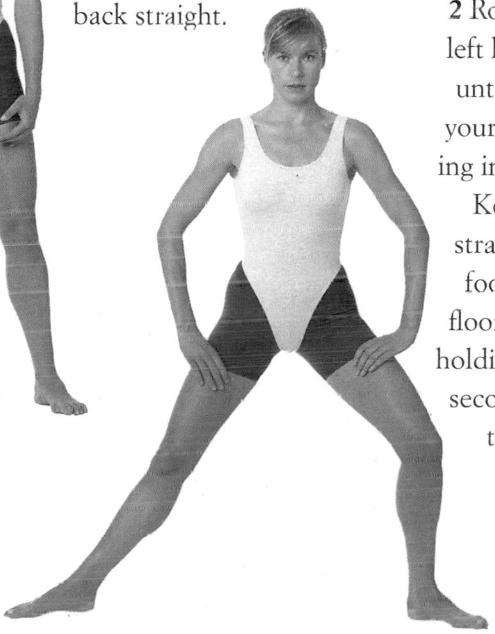

2 Rotate and bend your left leg out from the hip until your knee is over your left foot and pointing in the same direction. Keep your right leg straight and your right foot pressed into the floor. Repeat five times, holding the position for 5 seconds, swap leg positions and repeat.

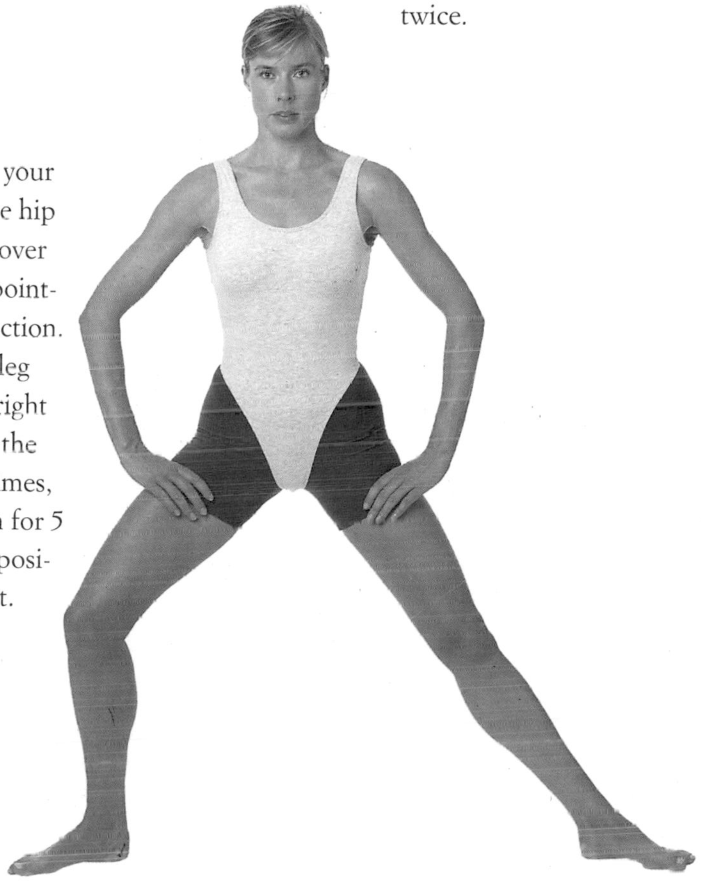

THE GENERAL EXERCISES

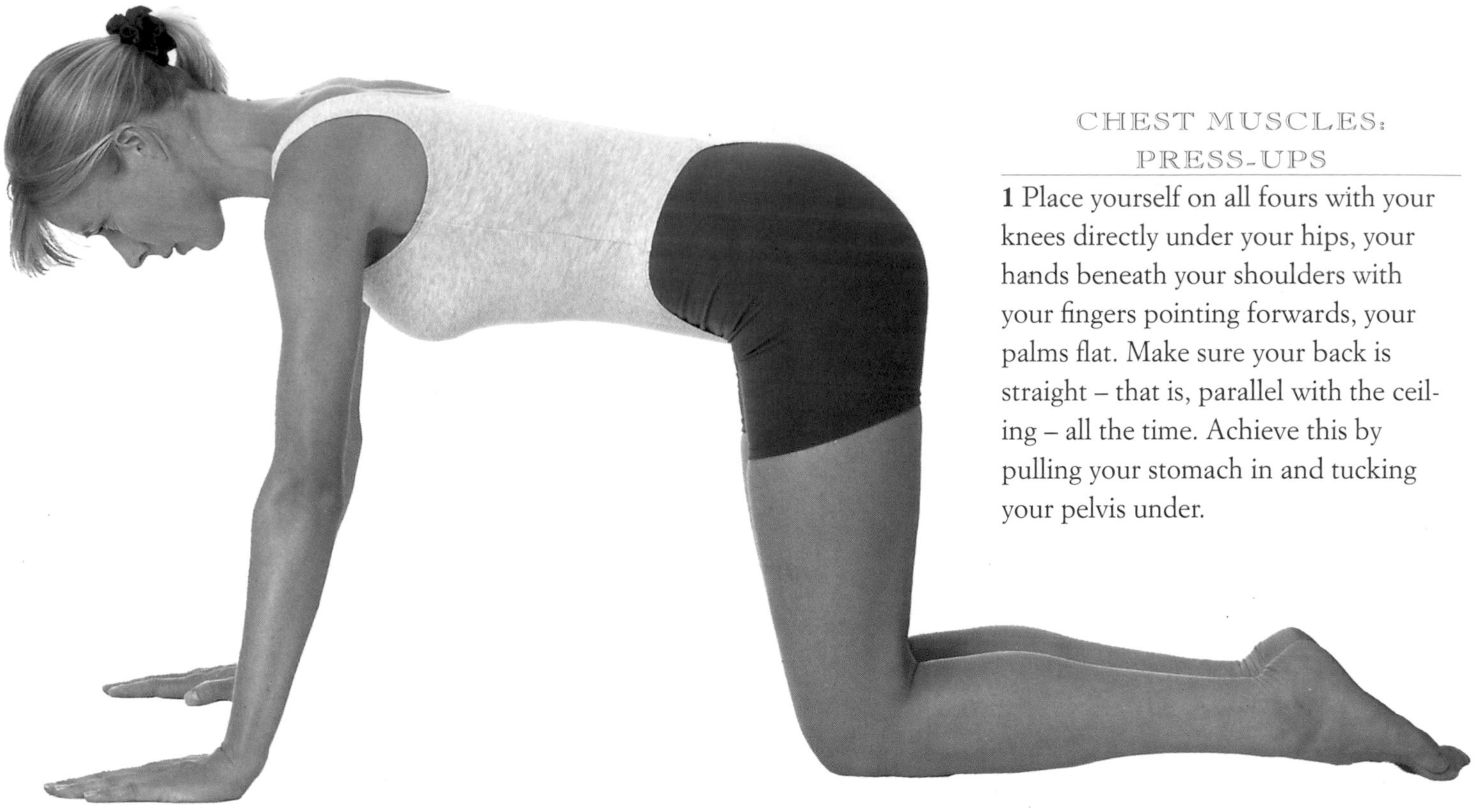

CHEST MUSCLES: PRESS-UPS

1 Place yourself on all fours with your knees directly under your hips, your hands beneath your shoulders with your fingers pointing forwards, your palms flat. Make sure your back is straight – that is, parallel with the ceiling – all the time. Achieve this by pulling your stomach in and tucking your pelvis under.

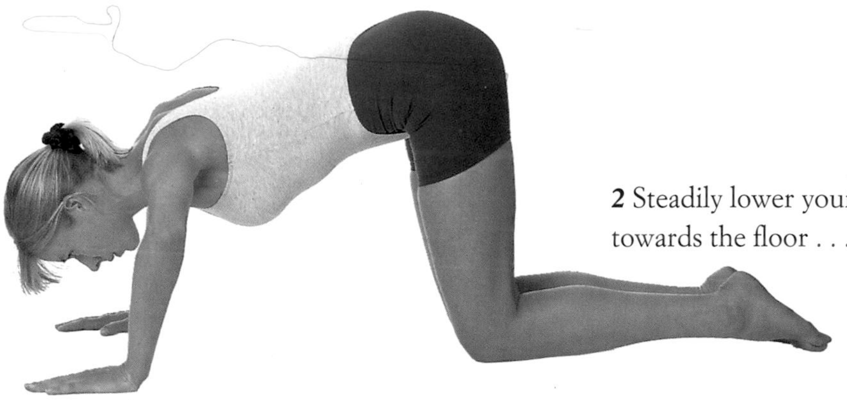

2 Steadily lower yourself – nose first – towards the floor . . .

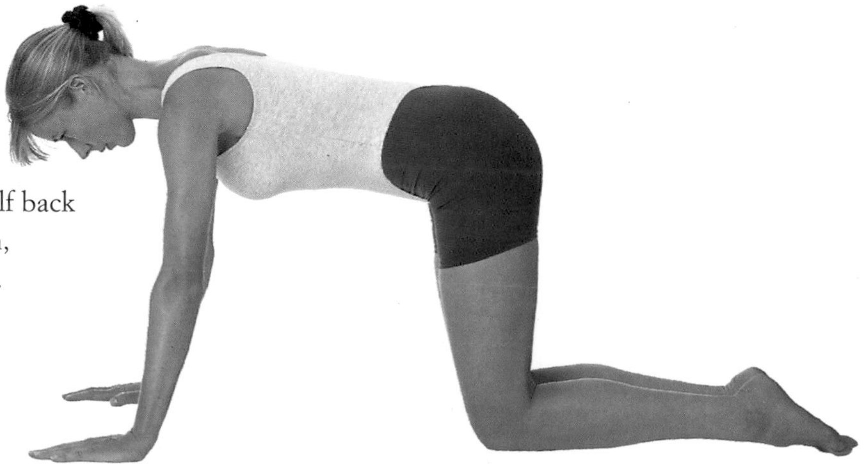

3 . . . then raise yourself back to the starting position, breathing in as you go.

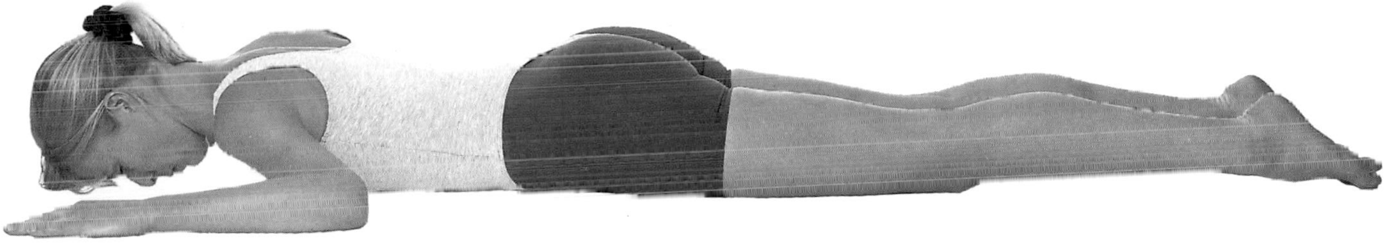

UPPER BACK MUSCLES: LYING FLIES

1 Lie on your front on the floor with your hips down, and keep your body relaxed. Rest your forehead on the floor, your arms out on each side at right angles to your body, elbows bent.

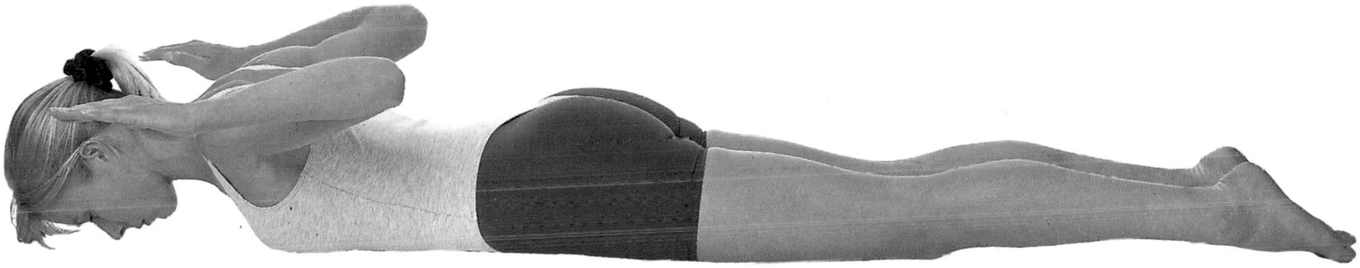

2 Keeping your elbows bent, steadily lift both arms, making sure they are parallel to the floor.

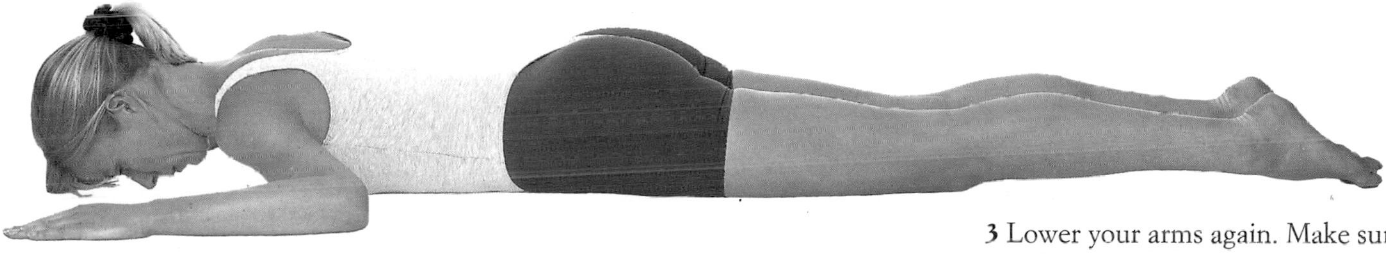

3 Lower your arms again. Make sure you do not pull your elbows back; keep them in line with your shoulders and keep your hips and feet in contact with the floor all the time.

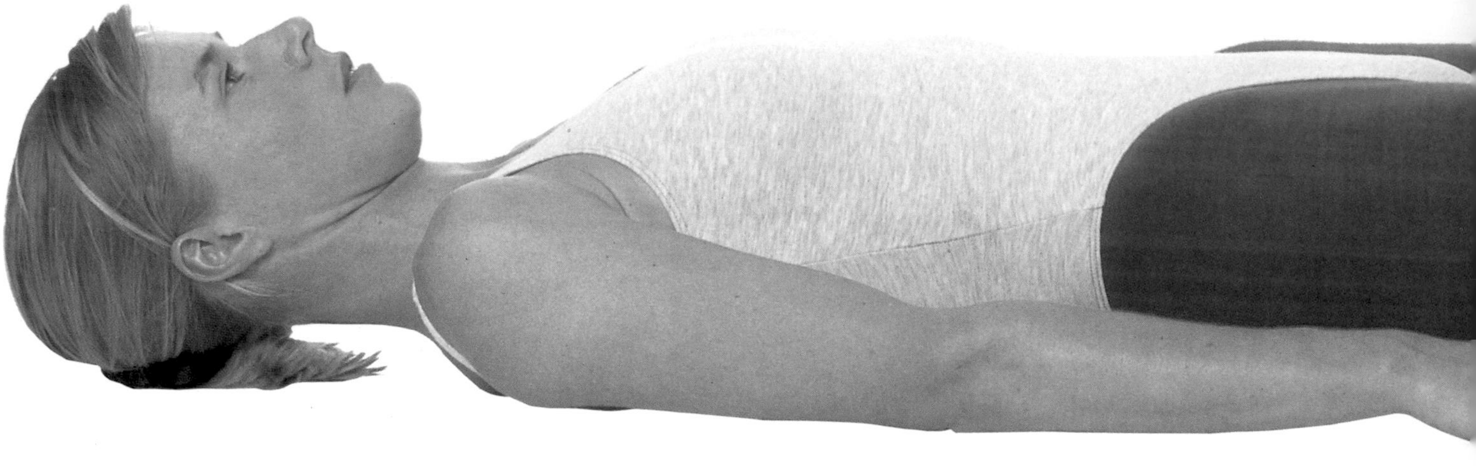

ABDOMINAL MUSCLES

When you do these exercises, keep your lower back pressed into the floor throughout and work slowly, with total control. In the Upper Abdominals exercise, lift your head and shoulders as one unit, never separately; roll up from the top of your head; imagine you are holding a peach between your chin and your chest and keep this gap constant throughout. Make sure your face muscles are relaxed all the time.

LOWER ABDOMINALS: REVERSE CURLS

1 Lie flat on your back on the floor, arms by your sides, palms flat on the floor beside you.

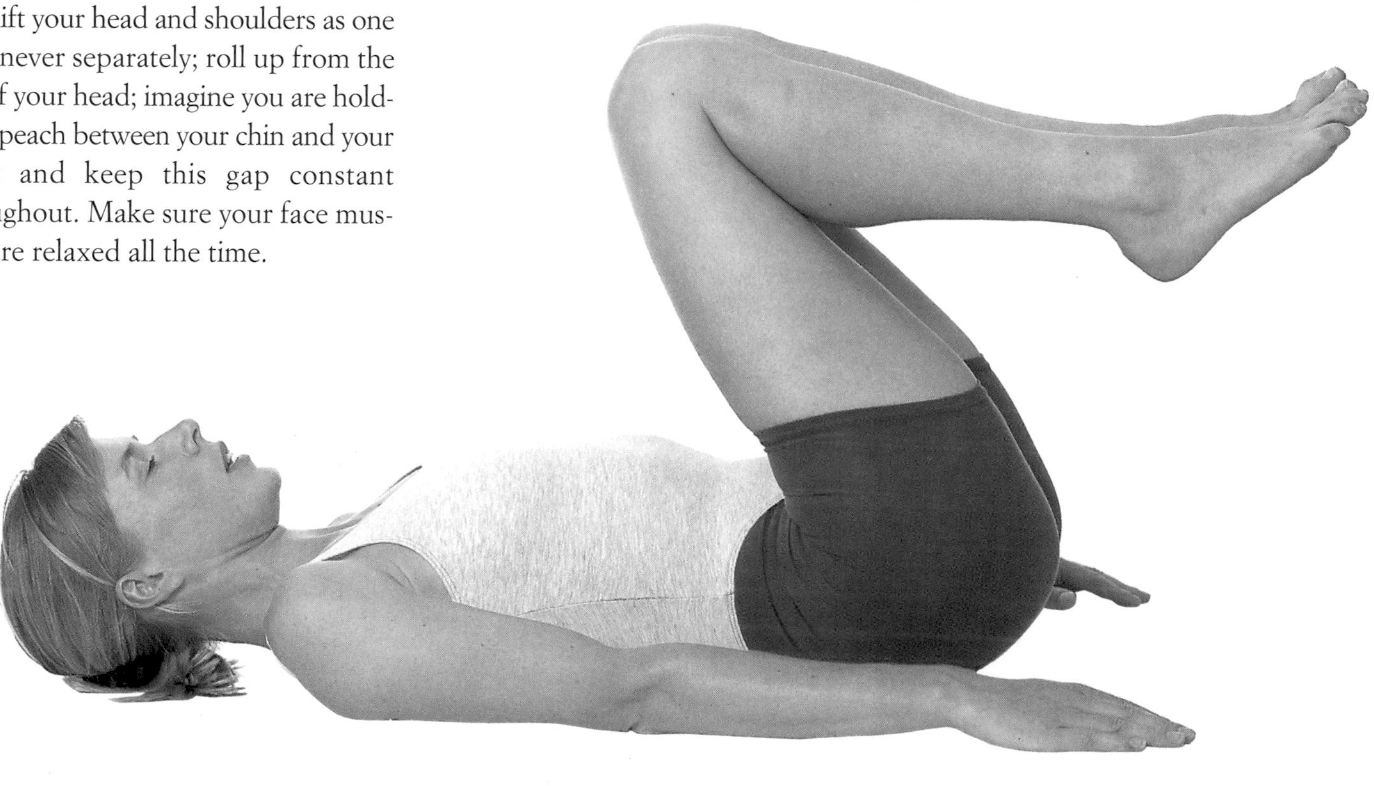

2 While keeping your arms and hands flat on the floor, bring your knees in towards your chest one at a time, and once there, keep both knees together in the bent position.

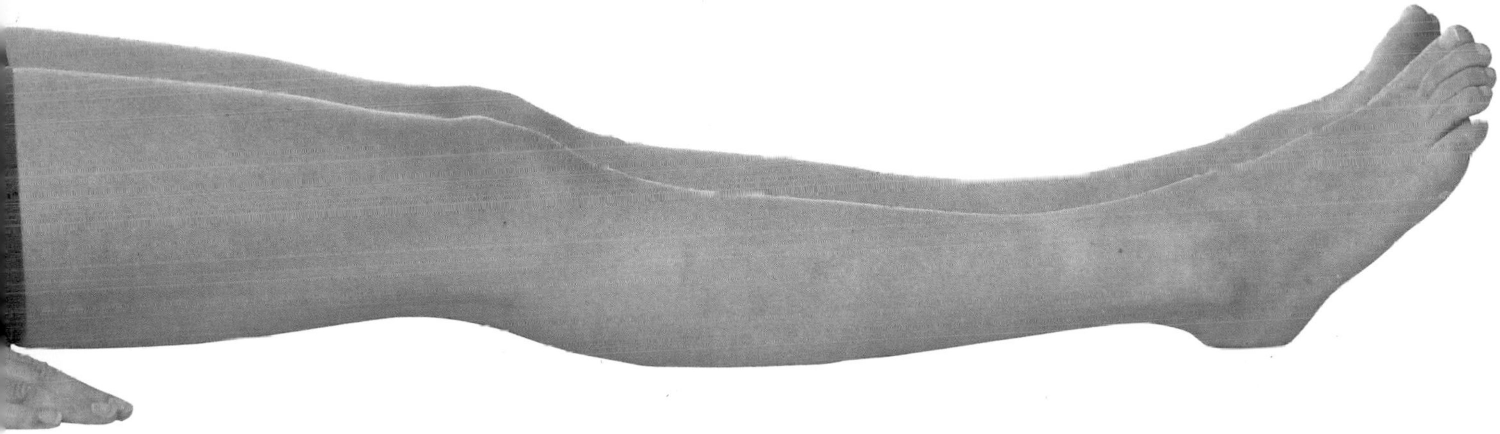

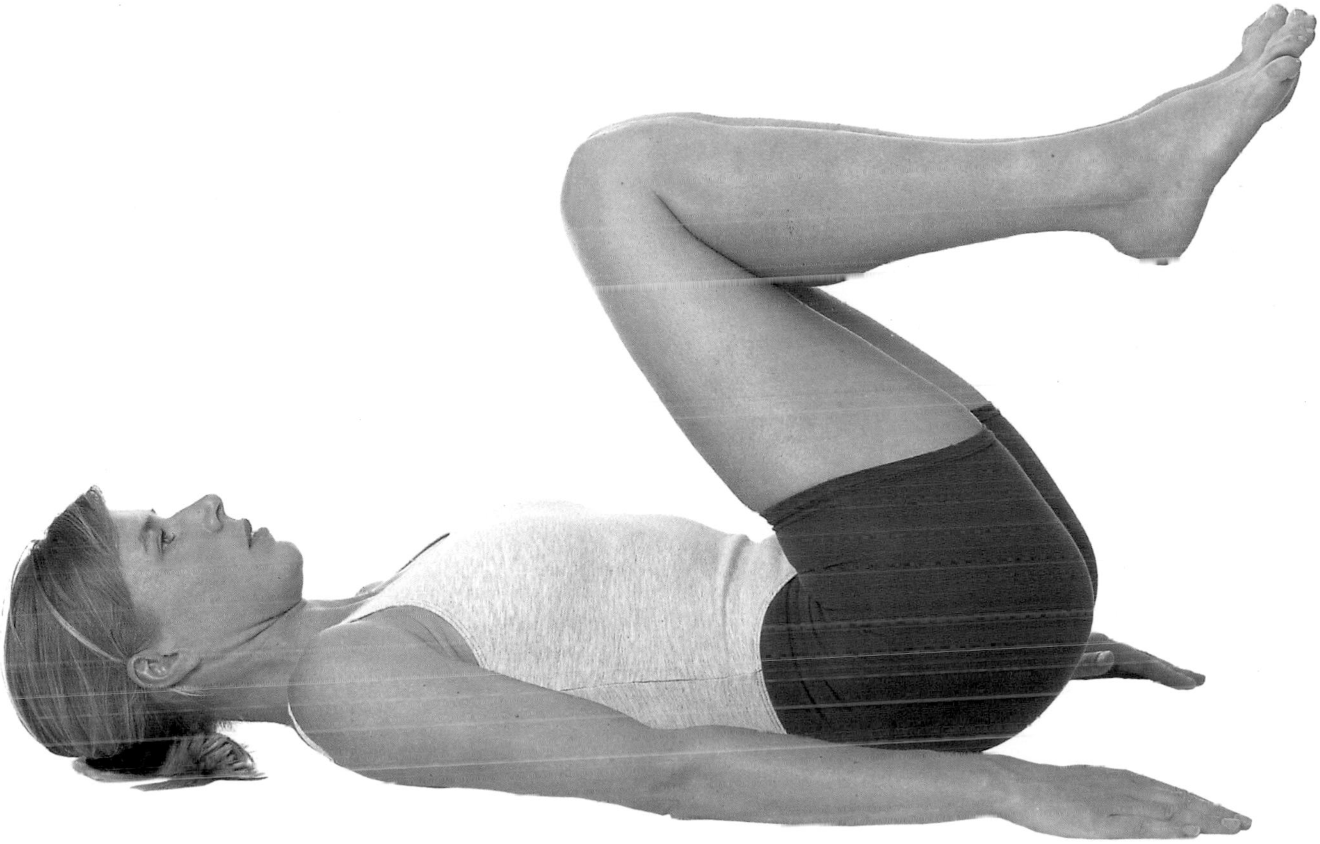

3 Breathe in and, keeping your spine pressed into the floor, pull in your abdominal muscles while at the same time curling up your coccyx (tail bone) to bring your knees closer to your chest. Keep your feet relaxed throughout. Lower your body to the starting position, exhaling as you go down.

UPPER ABDOMINALS: SIT UPS

1 Lying flat on the floor with your arms by your side, palms flat on the floor, bend your knees and keep your feet flat on the floor, a little distance apart in line with your hips.

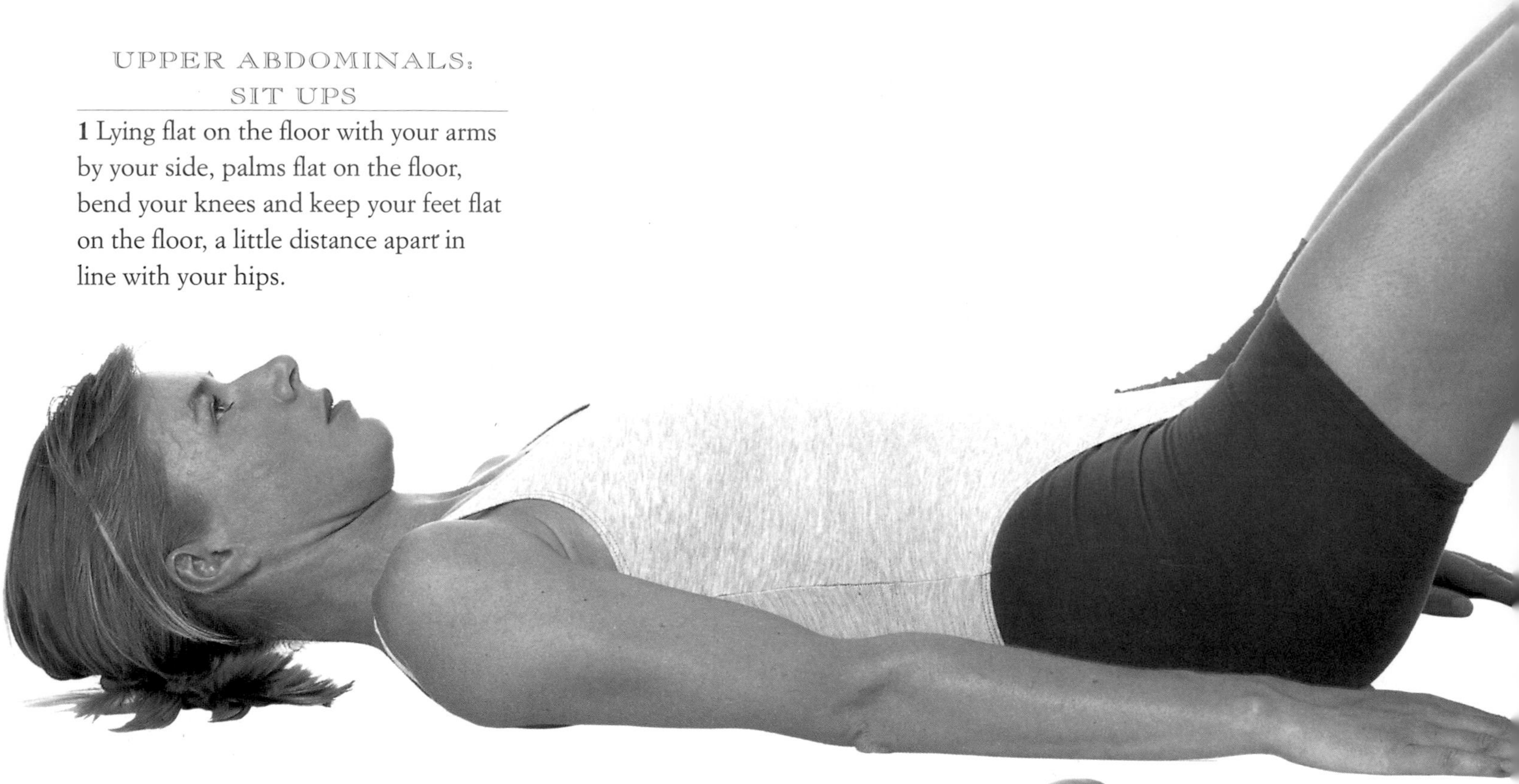

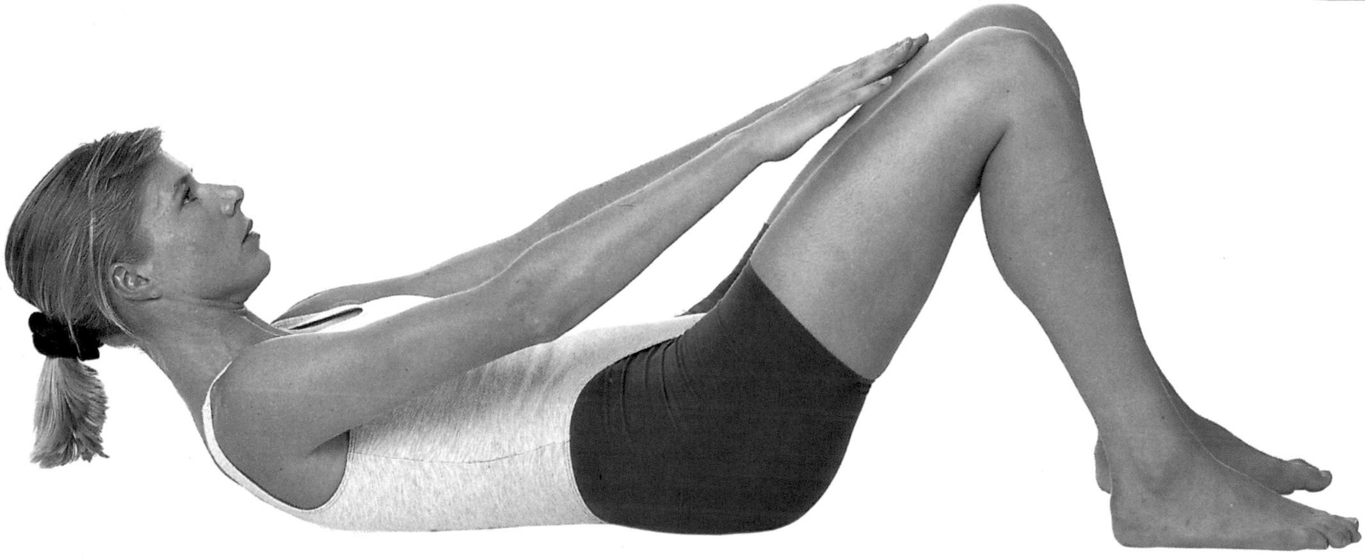

2 Lift your head and shoulders – inhaling as you move up – and push your fingertips towards your knees, keeping your arms straight.

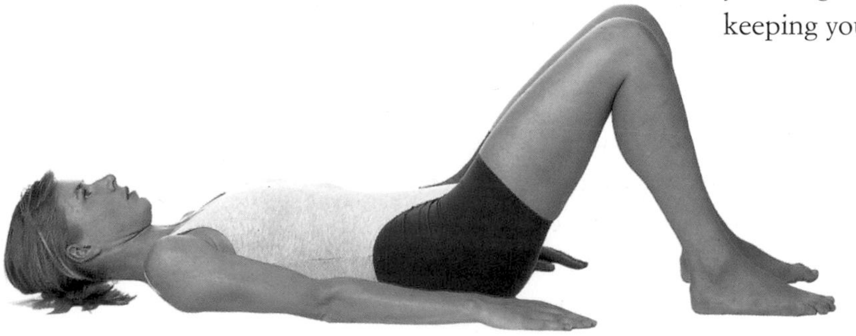

3 Lower your body back to the starting position, exhaling as you go down. Repeat the movement.

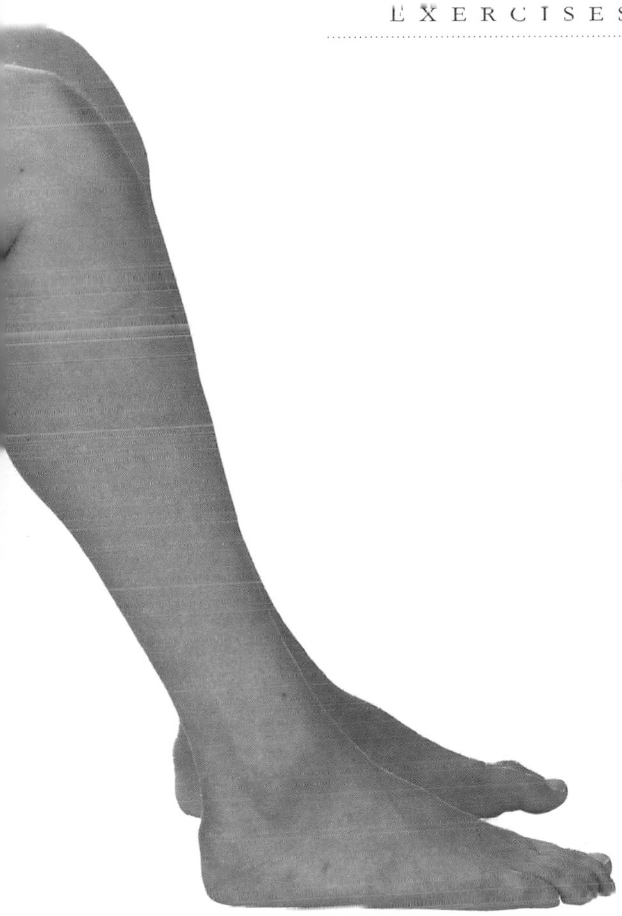

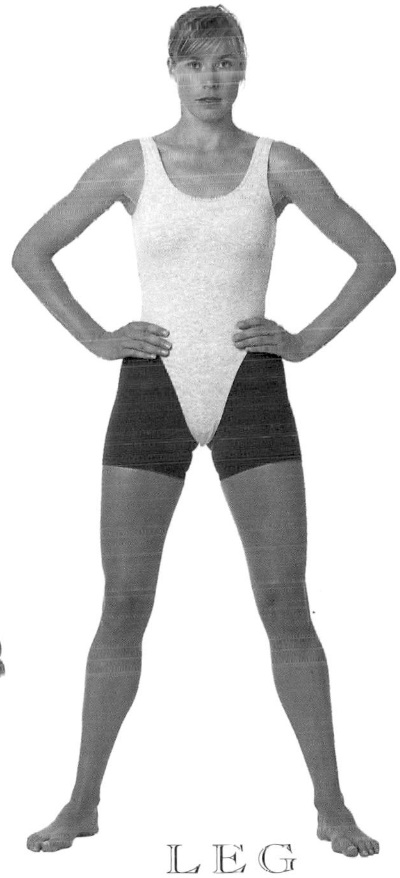

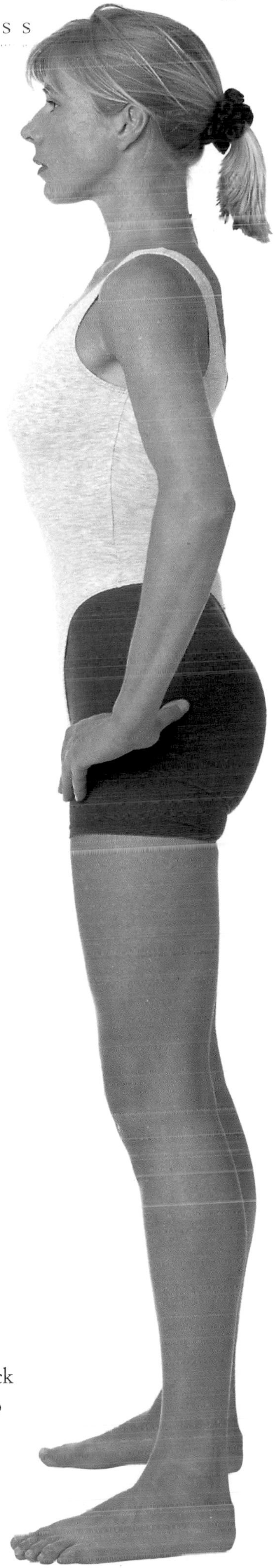

LEG MUSCLES: SQUATS

1 Stand up straight with your feet a little wider than shoulder-width apart. If you stand on tiptoe, this exercise tones your calf muscles and your quadriceps, the muscles on the front of your thighs; if you angle your toes slightly outwards while on tiptoe, it benefits your inner thighs.

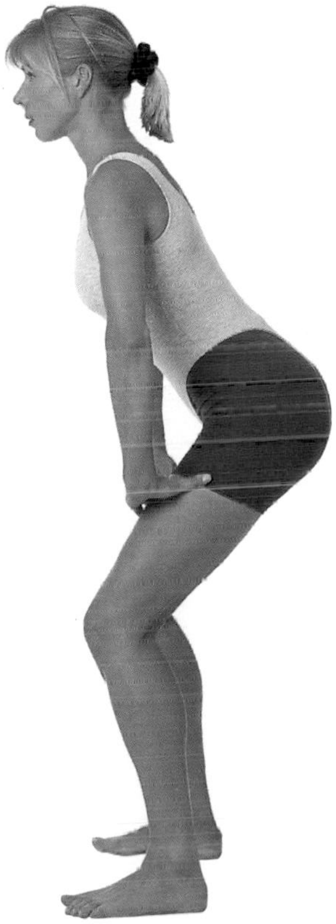

2 Resting your hands on the front of your thighs and keeping your arms straight, steadily bend your legs until you reach a squatting position, exhaling as you go down.

3 Then, inhale as you rise steadily back to the starting position. When you do this exercise, it is important to keep your back straight and your knees flexible. Do not let your knees bend further forward than your toes.

Sports Activities

Team sports and work-outs at the gym are not only fun, they also give you the chance to add to your exercise quota for the week, and therefore reach your self-improvement goals that much faster. The benefits of taking part in specific sports and of working out are given here.

BADMINTON:

Aerobic; improves joint flexibility, stamina, leg and shoulder tone and strength; 30–40 minutes continuous play burns up around 200–800 calories.

GOLF:

Improves arm, shoulder and leg tone, and strength (you walk four to five miles when you do a round of golf).

JOGGING:

Aerobic, improves stamina, leg strength and tone; an hour's jogging burns up 200–350 calories. If you think that jogging or running will suit your new active way of life, take the standard precautions before you start: check with your doctor and, as with all aerobic exercise, increase the pace gradually; always wear the right trainers (and support bandages if your joints are weak).

TENNIS:

Aerobic; boosts stamina and suppleness; strengthens and tones your shoulders, forearms, calves and thighs; play energetically (ideally twice a week) for an hour and you will burn up around 300–400 calories.

BRISK WALKING:

Aerobic; strengthens and tones your legs.

CYCLING:

Aerobic; builds stamina; tones your legs.

SKIPPING:

Aerobic; boosts stamina, strength and leg tone. Start by doing 3 skipping sets for 30 seconds a time with a 5-minute break after each set; build up to skipping for 2 minutes with a 10-minute break and also increase the repetitions.

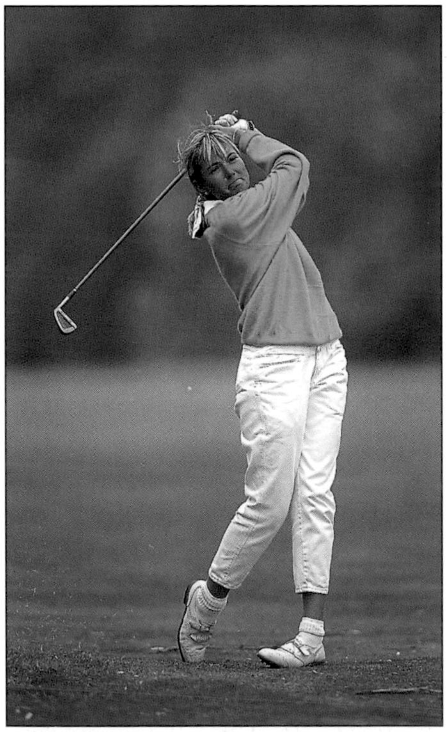

Golf is a sport that particularly benefits shoulders, arms, and legs. Playing a round involves a good deal of walking.

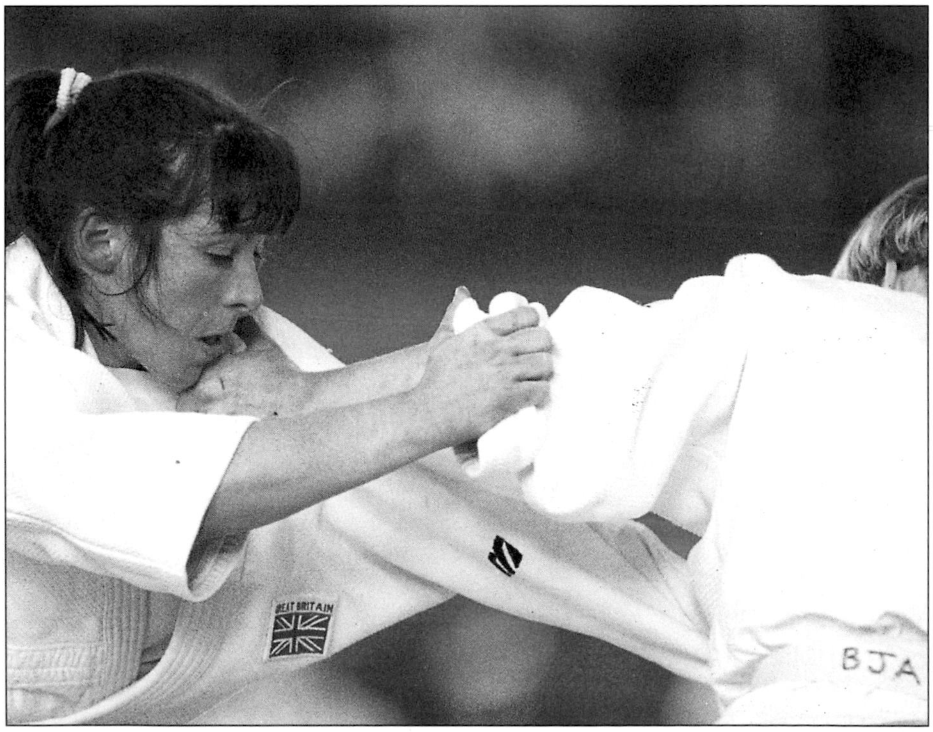

Judo is a body contact sport and one of the major martial arts. It requires a good deal of strength, agility, and physical courage.

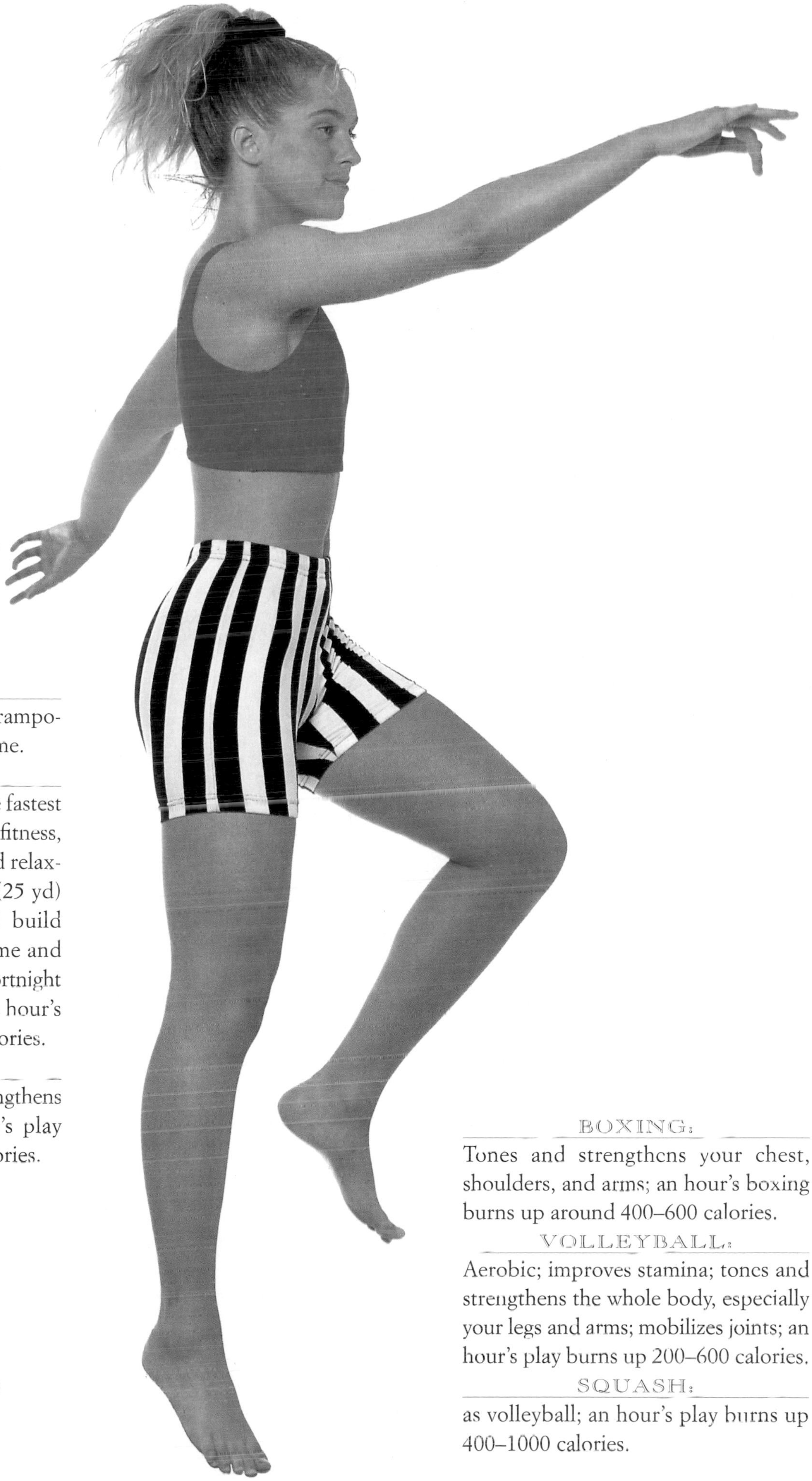

Gym-based Benefits

Aerobics: classes combine exercise with constant movement; they are fast fat-burners and ideal if you are after quick results.

Circuit, cross, resistance, or weight training: aerobic; increase stamina and strength; an hour of circuit training burns up between 350–550 calories.

Step classes: aerobic; improves stamina; tones and strengthens your lower torso; an hour-long class burns up between 500–800 calories.

Yoga: improves posture; tones, strengthens, and relaxes the body; loosens joints; an hour of yoga burns up about 200 calories.

REBOUNDING:

Aerobic; bounding on a mini trampoline is a fun way to get fit at home.

SWIMMING:

Aerobic; swimming is one of the fastest (and best) ways to boost overall fitness, muscle tone, joint flexibility, and relaxation. Do 4 lengths of a 25 m (25 yd) pool, rest for a minute and build endurance by reducing rest time and increasing swim time; within a fortnight you will be noticeably fitter; an hour's breaststroke burns 500–800 calories.

FOOTBALL:

Aerobic; improves stamina; strengthens and tones your legs; an hour's play burns up around 250–1000 calories.

Help for PMS

Exercise is the last thing you feel like doing when you are pre-menstrual. But if you do push yourself now, you will relieve the symptoms. If you cannot face an aerobics class, go for a swim; this will ease pre-menstrual cramp and put you in a better mood.

BOXING:

Tones and strengthens your chest, shoulders, and arms; an hour's boxing burns up around 400–600 calories.

VOLLEYBALL:

Aerobic; improves stamina; tones and strengthens the whole body, especially your legs and arms; mobilizes joints; an hour's play burns up 200–600 calories.

SQUASH:

as volleyball; an hour's play burns up 400–1000 calories.

Body Shape

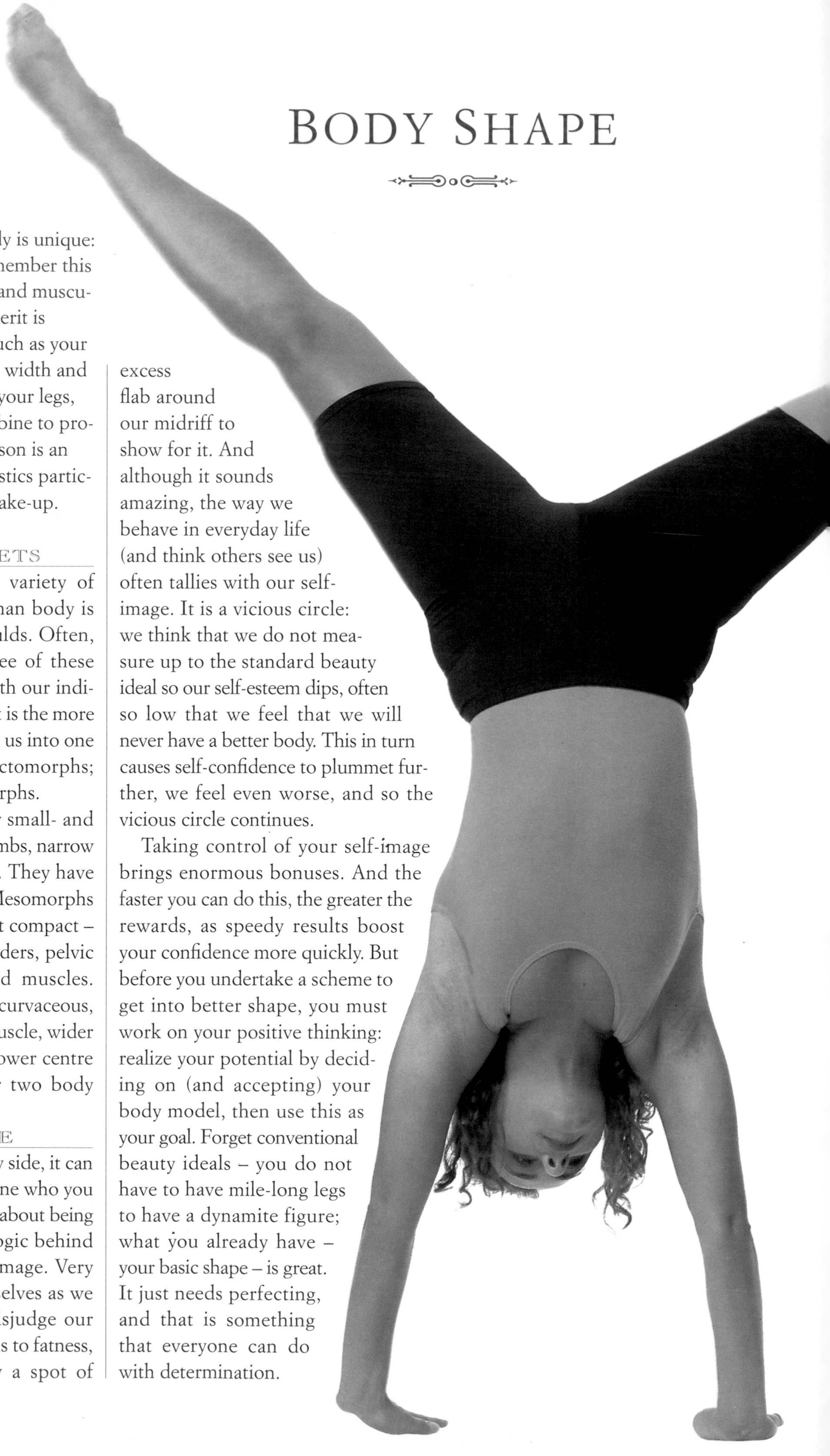

The shape of your body is unique: it is important to remember this because the basic skeletal and muscular form that you inherit is unchangeable. Features such as your height, foot size, shoulder width and the length and shape of your legs, nose, fingers and toes combine to produce a whole. Each person is an individual, with characteristics particular to their genetic make-up.

Body Brackets

Although we come in a variety of shapes and sizes, the human body is cast from three basic moulds. Often, features from two or three of these body types are jumbled with our individual characteristics, but it is the more dominant features that slot us into one of the following groups: ectomorphs; mesomorphs, and endomorphs.

Ectomorphs are usually small- and slender-framed with long limbs, narrow shoulders, hips and joints. They have little muscle or body fat. Mesomorphs have medium to large – but compact – frames with broader shoulders, pelvic girdle and well-developed muscles. Endomorphs are naturally curvaceous, with more body fat than muscle, wider hips, shorter limbs and a lower centre of gravity than the other two body types.

Self-Image

If you are a bit on the tubby side, it can be annoying to hear someone who you think is poker-thin whining about being overweight. But there is logic behind this that stems from self-image. Very few of us actually see ourselves as we really are. We tend to misjudge our bodies with sweeping claims to fatness, even when we have only a spot of excess flab around our midriff to show for it. And although it sounds amazing, the way we behave in everyday life (and think others see us) often tallies with our self-image. It is a vicious circle: we think that we do not measure up to the standard beauty ideal so our self-esteem dips, often so low that we feel that we will never have a better body. This in turn causes self-confidence to plummet further, we feel even worse, and so the vicious circle continues.

Taking control of your self-image brings enormous bonuses. And the faster you can do this, the greater the rewards, as speedy results boost your confidence more quickly. But before you undertake a scheme to get into better shape, you must work on your positive thinking: realize your potential by deciding on (and accepting) your body model, then use this as your goal. Forget conventional beauty ideals – you do not have to have mile-long legs to have a dynamite figure; what you already have – your basic shape – is great. It just needs perfecting, and that is something that everyone can do with determination.

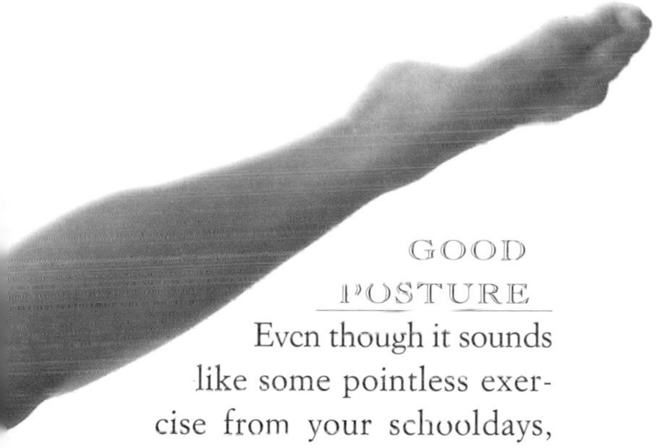

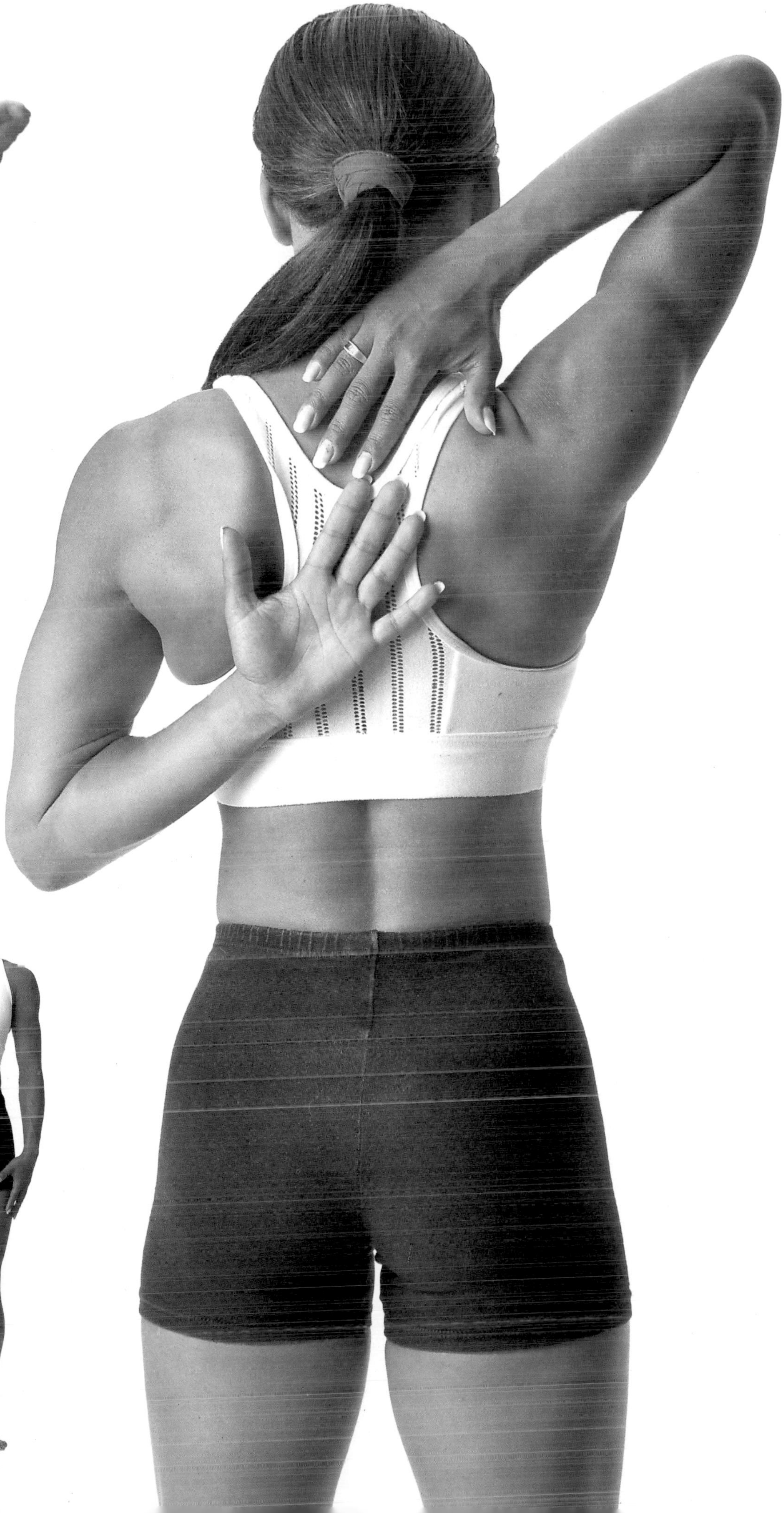

GOOD POSTURE

Even though it sounds like some pointless exercise from your schooldays, there is real wisdom in the old dictum "head up, shoulders back, bottom in". The difference that good posture makes to the look of our bodies is enormous, mainly because when we are standing properly our abdominal muscles are in their correct supporting role and the whole body is aligned so it looks leaner and taller. Good posture is also helpful to our mental and physical health; some alternative therapies (such as the Alexander Technique) are based on the principle of correct posture because it can ease back pain, stress, and even headaches.

Posture Exercise

Stand in front of a mirror, try these exercises and see what they do for the shape of your body:

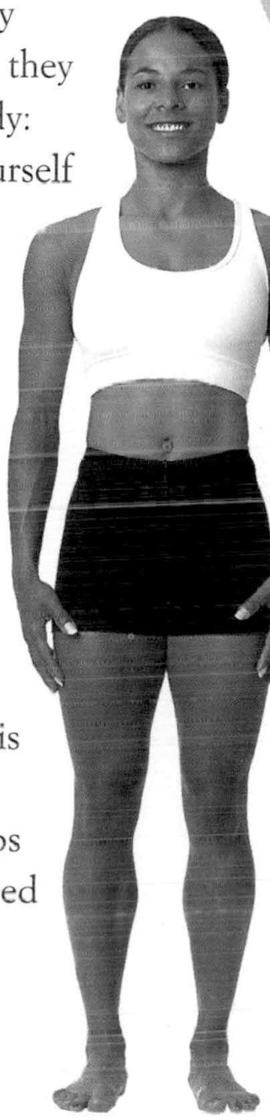

1 Do this exercise facing yourself first, then turn so you are sideways on:
Lift your head up and lengthen your spine.
Tuck in your chin and your bottom.
Bring your shoulders back and down.

2 Now stand with your legs slightly apart.
Check whether your weight is evenly spread.
Keep your shoulders and hips level and your weight balanced between the heel and ball of each foot.

Trouble Spots

Very few people are able to say honestly that they are totally happy with their body. Everyone has at least one gripe – if it is not big feet, it is thin hair or knobbly knees. All these perceived "flaws" can be improved or disguised, but as anyone who has ever tried (and failed) to move the fat that sits on strategic points such as hips, thighs, stomachs, and buttocks knows, it is much easier to hide the flaws than to tackle them. But it is possible to alter your outline with a combination of diet and exercise.

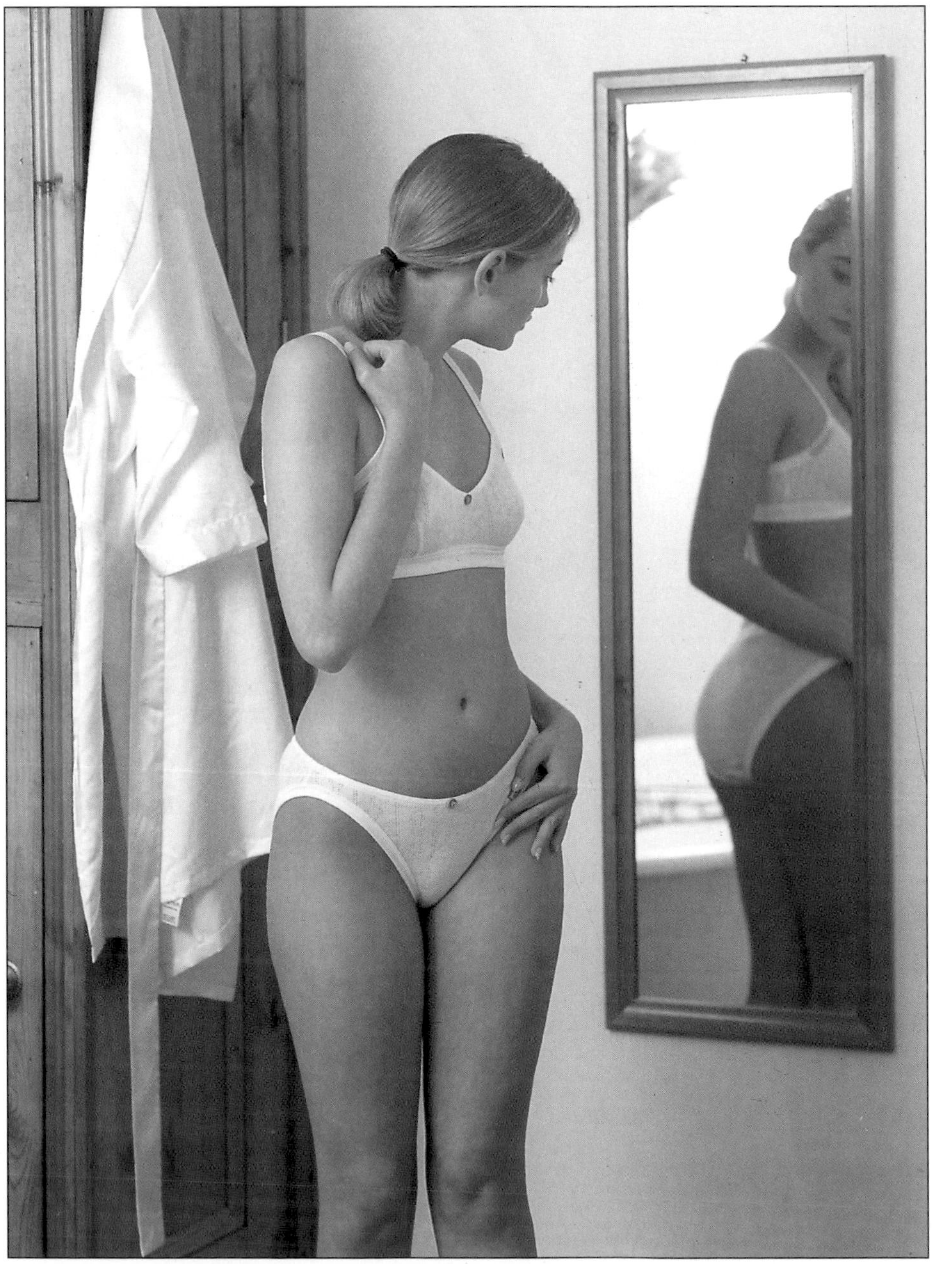

The best way to assess your figure is to stand in front of a full-length mirror. Be honest with yourself, and look for areas that need improving.

Finding and Improving Your True Form

Step 1: Confront Your Body
Go on, be brave. Strip to your underwear, stand in front of a mirror and have a good look at your body. Take your time and be tough but realistic. You may have disliked your thighs since you were 16 – and they will probably never be those of a super-model – but if you look hard enough you might just find that they are not as bad as you have always thought they were, and that improving them is not going to be that hard after all.

Step 2: Put Your Complaints in Writing
Note down all the things that irk you (and that you can do something about) as well as those that you like or do not mind. Then go through your list of dislikes, ticking the things that you really want to do something about. Also, make a mental note to start appreciating your good points: the more you focus on them the less you will notice the not-so-good zones.

Step 3: Action Checklist
Now, add a set of action points under the problem zones you have listed. If you want to firm up your arms for that sleeveless sundress you have been unable to wear for a decade of summers, make notes like this:

Flabby Upper Arms

- *Do Basic Exercises*
- *Check Diet*
- *Exfoliate/Moisturize*

Finally, add your goal(s) and your deadline to the top of the list and put it somewhere where you are going to see it frequently.

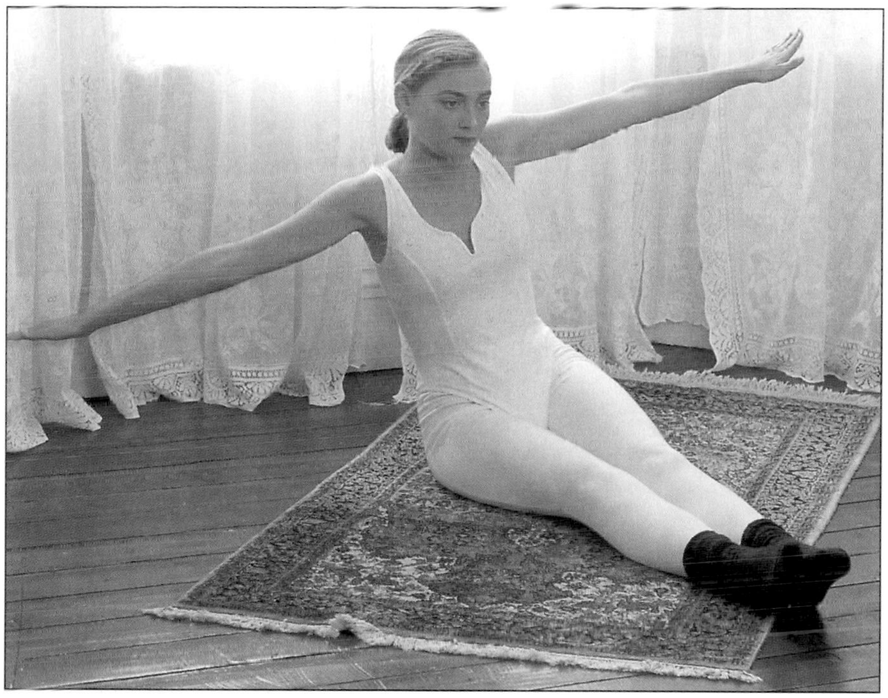

Two Quick Thigh-toners

If you do not have time to do a full exercise routine, grab 10 minutes in the morning.

Outer Thighs: sit on the floor with your legs straight out in front and hold your arms out to the sides as shown left. Roll sideways on to your bottom – go right over on to your outer thigh and then roll right over on to the other thigh.

Do this twenty times.

Inner Thighs: stand upright and consciously tighten – and hold – your buttock muscles for a slow count of 5. Repeat with your thigh muscles and then your calf muscles.

COMMON PROBLEMS

Any of the following can be discouraging, but remember – each problem has a solution.

Slack Stomachs

Our stomachs become flabby when the abdominal muscles slacken; this usually happens through lack of exercise. Your abdomen extends from just under the bustline to the groin, and it is packed with muscles that criss-cross to form a wall to hold the abdominal contents in place – a bit like a corset. Exercise is not the only way to keep your stomach flat: weight is also important and the long-term answer is diet and exercise.

Thunder Thighs

Thigh size and tone can certainly be altered with the right diet, correct body care and regular exercise. Sports such as cycling, skiing, tennis, squash, and riding (a great inner-muscle firmer) will tone your thighs, as will weight training for specific areas of the body.

Large Bottoms

There are three large muscles in our buttocks: *gluteus maximus, medius,* and *minimus*. These create the shape, but not the size, of our rear ends. It is the tone of these muscles and the fatty tissue around them that gives us the bottoms we have. The good news is that buttock muscles respond well to exercise, which means that any effort you put into bottom-toning exercises will be rewarded quite quickly.

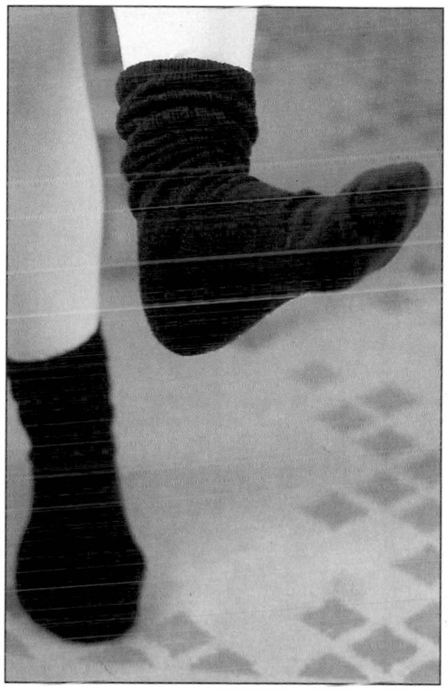

Ankle Exercises

Whenever you remember move your ankles around in a clockwise motion ten times, then repeat anticlockwise.

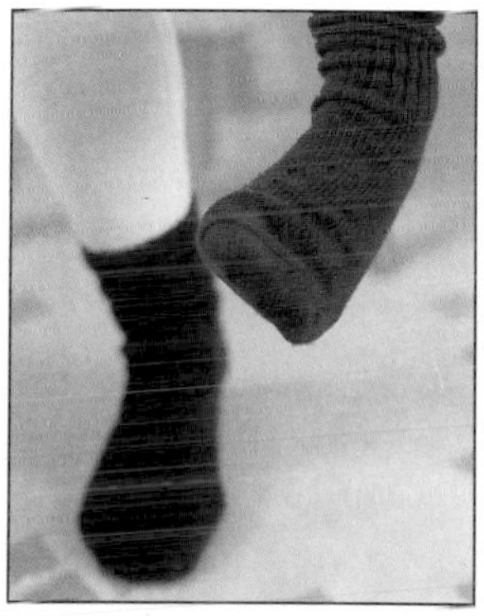

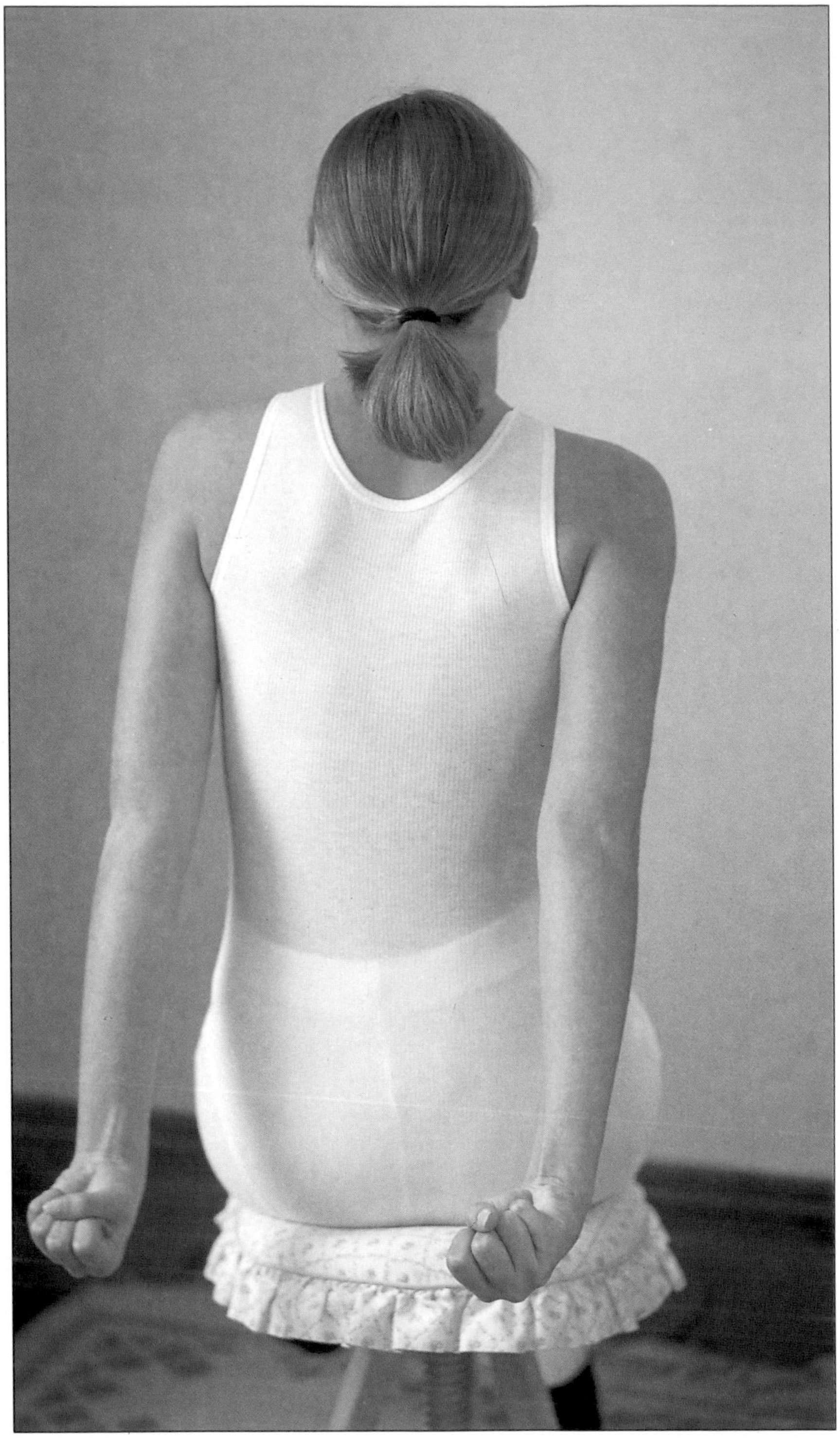

Flabby Arm Fixer

To firm up flabby arms, add this exercise to your daily exercise routine, or spend five minutes doing it twice a day. Sit on a chair holding your hands in loose fists, and, with your arms extended out behind, make downwards punching movements backwards and forwards.

Slack Upper Arms

Our arms do not really change shape much during our lives, unless we lose or gain a lot of weight. Muscle tone is the main problem, but, as in the case of thighs, exercise and specific weight training will tone up and re-shape flabby arms; very often, any changes in body shape that happen through exercise and diet are noticeable most quickly on your upper arms.

Droopy Breasts

Breast shape and size only really change when our weight swings dramatically, or during pregnancy, breast-feeding, menstruation, or if taking oral contraceptives. Gravity is the bust's enemy, especially if the breasts are not given proper support, because it literally drags the breasts down and slackens their tone. Although the breasts are supported by suspension ligaments, they do not contain any muscle (the milk glands are buffered by protective fatty tissue) so you cannot noticeably reverse lost tone. However, if you exercise the pectoral muscles beneath your armpits, you will give your breasts a firmer base and more uplift.

Thick Ankles

Trim and slender ankles that seem set to snap with every step are a great asset. But if you are not blessed with these, or if your ankles tend to become stiff and puffy from fluid retention, you need to master the art of deception and brush up on some ankle improving exercises.

Assess the flexibility of your ankles by sitting on a chair or stool with your feet on the floor and, while keeping your heel down, pull the rest of your foot up as far as it will go: if the distance between your foot and floor measures 12–15 cm (5–6 in) your joint flexibility is good; if it is between 10–12 cm (4–5 in) it is fair; and if it is less than that, your joint flexibility is poor.

The following exercises will help to improve the muscles that support your breasts.

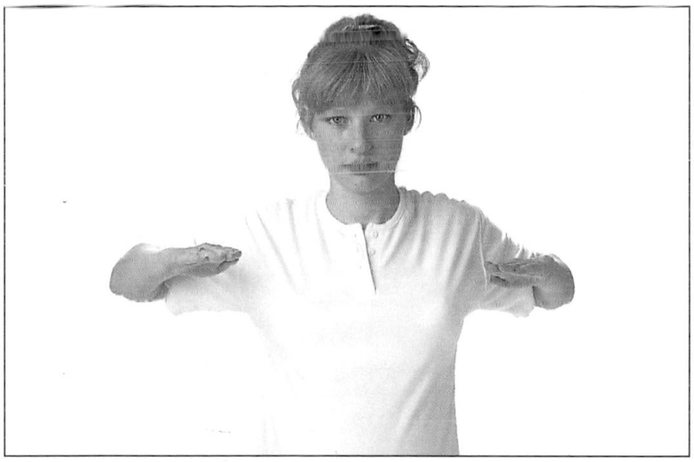

1 Stand erect and bend your arms at the elbows, holding your arms horizontally in front of your chest, with your fingertips touching. Move your elbows back as far as they will go, with a firm, quick movement. Return to the starting position and repeat as many times as you wish.

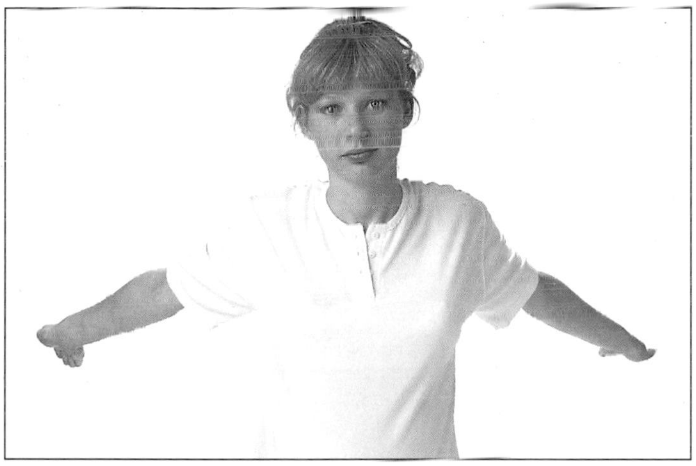

2 Resume the position you took in step 1, but this time, as you move your elbows back, straighten your arms, so that you fling them behind you. Repeat several times.

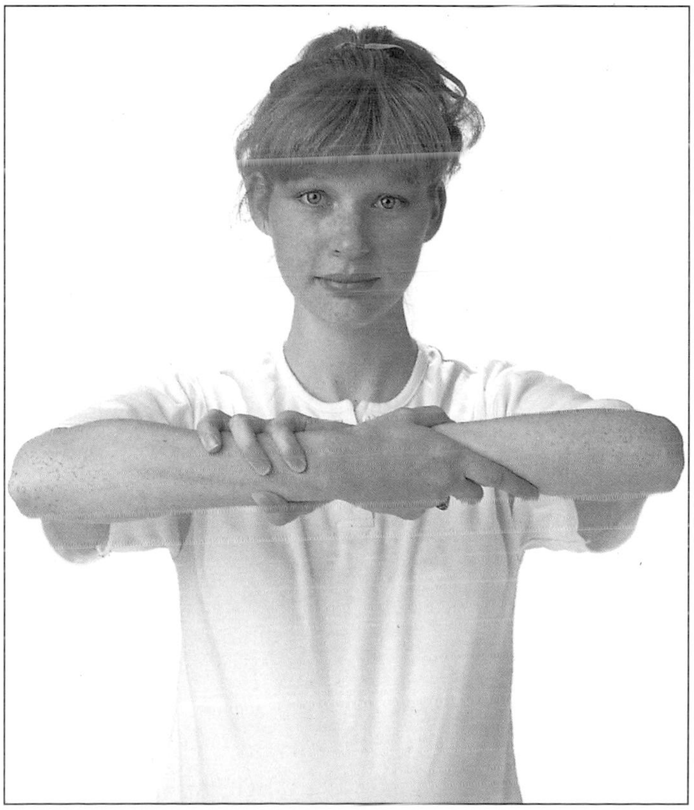

3 Stand erect and hold your arms in front of your chest, with elbows bent. Grasp your left arm just above the wrist with your right hand, and your right arm just above the wrist with your left hand. Now pull on each arm, as if you were trying to pull your hands apart, but maintain a tight grip. Hold for a few seconds. Relax your hands and then repeat several times.

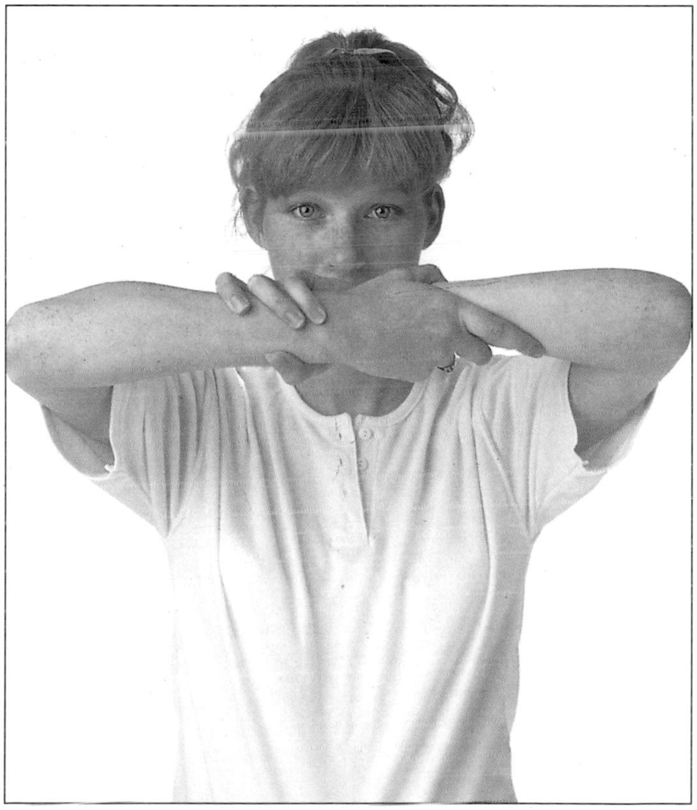

4 Now raise your arms and hold them out in front of your mouth, repeat step 3 in this higher position. If you wish, you can also do the exercise holding your arms just in front of your waistline.

BASIC EXERCISE ROUTINE

Add these basic exercises to your general fitness routine to give special problem areas extra work, or do them on their own as an isolated routine. If you do them on their own, use the abdominal muscle exercises from the general fitness plan for your stomach.

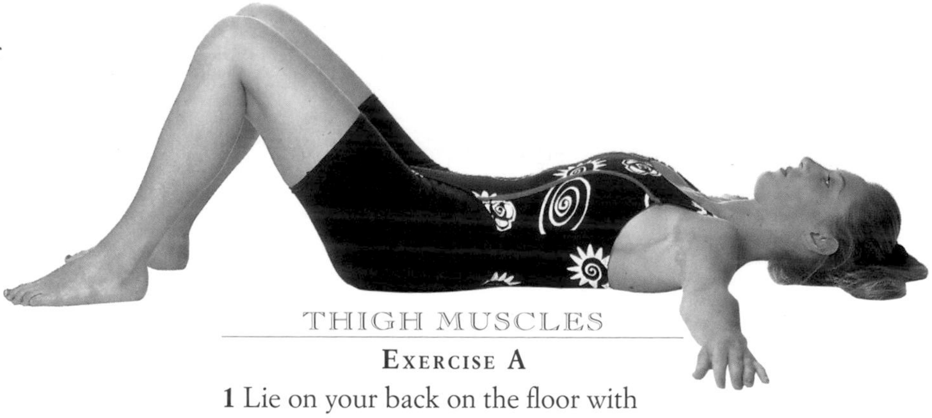

THIGH MUSCLES

EXERCISE A

1 Lie on your back on the floor with your arms resting straight out at right angles to your body and your feet apart, in line with your hips.

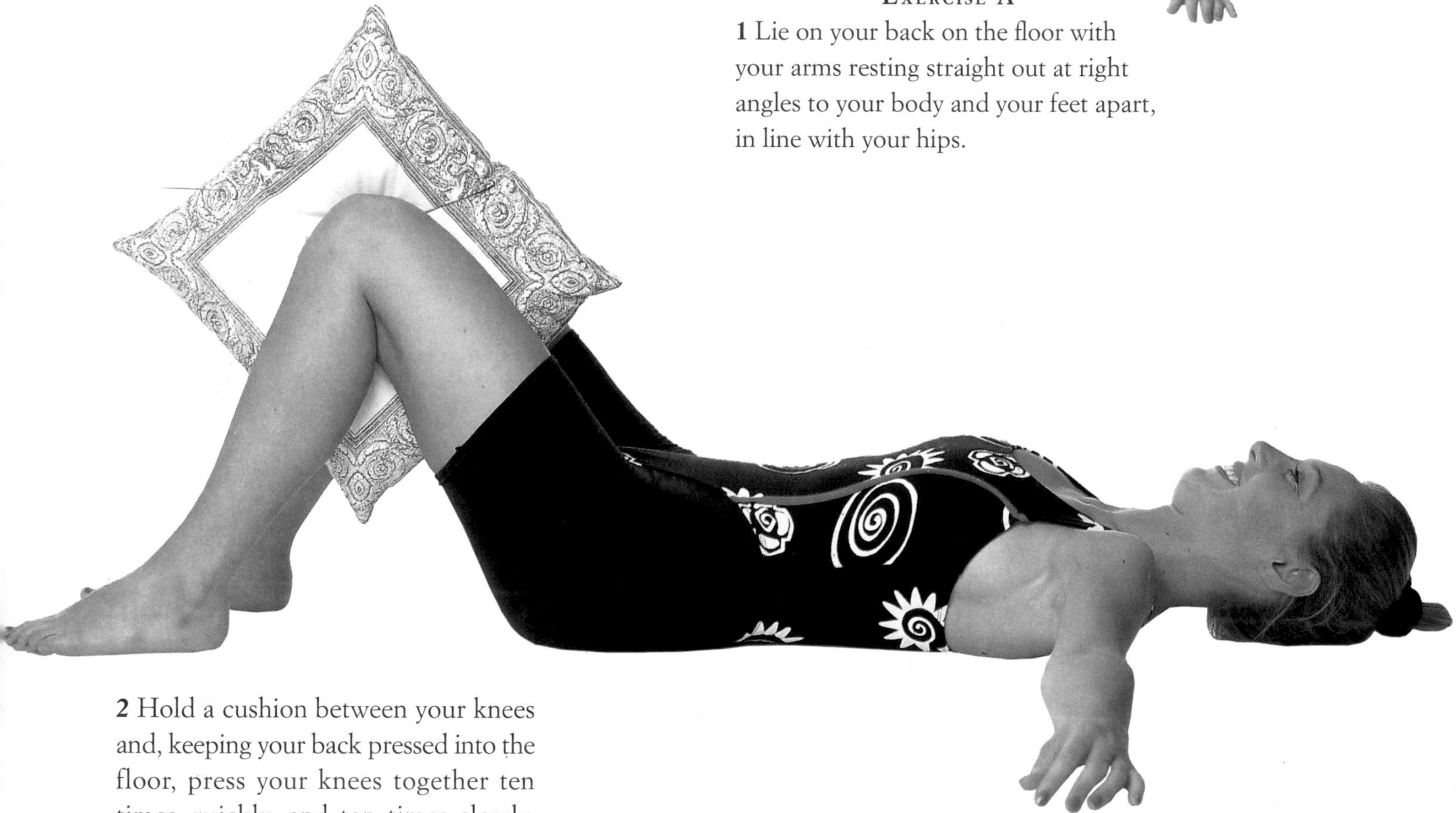

2 Hold a cushion between your knees and, keeping your back pressed into the floor, press your knees together ten times quickly, and ten times slowly, keeping the cushion in place throughout.

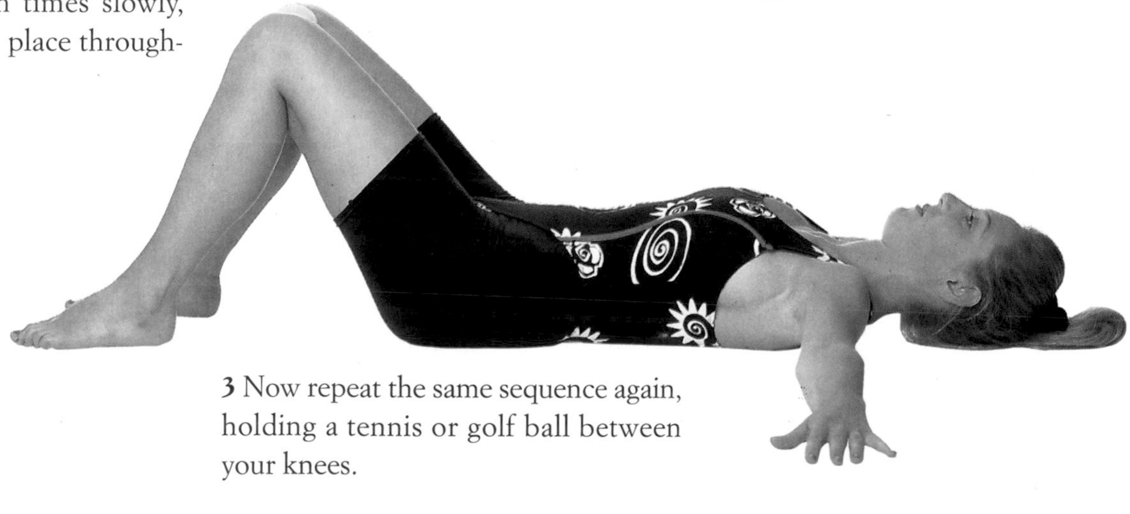

3 Now repeat the same sequence again, holding a tennis or golf ball between your knees.

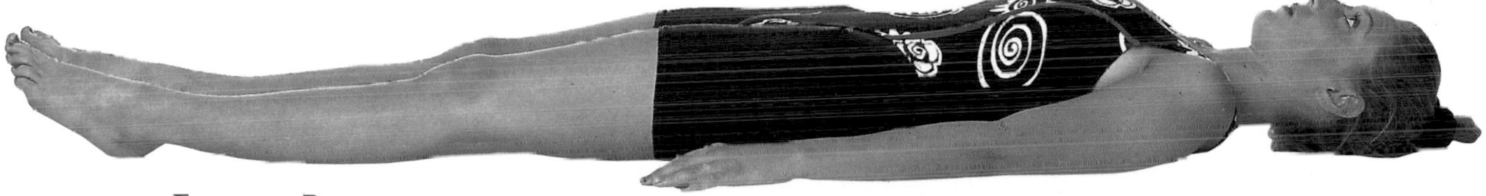

EXERCISE B

1 Lie on your back on the floor with your legs straight, and your lower back pressed to the floor. Put your arms along your sides, palms to the floor.

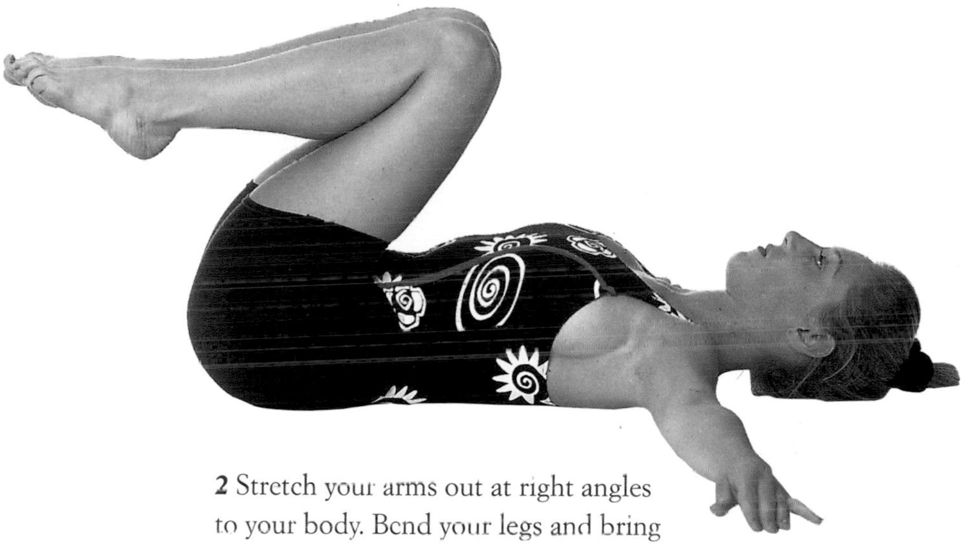

2 Stretch your arms out at right angles to your body. Bend your legs and bring your knees up to your chest.

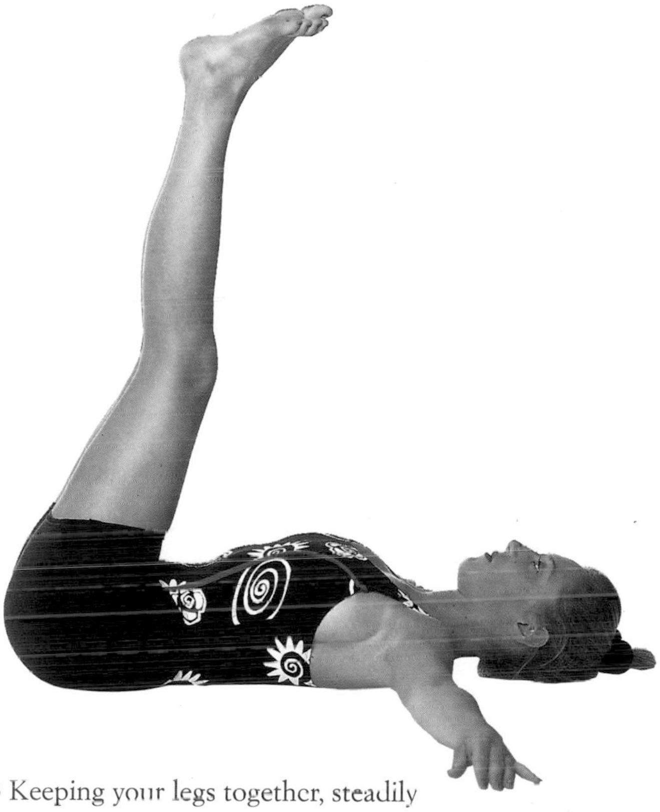

3 Keeping your legs together, steadily straighten them so that they are pointing up towards the ceiling. Keep your feet relaxed.

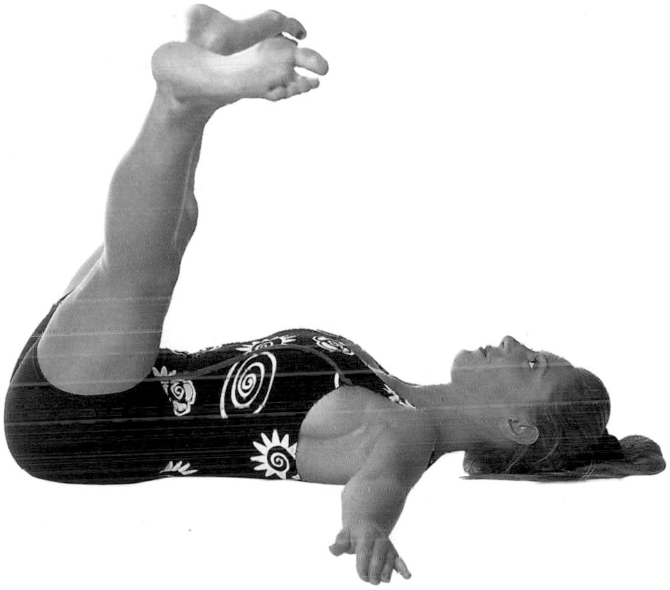

4 Slowly open your legs out sideways – as wide as you can – then close them again. Repeat the exercise (steps 2–4) four times. When you get used to the exercise, you can do it with small weights tied to your ankles.

Exercise C

1 Stand sideways on to a chair or table (lightly holding the edge to maintain your balance) with your shoulders down and relaxed, and with your knees bent and your feet facing forwards.

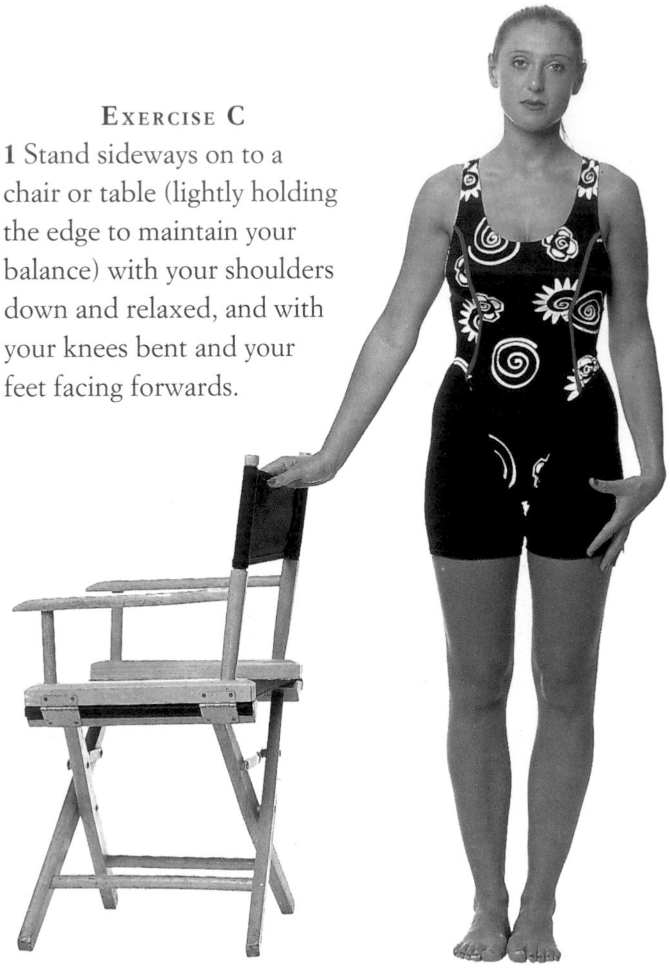

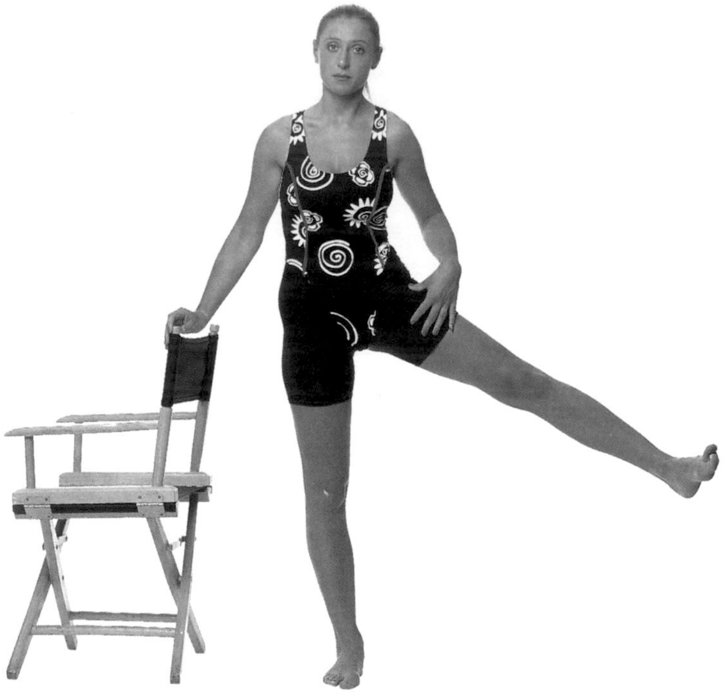

2 Lift your left hip slightly and slowly move your leg out and up (no higher than 45°), keeping your foot and knee facing forwards. Make sure you do not let your body tilt – keep it as straight as possible. Carefully lower your leg. Repeat the whole exercise ten times, then turn and repeat with the other leg.

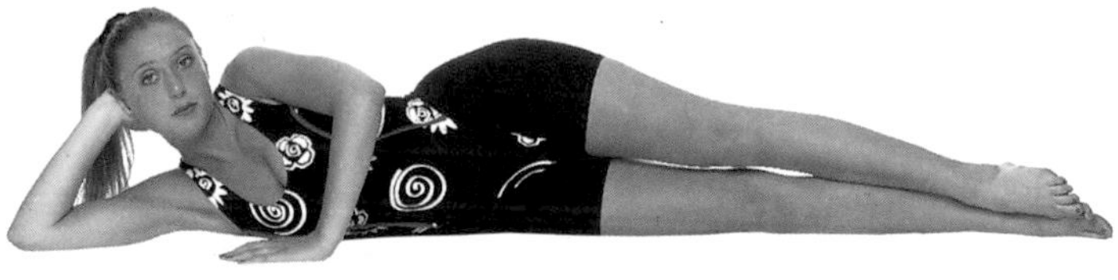

Exercise D

1 Lie on your right side on the floor with your legs out straight. Support your head with your right hand.

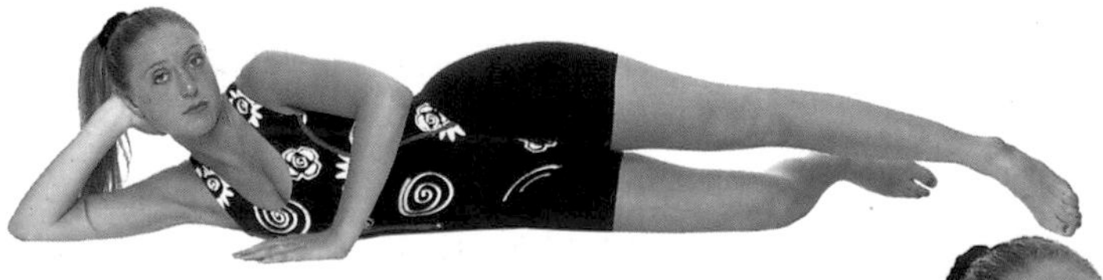

2 Bend your lower leg behind you to maintain balance and tilt your hips slightly towards the floor; your head, hips, knees, and feet should all be facing forwards. Balance yourself with your left hand on the floor.

3 Slowly lift your upper leg, then bring it down to touch the lower one; raise it again and repeat this action six times. Turn over and repeat steps 1–3 on the other side.

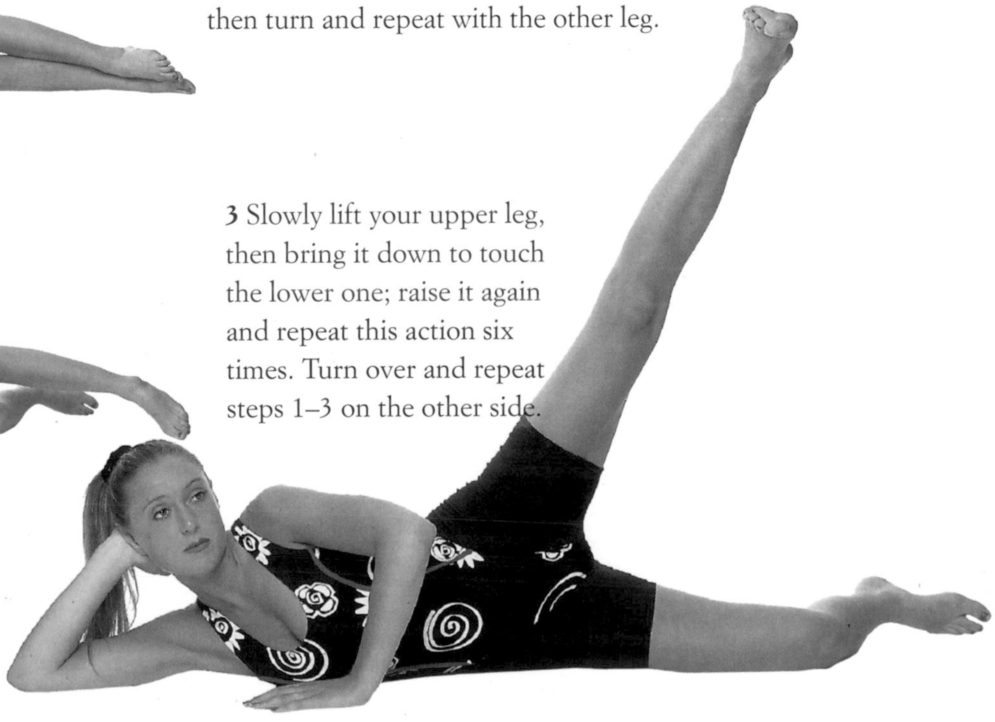

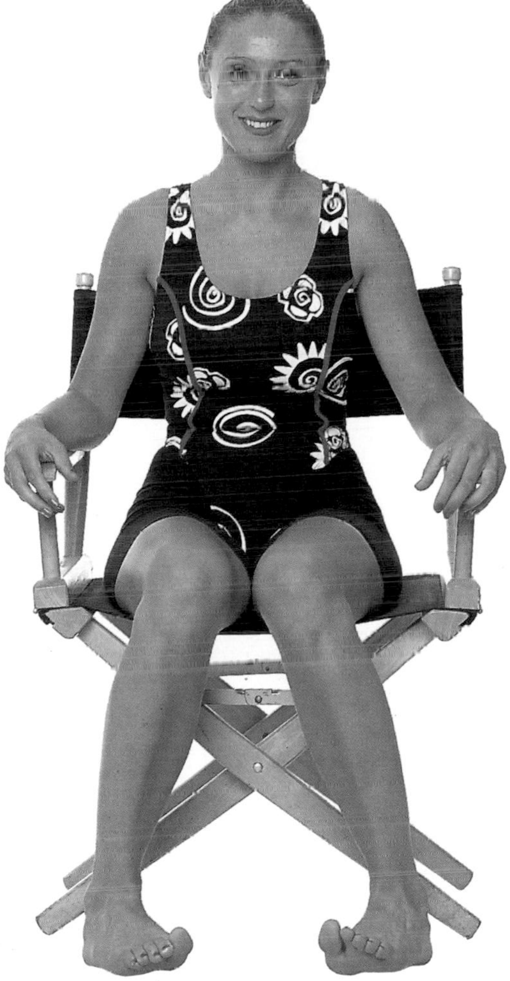

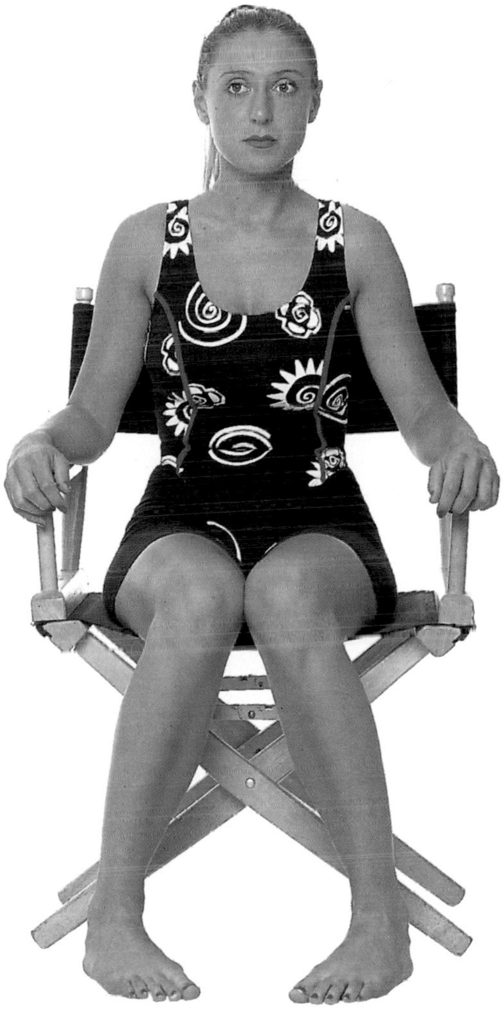

ANKLES AND CALF MUSCLES

Exercise A

1 Sit up straight on a chair, with your knees together and heels on the floor and slightly apart, in line with your hips. Bring your big toes up and roll your feet in towards each other.

2 Now tilt and move both feet down and outwards from the ankle, keeping your big toes raised as much as possible as you roll your feet on to their outer edges. Repeat ten times.

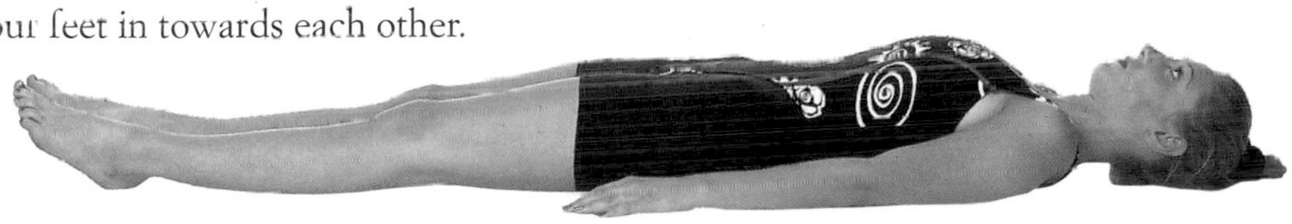

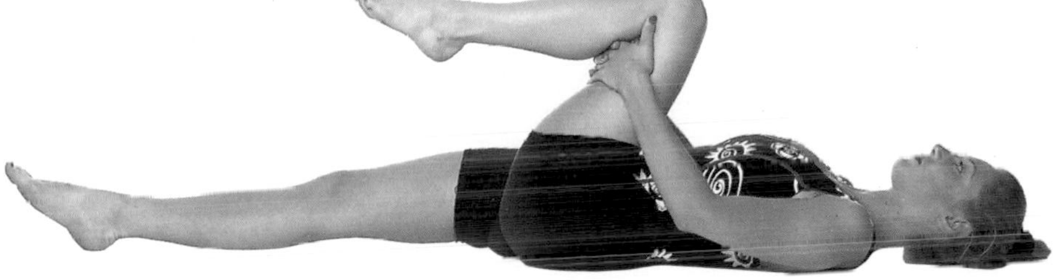

Exercise B

1 Lie flat on your back on the floor with your legs straight.

2 Bring one leg up and hold it beneath the back of your thigh so that it is pulled towards your chest. Rotate your foot ten times in a clockwise direction and ten times anti-clockwise. Repeat with the other leg. Increase the number of repeats to twenty for each foot, working alternatively in groups of 7.

BUTTOCK MUSCLES

Exercise A

1 Stand upright and lightly hold the back of a chair or the edge of a table to maintain your balance. Put your weight on your right leg and turn your left leg out from the hip.

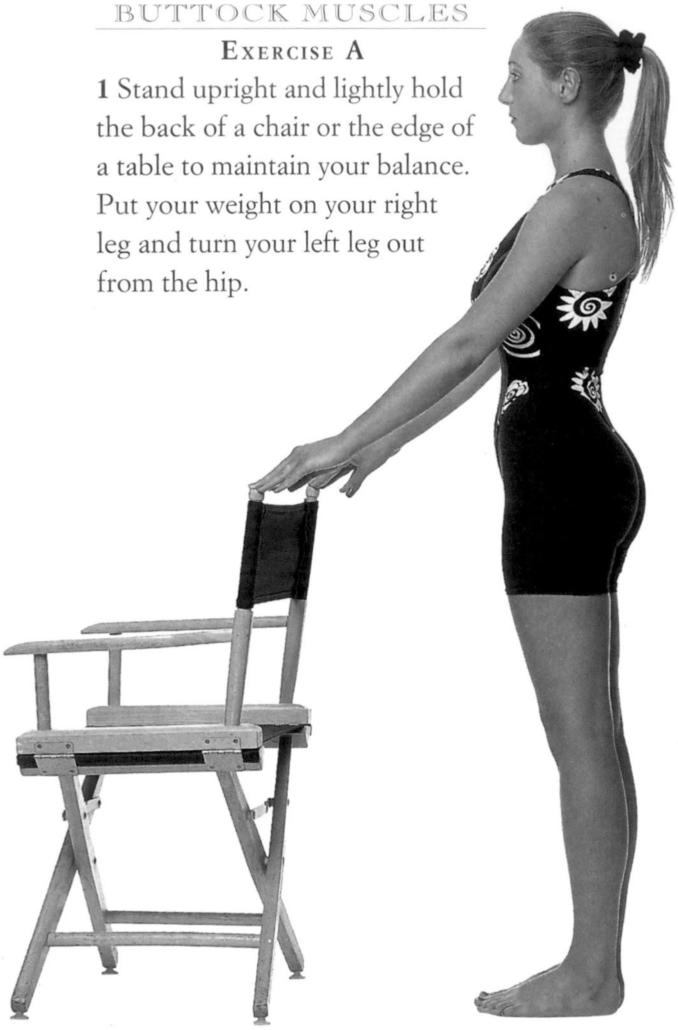

2 Keeping your foot flexed, take your left leg back as far as you can without bending it at the knee, forcing the movement or over-arching your back. Repeat with the other leg. Repeat five times for each leg and gradually build up to twenty repetitions.

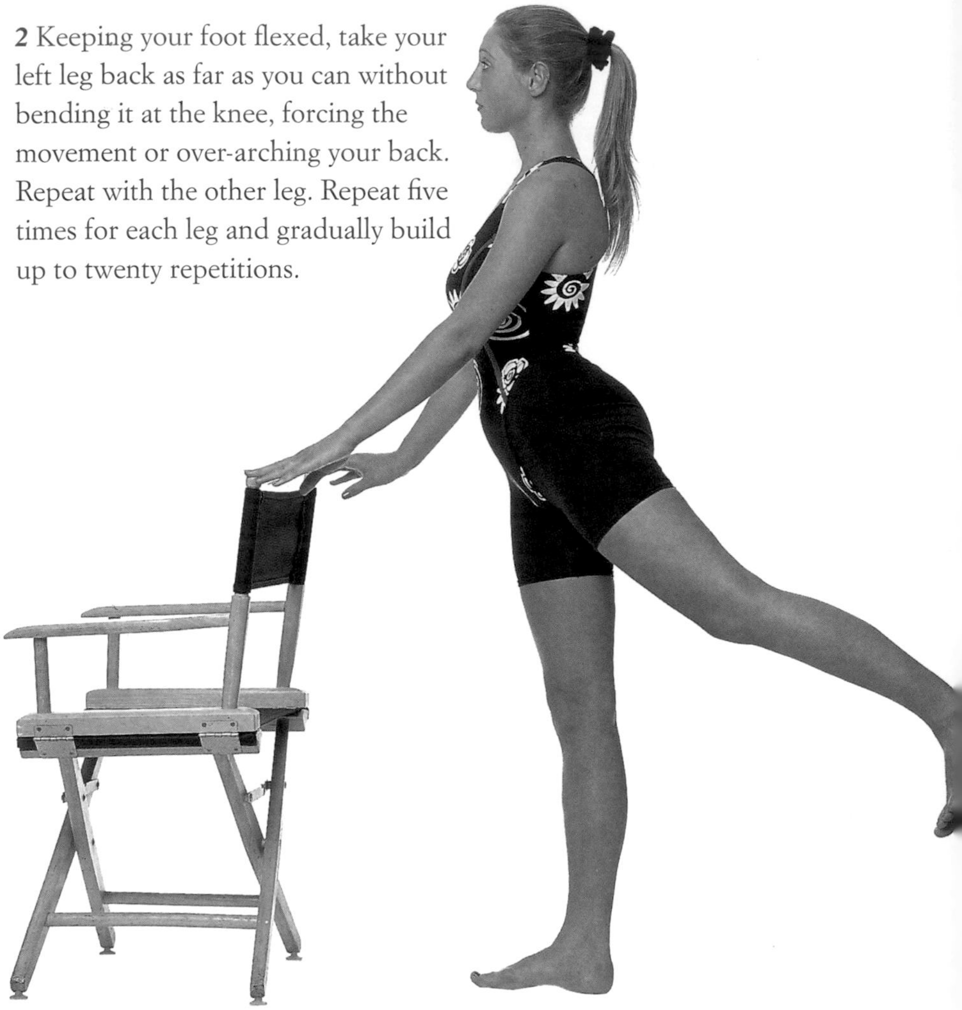

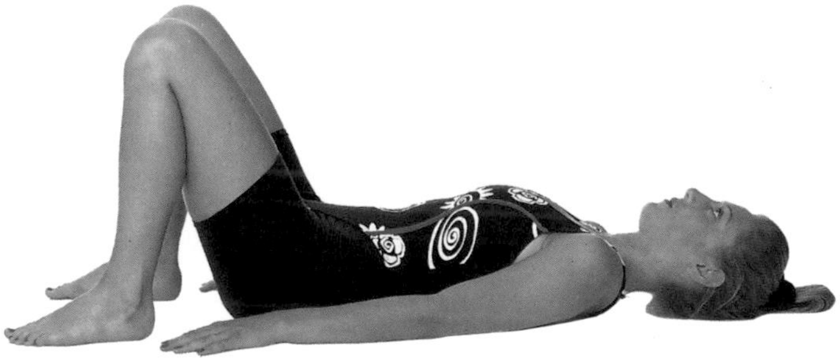

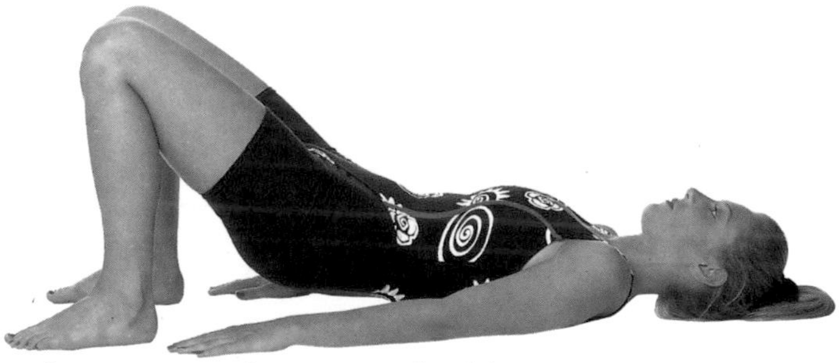

Exercise B

1 Lie on your back with your knees bent and your feet slightly apart, in line with your hips. Place your arms by your sides, palms flat on the floor.

2 Place your weight on your shoulders and upper back (not your neck), raise your bottom and tighten your buttock muscles, keeping your feet flat on the floor and your arms by your sides. Hold for several seconds. Lower your bottom to the floor. Repeat five times, building up to twenty repetitions.

Exercise C

1 Kneel on all fours with your knees slightly apart, in line with your hips, but keeping them tucked right under your hips. Place your hands in front of you, a shoulder-width apart and facing forwards. Bend your elbows so that you are leaning on your forearms.

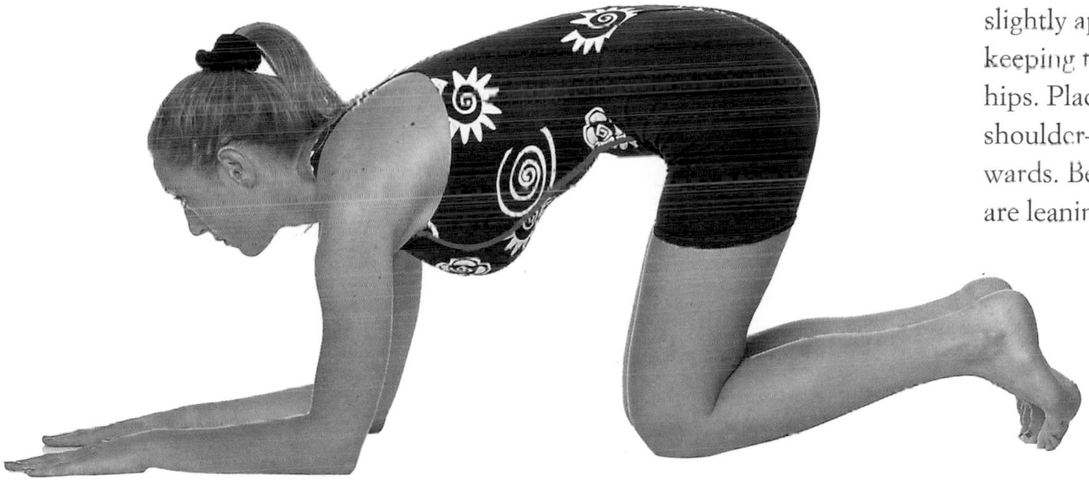

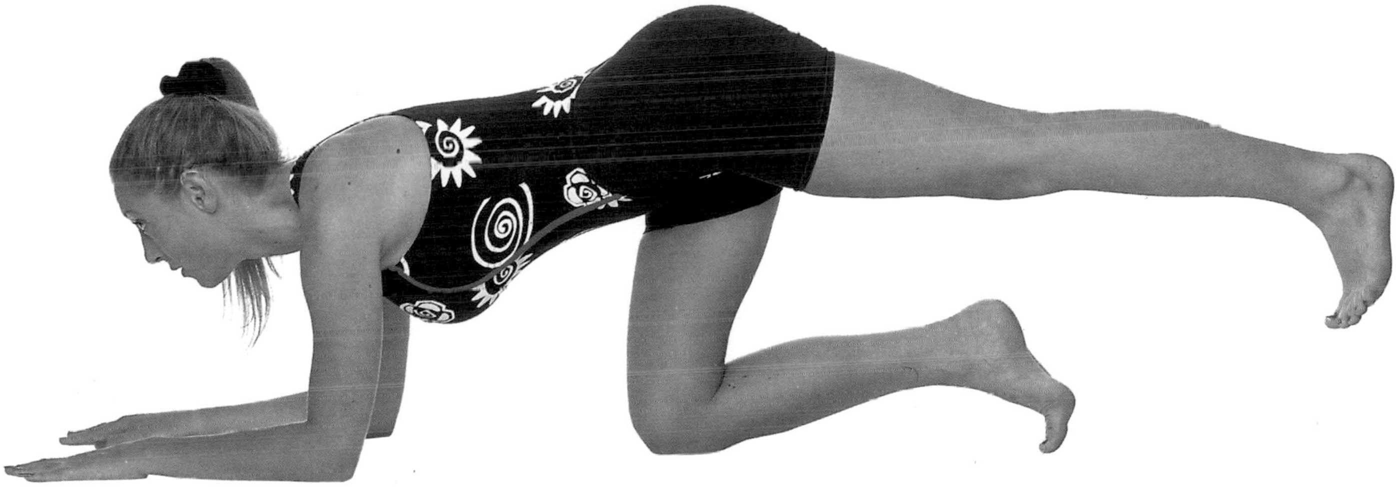

2 Keeping your foot flexed, push your left leg out straight behind you, keeping your back and hips parallel.

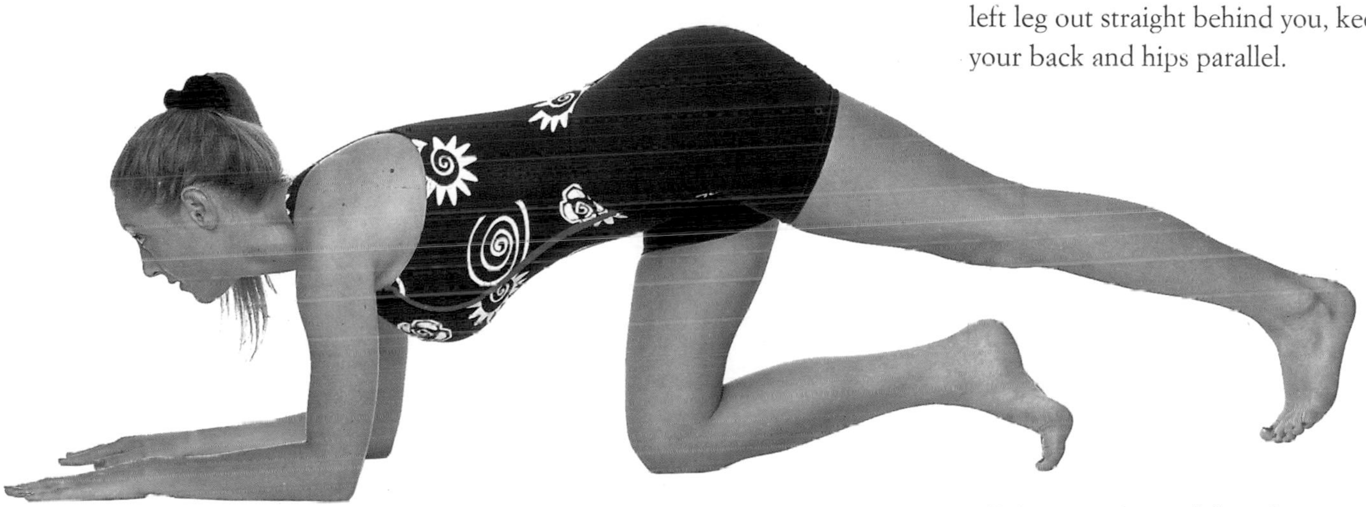

3 Bring your leg and foot down to the floor, keeping your foot flexed and your leg straight. Repeat steps 2 and 3 twelve times. Return to the original position, then repeat the exercise with your other leg. Build up to twenty repetitions.

GLOSSARY

ACUTE CONDITION: Arising suddenly and with intense severity, but only running a short course. (See chronic condition)
ALLOPATHIC: The conventional method of combating disease by using active ingredients specifically against the disease.
ANAEMIA: A deficiency in red blood cells, or in the haemoglobin carried by them. The resultant lack of oxygen carried around the body produces pallor, breathlessness and no energy.
ANALGESIC: Relieves pain.
APERIENT: A mild laxative.
ATROPHY: The shrinking or wasting away of muscles, glands or tissues due to disease or malnutrition.
BILE: A bitter green to brown alkaline fluid produced by the liver and stored in the gall bladder.
BILIOUS: Any disorder which results in the production of an excess amount of bile.
CHRONIC CONDITION: A disease or ailment that develops slowly and persists over a long period of time. (See acute condition)
DEMULCENT: Oily substance used to soften and soothe damaged surfaces such as the skin, or mucous membranes.
DILUENT: A substance used for dilution, e.g. water, base oil.
DIURETIC: Encourages urination.
DYSPEPSIA: Indigestion.
EMETIC: Causes vomiting.
EMOLLIENT: Softens and soothes the skin.
ENDOGENOUS: Caused or produced by factors within the organism or system.
FEBRIFUGE: Reduces fever.
FEBRILE: Feverish, or relating to a fever.
FIBROIDS: A structure resembling or consisting of fibrous tissue.
FOMENTATION: The act of applying heat and moisture to relieve inflammation and pain.
LEUCORRHEA: White to yellowish vaginal discharge.
MUCOUS MEMBRANE: Soft tissue lining most of the body's cavities and tubes.
PAROXYSMAL: A sudden attack or occurrence of a disease.
PERISTALSIS: Waves of contractions passing along the walls of hollow muscular organs, forcing the contents forwards.

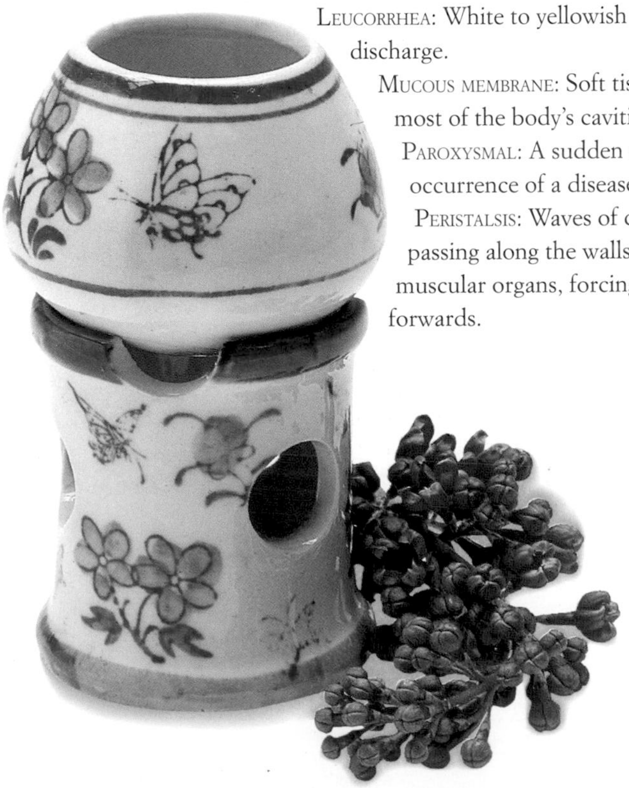

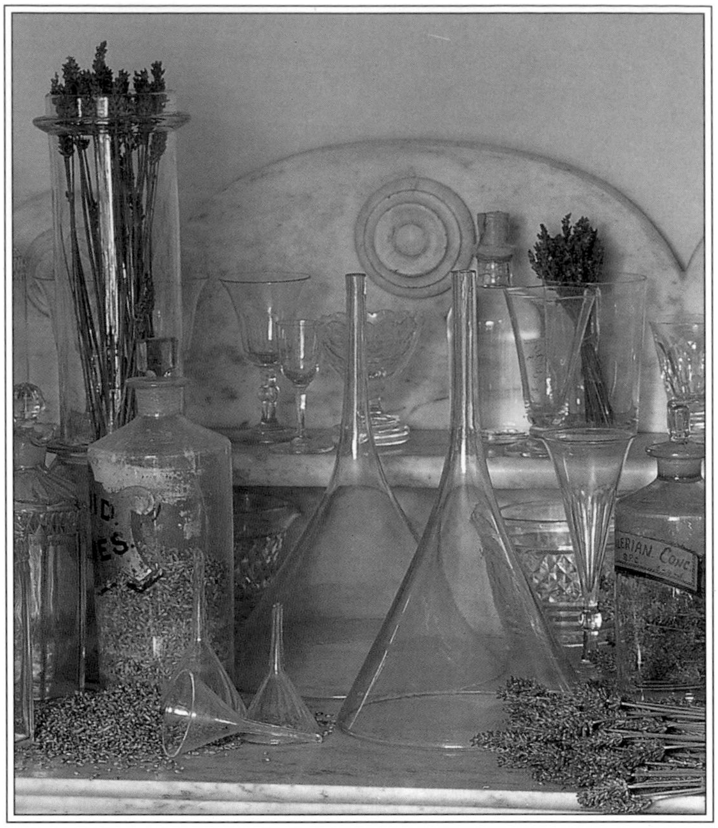

PHARMACOPOEIA: An authoritative written guide to medicinal drugs and their uses.
PROGESTERONE: A natural hormone that prepares the uterus to receive and develop the fertilized egg.
PROPHYLACTIC: Preventing or protecting from disease.
SALICYLATES: Salts of salicylic acid.
SALICYLIC ACID: A white crystalline substance used in the manufacture of aspirin.
SUCCUSS: A special way of shaking a homeopathic remedy in order to extract its medicinal properties.
SUPPURATING: Oozing.
SYNOVIAL MEMBRANE: Soft tissues lining joints and tendon sheaths.
TONIC: Invigorates and tones the body and promotes well-being.
TRIGEMINAL NERVES: Either of the fifth pair of cranial nerves which supply the muscles of the upper and lower jawbone.
WATERBRASH: Gas being brought up into the mouth with acidic fluid.

BIBLIOGRAPHY

Charles, Rachel. *Mind, Body and Immunity,* Methuen, London, England, 1990
Davis, Patricia. *Aromatherapy, An A-Z,* C.W. Daniel, Saffron Walden, England, 1988
Davis, Dr Stephen and Stewart, Dr Alan *Nutritional Medicine,* Pan Books Ltd, London, England, 1987
Editors of the Prevention Magazine Health Books, *The Doctor's Book of Home Remedies,* Bantam, New York, USA, 1991
Evans, Mark. *A Guide to Herbal Remedies,* C.W. Daniel, Saffron Walden, England, 1990
Evans, Mark. *Instant Aromatherapy for Stress Relief*, Lorenz Books, London, England, 1996
Evans, Mark. *Instant Massage for Stress Relief*, Lorenz Books, London, England, 1996
Evans, Mark. *Instant Stretches for Stress Relief*, Lorenz Books, London, England, 1996
Grieve, Mrs M. *Modern Herbal*, Penguin, London, England, 1984
Hanssen, Maurice. *E For Additives,* Thorsons, London, England, 1990
Hudson, John. *Instant Meditation for Stress Relief*, Lorenz Books, London, England, 1996
Hawkey, Susan. *Herbalism*, Lorenz Books, London, England, 1997
Kusick, James. *A Treasury of Natural First Aid Remedies From A-Z,* Reward Books, Prentice Hall Inc., New York, USA, 1995
Leung, Albert Y. *Encyclopaedia of Common Natural Ingredients used in Food, Drugs and Cosmetics*, John Wiley & Sons, New York, USA, 1980
Maybey, Richard. *The Complete New Herbal*, Elm Tree Books, London, England, 1988
McIntyre, Anne. *Herbs for Common Ailments*, Gaia Books, London, England, 1988
McVica, Jekka. *Jekka's Complete Herb Book,* Kyle Cathie, London, England, 1994
Maxwell-Hudson, Clare. *Aromatherapy Massage Book,* Dorling Kindersley, London, England, 1995
Mellor, Contance. *Natural Remedies for Common Ailments*, Granada Publishing Ltd, London, England, 1975
Mervyn, Leonard. *The Complete Guide to Vitamins and Minerals,* Thorsons, London, England, 1990

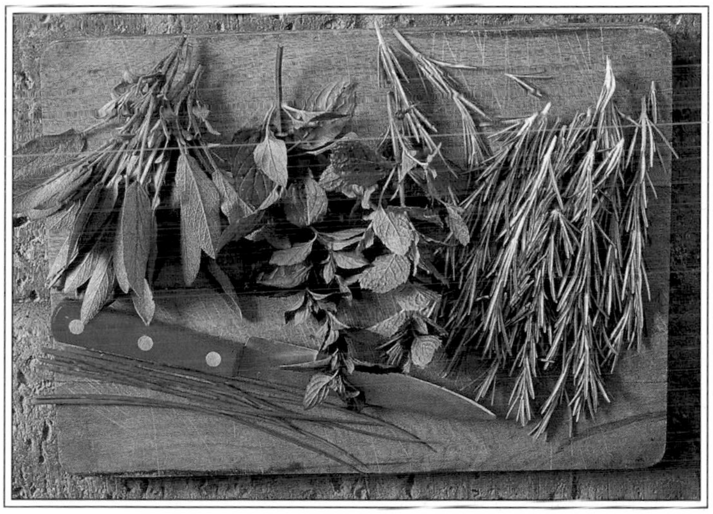

Messegne, Maurice. *Health Secrets of Plants and Herbs*, Collins, London, England, 1979
Mills, Simon (ed). *Alternative in Healing,* Macmillan, London, England, 1988
Newman Turner, Roger. *Naturopathic Medicine,* Thorsons, London, England, 1989
Ody, Penelope. *The Herb Society's Complete Medicinal Herbal,* Dorling Kindersley, London, England, 1993
Oxenford, Rosalind. *Reflexology*, Lorenz Books, London, England, 1997
Shepherd, Dr Dorothy. *Magic of the Minimum Dose.* C.W. Daniel, Saffron Walden, England, 1990
Tisserand, Robert. *The Art of Aromatherapy,* C.W. Daniel, Saffron Walden, England, 1977
van Straten, Michael. *The Complete Natural Health Consultant,* Ebury Press, London, England, 1987
various. *Homeopathy, The Family Handbook,* Unwin, London, England, 1987
Worwood, V. *The Fragrant Pharmacy*, Bantam Books, London, England, 1991

PUBLISHER'S ACKNOWLEDGEMENTS

The Publishers would like to thank the following contributors for additional text: John Hudson (Hypnotherapy), Andrew Oldroyd (Moxibustion), Susanne Franzen (Shiatsu), Karine Butchart (Makko Ho), Felicity Roma Bowers (Meditation), Paul Harvey (Yoga), Anne Gains, Nutritionist (Healthy Eating Plan), Clare Harris (Massage).

The Publishers would like to thank Jekka McVica for supplying herbs for photography.

Jekka McVica at
Jekka's Herb Farm, Rose Cottage, Shellards, Aleveston,
Bristol BS12 2SY
Tel: 01454 418878
(mail-order suppliers of herbs)

PHOTOGRAPHY CREDITS
The majority of photographs taken in this book were by Lucy Mason and Don Last.
The publishers would also like to credit the following photographers: Deni Bown; Gary Brettnacher; Jean-Loup Charmet, Paris; Liz Edison; Jacqui Hurst; Michelle Garrett; John Glover; Angela Hampton; Mary Evans Picture Libray; Debbie Patterson; Reflections, Jo Browne; Steve Satushek; Timothy Shonnard; The Image Bank: Chris Close; Tony Stone: Bruce Ayres; Jennie Woodcock; Zefa Norman; Harry Smith.

USEFUL ADDRESSES

UK

AROMATHERAPY
International Society of Professional Aromatherapists
The Hinckley and District Hospital
The Annex
Mount Road
Hinckley
Leicestershire LE10 1AG
(For information about courses, and essential oils)

International Federation of Aromatherapists
4 Eastmearn Road
Dulwich
London SE21 8HA
(Provides a list of professional aromatherapists)

GENERAL
Natural Childbirth Trust
Alexandra House
Oldham Terrace
Acton
London W3 6NH

Registry of Traditional Chinese Medicine
19 Trinity Road
London N2 8JJ

Research Council for Complementary Medicine
60 Great Ormond Street
London WC1N 3JF

Women's Health Concern
83 Earl's Court Road
London W8 6EF

Women's Health Information Centre
52 Featherstone Street
London EC1Y 8RT

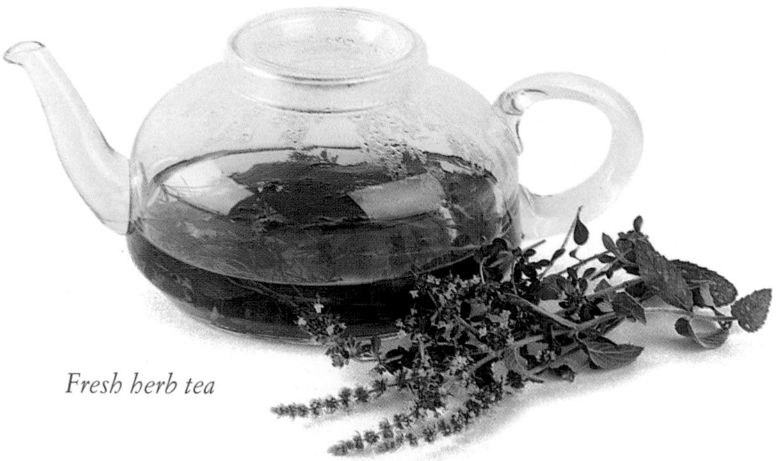

Fresh herb tea

HERBALISM
General Council & Register of Consultant Herbalists
18 Sussex Square
Brighton
East Sussex BN2 5AA

National Institute of Medical Herbalists
56 Longbrook Street
Exeter
Devon EX4 6AH
(Provides a list of professional herbalists and information about training courses)

Natural Medicine Society
Edith Lewis House
Black Lane
Ilkeston
Derbyshire DE7 8EJ

The Herb Society
134 Buckingham Palace Road
London SW1W 9SA
(For information about herbs and training courses)

The School of Phytotherapy/Herbal Medicine
Buckstreep Manor
Bodle Street Green
Hailsham
East Sussex, BN27 4RJ
(For information about training courses)

HOMEOPATHY
The Homeopathic Society
2 Powis Place
Great Ormond Street
London WC1N 3HT
(Provides a list of medically qualified homeopaths)

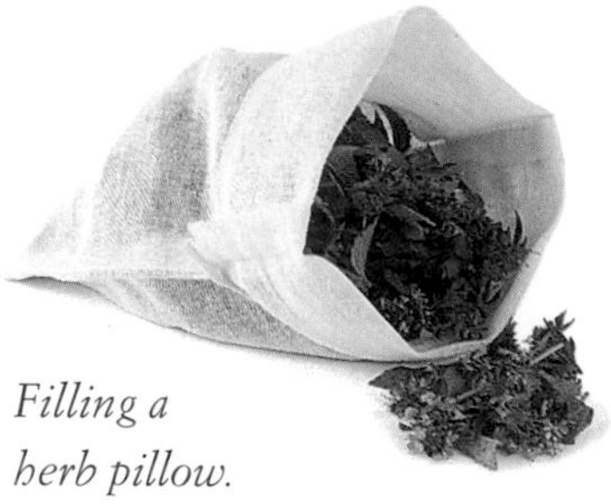

Filling a herb pillow.

The Society of Homeopaths
2 Artizan Road
Northampton NN1 4HU

Bach Flower Remedies
Dr. Edward Bach Centre
Mount Vernon Sotwell
Wallingford
Oxon, OX10 0PZ

HYPNOTHERAPY
National Council of Psychotherapists and Hypnotherapy
Registry
Steam Cottage
98 Wish Hill
Willingdon
East Sussex BM20 9HQ

The School of Meditation
158 Holland Park Avenue
London W11 4UH

NATUROPATHY
British Naturopathic and Osteopathic Association
6 Netherhall Gardens
London NW3 5RR
(Provides a list of practising naturopaths)

British Society for Nutritional Medicine
The Journal of Nutritional Medicine
P.O. Box 3AP
London

Eating Disorder Association
Sackville Place
44-46 Magdalen Street
Norwich
Norfolk NR3 1JE

The Secretary
The Incorporated Society of Registered Naturopaths
293 Gilmerton Road
Edinburgh EH16 5UQ

Institute for Optimum Nutrition
5 Jerdan Place
London SW6 1BE

The Mc Carrion Society
Institute of Brain Chemistry and Human Nutrition
Queen Elizabeth Hospital for Children
Hayward Building, 3rd Floor
Hackney Road
London E2 8PS

HERBAL SUPPLIERS
Culpeper Ltd (head office)
Hadstock Road
Linton
Cambridge
CB1 6NJ

East-West Herbs Ltd.
Langston Priory Mews
Kingham
Oxon, OC7 6UW

Gerard House Ltd.
475 Capability Green
Luton LU1 3LU

Midsummer Cottage Clinic
Nether Westcote
Nr Kingham
Oxon OX7 6SD

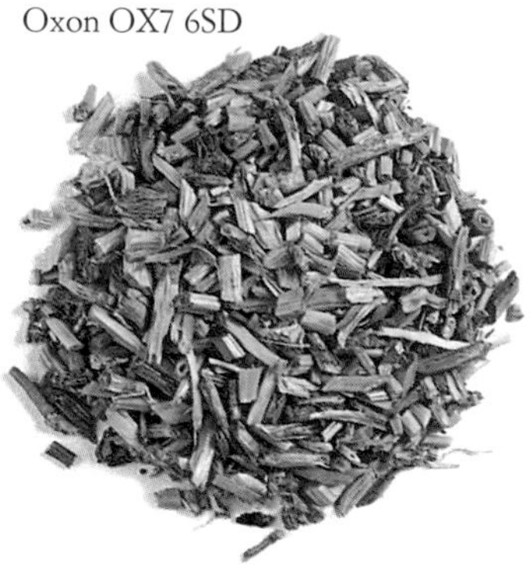

COUCH GRASS
(Agropyron repens)

Neal's Yard Apothecary
15 Neal's Yard
Covent Garden
London WC2H 9DP

Optimum-Phoenix
The Barn
Higher Trickeys
Morebath
Nr Tiverton
Devon EX16 9AL

The Herbal Apothecary
120 High Street
Syston
Leics IE7 8GC

ESSENTIAL OILS SUPPLIERS
Essence by Empress
P.O. Box 92
Penzance
Cornwall TR18 2XL

Fragrant Earth
P.O. Box 182
Taunton
Somerset TA1 1YR

Hartwood Aromatics
Hartwood House
12 Station Road
Hatton
Warwicks CV35 7LG

Shirley Price Aromatherapy
Wesley House
Stockwell Road
Hinckley
Leics LE10 1RD

SUPPLIERS OF HOMEOPATHIC REMEDIES
Most chemists and health food shops will stock a limited supply of homeopathic remedies. The list below will stock a complete range.

Buxton and Grant
176 Whiteladies Road
Bristol BS8 2XU

Freeman's Pharmacy
7 Eaglesham Road
Clarkston,
Glasgow G76 7BU

Goulds the Chemist
14 Crowndale Road
London NW1 1TT

Helios Pharmacy
97 Camden Road
Tunbridge Wells
Kent TN1 2QR

US

ASSOCIATIONS
American Association of Naturopathic Physicians (AANP)
2366 Eastlake Avenue
Suite 322
Seattle, WA 98102

American Holistic Medical Association (AHMA)
4101 Lake Boone Trail
Suite 201
Raleigh, NC 27607

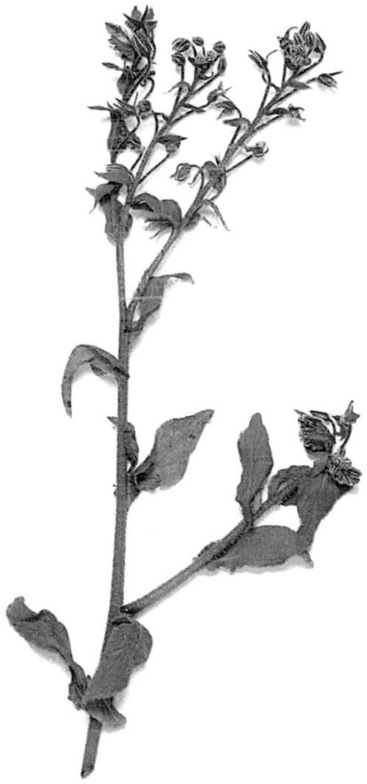

BORAGE *(Borago officinalis)*

American Botanical Council (ABC)
P.O. Box 201660
Austin, TX 78720

College of Maharishi Ayur-Veda Health Center
P.O. Box 282
Fairfield, IA 52556

American Chiropractic Association (ACA)
1701 Clarendon Blvd.
Arlington, VA 22209

American Osteopathic Association (AOA)
142 East Ontario St.
Chicago, IL 60611

Aveda
140 5th Avenue
New York, NY 10011

California School of Herbal Studies
Forestville, CA

Eastern Acupuncture & Natural Herb Center
8 Spring Street
New York, NY 10009

New Life Resource Center
938 8th Avenue
New York, NY 10019

Tom Thumb Workshops
P.O. Box 357
Mappsville, VA 23407

NEWSLETTERS
Alternatives
Mountain Home Publishing
(210) 367-4492. By David W. Williams, a chiropractor

Naturally Well
Phillips Publishing Inc.
(301) 424-3700. By Marcus Laux, M.D., a homeopathic specialist.

Alternative Medicine: The Definitive Guide and Alternative Medicine Yellow Pages. Compiled by The Burton Goldberg Group, Future Medicine Publishing, 1994

OUTLETS FOR HERBS
Cameron Park Botanicals
Highway 64 East
Raleigh, NC 27610

Caprilands Herb Farm
Silver Street
North Coventry, CT 06238

Flower Power Herbs and Roots Inc.
406 East 9th Street
New York, NY 10009

Herb Shoppe
215 West Main Street
Greenwood, IN 46142

San Francisco Herb Co.
250 14th Street
San Francisco, CA 94103

Seeds Blum
Idaho City State
Boise, ID 83706

Richter's Herb Catalog
Goodwood
Ontario
Canada, LOC 1AO

ESSENTIAL OILS SUPPLIERS
Bonny Doon Farm
600 Marin Road
Santa Cruz, CA 95060

Kiehl's
109 Third Avenue
New York, NY 10003

Lorann Oils
4518 Aurelius Road
P.O. Box 22009
Lansing, MI 48909-2009

AUSTRALIA

AROMATHERAPY
International Federation of Aromatherapists
Information Line: 190 2240 125

HERBALISM
National Herbalist Association
P.O. Box 61
Broadway, NSW 2066

HOMEOPATHY
Australian Institute of Homeopathy
P.O. Box 122
Roseville, NSW 2069

Blackmores Ltd
23 Roseberry Street
Balgowlah, NSW 2093

Newton's Pharmacy
119 York Street
Sydney, NSW 2000

Manuka Pharmacy
Manuka Arcade
Manuka, ACT 2603

Martin and Pleasance
135 Swan Street
Richmond, Vic 3000

Bach Flower Shop
309 Little Collins Street
Melbourne, Vic 3000

Ahimsa
Drivers Court
Samsonvale, Qid 4520

Brauer Biotherapies Pty Ltd
1 Para Road
Tanunda, SA 5352

Fitch's Pharmacy
731 Hay Street
Perth, WA 9000

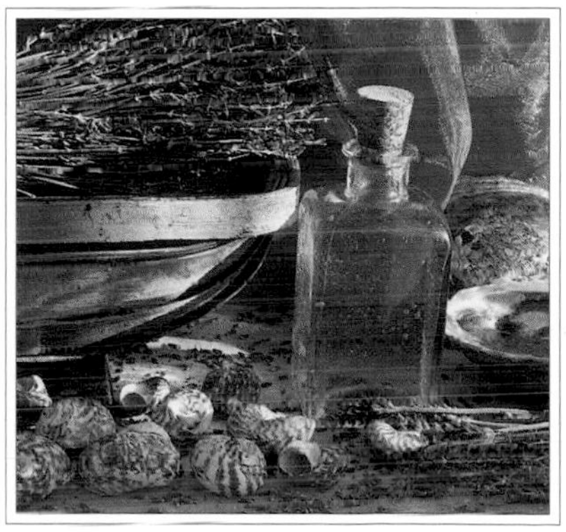

SAW PALMETTO
(Serenoa serrulata)

INDEX

Entries in **bold** type refer to illustrations

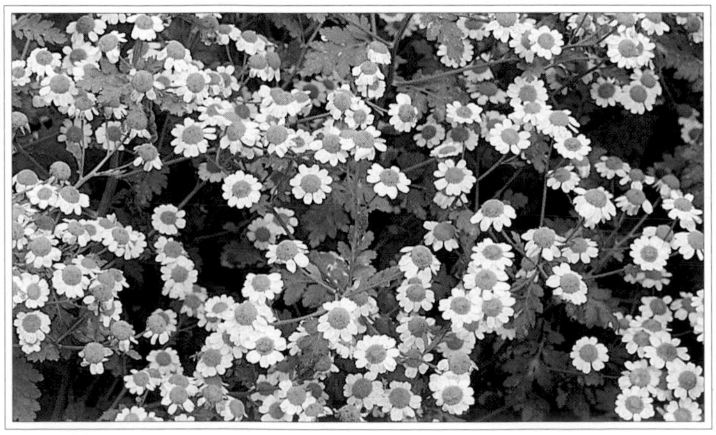

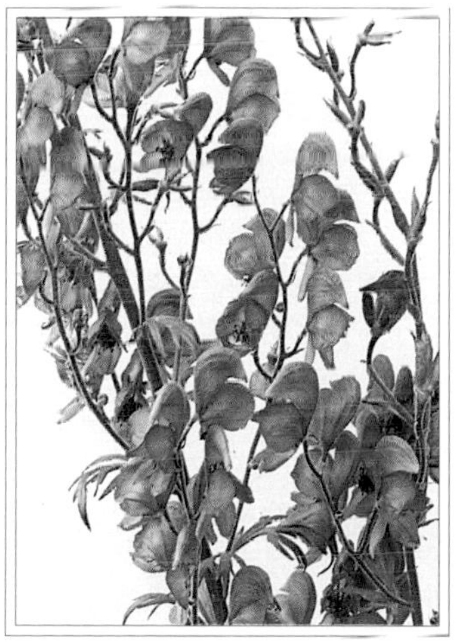

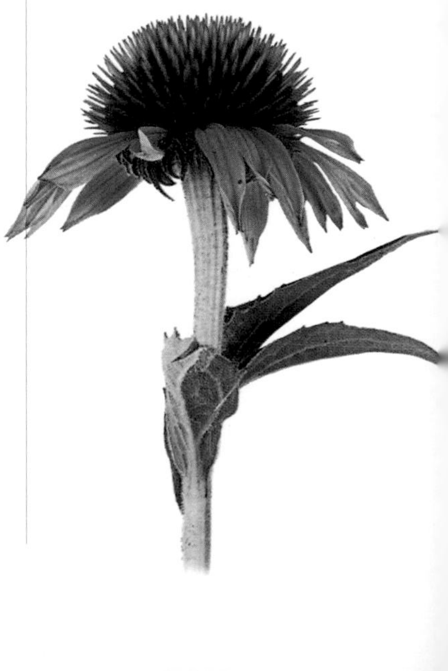

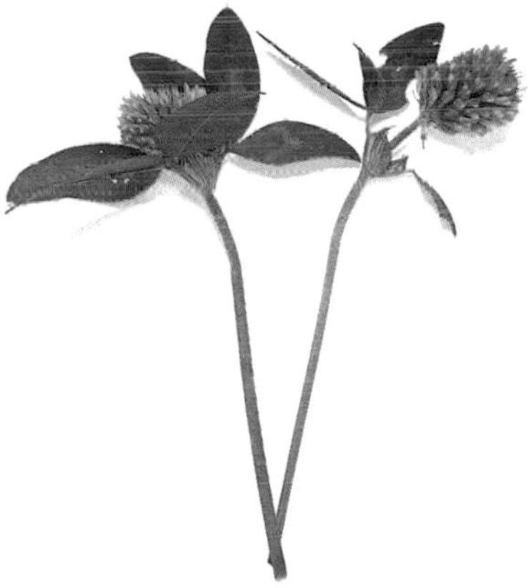

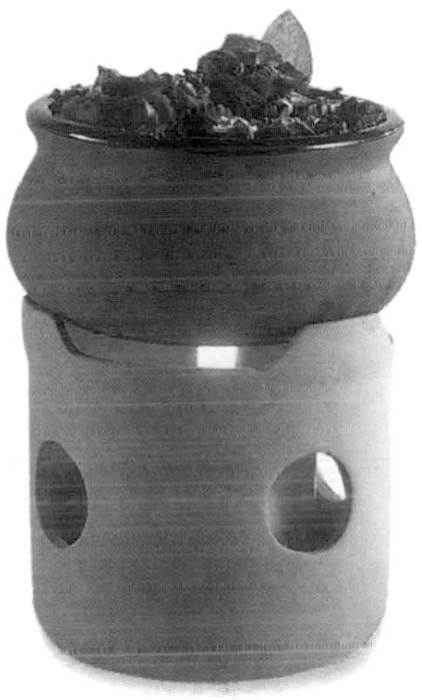

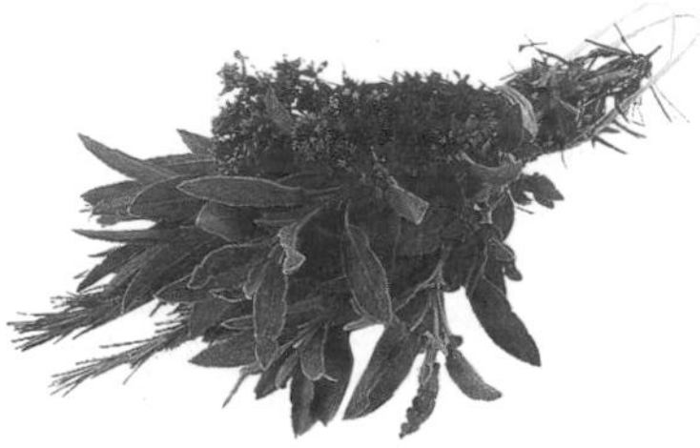

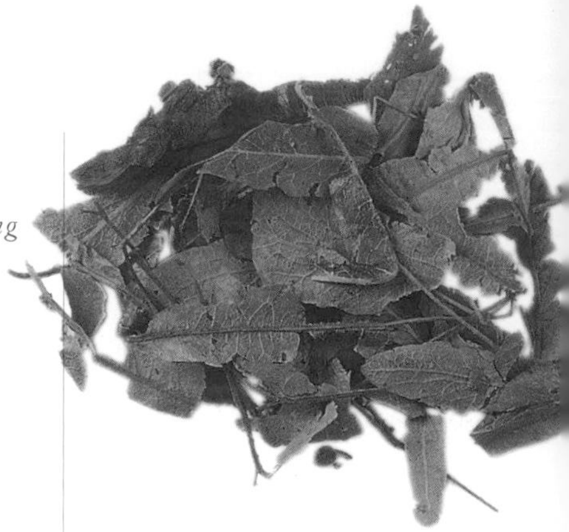

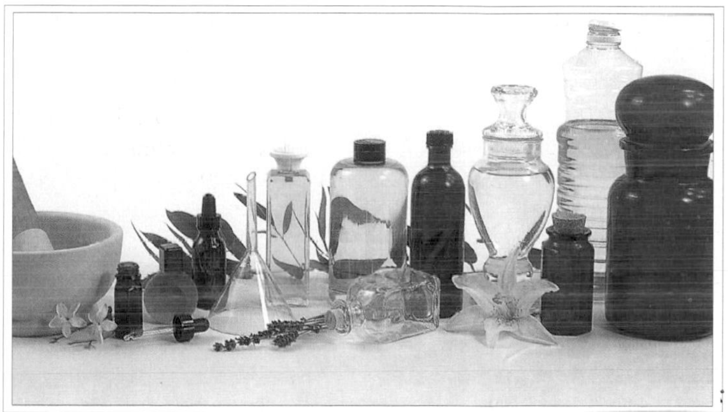

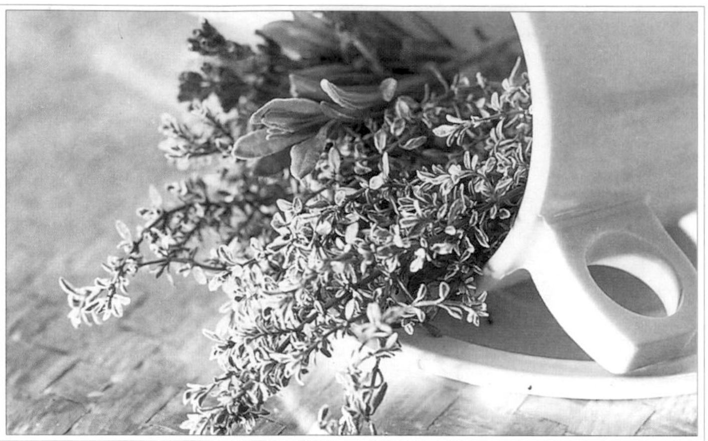